# Find videos for *Reconstructive Plastic Surgery of the Head and Neck* online at MediaCenter.thieme.com!

**Simply visit MediaCenter.thieme.com and, when prompted during the registration process, enter the code below to get started today.**

5Y7U-LMCA-D976-Z8JF

| | WINDOWS | MAC | TABLET |
|---|---|---|---|
| **Recommended Browser(s)**** | Recent browser versions on all major platforms and any mobile operating system that supports HTML5 video playback<br>*** all browsers should have JavaScript enabled* | | |
| **Flash Player Plug-in** | Flash Player 9 or Higher*<br>** Mac users: ATI Rage 128 GPU does not support full-screen mode with hardware scaling* | | Tablet PCs with Android OS support Flash 10.1 |
| **Recommended for optimal usage experience** | Monitor resolutions:<br>• Normal (4:3) 1024×768 or Higher<br>• Widescreen (16:9) 1280×720 or Higher<br>• Widescreen (16:10) 1440×900 or Higher<br>DSL/Cable internet connection at a minimum speed of 384.0 Kbps or faster WiFi 802.11 b/g preferred. | | 7-inch and 10-inch tablets on maximum resolution.<br><br>WiFi connection is required. |

Thieme

# Reconstructive Plastic Surgery of the Head and Neck

## Current Techniques and Flap Atlas

**Matthew M. Hanasono, MD**
Professor and Fellowship Program Director
Department of Plastic Surgery
The University of Texas MD Anderson Cancer Center
Houston, Texas

**Geoffrey L. Robb, MD**
Professor
Department of Plastic Surgery
The University of Texas MD Anderson Cancer Center
Houston, Texas

**Roman J. Skoracki, MD, FRCSC, FACS**
Professor and Division Chief of Reconstructive Oncologic Plastic Surgery
Department of Plastic Surgery
The Ohio State University Wexner Medical Center
Columbus, Ohio

**Peirong Yu, MD, FACS**
Professor
Department of Plastic Surgery
The University of Texas MD Anderson Cancer Center
Houston, Texas

765 illustrations

Thieme
New York • Stuttgart • Delhi • Rio de Janeiro

Executive Editor: Timothy Y. Hiscock
Managing Editor: Elizabeth Palumbo
Director, Editorial Services: Mary Jo Casey
Production Editor: Kenneth L. Chumbley
International Production Director: Andreas Schabert
Vice President, Editorial and E-Product Development:
Vera Spillner
International Marketing Director: Fiona Henderson
International Sales Director: Louisa Turrell
Director of Sales, North America: Mike Roseman
Senior Vice President and Chief Operating Officer:
Sarah Vanderbilt
President: Brian D. Scanlan

**Library of Congress Cataloging-in-Publication Data**

Names: Hanasono, Matthew M., author. | Robb, Geoffrey L., author. | Skoracki, Roman J., author. | Yu, Peirong, author.

Title: Reconstructive plastic surgery of the head and neck : current techniques and flap atlas / Matthew M. Hanasono, Geoffrey L. Robb, Roman J. Skoracki, Peirong Yu.

Description: New York : Thieme, [2016] | Includes bibliographical references and index.

Identifiers: LCCN 2015048818| ISBN 9781604068078 (hardcover) | ISBN 9781604068139 (eISBN)

Subjects: | MESH: Reconstructive Surgical Procedures--methods | Head--surgery | Neck--surgery | Head and Neck Neoplasms--surgery | Surgical Flaps

Classification: LCC RD119 | NLM WE 700 | DDC 617.9/52--dc23 LC record available at http://lccn.loc.gov/2015048818



Thieme Publishers New York
333 Seventh Avenue, New York, NY 10001 USA
+1 800 782 3488, customerservice@thieme.com

Thieme Publishers Stuttgart
Rüdigerstrasse 14, 70469 Stuttgart, Germany
+49 [0]711 8931 421, customerservice@thieme.de

Thieme Publishers Delhi
A-12, Second Floor, Sector-2, Noida-201301
Uttar Pradesh, India
+91 120 45 566 00, customerservice@thieme.in

Thieme Publishers Rio de Janeiro, Thieme Publicações Ltda.
Edifício Rodolpho de Paoli, 25º andar
Av. Nilo Peçanha, 50 – Sala 2508
Rio de Janeiro 20020-906 Brasil
+55 21 3172 2297

Cover design: Thieme Publishing Group
Typesetting by Prairie Papers
Medical Illustrator: Hyun-Hang Lee

Printed in China by Asia Pacific Offset 5 4 3 2 1

ISBN 978-1-60406-807-8

Also available as an e-book:
eISBN 978-1-60406-813-9



FSC
www.fsc.org
MIX
Paper from responsible sources
FSC® C012521

We dedicate this book to our mentors, colleagues, and patients for their inspiration, commitment, and courage. We also dedicate this work to our families for their patience, support, and love. We have written this book for our students, residents, and fellows. We hope that the information contained herein will capture your imagination and that you will one day take head and neck reconstruction far beyond anything we can imagine.

*Matthew M. Hanasono*
*Geoffrey L. Robb*
*Roman J. Skoracki*
*Peirong Yu*

# Contents

# Videos

# Preface

Concurrent with advances in the treatment of head and neck malignancies, head and neck reconstruction has flourished in recent years. Not only have we made great strides in restoring form and function to patients suffering from head and neck cancer, but the ability to reliably reconstruct surgical defects has also helped to improve cancer control by allowing more aggressive and complete oncologic ablation and facilitating timely administration of adjuvant therapies. As experience has enabled reconstructive surgeons to achieve consistently high flap success rates with predictably good functional and aesthetic results, the complexity of the surgical defects that we feel comfortable addressing has increased. Moreover, as survival from head and neck cancer has improved, we have observed an increase in second (or even third) primary cancers as well as long-term complications of treatment (such as osteoradionecrosis) in cancer survivors that frequently present even greater reconstructive challenges than the original cancer. To meet these challenges, reconstructive surgeons have explored new flaps and combinations of flaps, while seeking to minimize donor site morbidity with refined flap selection and muscle-sparing perforator dissection. Furthermore, we have reached beyond the boundaries of traditional surgical methods by embracing new techniques, such as composite tissue allotransplantation, and incorporating cutting-edge technologies, such as computer modeling, advanced imaging, and robotics, into our operative workflow.

The goal of this book is to provide an up-to-date guide to every aspect of head and neck reconstruction. We felt the need to fill a void since few recent texts are devoted solely to this broad and complicated field that is rich enough to be its own surgical specialty. We made every effort to make this book practical and complete. We believe trainees and young surgeons, as well as seasoned veterans, will benefit from the material presented, as both basic concepts and advanced techniques are discussed. Without a doubt, the coming years will see even more advances in head and neck reconstruction as surgeons continue to strive toward perfect and total restoration. We welcome such advances and hope that you, our readers, will be inspired by this book to contribute to them.

This book is divided into two parts. The first part is dedicated to various topics pertinent to modern head and neck reconstruction. Our goal in these chapters is to provide anatomic, functional, and oncologic information for a specific head and neck region and to present a reconstructive algorithm for that region based on our experience with the many thousands of head and neck reconstructions performed at MD Anderson Cancer Center over the past three decades. However, we set out to do much more than write a "how we do it" book. To give a balanced view, we invited many of the top reconstructive surgeons in the world to comment and expand upon our text. In many instances, these commentaries demonstrate that there is often more than one way to achieve excellent outcomes. In others, it shows that, as far as we have come, there is much yet to discover and learn.

Also in this section are a number of chapters dealing with specific aspects of the comprehensive care of the head and neck reconstruction patient, including a broad overview of head and neck cancer treatment, management of complications, and prosthetic rehabilitation, which may, in some cases, be the best reconstructive option for a given patient. Keeping with the spirit of discovery and innovation, we have also included chapters on robotic surgery, composite tissue allotransplantation, and imaging and computer modeling, which we feel are important new directions within the field of head and neck reconstruction.

The second part describes how to perform what we feel are the most important pedicled and free flaps for the head and neck reconstructive surgeon to have in his or her toolbox. Here, too, we acknowledge that there is more than one "right" way to perform the surgery, but hope that the reader will find the techniques we present, which have been refined by countless hours in the operating room, to be practical and reliable. Throughout both parts of the book, we have tried to illustrate the principles of reconstruction with clinical examples, featuring high quality photographs and illustrations. Further personalizing this text, we have added "Pearls and Pitfalls" sections that outline key concepts and critical nuances in surgical technique or patient management wherever they are pertinent.

We sincerely thank all of our contributors for their excellent work. In addition to the many expert commentaries included in our book, we humbly sought out the help of some extraordinary surgeons for chapters that could only be written by the leading authority on certain topics, such as facial and tracheal transplantation, as well as for the supraclavicular artery island flap and the thoracodorsal artery perforator flap. We are even more appreciative of our patients who have given us permission to share experience gained from their surgeries and photos taken during the course of their care so that others may benefit from their hardships. We welcome feedback and the chance to one day completely rewrite this work based on further innovation and evidenced-based research.

*Matthew M. Hanasono*

# Contributors

**James S. Brown, MD, FRCS, FDSRCS**
Professor
Department of Head and Neck Surgery
Aintree University Hospital
Liverpool University
Liverpool, England

**Ericka M. Bueno, PhD**
Scientific Director
Department of Plastic Surgery
Brigham and Women's Surgery
Boston, Massachusetts

**Richard C. Cardoso, DDS, MS, FACP**
Assistant Professor
Department of Head and Neck Surgery
Section of Oral Oncology and Maxillofacial Prosthetics
The University of Texas MD Anderson Cancer Center
Houston, Texas

**Edward I. Chang, MD, FACS**
Assistant Professor
Department of Plastic Surgery
The University of Texas MD Anderson Cancer Center
Houston, Texas

**Steven S. Chang, MD, FACS**
Director, Head and Neck Cancer Program
Josephine Ford Cancer Institute
Department of Otolarygnology–Head and Neck Surgery
Henry Ford Health System
Detroit, Michigan

**Albert Chao, MD**
Assistant Professor
Department of Plastic Surgery
The Ohio State University
Columbus, Ohio

**Ming-Huei Cheng, MD, MBA, FACS**
Professor
Department of Plastic and Reconstructive Surgery
Chief, Center for Tissue Engineering
Chang Gung Memorial Hospital
Linkou, Taiwan

**Ernest S. Chiu, MD, FACS**
Associate Professor of Plastic Surgery
Director, Helen L. and Martin S. Kimmel Hyperbaric and Advanced Wound Healing Center
Hansjörg Wyss Department of Plastic Surgery
New York University Langone Medical Center
New York, New York

**Sydney Ch'ng, MBBS, PhD, FRACS**
Institute of Academic Surgery at RPA Hospital
University of Sydney
Sydney, Australia

**Michael W. Chu, MD**
Assistant Professor
Department of Plastic and Reconstruction Surgery
Indiana University School of Medicine
Indianapolis, Indiana

**Joseph J. Disa, MD, FACS**
Attending Surgeon
Memorial Sloan Kettering Cancer Center
Plastic and Reconstructive Surgery Service
Professor of Surgery
Weill Cornell Medical College
New York, New York

**Ryan Michael Gobble, MD**
Assistant Professor of Plastic Surgery
Department of Surgery
University of Cincinnati College of Medicine
Cincinnati, Ohio

**Lawrence J. Gottlieb, MD, FACS**
Professor
Director, Burn and Complex Wound Center
Department of Surgery
University of Chicago Medicine and Biological Sciences
Chicago, Illinois

**Matthew M. Hanasono, MD**
Professor and Fellowship Program Director
Department of Plastic Surgery
The University of Texas MD Anderson Cancer Center
Houston, Texas

**Theresa M. Hofstede, BSc, DDS, FACP**
Associate Professor
Department of Head and Neck Surgery
The University of Texas MD Anderson Cancer Center
Houston, Texas

**F. Christopher Holsinger, MD, FACS**
Professor and Chief
Division of Head and Neck Surgery
Stanford University
Palo Alto, California

**Katherine A. Hutcheson, PhD**
Associate Professor
Department of Head and Neck Surgery
The University of Texas MD Anderson Cancer Center
Houston, Texas

**Amir Ibrahim, MD**
Assistant Professor in Plastic Surgery
Department of Surgery
Division of Plastic Surgery
American University of Beirut Medical Center
Beirut, Lebanon

**Michael Klebuc, MD**
Associate Professor of Clinical Plastic and Reconstructive Surgery
Weill Medical College, Cornell University
Institute for Reconstructive Surgery
Houston Methodist Hospital
Houston, Texas

**Evan Matros, MD, MMSc, MPH**
Assistant Professor
Plastic and Reconstructive Surgery Service
Memorial Sloan Kettering Cancer Center
New York, New York

**Patricia C. Montgomery**
Senior Anaplastologist
Department of Head and Neck Surgery
Section of Oral Oncology and Maxillofacial Prosthodontics
The University of Texas MD Anderson Cancer Center
Houston, Texas

**Goo-Hyun Mun, MD, PhD**
Associate Professor
Department of Plastic Surgery
Samsung Medical Center
Sungkyunkwan University School of Medicine
Seoul, Republic of Korea

**Peter C. Neligan, MB, FRCS(I), FRCSC, FACS**
Professor
Department of Surgery
University of Washington Medical Center
Seattle, Washington

**Bohdan Pomahac, MD**
Director, Burn Center
Director, Plastic Surgery Transplantation
Division of Plastic Surgery
Brigham and Women's Hospital
Boston, Massachusetts

**Geoffrey L. Robb, MD**
Professor
Department of Plastic Surgery
The University of Texas MD Anderson Cancer Center
Houston, Texas

**Karim A. Sarhane, MD, MSc**
Department of Surgery
University of Toledo
Toledo, Ohio

**Jesse C. Selber, MD, MPH**
Associate Professor
Department of Plastic Surgery
The University of Texas MD Anderson Cancer Center
Houston, Texas

**Roman J. Skoracki, MD, FRCSC, FACS**
Professor and Division Chief of Reconstructive Oncologic Plastic Surgery
Department of Plastic Surgery
The Ohio State University Wexner Medical Center
Columbus, Ohio

**Jan Jeroen Vranckx, MD, PhD, FCCP, FAAPS**
Chief, Department of Plastic and Reconstructive Surgery
Professor of Surgery
KU-Leuven University
PI Lab of Plastic Surgery and Tissue Engineering Research
UZ-Gasthuisberg, KU-Leuven University Hospitals
Leuven, Belgium

**Randal S. Weber, MD, FACS**
Professor and Chair
John Brooks Williams and Elizabeth Williams Distinguished University Chair in Cancer Medicine
Department of Head and Neck Surgery
The University of Texas MD Anderson Cancer Center
Houston, Texas

**Peirong Yu, MD, FACS**
Professor
Department of Plastic Surgery
The University of Texas MD Anderson Cancer Center
Houston, Texas

**Michael R. Zenn, MD, MBA, FACS**
Professor
Department of Plastic and Reconstructive Surgery
Duke University
Durham, North Carolina

# I

# Topics in Head and Neck Reconstruction

# 1 Lip Reconstruction

*Matthew M. Hanasono*

## Introduction

The challenge of lip reconstruction is to maintain oral competence while still providing adequate mouth opening, and to do so in an aesthetically pleasing way. Oral competence is needed for speech articulation, for preventing loss of foods and liquids, and for containing saliva, as well as for sucking, whistling, and kissing. Too small of an oral aperture results in problems with eating as well as oral hygiene and can make use of dentures impossible. If the lips do not oppose, the patient will drool, and speech and swallowing can be impaired. Aesthetically, even small abnormalities of the vermilion line, Cupid's bow, the philtral columns, or the oral commissures can be noticeable from a distance.

Numerous techniques have been described over the years for lip reconstruction, each with specific indications as well as advantages and disadvantages. While free flap reconstructions for large defects continue to evolve, most recent local flap techniques are modifications of tried and true methods. Several reviews have proposed algorithms for flap selection based on location and defect size. The exact method chosen for a given patient depends not only on the size and extent of the defect, but also on the quality of tissues, the patient's needs and expectations, and the surgeon's experience. A practical and reliable approach that addresses both local and free flap techniques is outlined below.

## Anatomy

The lips are each ~ 5 to 6 cm long. The blood supply comes from the paired superior and inferior labial branches of the facial artery. These arteries run submucosally on the intraoral side of the lip. The motor supply comes primarily from the buccal and marginal mandibular nerve branches. Sensory innervation comes from branches of the trigeminal nerve (the superior labial branches of $V_2$ for the upper lip and the mental branches of $V_3$ for the lower lip).

The sphincter function of the lips is provided by the orbicularis oris muscle, which is arranged circularly around the mouth and has no bony attachments. The orbicularis oris muscle has superficial fibers that hold the lips away from the face and deep fibers that approximate the lips to the alveolar arches. Ideally, the sphincteric ring is restored during lip reconstruction, although many defects are too large for this goal to be met. Several muscles dilate the mouth and provide support to the central ring, including upper lip dilators (zygomaticus major, zygomaticus minor, levator labii superioris, and levator labii superioris alaeque nasi), elevators of the oral commissure (levator anguli oris, buccinators, and risorius), and lower lip depressors (depressor labii inferioris, depressor anguli oris, mentalis, and platysma).

The vermilion is the exposed dry mucosal transition zone between the wet lip, which is supplied by salivary glands, and the skin. Its red color is due to the rich blood supply to the region. A thin, pale, junctional zone of skin, known as the white line, marks the boundary of the vermilion where it meets the cutaneous lip. Correct alignment of the white line is necessary to achieve an optimal aesthetic result in lip reconstruction.

## Small Lip Defects

Full-thickness defects approaching one-third the width of the lower lip can be closed directly as a wedge (**Fig. 1.1**). Smaller defects can be closed as a V-shaped wedge. As the size of the defect increases, the wedge can be modified to a W-shape, to avoid crossing the mental crease onto the chin. For larger defects, closer to one-third of the lip width (or even slightly larger in patients with sufficient tissue laxity), releasing incisions can be made along the mental crease to permit advancement of the lateral lip tissues for closure, which will usually produce a

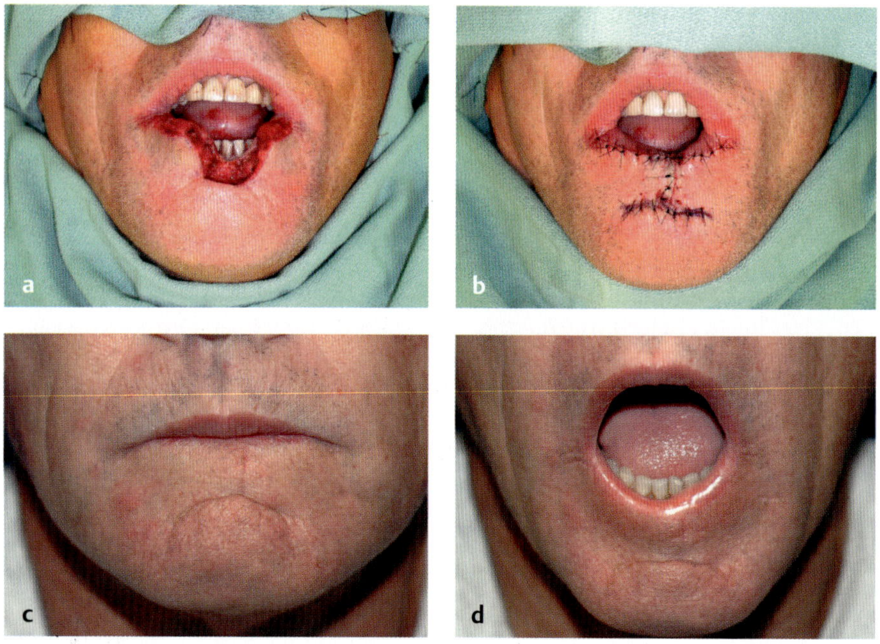


**Fig. 1.1** **(a)** Defect encompassing approximately one-third of the width of the lower lip. A vermilionectomy has also been performed. **(b)** Bilateral lip advancement flaps were performed and the labial mucosa was advanced to replace the missing vermilion lip epithelium. **(c)** The postoperative result, **(d)** with excellent mouth opening.

superior result **(Fig. 1.2)**. All lip closures should be performed in three layers, including the mucosa, the orbicularis oris muscle, and the skin, with care taken to precisely realign the white line. Notching of the lip due to contracture of the incision line can occur, especially in an irradiated field. Primary or secondary z-plasty may help to lengthen the scar. Use of a pentagonal excision rather than a V-shaped wedge may also be of benefit for small defects.

The upper lip is less accommodating, and wedge closures should be reserved for defects involving less than about one-fourth of the width of the lip. Wedge closure of larger defects will result in excessive tightness, causing the upper lip to sit posterior

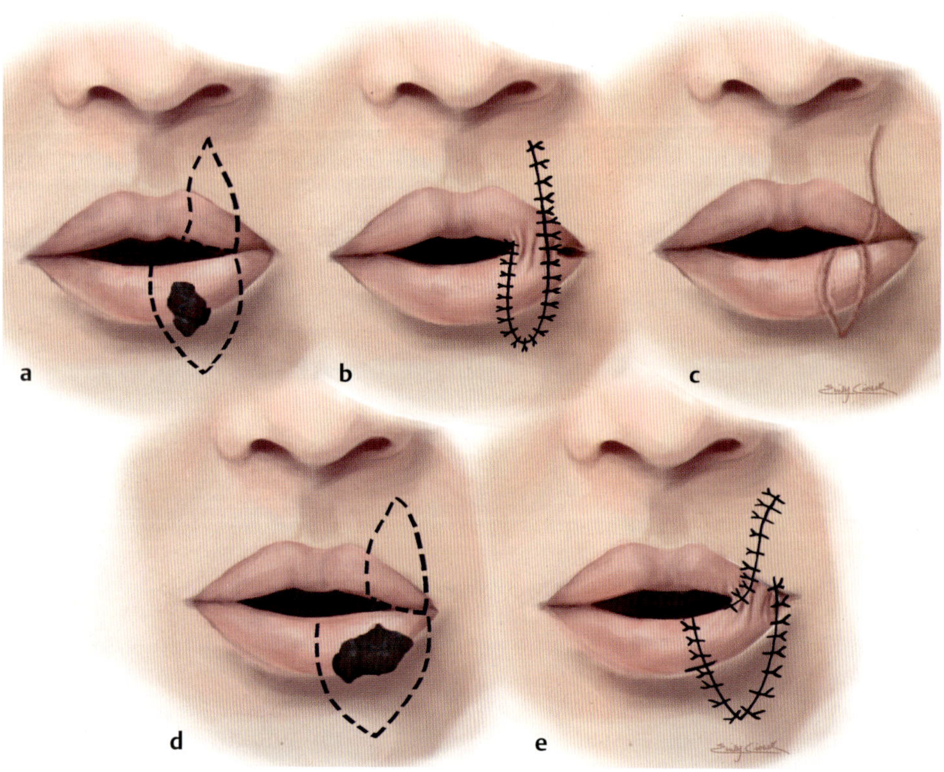


**Fig. 1.2** Diagram demonstrating **(a–c)** Abbe and **(d,e)** Estlander cross lip flaps for intermediate-size lip defects. The Abbe flap pedicle is divided ~ 14 to 21 days after the initial surgery.

to the lower lip. An advancement flap, with an incision made along the junction of the upper lip and the floor of the nose, as well as a perialar crescentic excision that permits further movement, can decrease the tightness of closure.[1] Defects that involve the philtrum can be closed with direct closure or bilateral advancement flaps, although the result will not restore the philtral columns and Cupid's bow shape of the vermilion border. A more aesthetic reconstruction of the philtrum usually requires utilization of the Abbe cross lip flap, discussed below.

## Intermediate Lip Defects

Most defects of the upper and lower lip, up to about two-thirds of the lip width (often even slightly more in the lower lip), are best managed with either lip switch flaps (Abbe or Estlander flaps) or circumoral advancement-rotation flaps (Karapandzic flaps). The lip switch flap, known as an Abbe flap[2] when used to reconstruct the central lip, and an Estlander flap[3] for commissural reconstruction, involves transferring full-thickness lip tissue from the opposing lip based on a labial artery pedicle **(Fig. 1.3)**. The width of the flap should be about one-half of the width of the excised tissue, which will reduce the size of the upper and lower lip by the same amount. For practical purposes, the maximum width of a lip switch flap is ~ 2 cm. The height of the flap should be the same as the height of the defect.

The Abbe flap should be designed so that its pedicle is centered on the defect, although it is best not to include either of the philtral columns when the flap originates from the upper lip, if possible.[4] The Estlander flap should utilize the melolabial crease as one border.

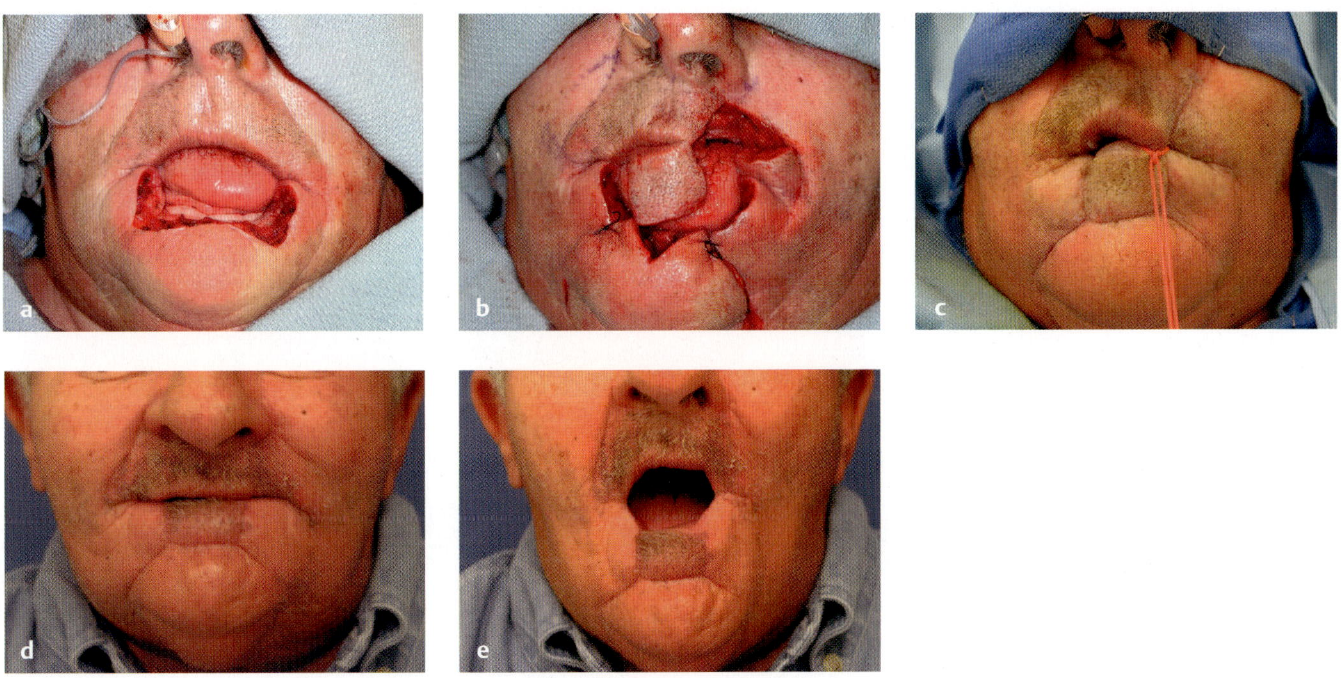

**Fig. 1.3** **(a)** A defect encompassing about one-half of the width of the lower lip in an older patient with substantial tissue laxity. **(b)** A rectangular Abbe flap, based on the right superior labial artery, is elevated and rotated into the defect. **(c)** Approximately 3 weeks after the initial surgery, the pedicle is divided. A vessel loop acting as a tourniquet around the pedicle demonstrates viability of the flap based on vascular ingrowth from the wound edges. **(d)** The postoperative result, **(e)** with good mouth opening.

Although traditionally the Abbe flap is thought of as triangular in shape, it may be designed to fit in W-shaped or rectangular defects. It is particularly useful for restoring the philtral subunit of the upper lip. The Abbe flap requires maintaining a bridge of tissue containing the arterial pedicle between the donor lip and the recipient lip for a period of 14 to 21 days. During that time, oral intake is compromised. The flap can be injured if the mouth is opened widely, so patients are usually limited to taking in liquids with a straw, or a nasogastric feeding tube can be placed.

The Estlander flap does not require pedicle division, although the patient can often benefit from revision to eliminate blunting and medialization of the commissure. Commissuroplasty can be performed to improve cosmesis and mouth opening after spontaneous remodeling is allowed for a period of at least 4 to 6 months following initial lip reconstruction with an Estlander flap. A simple method is to incise or remove a wedge of skin lateral to the commissure, then evert the buccal mucosa to simulate the vermilion lip (**Fig. 1.4**). Only a very modest amount of commissural movement should be performed by this method to avoid oral incontinence, although the procedure can be repeated to widen the commissure a little bit at a time. Alternatively, commissuroplasty can be performed by rotation and advancement of a superiorly based vermilion-mucosa flap following an incision of the cheek just lateral to the commissure (**Fig. 1.5**).[5] The resulting vermilion defect is reconstructed by advancing labial mucosa toward the white line.

An alternative to Abbe and Estlander flaps is the Karapandzic technique, which involves circumoral rotation-advancement flaps.[6] The Karapandzic technique is similar to the circumoral advancement-rotation flaps originally described by von Bruns[7]

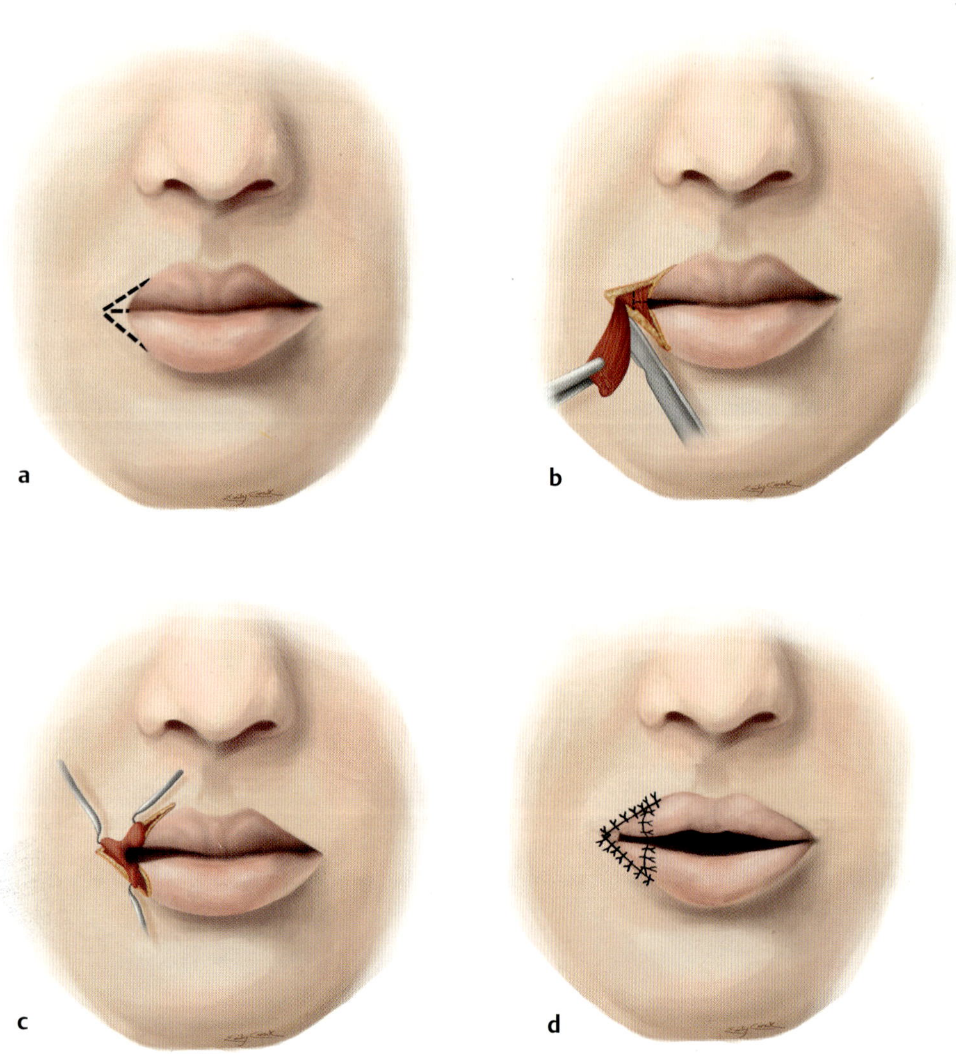


**Fig. 1.4** Commissuroplasty to improve mouth opening and to lateralize the oral commissure following initial lip reconstruction. **(a)** Planned incisions. **(b)** Removal of a triangle of skin and markings for muscle and mucosal incisions. **(c)** Eversion of the mucosa. **(d)** Completed commissuroplasty.

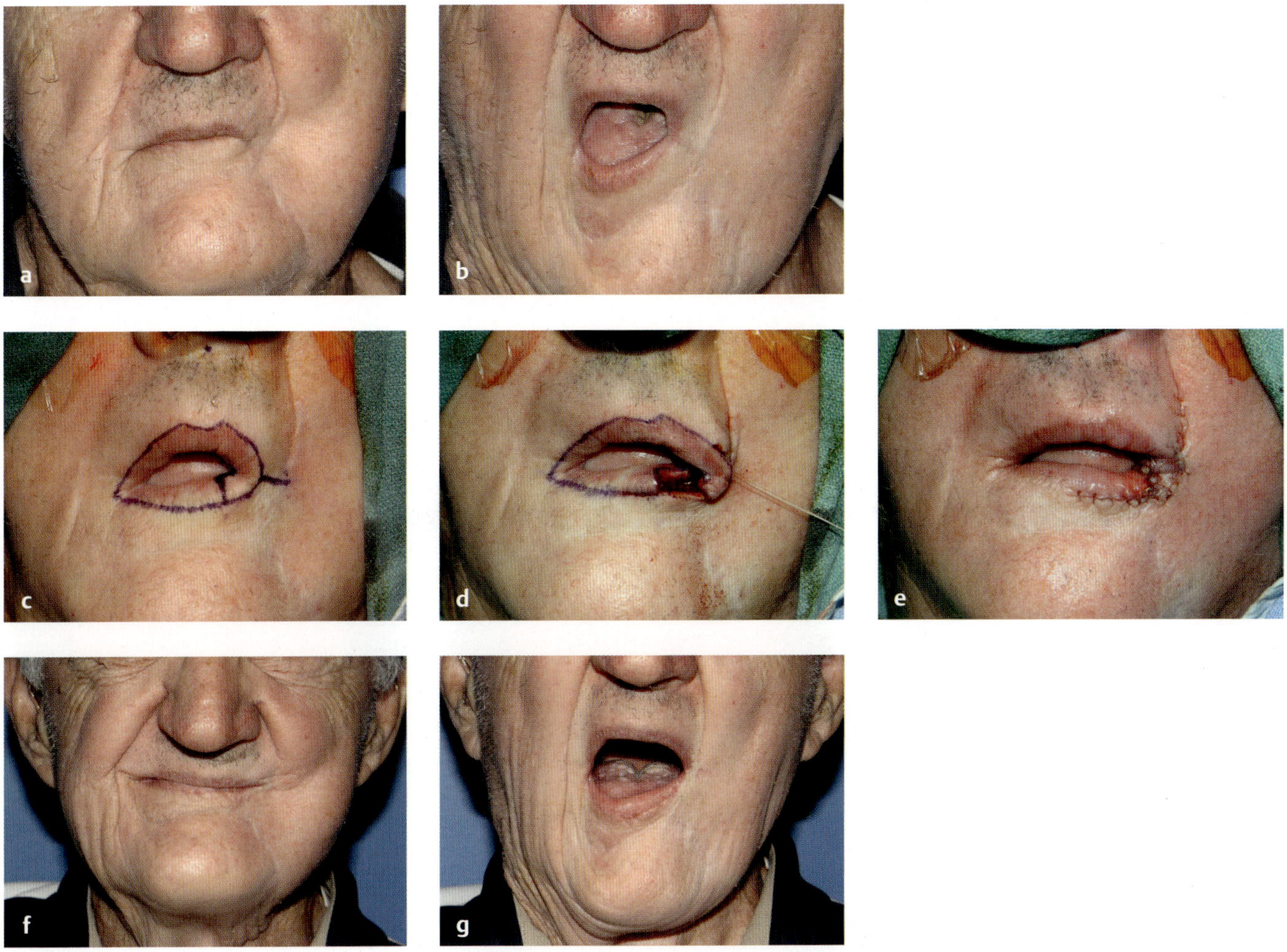


**Fig. 1.5 (a,b)** Alternative technique for commissuroplasty in a patient who had undergone lip reconstruction that resulted in a small oral aperture with a medialized oral commissure. **(c,d)** A skin incision is made lateral to the commissure and a vermilion flap is rotated into the new commissure location. Orbicularis oris muscle is also lateralized using a deep buried suture. **(e)** The labial mucosa is everted to cover the vermilion defect. **(f,g)** The postoperative result shows the left oral commissure in a more favorable, although not perfectly symmetrical, position, with improved mouth opening.

in 1857, but preserves the neurovascular supply to the lip flaps, making them more reliable as well as functional and sensate. In this technique, skin incisions are planned so that the height of the flaps is equivalent to the height of the lip defect, not necessarily staying within the melolabial crease laterally (**Fig. 1.6**). Deep to the skin, perioral muscles are selectively lysed while preserving nerves and blood vessels to the remaining lip until adequate flap mobility is achieved. Finally, the mucosal incisions are made in a "cut as you go" fashion; typically, the incision is shorter than the skin length required due to the more distensible nature of the mucosal tissues. Leaving adequate mucosa along the gingiva is important not only for having enough tissue to sew to, but also for preserving a gingivolabial sulcus in denture users.

A unilateral Karapandzic flap can reconstruct smaller defects, up to nearly 50% of the lip width, while bilateral Karapandzic flaps can be used for defects spanning two-thirds the width of the lip or even slightly more. The larger the defect, the greater the risk for microstomia, since no lip tissue is added, just as with other local lip flaps mentioned thus far. Blunting or rounding of the commissures can also occur but usually improves with time. The various lip flaps, including advancement, Abbe, Estlander, and Karapandzic flaps, can also be combined, depending on the defect and the location of donor lip tissue (**Fig. 1.7**).

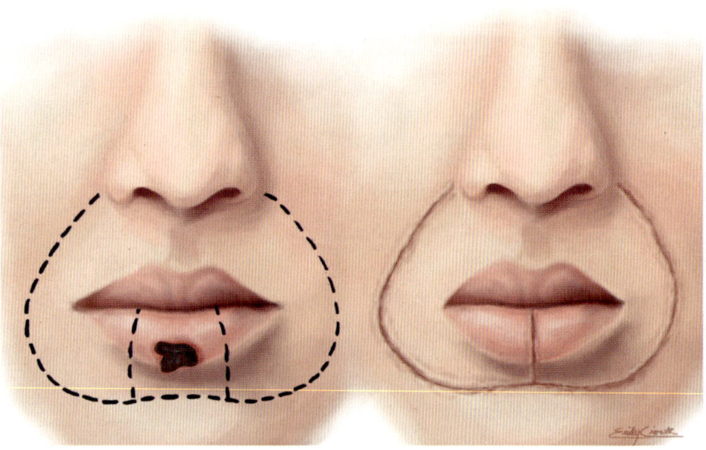

**Fig. 1.6** Diagram demonstrating the Karapandzic technique of circumoral neurovascular flap reconstruction for intermediate to large lip defects. This technique can be applied to both lower and upper lip defects, although it does not restore the philtral columns or the Cupid's bow shape of the upper lip vermilion border.

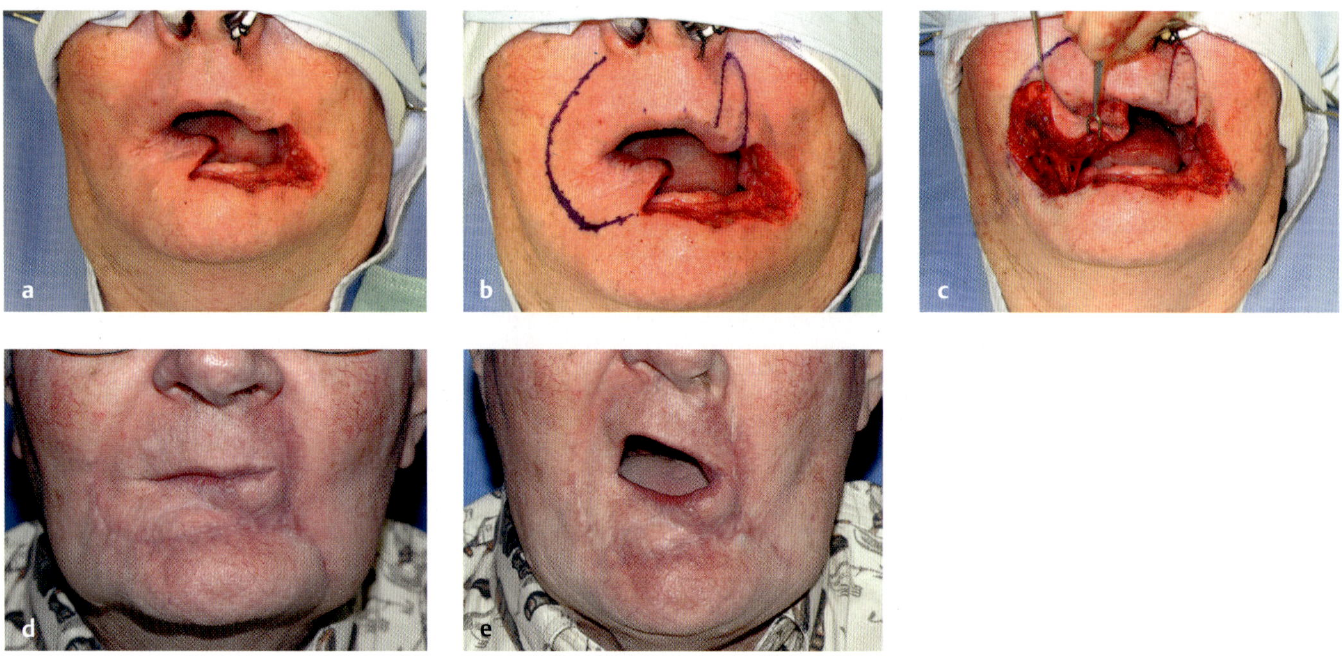


**Fig. 1.7** **(a)** A defect involving nearly two-thirds of the lower lip width, including the left oral commissure. **(b)** A right Karapandzic flap is combined with a left Estlander flap, which is used to restore the commissure. **(c)** Note that the nerves and blood vessels supplying the Karapandzic flap are preserved. **(d,e)** Postoperative result.

## ■ Near-Total and Total Lip Defects

Reconstruction of near-total and total defects is especially challenging. Local tissue techniques for lower lip reconstruction include use of nasolabial flaps (e.g., "gate flaps" described by Fujimori[8]) or cheek advancement techniques (e.g., Webster modification of the Bernard-Burrow repair[9,10]) **(Fig. 1.8)**. Similarly, inferiorly based nasolabial flaps or cheek advancement flaps with perialar crescentic excisions can be performed for upper lip reconstruction. None of these procedures provides a functional lip segment because the motor innervation is divided and/or the muscle fibers transferred are perpendicular to the orbicularis oris fibers. An Abbe flap from the lower lip to the central portion of the reconstructed upper lip to restore the appearance of the philtrum and to supply additional tissue can augment upper lip repairs. When using an Abbe flap to reconstruct the philtrum,

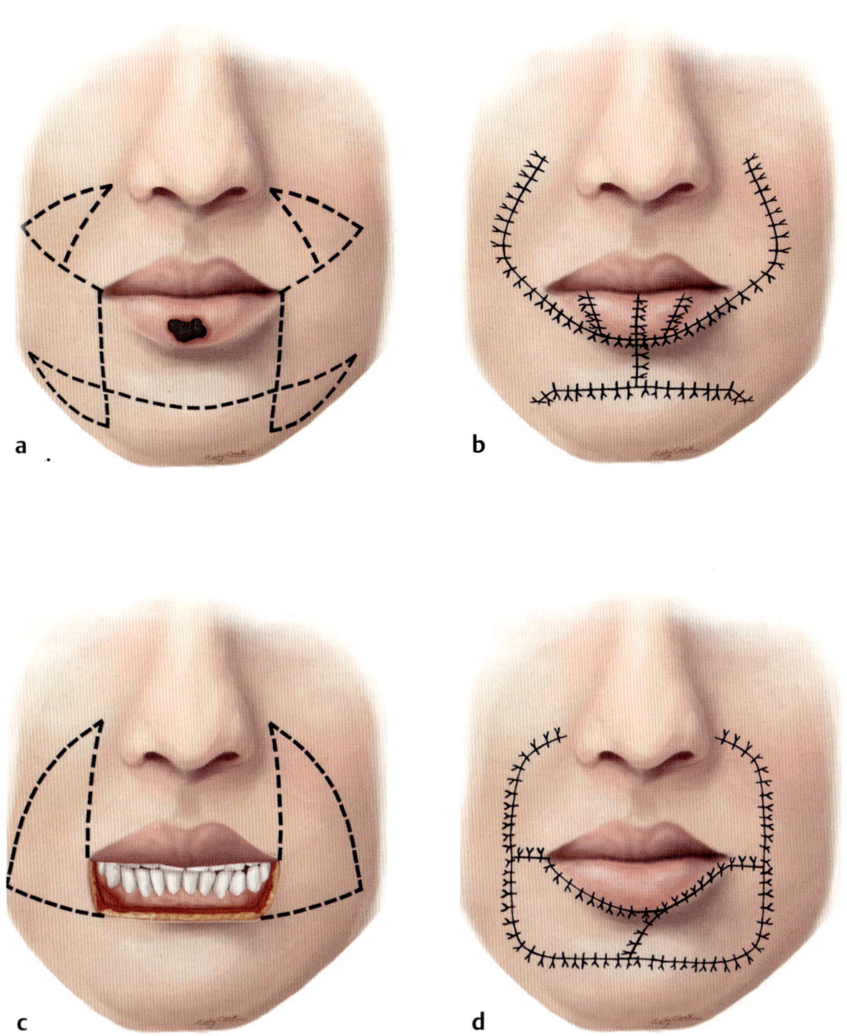

Fig. 1.8 Techniques for total lower lip repair. **(a)** Planned incisions for total lower lip repair with cheek advancement flaps (Webster modification of the Bernard-Burrow repair). The four triangles indicated by the dashed lines are excised and the cheeks are advanced medially toward each other. **(b)** Completed repair in which the buccal mucosa has been everted to replace the missing vermillion lip. **(c)** Planned incisions for total lower lip repair with nasolabial or "gate" flaps. The two gate flaps are rotated medially and the buccal mucosa is everted to replace the missing vermillion lip. **(d)** Completed repair in which the nasolabial flap donor sites have been closed primarily.

the width of the flap should be the same as the width of the original philtrum. Local tissue reconstruction may be satisfactory in patients with significant cheek tissue redundancy but often results in substantial microstomia and an adynamic, insensate lip.

An alternative to local tissue repair for near-total and total lip reconstruction is free tissue transfer. Most frequently, the radial forearm fasciocutaneous free flap is chosen because of its thinness and pliability.[4,11] When used for lower lip reconstruction, the flap is suspended over a palmaris longus tendon sling to help prevent oral incompetence. The tendon is either suspended to the zygomatic bones via screw-anchored sutures or woven into the remaining perioral muscles at the modioli. The width of the flap is also restricted to about half of the width of the defect to provide resting tension in an effort to minimize ptosis and eversion of the flap. On the other hand, the height of the flap should be as great as, or slightly greater than, the original lip height, since postoperative tissue contracture usually reduces the height of the reconstructed lip. The aesthetic result of free flap reconstruction is usually best when the entire facial subunit of the lip is replaced, which may require converting a near-total defect into a total defect. The lateral antebrachial cutaneous nerve and the cut end of the mental nerve can be anastomosed to provide sensation. A ventral tongue flap or a facial artery myomucosal (FAMM) flap can be performed secondarily to restore the vermilion color of the lip to a de-epithelialized portion of the free flap.[12] Medical tattooing can also be used.

The advantage of free flap reconstruction over cheek advancement and nasolabial flap reconstruction is that wound tension is greatly decreased by supplying a large quantity of tissue that is also well vascularized, which can be particularly important in a previously irradiated patient. Like the local tissue flap options for near-total and total lower lip reconstruction, the free flap is adynamic. When used for lower lip reconstruction, a folded free flap works as a dam to prevent drooling, but it can still be associated with major problems with eating. When used for upper lip reconstruction, a folded free flap is usually functionally more successful, since it mainly serves as a drape to cover the maxillary teeth, while the native lower lip provides oral competence. In both cases, the color match with the rest of the face may be poor, and the free flap usually results in the facial appearance of a ventriloquist's dummy.

Recently, we described a modification of the Karapandzic technique that can be used for near-total and total lower lip defects.[13,14] In this technique, lower cheek flaps are cantilevered on traditional Karapandzic neurovascular rotation-advancement flaps (**Fig. 1.9**). The buccal mucosa is everted onto the lower cheek flaps to restore the appearance of the vermilion lip. In contrast to the traditional Karapandzic technique, this technique uses additional tissue from the cheeks and recruits opposing lip tissue to restore the missing lip, reducing the risk for postoperative microstomia. In fact, the amount of lip that is typically restored by the extended Karapandzic flaps usually permits a generous amount of mouth opening postoperatively.

Although a small portion of the reconstructed lip will be adynamic, it does not seem to have a significant effect on oral competence, just as it does not with Abbe and Estlander flaps, which involve a similar amount of adynamic tissue. Compared with cheek advancement flaps, nasolabial flaps, and free flaps, the extended Karapandzic flap lip reconstruction yields superior sphincteric function of the lip. Sensation is preserved, and the cosmetic outcome is usually superior to free flap reconstruction. For less than total defects that are eccentrically located to one side or another, a combination of a traditional Karapandzic flap that takes advantage of remaining adjacent lip tissue and an extended Karapandzic flap on the side of the greater defect can be used (**Fig. 1.10**). Because of these advantages, the extended Karapandzic technique is our preferred method of addressing near-total and total lip defects, with free flaps being the secondary choice when the extended Karapandzic flaps are precluded by lack of adjacent tissue or prior surgery that might compromise flap reliability.

Our algorithm for selecting lip reconstruction techniques is summarized in **Fig. 1.11**.

## ■ Composite and Extended Lip Defects

For some head and neck cancers, the lip is involved secondarily by direct spread, such as from tumors of the floor of mouth or gingiva. On the other hand, some lip cancers spread to adjacent structures. In these cases, although it is sometimes tempting to use a single flap, it is usually best to reconstruct each structure separately.[15]

Cancers of the lower lip, for example, may involve the mandible by direct spread or via invasion of the mental nerve (**Fig. 1.12**). In such cases, the mandible is reconstructed with an osseous or osteocutaneous free flap and the lip is reconstructed with local flaps if possible. If the facial artery remains intact following the resection, it is probably prudent not to utilize it as a recipient blood vessel for a free flap, although blood flow to the lips usually remains sufficient to perform local flap reconstruction even after loss of one or both facial arteries due to col-

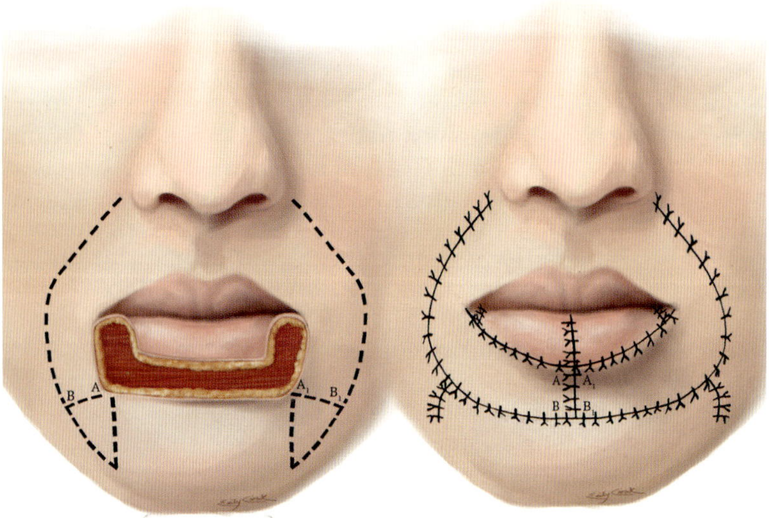

**Fig. 1.9** Total lower lip reconstruction with extended Karapandzic flaps. Traditional Karapandzic flaps are extended by lower cheek tissue, which is rotated medially an additional 90 degrees to reconstruct the central lower lip. **(a)** Planned incisions. Note that the triangles of skin indicated by the dashed lines are discarded. **(b)** Completed reconstruction in which point A is sutured to point $A_1$ and point B is sutured to point $B_1$ after rotation of the lower cheek tissue as well as circumoral advancement of the Karapandzic flaps.

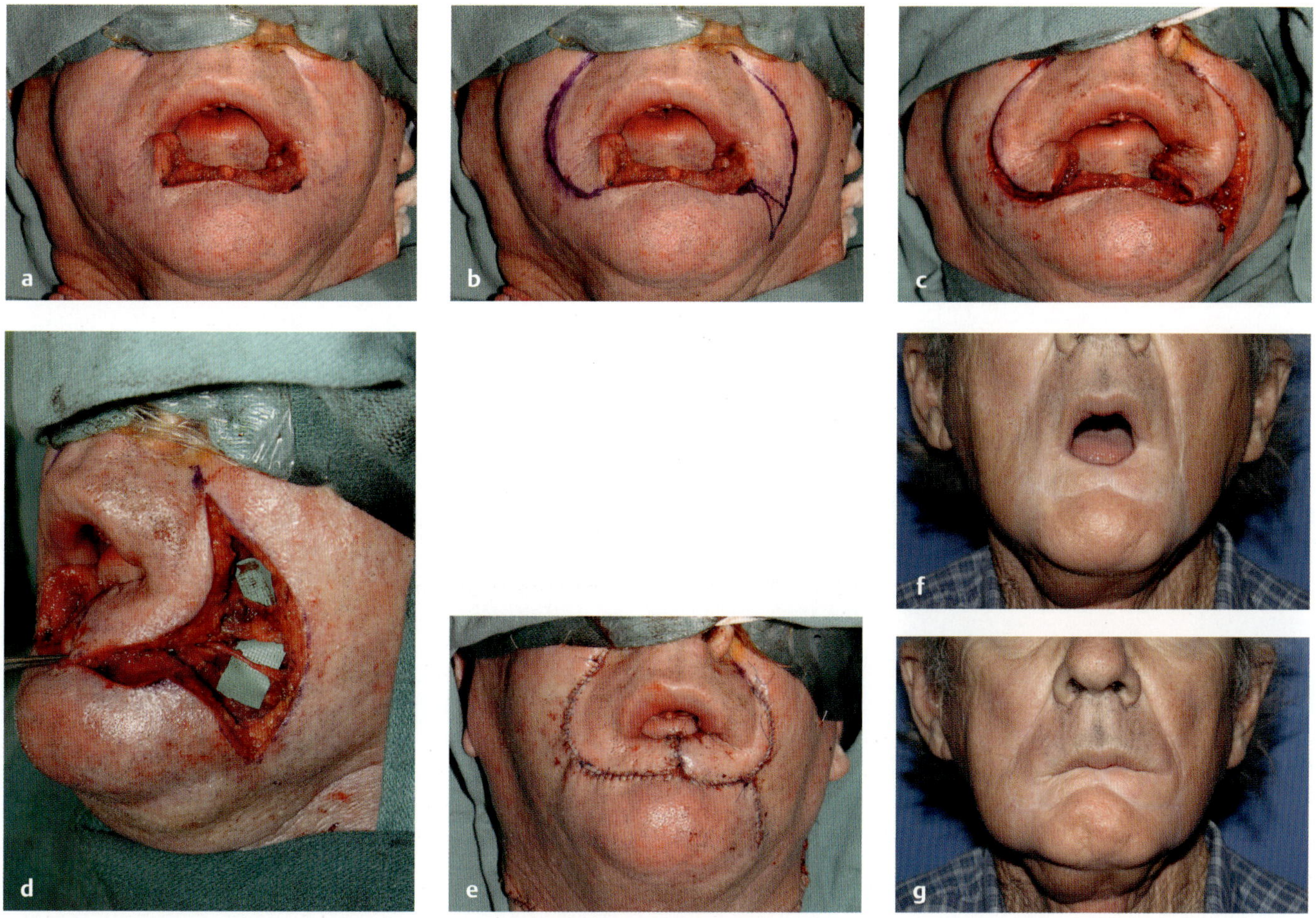

**Fig. 1.10** **(a)** A near-total lower lip defect sparing the right oral commissure. **(b)** A right Karapandzic flap and a left extended Karapandzic flap are designed. **(c,d)** Circumoral incisions are made, and the neurovascular supply to the flaps is carefully preserved. The left buccal mucosa is everted to replace the vermilion portion of the lip. **(e)** Appearance at the completion of surgery and **(f,g)** at 1 year postoperatively.

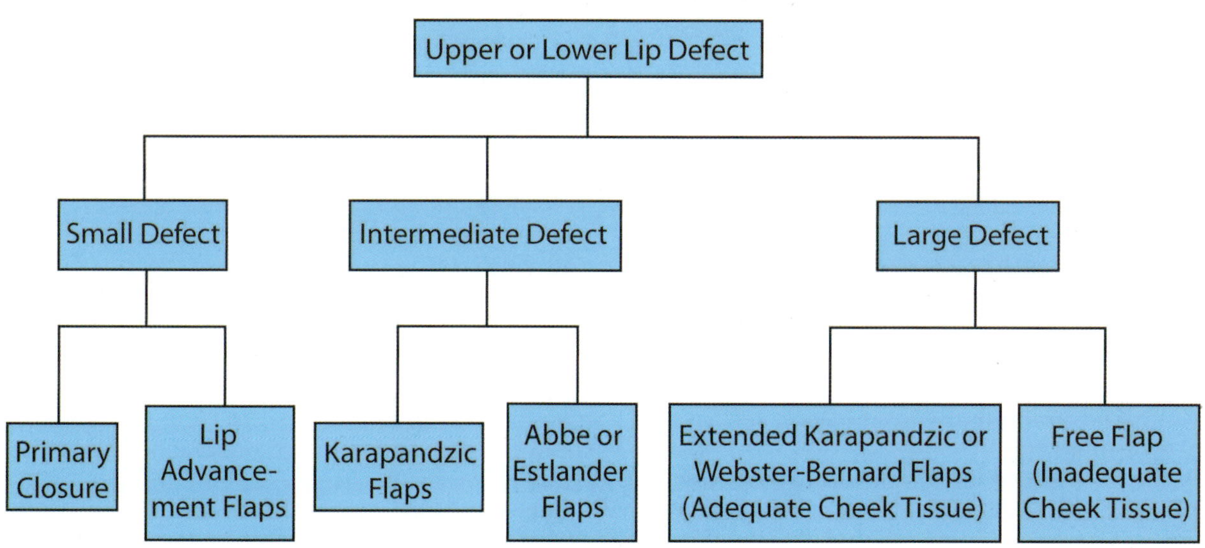


**Fig. 1.11** Algorithm for upper and lower lip reconstruction.

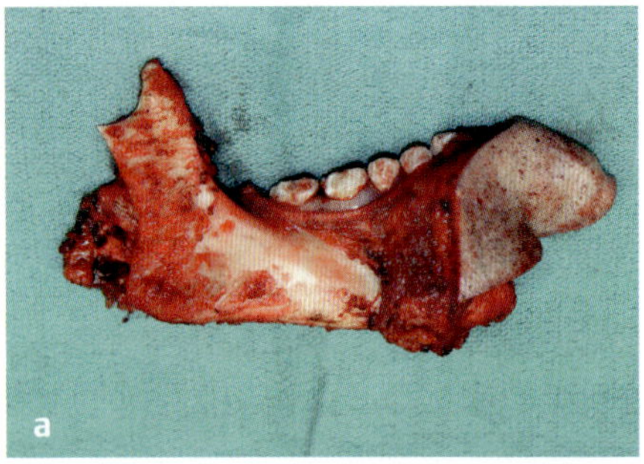

**Fig. 1.12** **(a)** A right lower lip cancer invading the mental nerve, requiring a hemimandibulectomy and two-third lower lip resection. **(b)** A fibular osteocutaneous free flap was used to reconstruct the mandibular defect. **(c,d)** The lip defect was reconstructed with bilateral Karapandzic flaps. **(e,f)** Postoperative result.

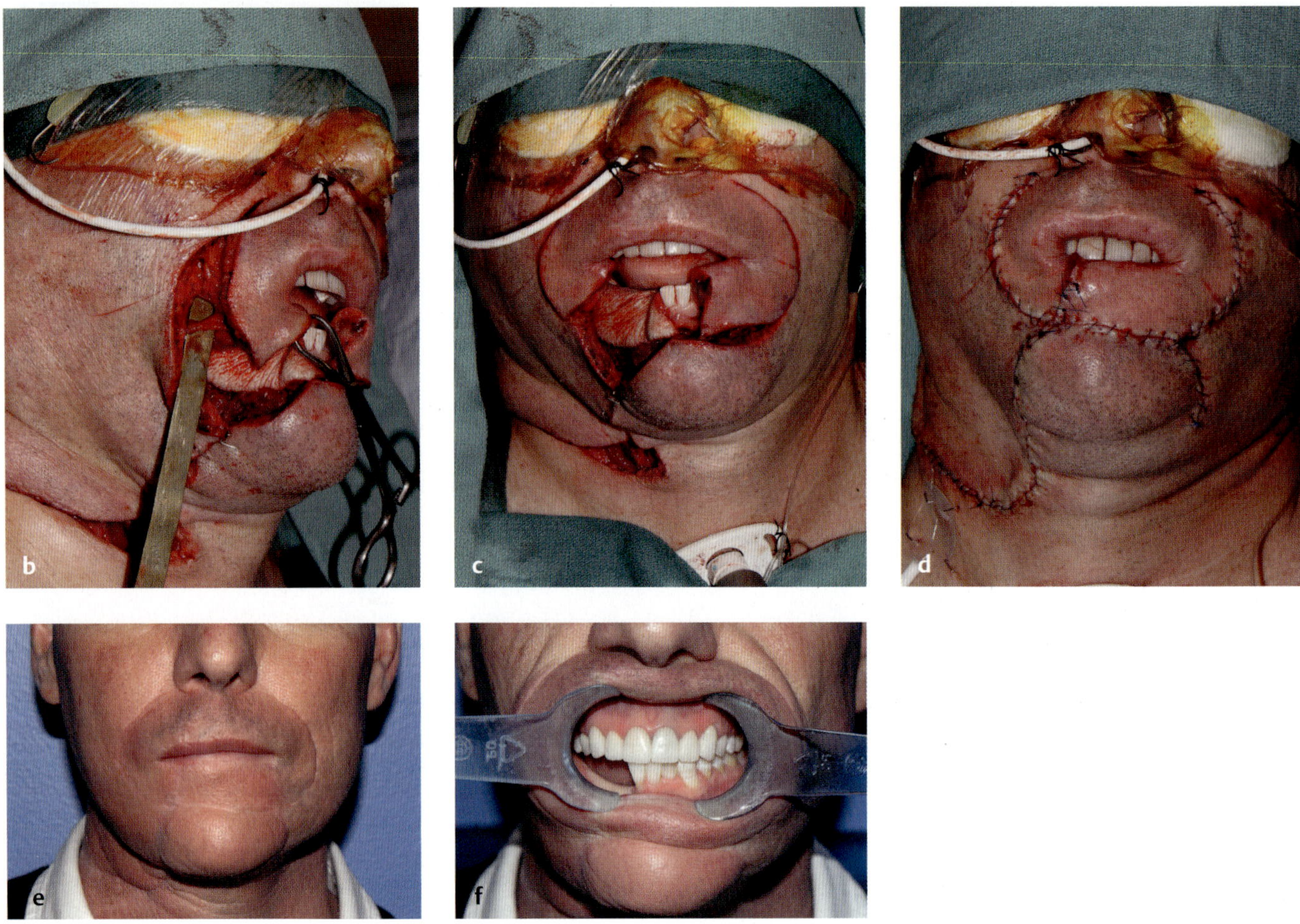

lateral circulation coming from the angular artery, which is a terminal branch of the internal carotid artery. When a very large defect leaves insufficient local tissues for reconstruction of the lower lip, the skin paddle from an osteocutaneous free flap may also serve to reconstruct the floor of the mouth and the lip, but the functional and aesthetic results are usually disappointing.

Upper lip cancers may spread to the maxilla as well as to the nose by direct extension. In these cases, staged nasal reconstruction should be performed separate from lip reconstruction. When postoperative radiation therapy is planned, it is usually best to perform delayed nasal reconstruction, because delicate reconstructions of the nose that involve multiple layers, including bone or cartilage grafts for support, do not tolerate radiation well. Small defects of the premaxilla can be obturated or reconstructed with an osteocutaneous free flap; however, this should be done immediately at the time of resection. Otherwise, the upper lip reconstruction, whether performed with local tissues or a folded fasciocutaneous free flap, will contract and make later attempts to restore midfacial projection very difficult. Large defects of the anterior maxilla require osteocutaneous free flap reconstruction.

## ■ Postoperative Care

Patients are restricted to a liquid diet or kept NPO and fed via a nasogastric feeding tube for several days after lip reconstruction. Incisions should be cleansed gently with soap and water or dilute hydrogen peroxide beginning the first postoperative day and antibiotic ointment should be applied twice daily for ~ 1 week. Wide mouth opening should be avoided until the incisions are well healed, which may take many weeks in previously irradiated patients. After the wounds are completely healed, mouth stretching and scar massage are encouraged. For defects that involve the commissure, patients should be instructed to perform finger retraction laterally to widen the oral aperture. For cases with functionally significant microstomia, a prosthedontist may be able to help create oral appliances that passively stretch the reconstructed lips.

## ■ Complications

Local flaps need to be designed so that their pedicle blood supply is not compromised. In cases where bilateral neck dissections have been performed, the facial arteries will likely have been ligated and flaps need to be checked for adequate vascularity, as evidenced by brisk bright red bleeding from the cut edge of the distal flap and pulsations from the ligated labial artery. Aggressive trimming of the pedicled portion of the Abbe and Estlander cross lip flaps in particular may need to be avoided. In such cases, refinement can be postponed until a second stage. Previously irradiated patients are at increased risk for fistula formation, and small fistulas can be managed by keeping the patient on NPO status and by placing a nasogastric feeding tube, facilitating spontaneous healing.

To some extent, all patients undergoing lip reconstruction with local flaps are at risk for microstomia. In some cases, commissuroplasty can help increase the size of the oral aperture following reconstruction of a lateral defect. A central lip defect may be improved by secondary reconstruction with an Abbe flap. Reconstructions with free flaps or larger denervated local flaps often result in loss of oral competence, causing drooling as well as difficulties with feeding and speech. Notching of the lip at incision lines can also occur. In many cases, the defects can be improved by excision of the scar and by closure that incorporates z-plasty flaps on the mucosal side.

## Pearls and Pitfalls

- V-shaped or W-shaped defects involving a third of the lower lip and a quarter of the upper lip can usually be closed primarily, while slightly larger defects can be closed with unilateral or bilateral lip advancement flaps.
- Central defects involving two-thirds of the lip width can be closed with an Abbe cross lip flap; lateral defects involving the oral commissure and two-thirds of the lip width can be closed with an Estlander cross lip flap.
- Blunting and medialization of the oral commissure is not uncommon with the Estlander cross lip flap but can be improved with secondary commissuroplasty.
- The Karapandzic technique of creating circumoral neurovascular flaps is often the best method of maintaining the oral sphincteric function in defects of up to two-thirds of the lip or even slightly more.
- Extended Karapandzic flaps can be used to reconstruct near-total or total lip defects, recreating the oral sphincter with sensate, well-vascularized tissue.
- Free flaps may be the best or only option for near-total or total lip reconstruction but are often suboptimal due to oral incompetence and skin color and texture mismatch.
- Composite or extensive defects should be reconstructed in a way that respects facial subunits, if possible.
- Free flaps for mandibular and maxillary reconstruction can be combined with local flaps for lip reconstruction to give optimal results.

## Expert Commentary *by Lawrence J. Gottlieb*

The lips are the most prominent feature of the lower third of the face and have significant functional, aesthetic, and social importance. They facilitate the articulation of certain sounds, the maintenance of oral competence during eating, drinking, sucking, and speaking, and the expression of emotions via smiling and kissing. In concert with motion of the mandible, they allow access to the mouth, not only for food intake but also for oral and dental hygiene, as well as for insertion and removal of dentures. The oral mucosal lining keeps its inner surface moist and serves incredibly complex immune functions as a "barrier organ" with the ability to distinguish between commensal and pathogenic microorganisms.

When we think of a functional lip, we should think not only of the skin covering but also of all the components beneath the skin that give human lips their three-dimensional characteristics that allow for communication, expression of emotions, and all the functions mentioned above. Therefore, the functional unit of the lips is the three-dimensional aesthetic unit. Ideally, reconstruction of the functional unit of the lip restores all missing components and results in a skin surface similar to the surface that was lost, with its borders hidden by natural skin folds, shadows, or hair, while maintaining an adequate stomal aperture and at the same time ensuring lip competence.

Restoration of the lips is complicated by the fact that the lips are mobile structures that function (aesthetically and mechanically) differently when in repose than when animated, since function and aesthetics are inextricably linked in the lips' functional units. In addition, as mobile structures, the lips are subjected to distortion by gravity, scar, and possibly radiation and denervation. Functional and aesthetic reconstruction of the mobile lip is further complicated when an adjacent facial unit's function is compromised by scars, trauma, radiation, and muscular dysfunction.

Lip reconstruction may be indicated for loss or abnormality of mucosa, vermilion, skin, subcutaneous tissue, muscle (denervation), or a combination of some or all of these components. The description of repair for each of these components is beyond the scope of this commentary. By and large, the most frequent circumstances requiring lip reconstruction are partial-thickness defects (loss of skin and subcutaneous tissue) or full-thickness defects from trauma or tumor extirpation.

Partial-thickness defects can generally be closed primarily (if small enough), or with a skin graft or flap (if too large to close primarily). In most situations, skin grafts provide a less than optimal aesthetic result, with discrepancies of color, texture, composition, and elasticity. When dealing with a partial or complete loss of a portion of the lip, adjacent "like" tissue will usually provide the best replacement, particularly when considering the qualities of skin cover. Although small skin cancers of the lips can be excised as a simple wedge, V-shaped wedge, or W-shaped wedge, as nicely described in the chapter, I rarely excise in such a fashion. Rather, for lower lip excisions, I excise the skin below the white line with an angulated V dictated by the direction of skin rhytids. Closure requires meticulous approximation of each layer, with particular attention to lining up the vermilion border and white roll. Breaking up the closure below the white roll by adding a small z-plasty or other interdigitations helps restore the gentle curve of the lip and avoids notching of the incision line (**Fig. 1.13** and **Fig. 1.14**).

For all but the smallest lateral upper lip defects, primary closure frequently causes distortion of the philtrum. Therefore, for larger lateral defects, I usually close with a crescent-shaped V-Y flap, reconstructing the aesthetic unit and paying particular attention to the small triangular portion of the lip just lateral to the nasal ala (**Fig. 1.15**). When lip defects are too large to close with "like" adjacent tissue, then a lip switch type procedure (Abbe or Estlander) or circumoral rotation-advancement (Karapandzic) flap should be considered. These procedures are paradigmatic of the restoration of the functional unit, in that they restore all the components (skin, muscle, and mucosa) of the missing portion of the lip. Although denervated when transferred, the transferred muscle within these lip segments generally regains some function through direct neurotization. The advantages, disadvantages, and limitations of these procedures as well as the various cheek-based flaps are well covered in the chapter, and they are not reiterated here other than to say that, as we push these concepts to larger and larger defects, one must balance the advantages of having like tissue and competent lips with the disadvantages of the addition of a significant amount of facial scars, the distortion seen with animation, and the relative microstomia produced.

When the defect is too large to close with "like" tissue, then regional or distant tissue is required. Invariably, if distant skin is used for reconstruction, the result is less than ideal, as skin from different parts of the body and even from different parts of the face, head, and neck has different qualities of color, texture, composition, pliability, and elasticity, as well as different attachments to deeper tissue, whether they be subcutaneous fat or muscle

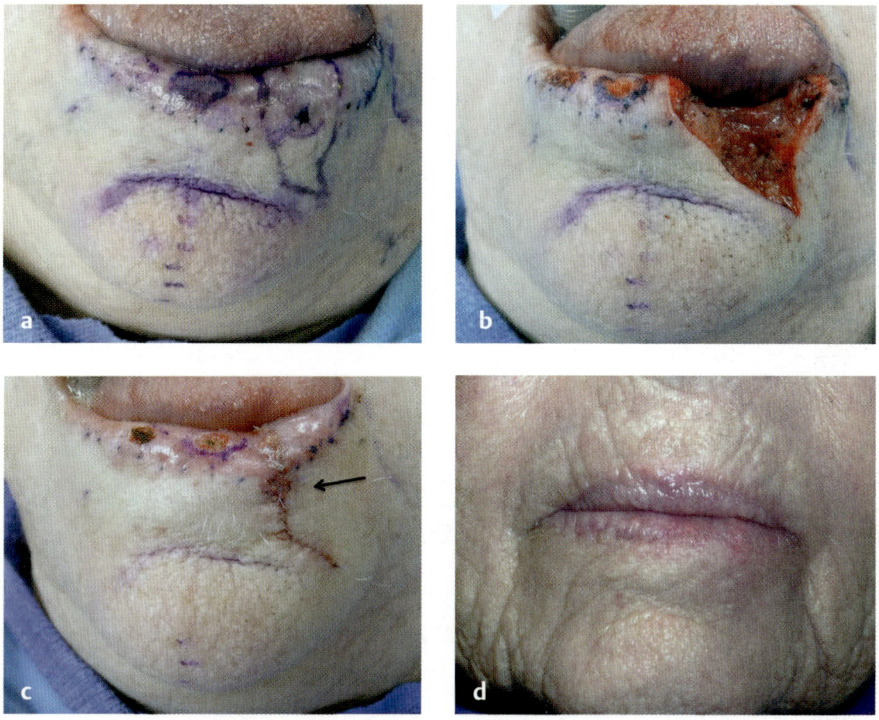

**Fig. 1.13** **(a)** An 85-year-old female with basal cell carcinoma, with excision planned as an angulated "V." **(b)** Defect after excision. Note that the vermilion border was previously tattooed to facilitate precise approximation. **(c)** Closure in layers. *Arrow* points to small z-plasty to break up the scar. **(d)** Postoperative result.

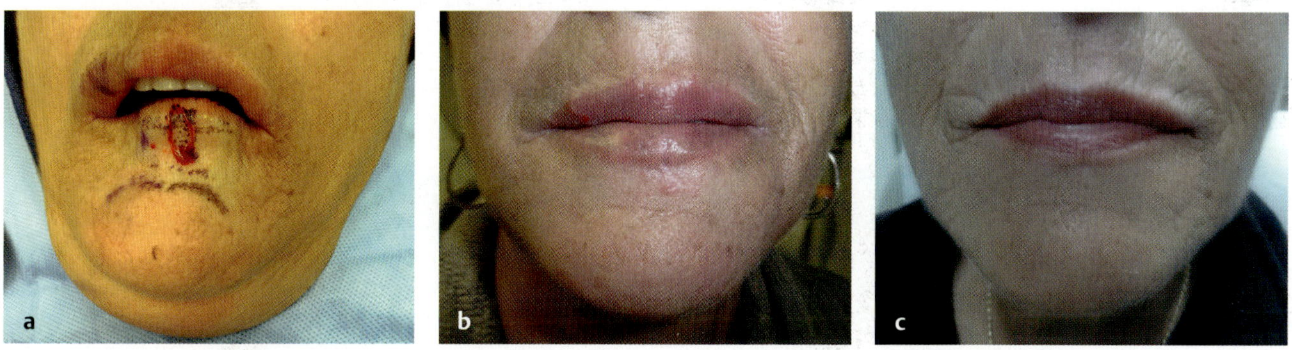

**Fig. 1.14** **(a)** A 61-year-old female undergoing re-excision of previously biopsied lesion. **(b)** Postoperative appearance at 2 weeks. Note angulation and interdigitation of incision below precisely approximated white roll. **(c)** Postoperative appearance with a barely perceptible scar.

fibers, and the different attachments lead to discrepancies in how well reconstructed lips look in animation versus repose.

Distant tissue, frequently in the form of a free tissue transfer, is generally required to successfully reconstruct greater than 80% of the lip. For a successful functional reconstruction of the lower lip, the orbicularis sphincter needs to be reconstructed or spanned. This is most frequently accomplished with the palmaris longus tendon of a radial forearm free flap (or fascia from other flaps) spanning from modiolus to modiolus, or to mobilized lateral muscle components (i.e., internal Karapandzic technique).[16] Suspending the palmaris longus tendon to fixed points merely allows the flap to drape over the tendon as if it were a clothes line and produces an adynamic lip. The best functional reconstruction using free flaps suspends the reconstructed lip skin independently of orbicularis sphincter restoration. Others have bridged the orbicularis muscle loss with innervated muscle flaps, including a free gracilis muscle covered by a skin graft[17] or an innervated platysmal myocutaneous flap from the submental area of the neck.[18] Although many advocate neurorrhaphy with sensory nerves of cutaneous free flaps, this is not absolutely necessary, because the flaps generally regain sensation with time from spontaneous neurotization.

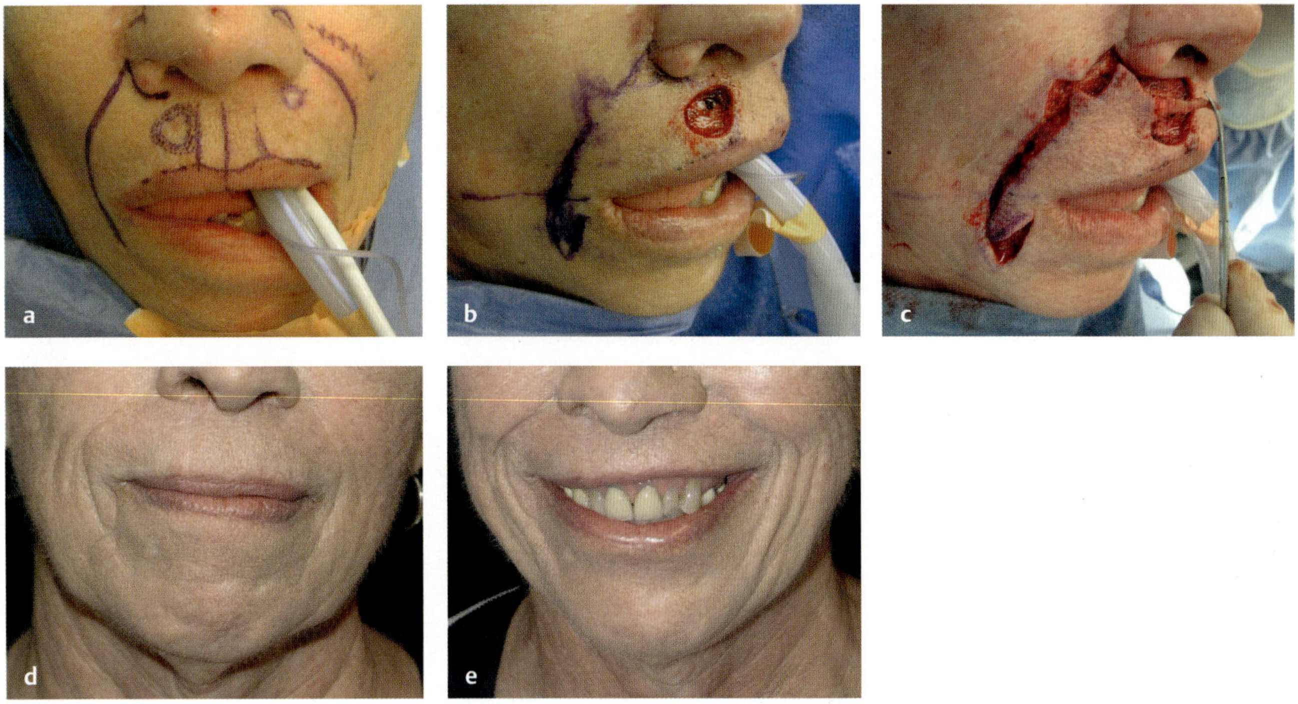

**Fig. 1.15** **(a)** A 64-year-old female with basal cell carcinoma of upper lip. Lesion and critical landmarks are marked. **(b)** Lesion excised and crescent V-Y flap marked. Note incorporation of a point to recreate triangular space lateral to the nasal ala. **(c)** De-epithelialized skin from above the lesion will be anchored to the nasal spine to limit any lateral pull or secondary distortion of scar. **(d)** Postoperative appearance, with a barely perceptible scar and without distortion of philtrum. **(e)** Minimal asymmetry noted with smiling.

Aesthetically pleasing reconstruction of large defects of the upper lip, with its gentle curves and delicate lines, is difficult, especially in women and children. Burget and Menick have successfully reconstructed large unilateral lateral defects with a large aesthetic subunit Abbe cross lip flap.[19] Overall, the best techniques for total or subtotal central upper lip reconstruction utilize bilateral lip or cheek advancement flaps complemented with an Abbe cross lip flap to create a semblance of a philtrum.

The advantage of free flap reconstruction of partial-thickness defects of the upper lip is the avoidance of any additional facial scars other than within the aesthetic unit or subunit; the disadvantage is the resultant abnormal color, texture, and composition of the transferred tissue **(Fig. 1.16)**. Full-thickness reconstruction of the upper lip tends to fare better in men if they are willing to wear a mustache. Hair-bearing fasciocutaneous flaps based on the superficial temporal vessels to resurface skin defects have been described, as have composite osteocutaneous flaps for more complex reconstructive needs **(Fig. 1.17)**.[16] Although using hair-bearing flaps to reconstruct the entire upper lip aesthetic unit successfully camouflages any irregularities of the reconstruction, if it is shaved, the lip looks like a "blob" and needs multistage revisions to look reasonable.

Whatever tissue is used to reconstruct the lip, one should try to hide scars along the borders of the aesthetic units or subunits of the lip or within (or parallel to) natural skin lines. In addition, although the lips may not be perfectly symmetrical, obtaining relative symmetry and avoiding distortion in repose, while minimizing distortion with animation, are essential to a successful reconstruction. The goal of lip reconstruction is for a casual observer not to be able to notice the scars (or the reconstruction) in normal social interactions.

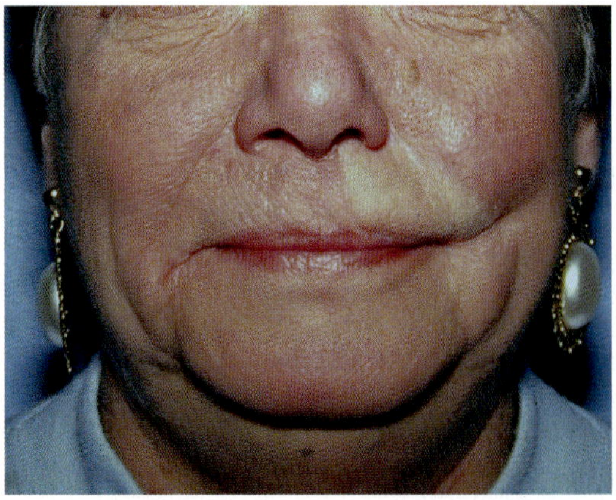

**Fig. 1.16** Abnormal color, texture, and thickness of radial forearm free flap aesthetic subunit reconstruction of left side of upper lip.

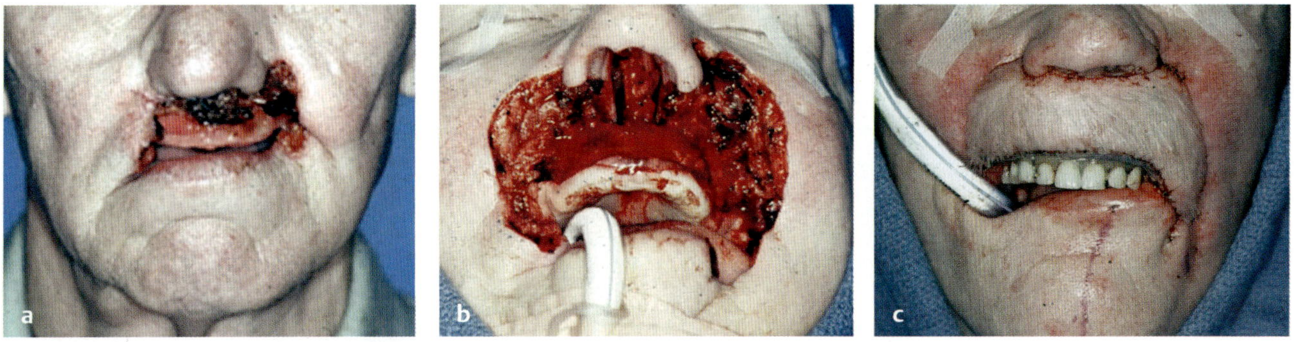

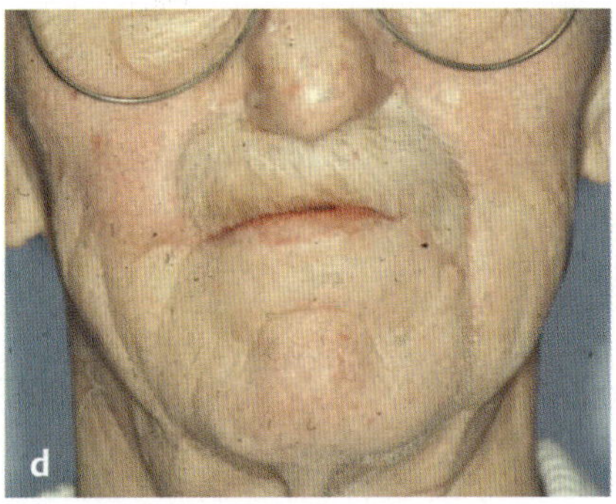

**Fig. 1.17** **(a)** A 72-year-old male with an indolent basal cell carcinoma of his upper lip. **(b)** Wide excision included the entire upper lip, extending into the medial aspects of the cheeks, a portion of the left lower lip, left commissure, a thin layer of the anterior portion of the maxilla, columella, nasal floor, and small portions of each nasal ala. **(c)** After negative pathological margins were obtained, the cheeks were advanced medially to each nasolabial fold and the upper lip was reconstructed with a hair-bearing osteofasciocutaneous temporoparietal free flap. **(d)** Postoperative result demonstrating the camouflage effect of the hair-bearing flap.

## References


1. Webster JP. Crescentic peri-alar cheek excision for upper lip flap advancement with a short history of upper lip repair. Plast Reconstr Surg (1946) 1955;16(6):434–464
2. Abbe R. A new plastic operation for the relief of deformity due to double harelip. Plast Reconstr Surg 1968;42(5):481–483
3. Estlander JA. A method of reconstruction loss of substance in one lip from the other lip. Arch Klin Chir 1872;14:622, reprinted in Plast Reconstr Surg 1968;42:361–366
4. Neligan PC. Strategies in lip reconstruction. Clin Plast Surg 2009;36(3):477–485
5. Kroll SS. Staged sequential flap reconstruction for large lower lip defects. Plast Reconstr Surg 1991;88(4):620–625, discussion 626–627
6. Hauben DJ. Victor von Bruns (1812–1883) and his contributions to plastic and reconstructive surgery. Plast Reconstr Surg 1985;75(1):120–127
7. Karapandzic M. Reconstruction of lip defects by local arterial flaps. Br J Plast Surg 1974;27(1):93–97
8. Bernard C. Cancer de la levre inferieure; restauration a l'aide de lambeaux quadratiares-latereaux. Scalpel (Brux) 1852;5:162–165
9. Webster RC, Coffey RJ, Kelleher RE. Total and partial reconstruction of the lower lip with innervated muscle-bearing flaps. Plast Reconstr Surg Transplant Bull 1960;25:360–371
10. Fujimori R. "Gate flap" for the total reconstruction of the lower lip. Br J Plast Surg 1980;33(3):340–345
11. Serletti JM, Tavin E, Moran SL, Coniglio JU. Total lower lip reconstruction with a sensate composite radial forearm-palmaris longus free flap and a tongue flap. Plast Reconstr Surg 1997;99(2):559–561
12. Pribaz JJ, Meara JG, Wright S, Smith JD, Stephens W, Breuing KH. Lip and vermilion reconstruction with the facial artery musculomucosal flap. Plast Reconstr Surg 2000;105(3):864–872
13. Langstein HN, Robb GL. Lip and perioral reconstruction. Clin Plast Surg 2005;32(3):431–445, viii
14. Hanasono MM, Langstein HR. The extended Karapandzic flap for total and near-total lip reconstruction. Plast Reconstr Surg 2011;127:1199–1205
15. Cordeiro PG, Santamaria E. Primary reconstruction of complex midfacial defects with combined lip-switch procedures and free flaps. Plast Reconstr Surg 1999;103(7):1850–1856
16. Gottlieb L, Agarwal S. Autologous alternatives to facial transplantation. J Reconstr Microsurg 2012;28(1):49–61
17. Ninkovic M, Spanio di Spilimbergo S, Ninkovic M. Lower lip reconstruction: introduction of a new procedure using a functioning gracilis muscle free flap. Plast Reconstr Surg 2007;119(5):1472–1480
18. Bauer T, Schoeller T, Rhomberg M, Piza-Katzer H, Wechselberger G. Myocutaneous platysma flap for full-thickness reconstruction of the upper and lower lip and commissura. Plast Reconstr Surg 2001;108(6):1700–1703
19. Burget GC, Menick FJ. Aesthetic restoration of one-half the upper lip. Plast Reconstr Surg 1986;78(5):583–593

# 2 Oral Cavity Reconstruction

*Peirong Yu*

## Introduction

The oral cavity is the most common site for squamous cell carcinoma of the head and neck. In the United States, the tongue and floor of the mouth are the most common sites for primary cancers, whereas in some regions of Asia, buccal cancer is most common. The organs in the oral cavity, particularly the tongue, play important roles in speech and swallowing, as well as in airway protection. The base of the tongue is more important for swallowing function, whereas the oral tongue is more important for speech and food manipulation. Proper reconstruction of these vital organs in the oral cavity may prevent life-threatening complications, restore function, and improve quality of life and patient self-image. Providing basic tissue coverage without taking into account these considerations is no longer acceptable in modern-day practice.

This chapter focuses on reconstruction of defects of the floor of the mouth, buccal surfaces and cheek, and tongue. The goal of reconstruction of the floor of the mouth is to provide thin and pliable lining so as not to obstruct lingual mobility. Similarly, buccal reconstruction also requires thin flaps to avoid bulk. Reconstructions after total or subtotal glossectomy require a large volume of tissue to provide enough bulk for better speech, swallowing, and airway protection. Conversely, the goal of reconstructing partial glossectomy defects is to preserve the mobility of the remaining tongue by providing a thin and supple flap. Sensory reinnervation is also an important part of oral cavity reconstruction. The patient and family should be made fully aware of potential functional sequelae of a total or subtotal glossectomy, including the possibility of long-term tube feeding and tracheostomy dependency.

## Regional Anatomy

The oral cavity consists of the the lips, buccal mucosa, mandibular and maxillary alveolar ridge, retromolar trigone, hard palate, floor of the mouth, and anterior (oral or mobile) tongue **(Fig. 2.1)**. Sensation in the oral cavity is provided by $V_2$ and $V_3$, branches of the fifth cranial nerve (CN). General sensation to the anterior two-thirds of the tongue is via the lingual nerve (CN $V_3$) and taste is via the chorda tympani (CN VII), accompanying the lingual nerve. Sensation

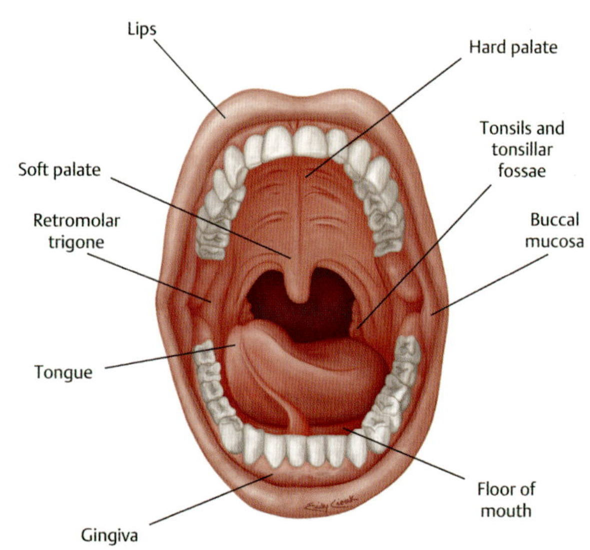


**Fig. 2.1** The oral cavity consists of the lips, buccal mucosa, mandibular and maxillary alveolar ridge, retromolar trigone (RMT), hard palate, floor of the mouth, and oral tongue. The main structures in the oral pharynx are the base of the tongue, tonsillar pillars, lateral and posterior pharyngeal walls, and soft palate.

in the oral cavity also contributes to the swallowing mechanism. Motor innervation of intrinsic oropharyngeal musculature is via the hypoglossal nerve (CN XII). Vascular supply to the tongue is via the lingual artery, a branch of the external carotid artery.

## ■ Reconstruction of Defects of the Floor of the Mouth

Defects of the floor of the mouth (FOM) are usually associated with a glossectomy or mandibulectomy. Isolated FOM defects that do not include the suprahyoid musculature may be repaired by skin graft or reconstructed with a local flap, such as a submental flap or facial artery myomucosal (FAMM) flap,[1,2] whereas combined defects resulting from glossectomy, mandibulectomy, or neck dissection require more substantial reconstruction.

### Isolated Floor of Mouth Defects

If no bone is exposed and the suprahyoid musculature is intact, FOM defects can be repaired by skin graft or they may be allowed to mucosalize spontaneously. When skin grafts are used, they are usually secured with a bolster dressing, which is removed 5 or 6 days after surgery. Partial skin graft loss is common for oral cavity reconstruction. No further management is necessary. Remucosalization can be expected.

FOM defects can also be reconstructed with local flaps, especially when a small area of bone is exposed or postoperative radiotherapy is planned. The submental flap or FAMM flap can reach the FOM easily with minimal donor-site morbidity. The FAMM flap is usually limited to a 2 cm width to allow primary closure of the donor site.[1] Therefore, its use is limited. The blood supply to the FAMM flap is provided by the facial artery. When a FAMM flap is elevated, a small amount of buccinator muscle is included in the flap, along with the buccal mucosa and the facial artery. Venous drainage depends mainly on the buccal venous plexus rather than the facial vein itself, which may not be included in the flap.[2] Although the FAMM flap can be superiorly based on the angular artery to repair palatal defects, the flap needs to be inferiorly based on the main facial artery to be rotated to the floor of the mouth with the pivot point near the retromolar trigone.

The submental flap can be harvested with a width of 4 to 6 cm, depending on the redundancy of the submental skin, while allowing primary closure of the donor site. This flap is vascularized by a branch of the facial artery. The anterior belly of the digastric muscle is usually included to ensure adequate perfusion.

Since the facial artery supplies both the FAMM flap and the submental flap, facial artery availability can be an issue when a neck dissection is required. The facial artery is commonly ligated and divided during a neck dissection. For immediate reconstruction, the submental flap can be raised first before neck dissection, if oncologically feasible, to ensure its blood supply. Therefore, good communication between the oncologic surgeon and reconstructive surgeon is essential.

### Extended Floor of Mouth Defects

When the FOM defect extends to the upper neck, with resection of part of the suprahyoid musculature along with a neck dissection, there is essentially a large connection between the oral cavity and neck, with exposure of the mandible, and a submandibular dead space. The goals of reconstruction are to seal the oral cavity from the neck and to eliminate the submandibular dead space while providing reliable lining for the FOM. Therefore, more extensive flap reconstruction is indicated. Local or regional flaps are usually not adequate or may not be the best choice to achieve functional and aesthetic reconstruction. Choices for flaps are discussed below.

#### The Radial Forearm Fasciocutaneous Free Flap

The radial forearm fasciocutaneous flap is a flap of choice because it provides a thin and supple lining that recreates the lingual sulcus once healed **(Fig. 2.2)**. The flap is reliable and has a robust blood supply. Flap elevation is straightforward and can usually be completed well within 1 hour. To obliterate the submandibular dead space, some adipofascial tissue in the upper arm is included during flap elevation **(Fig. 2.2c)**. This adipofascial tissue is proximal to the skin flap and is nicely positioned under the mandible during flap insetting.

A disadvantage of the radial forearm flap (RFF) is that, in thin patients, the flap is too thin to fill the upper neck dead space, thus increasing the risk of infection. The donor site requires skin grafting, with potential risks of tendon exposure, tendon adhesions, and unfavorable aesthetic results. Anesthesia in the proximal thenar area from sacrifice of the lateral antebrachial cutaneous nerve is common, and occasionally radial sensory nerve injury can occur, resulting in numbness in the radial aspect of the fingers.

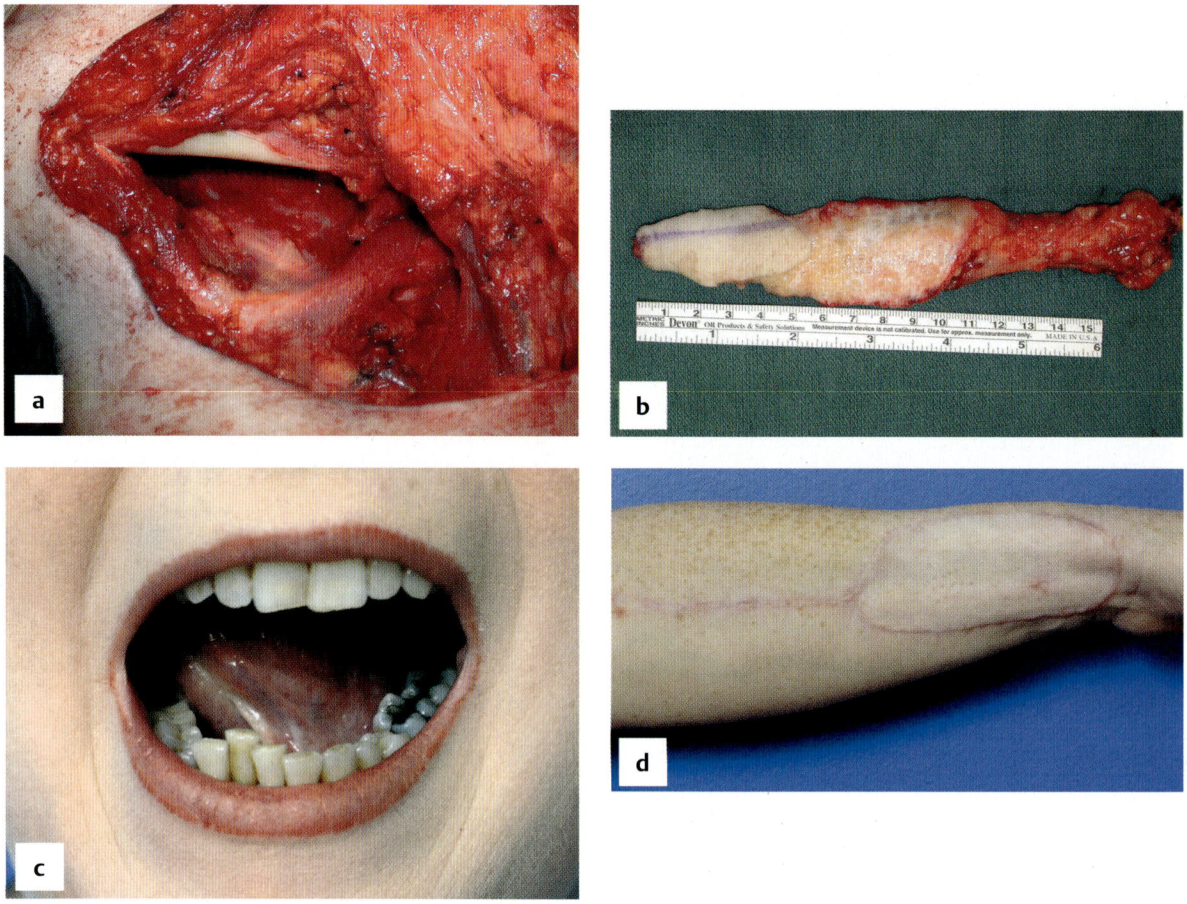


**Fig. 2.2** **(a)** A 35-year-old female underwent resection of a left floor of mouth tumor with a 2.5 × 4.5 cm mucosal defect in the left lingual sulcus. **(b)** A radial forearm flap was harvested with some adipofascial tissue to fill the upper neck dead space. **(c)** Six-month follow-up showing full range of mobility of the tongue with preservation of the lingual sulcus and **(d)** a well-healed donor site.

## The Ulnar Artery Perforator Flap or Ulnar Forearm Free Flap

The ulnar forearm flap is more distally based, similar to the RFF, whereas the ulnar artery perforator (UAP) flap is more proximally located to avoid tendon exposure above the wrist. The donor site is more hidden, and small defects can be closed primarily. The UAP flap is usually hairless and is as thin as the RFF. The author now prefers the UAP flap to the RFF. A small segment of the flexor carpi ulnaris muscle can be included to obliterate the dead space **(Fig. 2.3)** without compromising hand function.

The disadvantage of the UAP flap is that the pedicle is shorter, usually 4 to 5 cm long. Also, dissection along the ulnar nerve can be tedious. Furthermore, the UAP flap is a true perforator flap, with small perforating vessels, making it less robust than the RFF, and dissection is more technically demanding. However, in most head and neck reconstructions, the recipient vessels are within short reach. Therefore, a long vascular pedicle is not needed. In fact, a long pedicle will usually require careful looping and is less desirable.

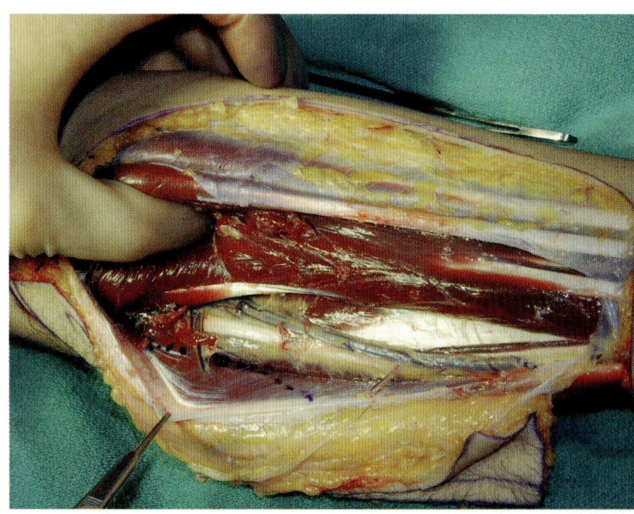

**Fig. 2.3** A small segment of the flexor carpi ulnaris muscle can be included in the ulnar artery perforator flap for small dead space filling.

## The Anterolateral Thigh Free Flap

The anterolateral thigh (ALT) free flap is a good choice for FOM reconstruction in patients with thin subcutaneous tissue in the thigh. In most Western patients, however, the ALT flap may be thicker than desired for FOM reconstruction **(Fig. 2.4)**. This is particularly true when the flap needs to cover the exposed mandible intraorally to replace gingival loss, although immediate flap thinning can be safely performed to reduce the bulk. Debulking can also be performed at a second stage several months later, even after radiotherapy **(Fig. 2.5)**. The advantage of the anterolateral thigh flap is the minimal donor-site morbidity, and flap elevation can be simultaneously performed with tumor resection by the primary surgical team, whereas the forearm flap is usually elevated after tumor resection. In addition, various amounts of the vastus lateralis muscle can be harvested to cover the mandible and to eliminate the submandibular and upper neck dead space. Replacing FOM defects with a bulky flap should be avoided because it may restrict tongue mobility and obliterate the lingual sulcus, causing drooling. In obese patients, even the RFF may be too bulky, and flap thinning is necessary.

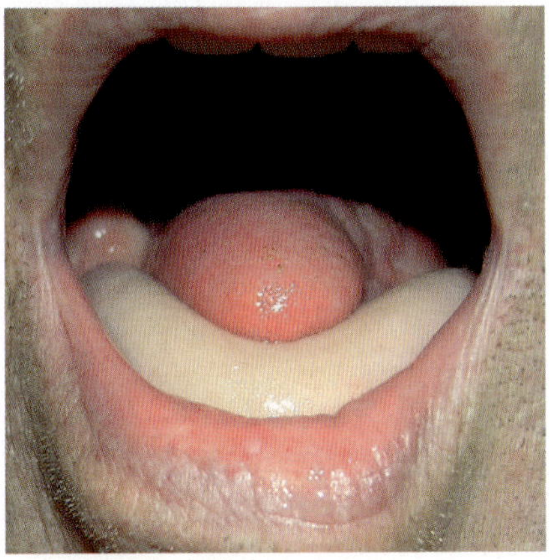

**Fig. 2.4** Following resection of the ventral tongue, closure of the remaining mobile tongue to itself may result in a "snake tongue," with loss of volume in the mobile tongue. A thick flap for floor of mouth reconstruction may obliterate the labial sulcus, causing drooling and obstruction of tongue mobility.

## The Pectoralis Major Pedicled Flap

The pectoralis major muscle flap can be harvested with ease and turned over the clavicle to reach the upper neck and floor of mouth. Whether to include a skin paddle is optional. The muscle placed in the FOM can remucosalize within 5 to 7 days, or it can be covered with skin grafts, although partial skin graft loss is common. Nevertheless, a skin graft can serve as a biological dressing for several days. In female patients, it is usually best not to include a skin paddle, due to its thickness as well as the distortion of the breast after harvest. The key to reconstruction of such defects is to obliterate the dead space in the FOM and upper neck to prevent infection. Therefore, a pectoralis major muscle alone may work well. To ensure easy reach to the FOM without tension and better aesthetic results, it is advisable to elevate the flap as an island flap. All the muscles around the vascular pedicle near the clavicle are divided to reduce the bulk and increase the arc of rotation. The transversely oriented clavicular portion of the pectoralis muscle is also divided to increase pedicle length. If necessary, a segment of the clavicle can be resected to allow the vascular pedicle to pass through and then can be replaced with mini titanium plates.

The disadvantages of using the pectoralis major flap include unfavorable aesthetic results in the neck and possible neck contracture from fibrosis of the muscle after radiotherapy. The flap also adds additional incisions in the chest. Therefore, it is not a good choice in young patients, especially in young women. In patients with a long neck and underdeveloped pectoralis major muscle, the muscle may not reach the FOM easily, and its pull-down force may compromise the reconstruction. In our practice, the pectoralis major flap is usually reserved for high-risk patients, such as those of advanced age and those with severe medical comorbidity. In young and more functional

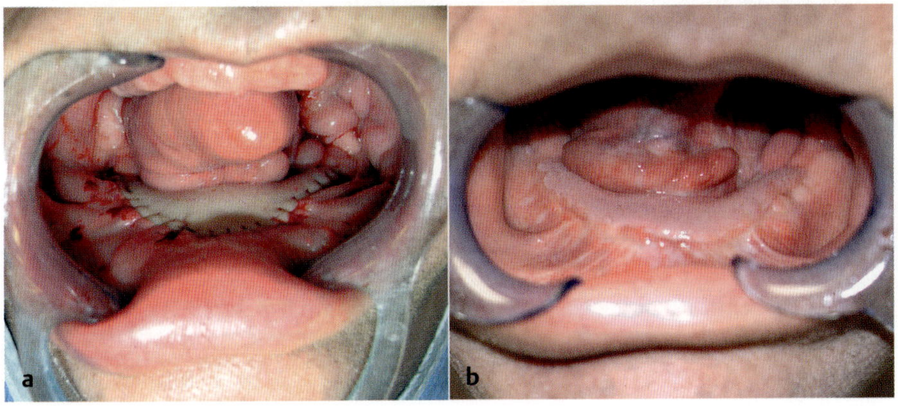


**Fig. 2.5** **(a)** Debulking of the thick flap used for floor of mouth reconstruction in **Fig. 2.4**. **(b)** A 6-week follow-up photograph shows a completely healed flap after thinning.

patients, a free flap is preferred to minimize neck deformity and to maximize functional and aesthetic outcomes. In the hands of experienced and efficient microsurgeons, a free flap reconstruction may not add much operating time, because elevation of a free flap can usually be done simultaneously with tumor ablation, while elevation of the pectoralis flap cannot start until tumor resection is completed.

### Reconstruction of Floor of Mouth Defects Involving the Ventral Tongue

When resection of the FOM involves the ventral tongue, it is common practice to close the tongue to itself by folding the lateral edges of the tongue ventrally and to reconstruct the FOM with a flap. With this technique, however, the bulk of the tongue is reduced significantly, producing a "snake tongue" deformity **(Fig. 2.4)** that results in impairment of speech and swallowing functions. An alternative approach, preferred by the author, is to resurface the ventral tongue and the FOM simultaneously with a thin radial forearm fasciocutaneous free flap or UAP flap **(Fig. 2.6)**. This technique preserves the volume and mobility of the tongue. Great care is taken to preserve the blood supply to the remaining tongue.

When the resection involves the mandibular gingiva and labial mucosa up to the vermilion border, it is important not to sew the flap all the way to the vermilion because this will obliterate the labial sulcus and push the lip downward, causing drooling and deformity. Instead, the flap edge should be sewn to the labial tissue at the base of the labial sulcus; the remaining labial mucosa defect is left to remucosalize spontaneously or is skin grafted. The remucosalization process takes approximately 1 week and heals well. The same principle applies to mandibular reconstruction with a fibular osteocutaneous flap in patients in whom the labial mucosa defects extend to the vermilion **(Fig. 2.7)**.

## ■ Reconstruction of Glossectomy Defects

The most common defects in the oral cavity requiring reconstruction are glossectomy defects. Glossectomy defects can be partial, subtotal, or total. Small defects of up to one-quarter or even one-third of the tongue with minimal resection of the FOM may be closed primarily or with a skin graft with maximum preservation of tongue mobility and function. However, resection of the FOM combined with neck dissection creates a connection between the oral cavity and the neck along the lingual cortex of the mandible. These defects, even if they involve less than one-third of the tongue, are best reconstructed with a flap to minimize the risk of infection and fistula formation, which can potentially delay crucial adjuvant therapy. The most common defects in our practice are hemiglossectomy defects, which account for 65% of all glossectomy defects that require reconstruction. Because the tongue is a highly functional organ responsible for speech and deglutition, every effort should be made to maximize its functional preservation while providing reliable coverage.

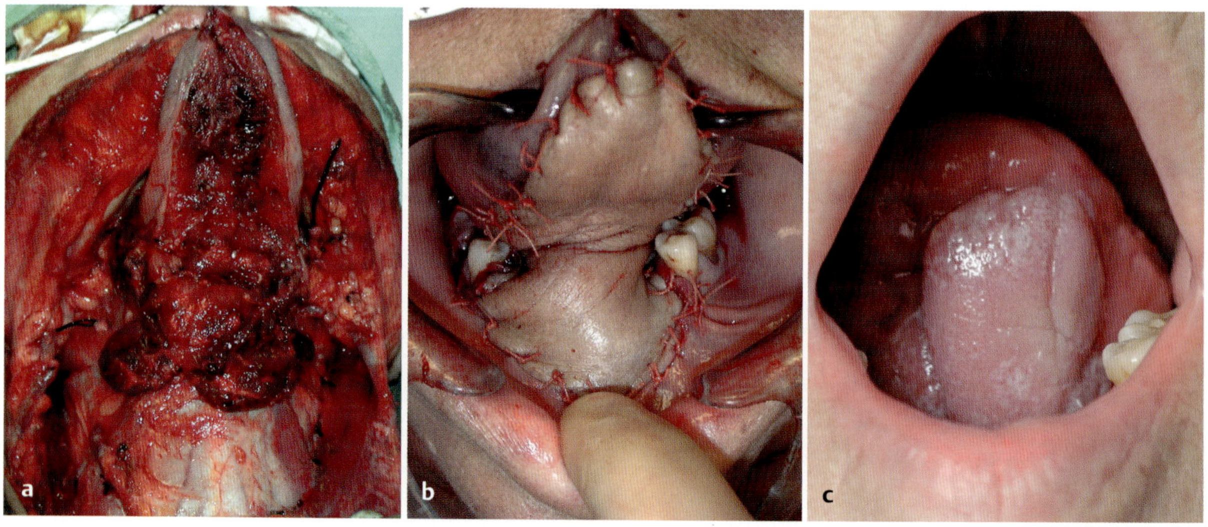


**Fig. 2.6** An alternative approach to reconstructing the ventral tongue defect is to use a thin forearm flap, which is also needed to reconstruct the floor of the mouth. Pictured are **(a)** the ventral tongue defect, **(b)** the RFF used to resurface the ventral tongue and to reconstruct the floor of the mouth, and **(c)** the healed flap at 3 months after surgery, showing good mobility of the remaining tongue with preservation of bulk.

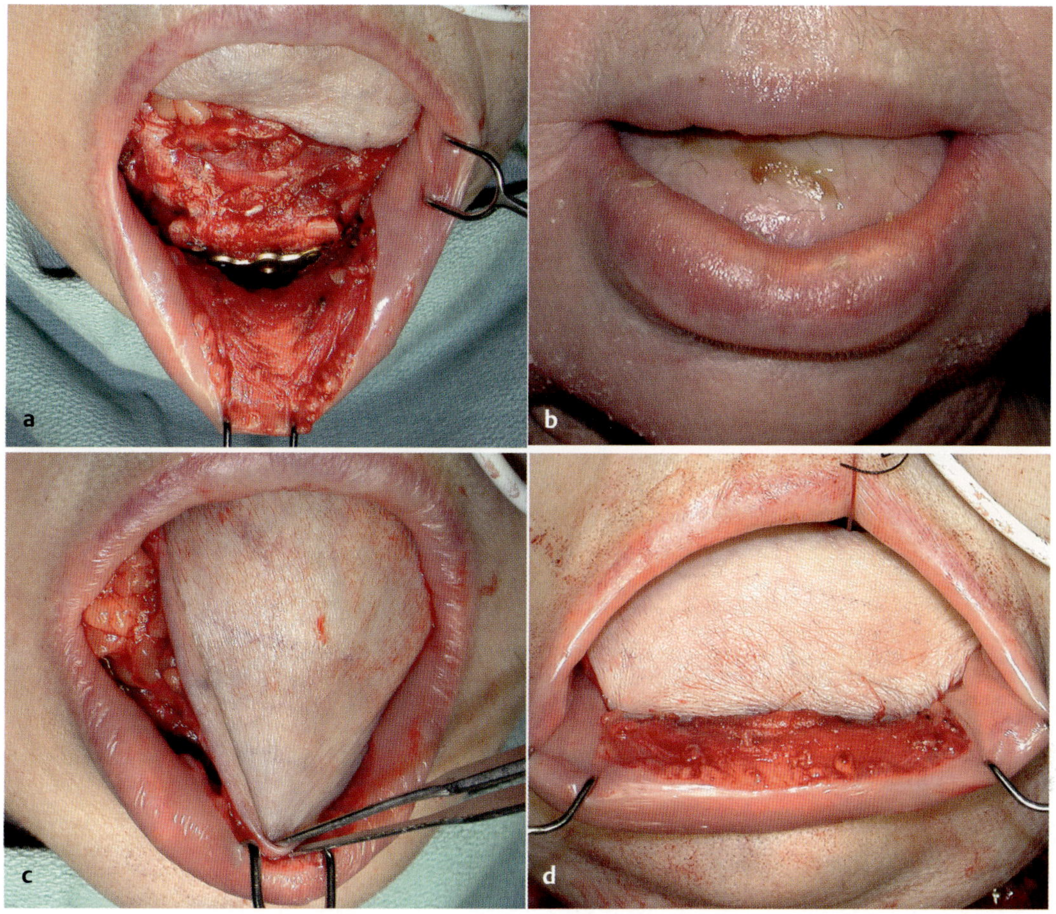


**Fig. 2.7** **(a)** When resection of labial mucosa approaches the vermilion border, **(b,c)** sewing the flap to the mucosal margin may obliterate the labial sulcus and push the lower lip down, causing drooling. **(d)** A better approach is to inset the flap to the bottom of the labial sulcus and to leave the raw surface on the lower lip to remucosalize spontaneously to preserve the labial sulcus and prevent drooling.

## Reconstruction of Partial (Hemi-) Glossectomy Defects

### Goals of Reconstruction

The tongue is a highly functional organ with complex mobility. After resection, the remaining tongue has the ability to produce intelligible speech and adequate food bolus manipulation as long as it is not tethered. Therefore, the goal of reconstruction is to preserve the mobility of the remaining tongue in addition to providing basic soft tissue coverage. Excess bulk in the oral cavity may impede the mobility of the remaining tongue, resulting in poor function. Thus, a bulky flap should be avoided in hemiglossectomy reconstruction. Consideration should also be given to sensory reinnervation.

### Choice of Flaps

A thin flap, such as the radial forearm fasciocutaneous free flap, UAP flap, or a thin ALT free flap, is usually the flap of choice. The radial and ulnar forearm free flaps are the author's preferred flaps for hemiglossectomy reconstruction because they provide thin and pliable tissue and allow for the possibility for sensory reinnervation. The ALT flap, which also has the potential for sensory reinnervation, is another excellent choice, and it may be the best option in thin patients due to its minimal donor-site morbidity. The lateral arm flap is also a good choice in thin patients, with the potential for sensory reinnervation and primary closure of the donor site. However, the more difficult dissection and smaller caliber (usually 1.5 mm) of the pedicle artery make this flap less popular.

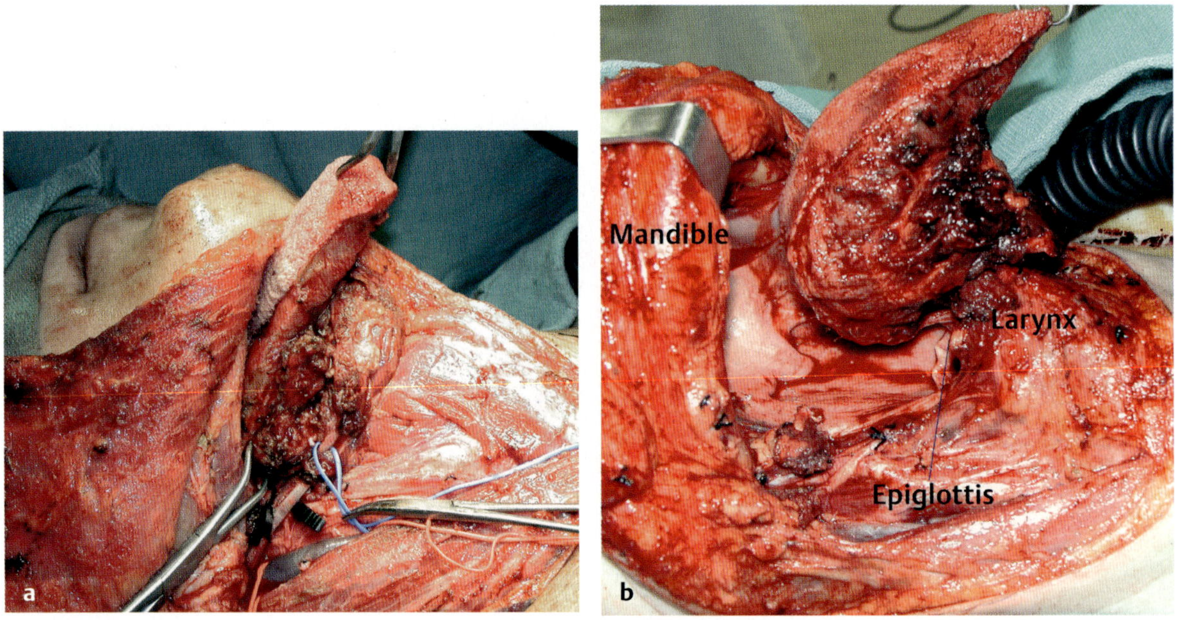


**Fig. 2.8** A hemiglossectomy defect **(a)** may extend only to the base of tongue or **(b)** involve the oropharyngeal wall, base of the tongue, and lateral pharyngeal wall down to the epiglottis.

The pectoralis major muscle or myocutaneous flap may provide basic coverage; however, its bulk and potential to result in tongue tethering and neck contracture are disadvantages for hemiglossectomy reconstruction, as discussed above. The functional outcomes following pectoralis major pedicle flap reconstruction are usually compromised. Therefore, this flap is usually reserved for salvage after a failed free flap reconstruction or for use in high-risk cases deemed unsuitable for free flap reconstruction.

## Surgical Techniques

### Evaluation of the Defect

The length of the surgical defect is measured from the tip of the remaining tongue to the posterior limit, which can be in the base of the tongue or immediately above the epiglottis. In the latter case, there will also be a defect in the lateral pharyngeal wall **(Fig. 2.8)**. The width of the defect is difficult to measure accurately because of the loss of three-dimensional structure. A flap width of 6 to 8 cm is usually required to adequately recreate the lateral sulcus (gutter) and provide enough surface area coverage. Neck dissection is commonly performed along with a glossectomy; therefore, extra soft tissue is included in the flap design to eliminate any submandibular/upper neck dead space. The cut end of the lingual nerve should be explored for potential sensory reinnervation. The lingual nerve is a better recipient nerve for sensory reinnervation of the neotongue in comparison to other nerves, such as the inferior alveolar nerve and the greater auricular nerve. The lingual nerve can be found along the lingual cortex and anterior to the angle of the mandible **(Fig. 2.9)**. It is usually 2 mm in diameter. After evaluation of the defect, a Dobhoff feeding tube is inserted into the stomach, if it has not been placed already by the ablative surgeons.

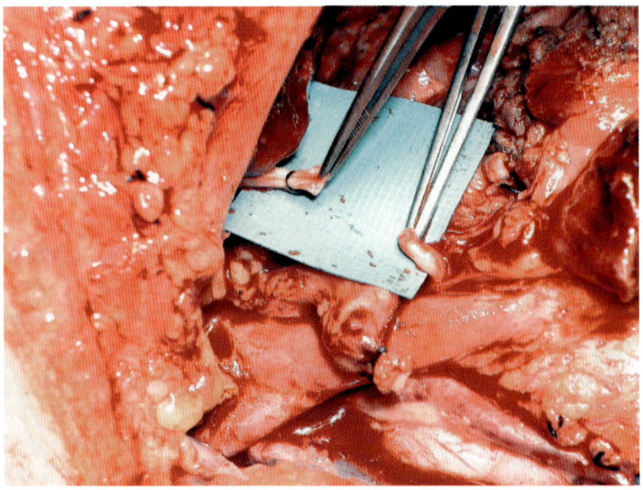

**Fig. 2.9** The cut end of the lingual nerve can be found along the lingual cortex of the mandible, just anterior to the mandibular angle.

## Exploring Recipient Vessels

After assessment of the defect, the recipient vessels are examined. The lingual artery is often exposed and divided during glossectomy. It has a diameter between 2 and 2.5 mm in most cases, making it an ideal recipient artery. The artery is dissected back to its origin from the external carotid artery and is brought under the posterior belly of the digastric muscle, which can be divided if necessary **(Fig. 2.10)**. To maximize the inflow of blood to the flap, the curved portion of the artery is removed, leaving only a 1 cm stump on the external carotid artery.

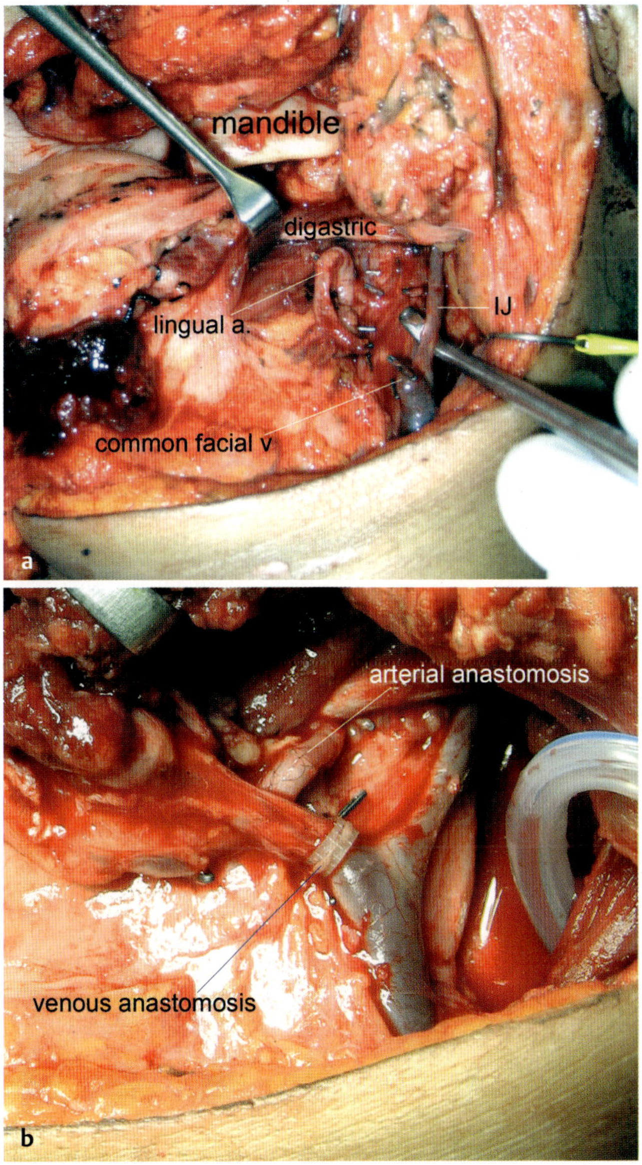


**Fig. 2.10 (a,b)** The lingual artery can be found underneath the posterior belly of the digastric muscle. It is trimmed back to remove the curvature. The common facial vein stump off the internal jugular vein (IJ) can be used for end-to-end anastomosis, commonly with a vein coupler.

The author's preferred recipient vein is the common facial vein stump, which drains into the internal jugular vein. It has a diameter of 3 to 5 mm. The second choice is to perform an end-to-side anastomosis on the internal jugular vein itself. If the internal jugular vein is also unavailable, the external jugular vein is the next choice if it is in good condition. Care must be exercised postoperatively if the external jugular vein is used to prevent tight tracheostomy ties from compressing this fairly superficial vein.

## Flap Harvesting: The Radial Forearm Flap

The flap design is based on the dimensions of the defect. Flap elevation is well described in the literature, with the following modifications. The author prefers to use the venae comitantes as vein outflow to the cephalic vein. In many patients, the cephalic vein is far away from the radial artery. Including the cephalic vein may unnecessarily increase the flap width. In most cases, the venae comitantes of the RFF are adequate for venous drainage. However, the venae comitantes can be extremely small and inadequate in some patients. Therefore, the author's approach is to tentatively outline the flap, centered on the radial vessels, and make a small transverse incision at the wrist crease to explore the venae comitantes first **(Fig. 2.11)**. If one of these veins is at least 1 mm in diameter, there is no need to include the cephalic vein. Otherwise, the flap design is shifted laterally to capture the cephalic vein. Suprafascial dissection is preferred,[3] and flap elevation is performed

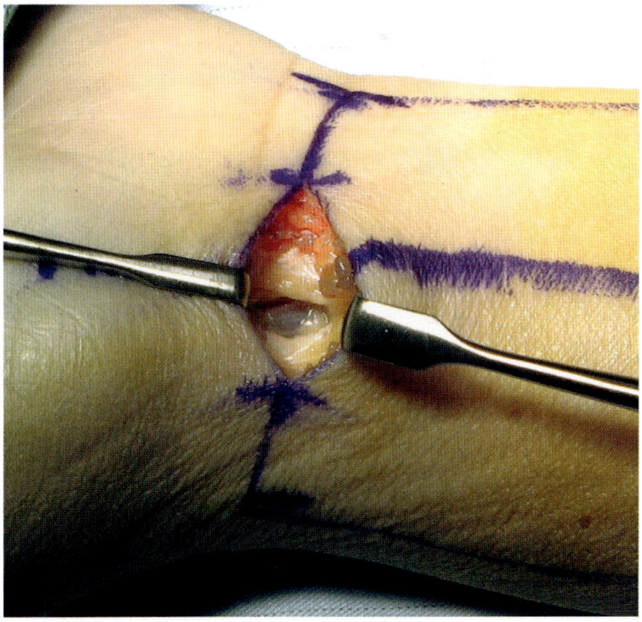

**Fig. 2.11** A small exploratory incision was made first at the wrist crease to confirm the size of the venae comitantes of the radial forearm flap vascular pedicle. If both venae comitantes are less than 1 mm in diameter, the flap design is shifted more laterally to include the cephalic vein.

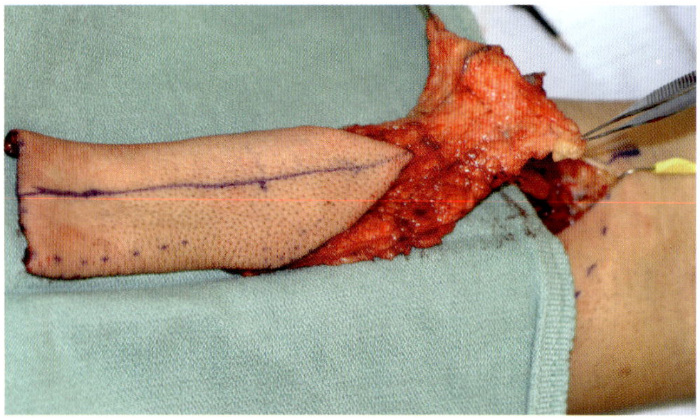

**Fig. 2.12** When bulk is needed to fill the dead space in the upper neck, the adipofascial tissue in the upper forearm can be included in the RFF.

under tourniquet control. The thenar branches of the superficial radial sensory nerve can be preserved with suprafascial dissection. At the midforearm level, the lateral antebrachial cutaneous nerve can be found near the midline. This nerve is included in the flap for sensory reinnervation. In most hemiglossectomy cases, there is a small dead space left under the mandible. Therefore, some adipofascial tissue from the proximal forearm is included in the flap to fill the dead space, which is an important measure to decrease the risks of infection and fistula formation. This is accomplished by elevating the proximal forearm skin flaps below the subdermal plexus, leaving the subcutaneous tissue attached to the flap and the vascular pedicle **(Fig. 2.12)**. The venae comitantes are usually no larger than 1.5 mm in diameter before they converge; therefore, the vein is usually taken above the convergence of the venae comitantes, where the diameter is greater than 2.5 mm in most cases. Once the flap and the vascular pedicle are completely dissected, the tourniquet is released to perfuse the flap and the hand for several minutes before dividing the pedicle.

## Flap Harvesting: The Ulnar Artery Perforator Flap

The ulnar artery perforator flap is now preferred by the author for reconstruction of hemiglossectomy defects. (Key points for flap design and elevation are discussed below under surgical techniques.) The distal border of the flap is usually 5 cm above the wrist crease to avoid tendon exposure **(Fig. 2.13)**. Dissection is performed under tourniquet control and begins on the radial side and proceeds toward the ulnar side. Suprafascial dissection is performed until the perforators are seen where the fascia is incised and subfascial dissection is performed. The perforators are small, thus meticulous dissection is required **(Fig. 2.14)**. The ulnar nerve is carefully separated from the ulnar artery and vein, and retraction of the nerve should be avoided. The medial antebrachial cutaneous nerve is included in the flap for sensory reinnervation **(Fig. 2.14)**. A small segment of the

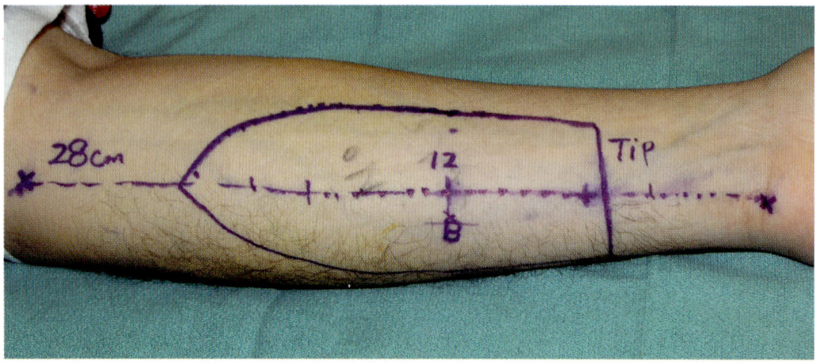


**Fig. 2.13** The ulnar artery perforator flap is designed over the ulnar artery, with the distal end of the flap ~ 5 cm above the wrist crease to minimize tendon exposure.

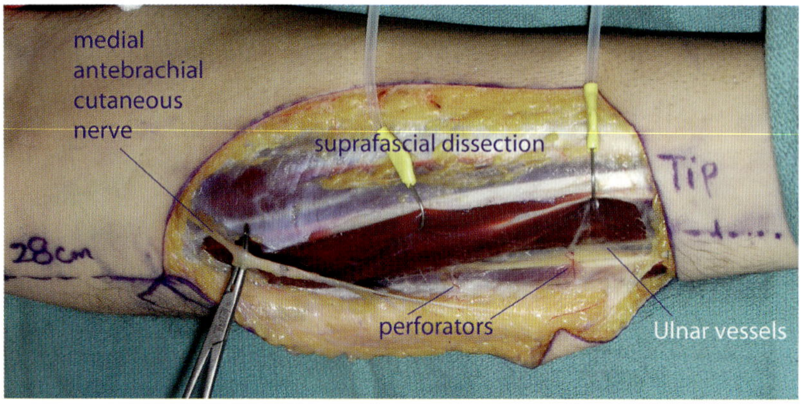


**Fig. 2.14** The medial antebrachial cutaneous nerve can be included in the ulnar artery perforator flap for sensory reinnervation. The perforators are usually small; therefore, meticulous dissection is required.

flexor carpi ulnaris muscle can be included for dead space filling **(Fig. 2.3)**.

## Flap Harvesting: The Anterolateral Thigh Flap

In thin patients, the ALT flap can also be used for hemiglossectomy reconstruction. (Key points for flap design and elevation are discussed below under surgical techniques.) To fill the submandibular dead space, a small segment of the vastus lateralis muscle is included in the flap. The periphery of the flap can be thinned to reduce the bulk, if necessary. The lateral femoral cutaneous nerve can be included in the ALT flap for sensory reinnervation.

## Flap Insetting

The distal end of the flap is oriented toward the tip of the remaining tongue. Flap insetting starts from the posterior end of the defect, either at the base of the tongue or above the epiglottis. This part of flap insetting is completed through the neck exposure, before vascular anastomoses are performed. When flap insetting reaches the mandible, one can either proceed with vascular anastomosis or continue the insetting intraorally depending on the surgeon's preference and the ischemia time. Intraorally, one lateral edge of the flap is sutured to the gingiva and the other to the cutting edge of the remaining tongue. A key step in flap insetting is to create the ventral sulcus of the neotongue to avoid tethering. The distal medial corner of the flap is sutured to the tip of the remaining tongue. The distal edge of the flap is then sutured to the ventral surface of the remaining tongue **(Fig. 2.15)**, thus creating a ventral sulcus and lateral gutter **(Fig. 2.16)**. A single layer of interrupted 3–0 absorbable sutures is preferred by the author, although some surgeons prefer horizontal mattress sutures. It is important, however, not to tie the horizontal mattress sutures too tightly so as to avoid flap edge necrosis and fistula formation. When there is no gingiva left to attach the flap to, it can be sewn to the teeth by tying the suture knots around the teeth.

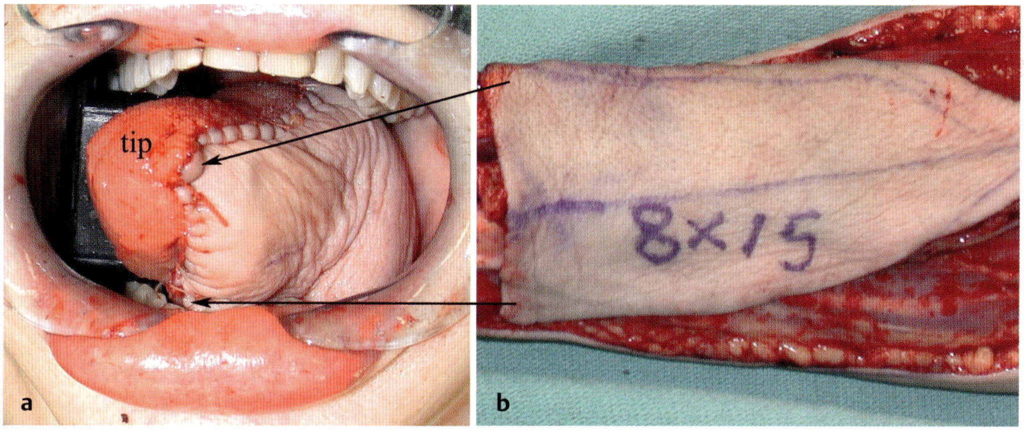


**Fig. 2.15** One important aspect of hemiglossectomy reconstruction is to preserve the mobility and avoid tethering of the remaining tongue. **(a)** The ventral sulcus from the tip of the tongue to the mandibular gingiva measures 6 to 8 cm. Therefore, a flap width of 6 to 8 cm is required to recreate the ventral sulcus of the mobile tongue. **(b)** One corner of the distal flap is sewn to the tip of the tongue, and the other, to the mandibular gingiva at the anterior midline.

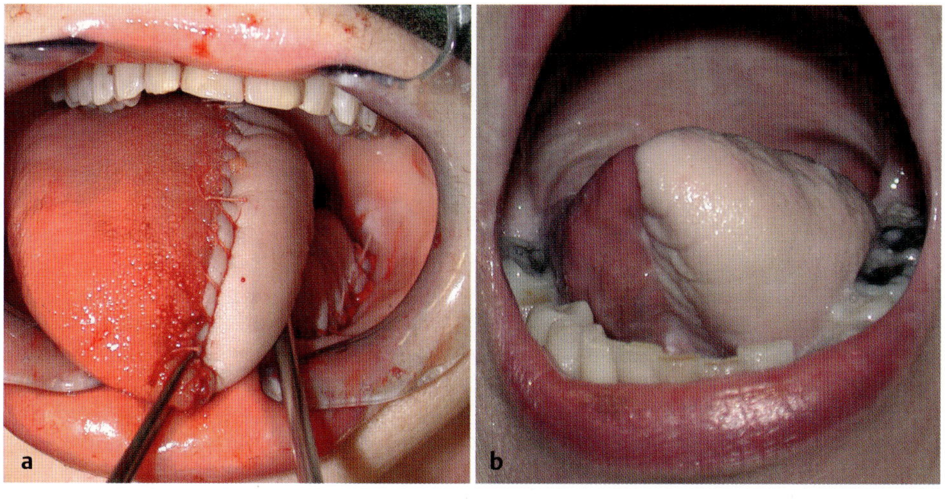


**Fig. 2.16** **(a)** Adequate width of the flap is needed to recreate the lateral gutter of the tongue. **(b)** Photograph taken 9 months after surgery showing good mobility of the reconstructed tongue.

### Revascularization and Reinnervation

Once the flap is partially or completely inset, the flap pedicle is brought under the mandible to the neck. Great care should be taken not to twist the pedicle. When the lingual artery and common facial vein are used, the vascular pedicle is usually longer than needed. The pedicle is then carefully positioned with a gentle curve to avoid kinking. Next, the cut end of the lingual nerve is freshened and the sensory nerve from the flap is anastomosed to the lingual nerve with several epineural 8–0 nylon sutures. This is usually done with loupe magnification, as the lingual nerve is inaccessible to the operating microscope. Sensory recovery of the flap with this technique has been well documented and, therefore, sensory reinnervation is strongly recommended. After the vascular and neural anastomoses are completed, the extra adipofascial tissue or muscle from the flap is carefully positioned to fill the submandibular space while avoiding pedicle compression.

Next, the oral cavity is irrigated with normal saline until clean. The neck wound is then irrigated with an ample amount of warm normal saline (2 or 3 L), taking care not to squirt the saline directly on the vascular pedicle to avoid vessel spasm. Meticulous hemostasis is essential to avoiding a postoperative hematoma, which can compress the vascular pedicle. All areas should be carefully examined, even if they have already been examined by the ablative surgeons. A 15 Fr Blake drain is placed on each side of the neck, lateral to the internal jugular vein. At this point, the neck is slightly flexed (take out the shoulder roll and flex the neck to a neutral position), and the vascular pedicle is examined again. Because the neck is usually hyperextended during surgery, flexing the neck to a normal position can significantly change the position of the vascular pedicle, causing kinking or compression. The pedicle is repositioned if necessary to avoid such problems. The neck incision is then closed. Finally, the reinforced endotracheal tube is replaced with a #6 Shiley tracheostomy tube, if this has not been done by the ablative surgeons.

## Reconstruction of Total or Subtotal Glossectomy Defects

### Goals of Reconstruction

Although functional outcomes after reconstruction for partial glossectomy defects are generally good, speech and swallowing functions after reconstruction for total and subtotal glossectomy defects remain disappointing. The extent of surgical resection may be the most important factor affecting function. The more tongue musculature that is left intact, the better the functional outcome will be. Unlike with hemiglossectomy, once most or all of the tongue is removed, mobility of the remaining tongue is no longer a concern. Therefore, the main goal of reconstruction is to provide enough tissue bulk. Tissue bulk is important for reconstructing large defects of the tongue for two reasons. First, it is needed to help the neotongue touch the palate to produce better speech and push food toward the hypopharyx. Second, the tissue bulk diverts saliva and food to the lateral pharyngeal gutters during swallowing to minimize aspiration.[4]

### Choice of Flaps

#### The Anterolateral Thigh Flap

To achieve adequate tissue bulk, large tongue defects are typically reconstructed with a myocutaneous flap. In Western patients, the ALT flap usually has the right amount of bulk for total or near-total tongue reconstruction[5,6] and has become the author's flap of choice. It also has the advantages of providing sensory and motor reinnervation and minimal donor-site morbidity. This is particularly important in high-risk patients. Also, a simultaneous two-team approach is easily accomplished with the ALT flap.

#### The Vertical Rectus Abdominis Myocutaneous (VRAM) Flap

The VRAM flap is a time-honored flap that is reliable and easy to harvest.[7] The subcutaneous fat in the VRAM flap is softer than that in the ALT flap, making it easier to inset. The included rectus abdominis muscle fills the upper neck defect nicely. However, the VRAM has several disadvantages. In elderly patients and those with significant chronic obstructive pulmonary disease with minimal pulmonary reserve, harvesting the VRAM may further compromise their pulmonary function due to incisional pain and abdominal weakness. Using muscle alone with skin grafting is not recommended because significant atrophy can occur quickly, especially after radiotherapy, resulting in a funnel shape that allows food to pour into the hypopharynx and larynx, causing aspiration. Furthermore, sensory and motor reinnervation with the VRAM flap is not satisfactory.

#### Other Free Flaps

For obese patients in whom ALT or VRAM flaps are too thick, the RFF, UAP flap, or the lateral arm flap may be thick enough to provide adequate bulk. The gracilis myocutaneous flap and the latissimus dorsi myocutaneous flap also have been used, with motor reinnervation.

## The Pedicled Pectoralis Major Flap

Free flap reconstruction is usually a much better option than pedicled flaps for total or subtotal glossectomy defects. The pedicled pectoralis flap, however, may be used in high-risk patients who are poor candidates for free flap reconstruction or in patients in whom a free flap has failed.

## Surgical Techniques

### Flap Design and Elevation: The ALT Flap

Most subtotal glossectomy defects involve the entire mobile tongue and 50% or more of the base of the tongue. The FOM musculature is usually removed during resection, with the hyoid bone as the distal extent of the defect **(Fig. 2.17)**. A flap 7 to 8 cm wide and 10 to 15 cm long is usually required. Details of ALT flap harvesting are discussed in a separate chapter.[6,7,8] It is important to remember that only the anterior incision is made first until all the perforators are dissected out. The posterior incision can then be redesigned according to the exact locations of the perforators if necessary. The lateral femoral cutaneous nerve of the ALT flap can be found at the proximal incision site of the flap, along the AP line, immediately above the deep fascia **(Fig. 2.18a)**. An additional 5 cm of nerve length can be obtained by subcutaneously dissecting the nerve in the upper thigh. Various amounts of the vastus lateralis muscle can be harvested with the flap to fill the upper neck dead space or to be used for motor reinnervation **(Fig. 2.18b)**.

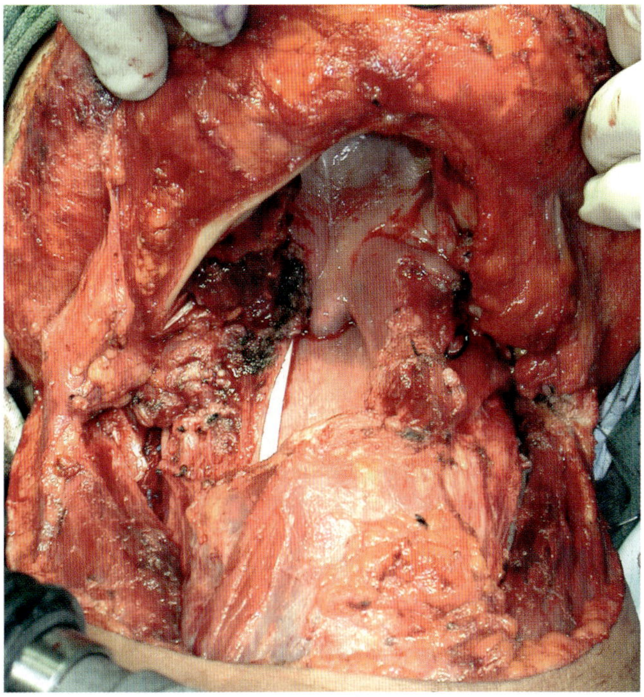

**Fig. 2.17** A total glossectomy defect with resection of all suprahyoid musculature.

### Flap Insetting

As in hemiglossectomy reconstruction, flap insetting begins at the base of the tongue or lateral pharynx. The tip and edges of the flap are sutured to the mandibular gingiva or around the teeth, since it is not possible to recreate the ventral sulcus. It may be helpful to inset the flap before revascularization because

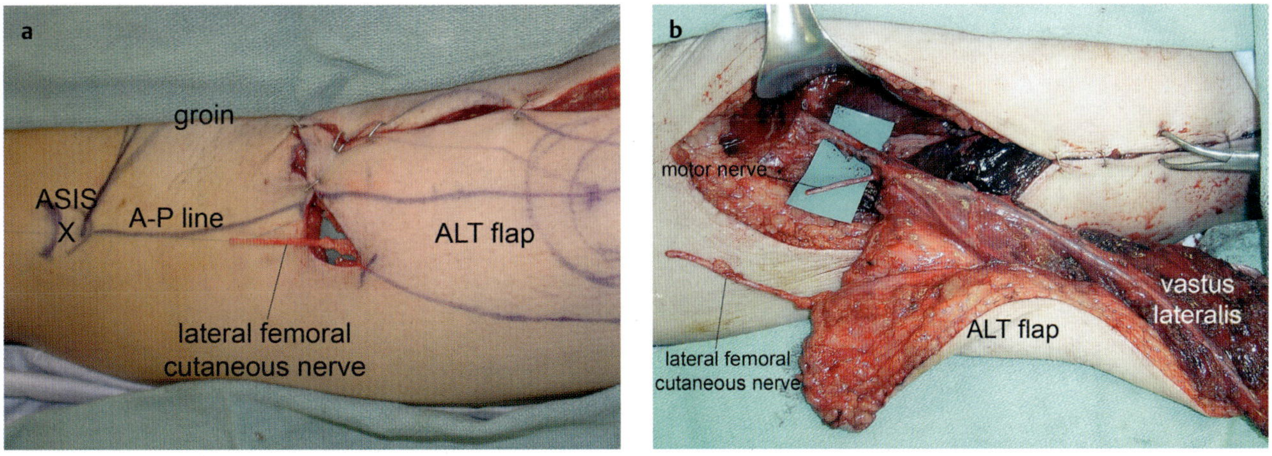


**Fig. 2.18** **(a)** The anterolateral thigh (ALT) flap was used for reconstruction. The lateral femoral cutaneous nerve, a sensory nerve of the ALT flap, can be found at the proximal incision of the flap above the deep fascia along the line connecting the anterior superior iliac spine (ASIS) and the superolateral corner of the patella (AP line). **(b)** The superficial half of the vastus lateralis muscle is included in the flap with its motor nerve, a branch of the femoral nerve, for motor reinnervation. (*Continued on page 30*)

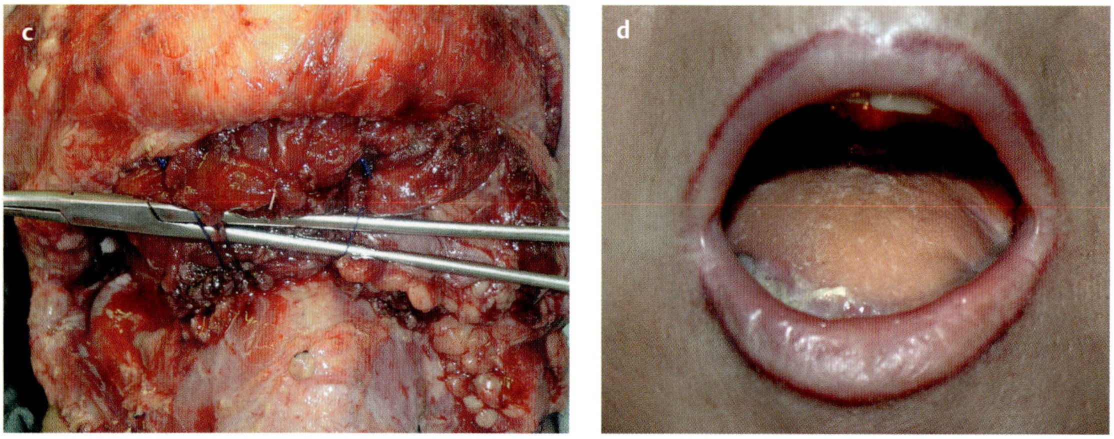


**Fig. 2.18** (*Continued*) **(c)** The muscle portion was placed in the upper neck, and transhyoid laryngeal suspension was performed with permanent sutures. **(d)** A healed neotongue 2 weeks after surgery.

a nonperfused flap is thinner and softer. Patients undergoing reconstruction for total or subtotal glossectomy defects often have a more advanced stage of cancer that requires bilateral neck dissection, which results in a skeletonized neck. In such cases, a segment of the vastus lateralis muscle is included in the ALT flap to fill the upper neck **(Fig. 2.18c)**. Such reconstruction may reduce the risk of orocutaneous fistula and wound infection. With the VRAM flap **(Fig. 2.19)**, the rectus abdominis muscle serves the same purpose. At the completion of flap insetting, the bulk of the flap should touch the palate with the mouth closed, as it will undergo significant atrophy over time **(Fig. 2.20)**.

## Choice of Recipient Vessels

The recipient vessels are the same as those used for hemiglossectomy reconstruction, with the lingual artery and common facial vein as the author's first

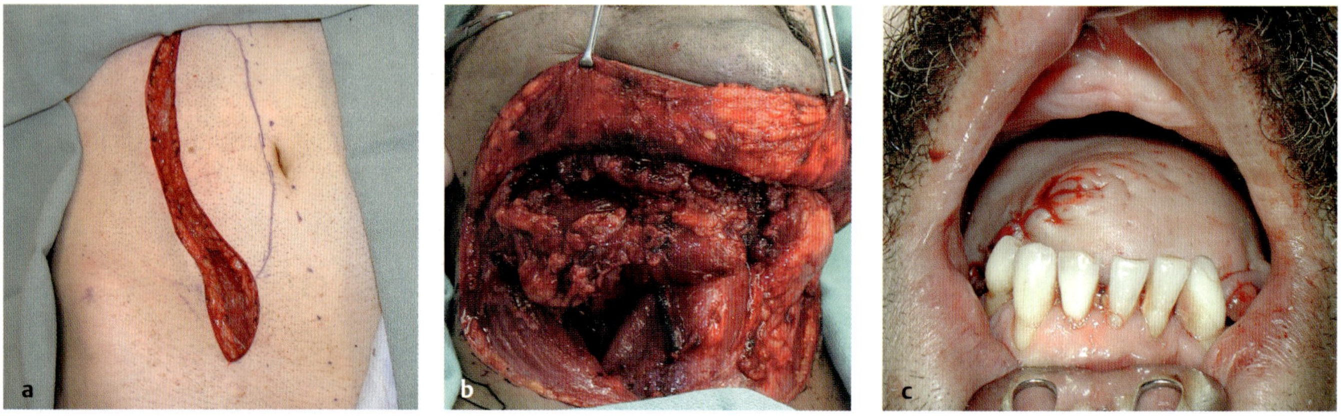


**Fig. 2.19** **(a)** A vertical rectus abdominis myocutaneous (VRAM) flap was harvested from the abdomen. **(b)** The muscle fills the large soft tissue defect of the upper neck nicely to obliterate dead space. **(c)** A bulky neotongue is created so that it can touch the palate.

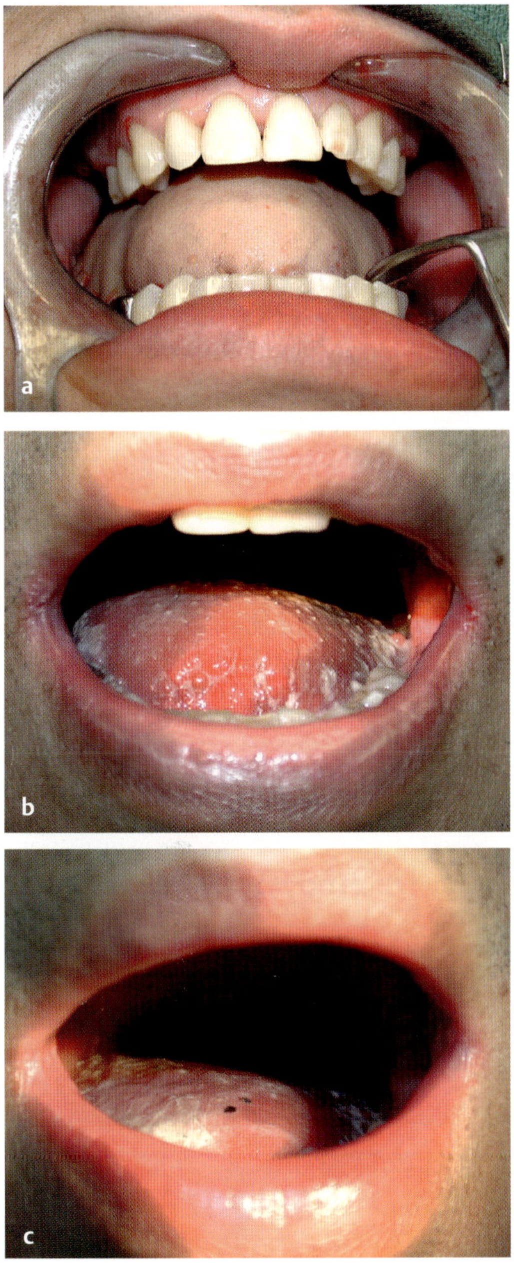


Fig. 2.20 With time, especially after radiotherapy, the flap will shrink considerably. **(a)** At the end of surgery. **(b)** 3 months postoperatively. **(c)** 1 year after surgery and radiotherapy.

choice. Both sides of the neck are usually exposed during surgery and are easily accessible. However, many patients who have undergone previous surgery and/or radiation therapy may have a frozen neck due to significant scarring. The availability of recipient vessels may be limited in these patients. The transverse cervical vessels, which are available in 92% of patients,[9] can be a good choice. The pedicle length of the ALT flap, VRAM, or the RFF is more than adequate to reach the transverse cervical vessels. In addition, using the transverse cervical vessels keeps the vascular pedicle straight.

Following vascular anastomoses, sensory reinnervation of the flap is accomplished by coapting the sensory nerve of the flap to the lingual nerve via the same procedure described for hemiglossectomy reconstruction.

### Laryngeal Suspension

Because the suprahyoid musculature is removed during total and subtotal glossectomy, the hyoid bone needs to be resuspended to the mandible to minimize the risk of aspiration. Laryngeal suspension from the mandible is performed with circumhyoid sutures (0-Prolene) placed through drill holes on both sides of the mentum.[10] The distance between the hyoid bone and the mentum is ~ 4.5 to 5 cm **(Fig. 2.18c)**. Care should be taken to avoid compression of the vascular pedicle by the suspension sutures. The muscle included in the flap provides excellent protection of the vascular pedicle.

## Motor Innervation: Functional Muscle Transfer

Functional muscle transfer has been successfully employed to restore upper extremity functions and for facial reanimation. However, its use in tongue reconstruction has been infrequent and produces uncertain results. It is technically impossible to recreate the complex movements of the tongue and restore all of its functions. The goals of reconstruction, therefore, are to improve airway protection and speech and swallowing functions.

Aspiration can be partially overcome by static, anterior suspension of the larynx from the anterior mandible with transhyoid sutures, as described above. The mobility of the larynx after surgery and radiotherapy is severely limited; therefore, attempting to orient the muscle flap vertically from the hyoid bone to the mandible to elevate the larynx may not be fruitful.

During speech, the tip of the tongue is mostly responsible for articulation. Since a mobile tongue cannot be recreated, speech will need to rely on the bulk of the reconstructed tongue touching the palate. Thus, the main goal of functional muscle transfer for total tongue reconstruction should be to improve swallowing function. It has been proposed that orienting the muscle horizontally as a sling with the ends anchored to the pharyngeal constrictors and the medial pterygoids may help to elevate the neotongue. However, the sling effect is minimal, since the placement of the muscle is quite flat, and not as dramatic as has been described.[11]

Various flaps have been used for functional tongue reconstruction, including the latissimus dorsi,[11] gracilis,[12] and VRAM flaps.[13] The author has used the transverse upper gracilis (TUG) myocutaneous flap and the ALT flap with the vastus lateralis muscle for motor reinnervation. The ALT flap with the vastus lateralis muscle has become the author's preferred method since it can provide both sensory and motor innervation as well as a large vascular pedicle. Usually only the superficial layer of the vastus lateralis muscle is harvested. The neurovascular pedicle travels within the muscle and separates the superficial and deep layers of the muscle. Dissection of the muscle is performed in the plane immediately deep to the neurovascular bundle **(Fig. 2.18b)**. The motor nerve to the muscle, a branch of the femoral nerve, is dissected out and is separated from the main motor nerve proximally.

The design of the TUG flap differs from the traditional gracilis flap in that the skin paddle is oriented in a transverse fashion in the proximal thigh **(Fig. 2.21)**. This design has the following advantages. First, the blood supply to the horizontally oriented proximal skin paddle is more reliable, since the cutaneous perforators are proximally located and horizontally oriented. Partial necrosis of the skin paddle is very rare, unlike the distal third of a traditional longitudinally oriented skin paddle. Second, the cross orientation between the muscle and skin is ideal for flap insetting, in which the muscle is oriented horizontally and the skin is oriented vertically. The skin paddle extends from the femoral vessels anteriorly to the posterior midline of the thigh. Flap dissection begins at the anterior edge of the skin paddle, proceeding in the subcutaneous plane medially until the gracilis muscle is seen. The vascular and neural pedicles are then dissected out as in the conventional gracilis flap. The rest of the skin paddle is then elevated and the muscle is transected. A flap width up to 8 cm can usually be closed primarily.

## Flap Insetting

The muscles are anchored horizontally to the pharyngeal constrictors and the medial pterygoids, as described previously,[11] in the hope that muscle contraction will elevate the neotongue to facilitate

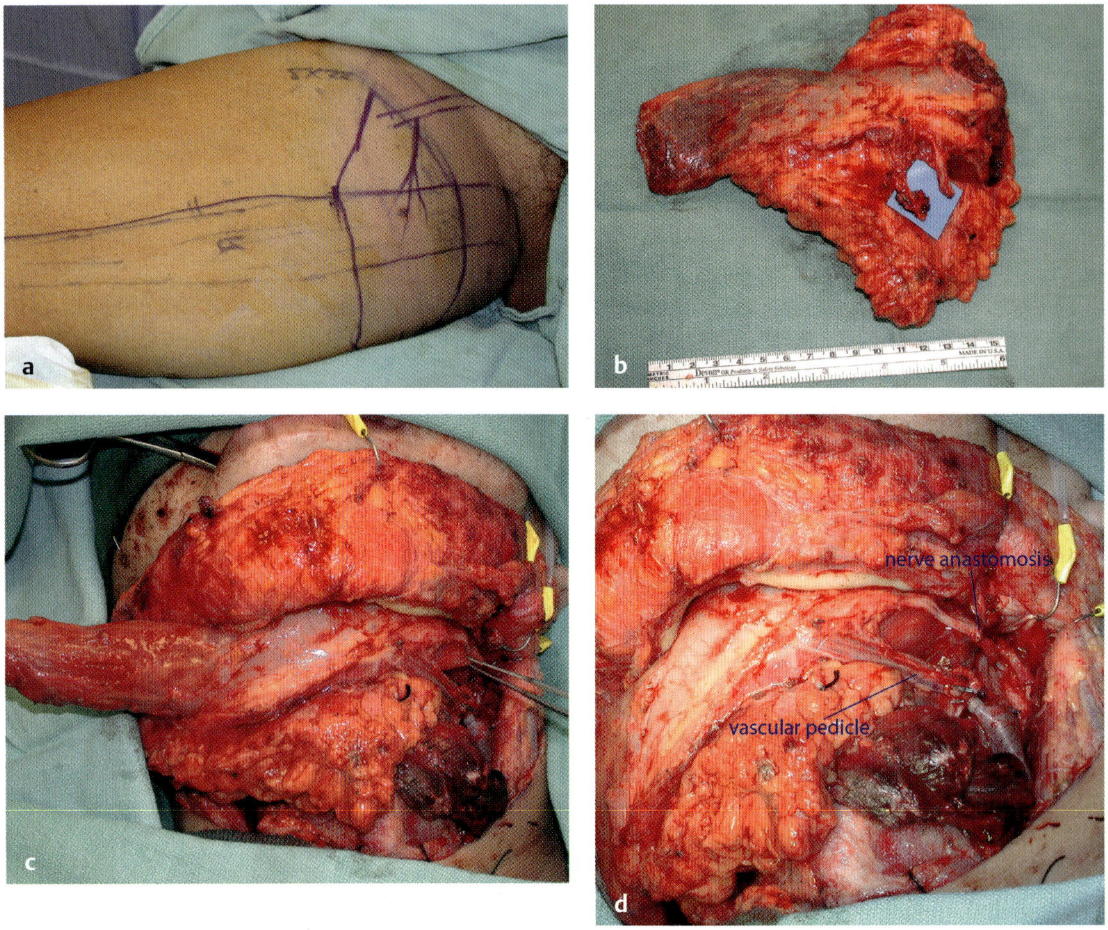


**Fig. 2.21** **(a)** A transverse gracilis myocutaneous flap is designed over the medial thigh with the skin paddle oriented transversely, perpendicular to the muscle direction, to increase the reliability of the skin paddle. **(b)** The flap is harvested with its vascular pedicle and motor nerve. **(c)** The muscle is oriented horizontally and the skin paddle is oriented vertically to create a neotongue. **(d)** The motor nerve is anastomosed to the hypoglossal nerve for motor reinnervation.

swallowing. The muscle is slightly stretched during insetting. The skin paddle is oriented vertically and sutured to the pharyngeal, buccal, and gingival mucosa as described above.

### Outcomes

Based on literature review and the author's own experience, meaningful muscle contractions and tongue mobility have not been achieved with motor reinnervation of the neotongue except for some minor muscle twitches. In the author's experience, one-third of patients are completely dependent on tube feeding, one-third are partially dependent on tube feeding, and the others do not require tube feeding. The oncologic outcomes for these patients are poor. The author's experience with flap revisions after radiotherapy in other areas suggests that complete fibrosis of the muscle flap can develop within 3 months. Thus, it is likely that muscle fibrosis may precede reinnervation after radiotherapy, making motor reinnervation less effective. In selected patients with a good prognosis and no need for postoperative radiotherapy, motor nerve reinnervation may achieve some degree of muscle movement and prevent muscle flap atrophy. At the very least, it serves as a noninnervated flap, providing coverage and bulk without adding much operating time. However, except for the ALT flap with the vastus lateralis muscle included, flaps used for motor reinnervation do not generally confer the possibility of meaningful sensory reinnervation. Therefore, the author's current approach is to reconstruct total glossectomy defects using the ALT flap and the superficial half of the vastus lateralis muscle, with both sensory and motor reinnervation. Functional muscle transfer is not indicated in partial glossectomy reconstruction because the function of the remaining tongue is far superior to that of the reinnervated muscle.

## Postoperative Care

After reconstructive surgery, patients are usually kept in the surgical intensive care unit (ICU) overnight, sedated, and placed on a ventilator, which they are weaned off the next morning, as tolerated. Patients are usually transferred to a flap-monitoring floor after an overnight ICU stay. However, the author has elected to wake up patients at the end of surgery and to skip the surgical ICU stay in an increasing number of cases in recent years. This approach has significantly expedited recovery and shortened the length of hospital stay. Patients with limited cardiopulmonary reserve benefit most from this protocol. Heavy sedation is usually required for ventilated patients in the ICU. It is not uncommon for these patients to develop hypotension after sedation and aggressive fluid resuscitation is required because the use of vasopressors is considered contraindicated after a free flap reconstruction. Many patients then develop fluid overload and subsequent cardiopulmonary complications. The rapid awakening protocol may eliminate this vicious cycle.

Delirium tremens prophylaxis should be given to patients who are known to be heavy drinkers, which is common among patients with head and neck cancer. In patients with a history of alcohol abuse and narcotic dependence, postoperative confusion and agitation are common and may cause hypertension, hematoma, anastomotic breakdowns, and avulsion of the vascular pedicle. Therefore, prompt management of these issues with neuropsychiatric staff is important.

Tube feeding is started on the first postoperative day. Ambulation usually starts on postoperative day 2. Broad-spectrum antibiotics, such as ampicillin-sulbactam, are usually continued for 3 days or longer, as indicated. The nursing staff checks the flaps every hour for 2 days. This can be reduced to every 2 hours for 2 days thereafter and then every 4 hours until discharge. A modified barium swallow (MBS) study is performed by a speech pathologist, usually on postoperative day 7, to evaluate swallowing function, possible leaks, and aspiration. In patients with no leaks or aspiration, a liquid diet is started and then quickly advanced to a soft or regular diet as tolerated. Patients should rinse their mouths frequently with saline or chlorhexidine mouthwash for several weeks. In patients with leaks or aspiration upon swallowing, oral intake is withheld, and an MBS study is repeated in 2 weeks or longer, as clinically indicated.

## Surgical Outcomes and Complications

### Functional Outcomes

Following hemiglossectomy reconstruction with the techniques described above, more than 90% of patients are able to resume an oral diet without the need for tube feeding, and most patients can tolerate a regular or soft diet, depending on their dental status. Tumor recurrence, a bulky flap, and aspiration can prevent resumption of an oral diet. Aspiration frequently occurs in patients when the surgical resection extends to the epiglottis. With proper training by speech pathologists, most motivated patients can relearn how to swallow. All patients who have undergone a hemiglossectomy and reconstruction should be able to have their feeding tubes removed and to speak intelligibly. Functional outcomes after total or subtotal glossectomy reconstruction remain disappointing. Overall, approximately half of the patients require partial or complete tube feeding.

## Surgical Complications

Common recipient-site complications include neck infection, leak, orocutaneous fistula, wound dehiscence, delayed healing, and hematoma. The most common medical complications are pneumonia and respiratory failure.

Neck wound infection is the result of prolonged wound exposure and oral contamination during surgery. Many patients with tongue cancer have poor oral hygiene because of pain. Prior chemoradiation therapy can also increase the risk of infection. Copious irrigation and obliteration of submandibular dead spaces are important for preventing postoperative wound infection, which often occurs 5 to 7 days after surgery. Once infection occurs, early drainage and thorough débridement and irrigation may enable primary wound closure over a drain. However, part of the wound should be left open for dressing changes if the wound is deemed compromised. If adequate vascularized tissue remains in the upper neck after débridement, no additional intervention is needed. However, any dead space in the upper neck should be covered with a muscle flap. The pectoralis major muscle flap is commonly used for this purpose and to protect the carotid artery, which is particularly important in patients who have had prior chemoradiation therapy. Early recognition of wound infection and intervention are crucial to avoiding delays in adjuvant therapy, as postoperative radiotherapy usually starts 4 to 6 weeks after surgery.

Intraoral leaks, dehiscence, or fistula can result from: (1) improper suturing technique; (2) compromised tissue quality, such as in the previously irradiated neck/oral cavity; and (3) wound infection. The gingival mucosa is thin and can be easily torn; therefore, meticulous tissue-handling techniques are essential. Unlike in skin closure, "big bites" are recommended when insetting the flap. Too many small stitches and tight knots may cause skin or mucosa edge ischemia, leading to dehiscence and leakage. The area behind the mandible is often difficult to sew and may require particular attention. As long as the submandibular/upper neck dead space is filled with well-vascularized tissue, leaks usually heal within 2 weeks with proper care. A dead space can lead to an orocutaneous fistula, in which case a pectoralis major muscle flap may be needed. A skin paddle is usually not necessary, as the exposed muscle will mucosalize within several days.

### Sensory Recovery After Reinnervation

Spontaneous sensory recovery can occur without sensory nerve reinnervation, as has been shown in several studies.[14,15,16] However, sensory recovery is usually not complete and depends on the residual nerve population.[17] Therefore, large noninnervated flaps may result in poorer sensory recovery than small, thin flaps.

Sensory recovery after reinnervation has been well documented. Boyd et al[14] observed near-normal sensory recovery in eight patients with partial glossectomy defects with the use of the radial forearm free flap transferred intraorally and reinnervated by coapting the lateral antebrachial cutaneous nerve to the lingual nerve. They also demonstrated that flap sensation was superior to that in the native forearm skin. This was due to the much larger cortical representation of the recipient nerve. Similar findings were reported in another study,[15] which also demonstrated that only the lingual and alveolar nerves, and not the posterior auricular nerve or the cervical plexus, provided adequate sensory recovery.

Sensory reinnervation for total or subtotal glossectomy reconstruction is infrequently performed.[7,18] Unlike the antebrachial cutaneous nerve of the RFF, which is a pure sensory nerve, the intercostal nerve of the commonly used rectus abdominis myocutaneous flap is composed of 70% motor and 30% sensory fibers,[19] resulting in inferior sensory recovery.[20] The ALT flap also has the potential for sensory reinnervation if the lateral femoral cutaneous nerve is used. Our results[7] showed that innervated ALT flaps achieved near-normal two-point discrimination and excellent protective (threshold testing) and temperature and pain sensation, whereas none of the noninnervated flaps achieved meaningful sensation. Postreconstruction radiotherapy resulted in delayed sensory recovery, but the end results were no different after 12 months. Swallowing function was also found to be better in patients with innervated flaps than in those without. A sensate neotongue also provides a higher degree of patient satisfaction. All patients expressed pleasure at the return of sensation after a long period of having a "woody flap."

## ■ Summary

Reconstruction of oral cavity defects should focus on function as well as reliable coverage. Consideration should also be given to minimizing donor-site morbidity and to maximizing aesthetic results.

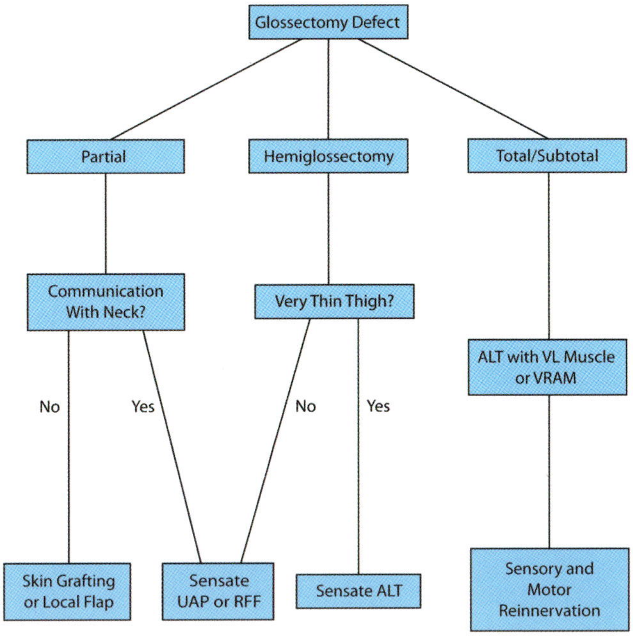


**Fig. 2.22** Algorithm for reconstruction of oral cavity defects.

Local flaps are often inadequate. A thin flap, such as the radial forearm or UAP flap, is best for hemiglossectomy reconstruction, whereas the ALT flap is preferred for total or subtotal glossectomy reconstruction. An algorithm is shown in **Fig. 2.22**. Careful planning and attention to detail during surgery may prevent many postoperative complications. Early recognition and intervention for complications may prevent delay in adjuvant therapy and disastrous consequences.

## Pearls and Pitfalls

- Small FOM defects with bone exposure may be amenable to closure with locoregional flaps, such as the submental flap or the facial artery myomucosal flap; larger defects will usually require a free flap.
- Small partial glossectomy defects can sometimes be reconstructed with a skin graft, as long as there is no communication with the neck and graft contracture will not inhibit tongue movement and compromise speech, swallowing, or oral hygiene.
- Hemiglossectomy defects are best reconstructed with a thin fasciocutaneous free flap, such as the radial forearm fasciocutaneous free flap or ulnar artery perforator flap.
- Subtotal and total glossectomy defects have a guarded prognosis for meaningful speech and swallowing, although with modern reconstructive techniques, the airway can be managed without laryngectomy.
- Subtotal and total glossectomy defects require reconstruction with bulky soft tissue free flaps so that the dead space of the mouth is obliterated and, with muscular contraction, the soft palate and pharyngeal walls can make contact with the flap to permit speech articulation and swallowing. The anterolateral thigh and vertical rectus abdominis myocutaneous flaps are our first choices if the body habitus is appropriate.
- Suture laryngeal suspension may be of benefit in preventing aspiration in near-total and total glossectomy reconstructive patients.

## Expert Commentary *by Ming-Huei Cheng*

This chapter provides very practical information for surgeons to follow and to apply to their own clinical cases. It comprehensively covers the assessment of oral defects, surgical planning, selection of the appropriate flap for different defects, surgical technique, functional outcome evaluation, and management of possible complications. The figures provide excellent illustrations of outcomes of oral cavity reconstruction.

We have performed oral and tongue reconstructions using approaches similar to those described in the chapter for recipient-site assessment and flap selection, with promising results. However, there are some differences in our practice, such as innervation of the transferred flap. We do not try to transfer a functional muscle at the primary tongue reconstruction stage, since the patients usually require postoperative radiation, which will compromise nerve regeneration and also result in fibrosis of the transferred muscle.[21] Second, movement of the innervated muscle flap, which can only contract in one direction, will likely not be in coordination with the movements of the residual native tongue, which can move in many more directions due to the multidirectional orientation of its intrinsic muscles.

Anastomosis of the lingual nerve may help with the rapid recovery of protective sensation in the transferred flap. We used to anastomose the sensory nerve in hemiglossectomy tongue reconstruction

15 years ago,[15] but we do not routinely anastomose any sensory nerve during oral and tongue reconstruction now. Most patients in our practice regain protective sensation by 6 to 8 months after surgery, depending on the depth of the defect. We have observed very few complaints or complications due to sensation, such as scald burn of the reconstructed tongue by food. On the other hand, by sparing the lateral antebrachial cutaneous nerve in the suprafascial dissection of the radial forearm flap, donor-site morbidity is minimized.

Another difference in our practice is that, for radial forearm free flap dissection, we do not take the additional proximal soft tissue for the obliteration of the submandibular dead space. We pay attention to watertight sutures at flap inset and check the closure by filling the oral cavity with saline and looking for leakage into the neck. We experience very few orocutaneous fistulas following oral cavity reconstruction, which is probably due to the complete survival of transferred free flaps.

For the ulnar forearm flap, which is not a true perforator flap according to the definition of perforator flap, we like a more distal flap design than Dr. Yu's design. The distal edge of the ulnar forearm flap may be located 1 cm proximal to the wrist crease. By performing a suprafascial dissection of the radial side of the flap, over the flexor digitorium superficialis muscle and tendons, tendon exposure can be usually avoided **(Fig. 2.23)**. The mean number of sizable cutaneous perforators of the ulnar forearm flap is 4.3, which makes this flap very reliable.[22] The disadvantage of the ulnar forearm flap is the smaller diameter of the ulnar venae comitantes, which may make anastomosis difficult due to size mismatch with the recipient vein.

The selection of recipient vessels varies in each case. We most commonly use the superior thyroid artery or the facial artery. The superior thyroid artery is our preferred recipient artery because of its size compatibility with the radial and ulnar arteries and its comfortable location for anastomosis. The superior thyroid vein or facial vein is usually used as the recipient outflow.

For flap inset in the hemiglossectomy reconstruction, we like to inset the most distal part (the most reliable circulation) of the radial forearm flap to the tongue base, since the cutaneous perforators are located more distally. In this setting, it is easy to débride the necrotic tissue anteriorly if there is partial necrosis of the proximal part of the transferred radial forearm flap.

Finally, we feel that the anterolateral thigh (ALT) free flap is the most versatile option for oral cavity reconstruction.[23] The thickness of the ALT perforator flap in thin patients is good for large oral cavity or hemi-tongue defects. The ALT myocutaneous free flap is suitable for subtotal or total tongue defects because it provides adequate soft tissue bulk to restore partial swallowing function. With a pentagon-shaped flap design, we may achieve good swallowing function even after total glossectomy.[21]

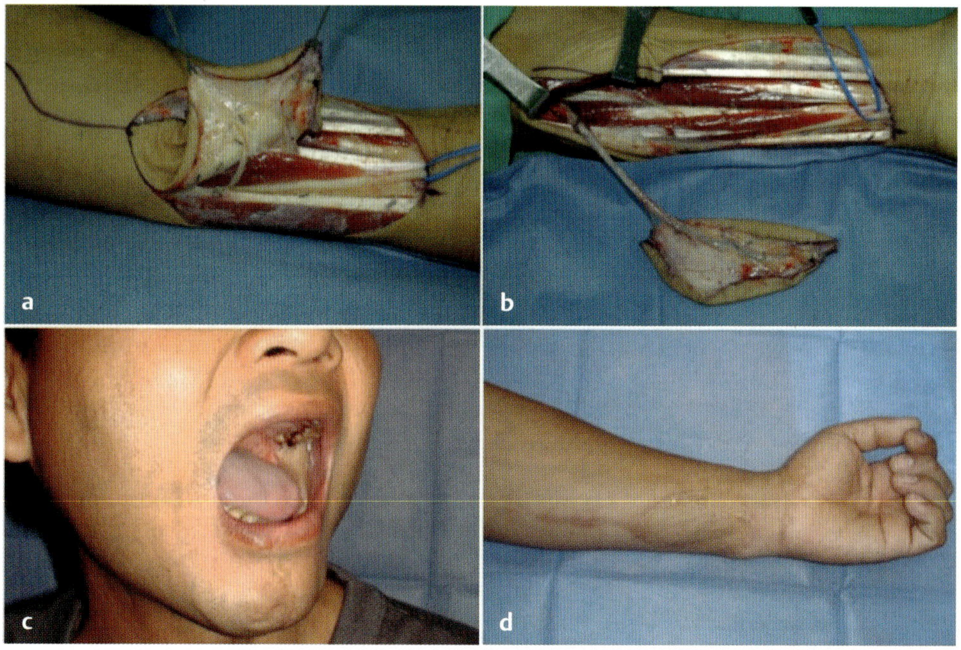


**Fig. 2.23** **(a)** Ulnar forearm free flap harvested suprafascially. A blue vessel loop is placed around the ulnar nerve. **(b)** Completed flap dissection from the left forearm. **(c)** Result following buccal reconstruction with an ulnar forearm free flap. **(d)** Appearance of the donor site.

## Speech Therapy Multidisciplinary Commentary *by Katherine A. Hutcheson*

As elegantly described, surgical and reconstructive techniques greatly influence postsurgical functional outcomes. The goal of this commentary is to highlight the complementary role of postsurgical rehabilitation practices that can also significantly alter functional outcomes.

### Small Resections

Oral resections represent a complex array of functional defects with diverse reconstructive and rehabilitation goals. For smaller resections confined to oral structures and treated with single-modality surgical therapy, oral functions are the primary concern. Expected functional issues in these cases include inefficient oral bolus preparation, incomplete oral bolus clearance, and articulation errors. It should be expected that successful surgery and rehabilitation will result in fully understandable speech with minor articulation errors at most, and mild, often temporary, inefficiency of oral preparatory (bolus formation, mastication) and transport functions. The primary reconstructive goal is to maximize range of motion of the mobile tongue and dynamic oropharyngeal structures by avoiding tethering to adjacent stationary structures.

Rehabilitation then focuses on maximizing agility and endurance of tongue movement, since patients often experience fatigue and functional deterioration with prolonged use as they tire from the "drag" of the immobile flap on the remaining mobile structures. Dysphagia therapy in this subgroup of patients with smaller oral resections focuses on ease and efficiency of oral transport. Special equipment is not typically required for oral bolus clearance, even in early postsurgical recovery. Dysphagia therapy typically combines oral manipulation exercise tasks with mass practice of functional swallows. After a brief period on a limited diet of liquids and blended foods, patients rapidly resume intake of chewable foods. Articulation therapy focuses on normalizing speech sound production, because for the most part, patients' speech is highly intelligible even very early after surgery. Articulation is normalized by adjusting tongue placement or by use of nonlingual compensations.

### Large Resections

For larger oral resections, such as near-total or total glossectomy, and resections extending to include more than one-quarter of the tongue base, both oral- and pharyngeal-phase functions must be considered. Chronic aspiration is expected in at least one-third of cases, but it can be decreased by laryngeal suspension and by reconstituting the bulk of the tongue base so that it provides distal driving pressure and directs the bolus toward natural lateral pharyngeal channels rather than the airway. Even more common than aspiration is extreme inefficiency of bolus transport through the oral cavity and pharynx. Postoperative speech is equally challenging. With the bulk of the mobile tongue resected, even the optimally reconstructed tongue no longer lifts and conforms the complex lingual-palatal contacts necessary to articulate words normally. Rather, articulation is approximated by exaggerated mandibular postures to push the neotongue against the palate. Functional outcomes after total glossectomy remain disappointing for many patients. But with optimal reconstruction and rehabilitation, a select minority of highly motivated patients can return to full oral nutrition of solid foods and can achieve fully intelligible, although noticeably distorted, speech after total glossectomy. In the experience of this author, 10% or less of patients achieve this high level of functional success. It is more common for the bulk of even successfully rehabilitated patients to remain on liquids or blended foods and to produce occasionally unintelligible words.

After large oral resections, dysphagia therapy focuses first on establishing a safe swallow that protects the patient against aspiration. Exercises facilitating airway protection and mass practice of safe swallows are the starting point for dysphagia therapy. Special equipment, sometimes referred to as adaptive equipment, such as glossectomy spoons, chopsticks, tongue blades, and zip/squeeze bags, is often required to assist with oral inefficiency. Adaptive equipment can be used to either bypass the oral cavity for direct placement of a bolus into the upper pharynx or to assist with push of thicker bolus consistencies posteriorly through the oral cavity. Articulation therapy consists of speech drills to master approximations of target phonemes. Understandability or intelligibility of speech is the major focus. Speech can be further improved by fitting of a palatal drop (palatal augmentation) prosthesis, particularly for patients who have had the majority of the mobile tongue resected, but the sensory feedback from the palate is disrupted when the prosthesis is in place, so many patients elect to eat with it removed.

## Radiotherapy and Chemoradiation

Adjuvant radiotherapy or chemoradiotherapy is the norm for most patients with advanced-stage disease necessitating oral reconstruction. Edema, fibrosis, and atrophy of structures that are important for swallowing in the irradiated field lead to irreversible, and, at times, progressive dysfunction of the constrictors, tongue base, and laryngeal apparatus. Even in the absence of major resections, head and neck radiotherapy can cause significant degrees of pharyngeal dysphagia. For instance, chronic aspiration is reported in up to 31% of patients treated with definitive chemoradiation for advanced stage oropharyngeal cancers, even when highly conformal intensity modulated radiation therapy (IMRT) planning is used to minimize the dose to nontarget, normal, swallowing-critical structures (e.g., the pharyngeal constrictors or larynx).[24]

We and others have demonstrated that patients who keep the swallow system active during radiotherapy have better acute and long-term swallowing outcomes.[25] Maintenance of oral intake through the duration of radiotherapy significantly and independently predicts for better function even years into survivorship. For patients with surgically treated oral cancers, this means that there is a critical, short interval of time between surgery and the start of adjuvant radiotherapy for the patient to regain swallowing function. In the experience of the author, patients who are still NPO postsurgically when they start adjuvant radiotherapy have very little chance of meaningful swallow recovery.

## Rehabilitation

Optimal rehabilitation is early rehabilitation. Atrophy and adverse remodeling of skeletal muscles begin just hours after immobilization. For this reason, patients should resume oral functions as early as possible after surgery. Temporary postsurgical immobilization is necessary to allow for sufficient healing. Early functional mobilization of oral structures should be a shared goal of the surgical and rehabilitation teams, and this goal should be communicated clearly with the patient and family. Rehabilitation is much more effective when the patient and family are engaged with a shared ownership in the recovery process. This begins by clearly articulating goals and timelines. Practical steps in swallowing therapy for the postsurgical oral cavity cancer patient are outline in **Table 2.1**.

Lymphedema management is an often forgotten component of postsurgical rehabilitation. Lymphedema is common and particularly severe in patients who require bilateral neck dissections and

**Table 2.1** Stepwise approach to dysphagia management after oral surgery and reconstruction

| | |
|---|---|
| Step 1: Saliva management | Saliva swallows are functional swallows. Immediately after surgery, encourage patients to begin swallowing their saliva. Decrease dependence on oral suction as quickly as possible. |
| Step 2: Start oral intake | As soon as they are adequately healed, patients begin oral intake of consistencies that are safe to swallow. We advocate for videofluoroscopy, also known as the modified barium swallow (MBS), to identify readiness for oral intake after oral surgery with reconstruction. Videofluoroscopy is ideal to test simultaneously for healing and swallow safety. The MBS has two goals: (1) to rule out suture line leaks and (2) to rule out aspiration. If aspiration is detected, MBS allows the clinician to establish the efficacy of swallowing strategies in real time. Oropharyngeal physiology is evaluated to understand the pathophysiology of postsurgical dysphagia and to define therapeutic targets. |
| Step 3: Mass practice with successful swallowing of nonchewable consistencies | Patients first master swallowing a limited range of textures. Patients are provided goals to systematically and rapidly increase the volume of oral intake in a narrow range of textures using any strategies necessary to prevent aspiration. This usually includes swallowing liquids and/or blended foods. Mass practice with these limited bolus types continues until the patient is consistently successful with nonchewable foods. |
| Step 4: Increase complexity of oral intake | Once the patient has mastered nonchewable foods, the focus changes to increasing the complexity of food types. Systematically, the speech pathologist helps the patient to identify techniques necessary to efficiently manipulate and move solid foods through the oral cavity and pharynx. Patients may initially require special utensils or preparations of foods. Therapy sessions navigate systematically along a hierarchy of more and more challenging foods. Special equipment and swallowing postures are forgone as much as possible to provide the most natural eating experience achievable for the patient. |

adjuvant radiotherapy. Both internal and external lymphedema are significantly correlated with self-rated swallowing impairment. Alongside conventional speech and swallowing therapies, head and neck lymphedema therapy offers comprehensive rehabilitation. Complete decongestive therapy (CDT) is the gold-standard nonsurgical therapy for lymphedema.[26] Hallmarks of CDT are manual lymphatic drainage massage coupled with compression bandaging. CDT can soften and shrink the interstitial filling, resulting in superior cosmetic and functional outcomes.

## Summary

Oral anatomy and physiology are exquisitely complex, and functional restoration requires the integration of multiple disciplines that share the common goal of complete functional restoration. Considerations of reconstruction for functional restoration are articulated clearly in the chapter. Functional outcomes are further optimized by dysphagia-optimized radiation planning, dental restoration, lymphedema management, and proactive speech and swallowing therapy with speech pathology.

## References


1. Pribaz J, Stephens W, Crespo L, Gifford G. A new intraoral flap: facial artery musculomucosal (FAMM) flap. Plast Reconstr Surg 1992;90(3):421–429
2. Dupoirieux L, Plane L, Gard C, Penneau M. Anatomical basis and results of the facial artery musculomucosal flap for oral reconstruction. Br J Oral Maxillofac Surg 1999;37(1):25–28
3. Chang SC, Miller G, Halbert CF, Yang KH, Chao WC, Wei FC. Limiting donor site morbidity by suprafascial dissection of the radial forearm flap. Microsurgery 1996;17(3): 136–140
4. Urken ML, Moscoso JF, Lawson W, Biller HF. A systematic approach to functional reconstruction of the oral cavity following partial and total glossectomy. Arch Otolaryngol Head Neck Surg 1994;120(6):589–601
5. Yu P. Characteristics of the anterolateral thigh flap in a Western population and its application in head and neck reconstruction. Head Neck 2004;26(9):759–769
6. Yu P. Reinnervated anterolateral thigh flap for tongue reconstruction. Head Neck 2004;26(12):1038–1044
7. Lyos AT, Evans GRD, Perez D, Schusterman MA. Tongue reconstruction: outcomes with the rectus abdominis flap. Plast Reconstr Surg 1999;103(2):442–447, discussion 448–449
8. Yu P, Youssef A. Efficacy of the handheld Doppler in preoperative identification of the cutaneous perforators in the anterolateral thigh flap. Plast Reconstr Surg 2006;118(4):928–933, discussion 934–935
9. Yu P. The transverse cervical vessels as recipient vessels for previously treated head and neck cancer patients. Plast Reconstr Surg 2005;115(5):1253–1258
10. Weber RS, Ohlms L, Bowman J, Jacob R, Goepfert H. Functional results after total or near total glossectomy with laryngeal preservation. Arch Otolaryngol Head Neck Surg 1991;117(5):512–515
11. Haughey BH. Tongue reconstruction: concepts and practice. Laryngoscope 1993;103(10):1132–1141
12. Yousif NJ, Dzwierzynski WW, Sanger JR, Matloub HS, Campbell BH. The innervated gracilis musculocutaneous flap for total tongue reconstruction. Plast Reconstr Surg 1999;104(4):916–921
13. Yamamoto Y, Sugihara T, Furuta Y, Fukuda S. Functional reconstruction of the tongue and deglutition muscles following extensive resection of tongue cancer. Plast Reconstr Surg 1998;102(4):993–998, discussion 999–1000
14. Boyd B, Mulholland S, Gullane P, et al. Reinnervated lateral antebrachial cutaneous neurosome flaps in oral reconstruction: are we making sense? Plast Reconstr Surg 1994;93(7):1350–1359, discussion 1360–1362
15. Santamaria E, Wei FC, Chen IH, Chuang DCC. Sensation recovery on innervated radial forearm flap for hemiglossectomy reconstruction by using different recipient nerves. Plast Reconstr Surg 1999;103(2):450–457
16. Vriens JPM, Acosta R, Soutar DS, Webster MHC. Recovery of sensation in the radial forearm free flap in oral reconstruction. Plast Reconstr Surg 1996;98(4):649–656
17. Shindo ML, Sinha UK, Rice DH. Sensory recovery in noninnervated free flaps for head and neck reconstruction. Laryngoscope 1995;105(12 Pt 1):1290–1293
18. Matloub HS, Larson DL, Kuhn JC, Yousif NJ, Sanger JR. Lateral arm free flap in oral cavity reconstruction: a functional evaluation. Head Neck 1989;11(3):205–211
19. Courtiss EH, Goldwyn RM. Breast sensation before and after plastic surgery. Plast Reconstr Surg 1976;58(1):1–13
20. Kimata Y, Uchiyama K, Ebihara S, et al. Comparison of innervated and noninnervated free flaps in oral reconstruction. Plast Reconstr Surg 1999;104(5):1307–1313
21. Engel H, Huang JJ, Lin CY, et al. A strategic approach for tongue reconstruction to achieve predictable and improved functional and aesthetic outcomes. Plast Reconstr Surg 2010;126(6):1967–1977
22. Huang JJ, Wu CW, Lam WL, et al. Anatomical basis and clinical application of the ulnar forearm free flap for head and neck reconstruction. Laryngoscope 2012;122(12):2670–2676
23. Ali RS, Bluebond-Langner R, Rodriguez ED, Cheng MH. The versatility of the anterolateral thigh flap. Plast Reconstr Surg 2009; 124(6, Suppl):e395–e407
24. Hutcheson KA, Lewin JS. Functional assessment and rehabilitation: how to maximize outcomes. Otolaryngol Clin North Am 2013;46(4):657–670
25. Hutcheson KA, Bhayani MK, Beadle BM, et al. Eat and exercise during radiotherapy or chemoradiotherapy for pharyngeal cancers: use it or lose it. JAMA Otolaryngol Head Neck Surg 2013;139(11):1127–1134
26. Smith BG, Hutcheson KA, Little LG, et al. Lymphedema outcomes in patients with head and neck cancer. Otolaryngol Head Neck Surg 2015;152(2):284–291

# 3 Mandibular Reconstruction

*Matthew M. Hanasono*

## ■ Introduction

Restoration of the mandible is among the most challenging and arduous surgeries in head and neck reconstruction. Mandibular defects frequently involve composite tissues, including oral mucosa and soft tissue structures, mandibular bone, and, in some cases, external skin. Many advances have been made in mandibular reconstruction in the past two to three decades, including: the development of vascularized bone flaps; the advent of low-profile, high-tensile-strength reconstruction plates; the ability to restore dentition with osseointegrated implants; and the incorporation of computer-aided design (CAD) and computer-aided manufacturing (CAM) into surgical planning.

Goals of mandibular reconstruction include reestablishing the shape of the lower third of the face, creating a surface for mastication or dental restoration, preventing deviation of the jaw leading to malocclusion, maintaining free movement of the temporomandibular joint, and providing a stable wound that does not result in an orocutaneous fistula. In addition, mandibular reconstruction should not result in tethering of the tongue in a way that affects speech or deglutition, or introduce redundant tissue that can obstruct the airway or compromise oral hygiene. The reconstruction must also be reliable and long lasting. Mandibular reconstruction that results in early fracture or extrusion of bone flaps or grafts, as well as reconstruction plates, results in a situation that is frequently even more difficult to treat than the initial defect.

## ■ Regional Anatomy

The mandible provides the bony support for the lower third of the face and bears the lower teeth. Each side of the mandible consists of a lateral horizontal portion, called the body; a perpendicular portion, called the ramus; an alveolar process along the upper border of the mandible, which bears the teeth; a condyle, which forms the temporomandibular joint with the temporal bone; and a coronoid process, which is a triangular bony projection, anterior to the condyle **(Fig. 3.1)**. The paired mandibular bones join anteriorly in the midline at the symphysis. The portion of the body just lateral to the symphysis is often referred to as the parasymphyseal region. It is in the parasymphyseal region that the mandible curves most acutely, in the vicinity of the canine tooth. The body and the ramus meet in a region termed the angle of the mandible (also known as the gonial angle). There are two foramina on each side of the mandible: the mandibular foramen, which is penetrated by the inferior alveolar nerve, a branch of the mandibular division of the trigeminal nerve (cranial nerve [CN] V); and the mental foramen, from which the mental nerve, a continuation of the inferior alveolar nerve, emerges inferior to the second premolar tooth and supplies sensation to the lower lip.

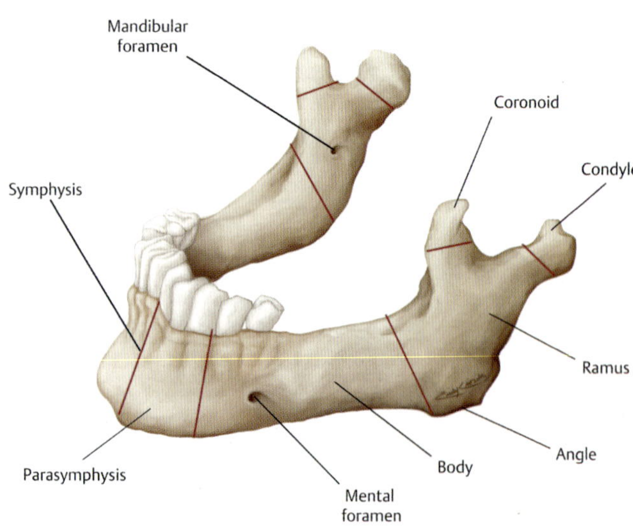


**Fig. 3.1** Bony anatomy of the mandible.

Many muscles attach to the bony mandible. Anteriorly, the paired genioglossus muscles attach to the inner surface of the mandible at the mental spines, just lateral to the lower part of the symphysis. Immediately below the attachment of the genioglossus muscles are the attachment points of the paired geniohyoid muscles. The mylohyoid, digastric, and superior pharyngeal constrictor muscles also attach to the inner surface of the mandible along its inferior, inner border. Loss of the anterior mandible, therefore, can have profound effects on swallowing and on protection from aspiration, due to posterior displacement of the tongue and limited laryngeal elevation, which can also contribute to airway obstruction. Because of this, close airway monitoring and strong consideration for prophylactic tracheostomy, at least temporarily, are indicated, especially following resection of the anterior mandible. Patients need to be counseled regarding potential impairment of swallowing and chronic aspiration following anterior mandibular resection. Speech can also be affected and the tongue will have limited protrusion. Efforts to suspend the larynx and the tongue to the reconstructed anterior mandible with sutures are reasonable, although the efficacy of this practice has not been proven.

The muscles of mastication insert along the posterior mandible. The temporalis muscle inserts mostly onto the coronoid process, while the masseter muscle inserts broadly along the lateral surface of the mandibular ramus and posterior body. The lateral pterygoid muscles attach to the condylar neck on each side, while the medial pterygoid muscles, which serve to depress the mandible and open the mouth, insert on the medial surface of the angle. Loss of the posterior portions of the mandible, therefore, results in impaired unilateral mandibular movement on the affected side. After unilateral resection of the posterior mandible, and even with bony restoration, mouth opening and closing will be dependent upon the actions of the contralateral muscles of mastication. Contraction of the remaining contralateral medial and lateral pterygoid muscles will tend to rotate the mandible toward the side of the resection.

## Reconstructive Options

Options for treating mandibular defects include performing no reconstruction, with primary closure of the oral soft tissues to themselves, and reconstruction with metal plates, nonvascularized bone grafts, osteomyocutaneous pedicled flaps, soft tissue pedicled or free flaps, and osseous or osteocutaneous free flaps.

### Mandibular Reconstruction with Reconstruction Plates

Mandibular reconstruction with a reconstruction plate that spans a segmental bony mandibular defect was a more popular technique prior to the development of microvascular free bone flaps. Some centers still rely at least partially on reconstructive plates when a patient is deemed unsuitable for a prolonged operative procedure involving free tissue transfer, or when microvascular expertise is not available. However, experience has shown that such reconstructions are at high risk for complications, including plate fracture and/or exposure, either intraorally or through the skin of the cheek or chin.

To help decrease the rate of exposure, many surgeons have combined reconstruction plates with a pectoralis major muscle or myocutaneous pedicled flap, or a soft tissue free flap. However, Wei et al,[1] in a series of 80 patients, still reported a complication rate of 69% when a reconstruction plate was combined with soft tissue free flaps, primarily the anterolateral thigh (ALT) fasciocutaneous free flap. Plate exposure was the most common complication, followed by soft tissue deficiency, deformity of the lateral face, intraoral contracture, trismus, and osteoradionecrosis. Thirty-one percent of the patients with complications ultimately underwent a secondary salvage procedure with a fibular osteocutaneous flap.

Overall, complication rates associated with a reconstructive plate and soft tissue flap are reported to be between 21% and 87%.[2] Anterior defects are associated with a higher rate of plate extrusion than lateral defects, as are defects in patients undergoing radiation treatment or with a history of prior irradiation. In addition, larger defects result in significantly higher failure rates than smaller defects.

Even when patients are reasonable candidates for a free flap, some surgeons advocate plate or combined plate and soft tissue flap reconstruction in patients with advanced cancers and a limited life expectancy, since surgery is usually shorter and recovery is usually faster. However, this approach must be carefully considered on a case-by-case basis, as the incidence of plate-related complications is high. In addition, the results are rarely ideal, due to persistent contour deformity and malocclusion. Secondary salvage of such complications with vascularized bone flaps can be performed, but salvage is much more difficult than reconstruction performed at the time of the resection. Additional difficulties at the secondary surgery include more challenging dissection of recipient vessels and greater difficulty restoring accurate occlusion due to postoperative and radiation-associated scar contracture.

## Nonvascularized Bone Grafts

Autogenous bone grafts can be used for mandibular reconstruction. The bone is revascularized by a process of creeping substitution. Sources of cortical bone graft include iliac crest, split calvarium, and rib. Nonvascularized bone grafts may be used in defects less than ~ 5 cm long. High failure rates are frequently seen in longer segments and in anterior defects. Preoperative or postoperative radiation therapy is usually considered a contraindication, due to high rates of extrusion, resorption, and infection, and, therefore, use of nonvascularized bone grafts for mandibular reconstruction is usually restricted to patients with benign disease or patients who require mandibular surgery for orthognathic rather than oncologic indications. Metallic mesh or Dacron trays filled with morselized cancellous bone have also been used for limited defects. This technique has been shown to be associated with a high rate of extrusion and bone graft dissolution, and it has generally fallen out of favor.

## Vascularized Bone Flaps

Mandibular reconstruction with vascularized bone flaps transferred by microsurgical anastomosis should be considered the gold standard in oncologic reconstruction. Vascularized bone flaps are associated with early bony union, generally within 6 weeks. Vascularized bone flaps demonstrate very little bony resorption, with ~ 90% of bone height being preserved long-term. Unlike nonvascularized bone grafts, bone flaps can be used to reconstruct large segmental bone losses and can tolerate radiation therapy without resorption, fracture, or extrusion. The commonly used bone flaps may be harvested with a cutaneous or muscular component that allows for simultaneous soft tissue reconstruction. Some flaps can be harvested simultaneously with oncologic resection or cervical vessel dissection by a second team to save time. Some vascularized bone flaps can reliably accept osseointegrated implants. A minimum of 6 to 7 mm of bone height is required for placement of osseointegrated dental implants.

Pedicled flaps, such as the pectoralis major muscle with rib or sternal bone and the trapezius muscle with scapula, have also been described.[3] The pectoralis osteomyocutaneous flap can be used for anterior defects and the trapezius osteomyocutaneous flap for lateral defects. The lack of reliability (particularly of the distal flap that supplies the bone), limited ability to shape and configure both the soft tissue and the bony flap components to fit the defect, restricted reach, and limited availability of bone make these two flaps secondary options after free bone flaps. Their use is primarily of historic significance.

### Fibula Free Flap

The fibular osteocutaneous flap is probably the most frequently used choice for mandibular reconstruction.[4,5] The fibula is primarily an ankle stabilizer and provides the origin for several muscles of the lower leg, but it is expendable provided the distal several centimeters of the bone, including the lateral malleolus, are spared. Generally, a 22 to 25 cm segment of fibula may be harvested in the adult patient, permitting reconstruction of near-total mandibular defects with a single flap.

The vascular supply of the fibula free flap is the peroneal artery and vein. It is important to examine both lower extremities and palpate for dorsalis pedis and posterior tibial pulses preoperatively. A patient with findings consistent with arterial insufficiency or venous stasis may not be a candidate for a fibula free flap. In addition to pathologic conditions, it is important to rule out the possibility of peroneal arteria magna, an anatomical variant in which the peroneal artery is the dominant arterial inflow to the distal lower extremity. When the pedal arteries are not palpable or the circulation to the lower extremity is questionable, additional studies may be required, such as conventional, magnetic resonance, or computed tomographic angiography of the lower extremities prior to performing fibula free flap harvest.

The choice of leg is based on the anticipated side of the recipient blood vessels and expected need for extra- or intraoral lining. In general, we prefer to use the leg that is contralateral to the side of the recipient blood vessels when intraoral lining is needed, based on the location of the septocutaneous perforators that travel along the posterolateral border of the fibula in its native position on the leg. The flap is oriented so that the pedicle is on the lingual side, to minimize external compression and to allow plate placement on the lateral aspect of the fibula, and, for posterior defects, it is usually placed posteriorly. Details regarding flap harvest are discussed in a separate chapter of this text.

Osteotomies may be completed while the flap is left in situ or during the inset of the flap into the mandibular defect. Performing the osteotomies while the pedicle is still attached to the leg has the advantage of minimizing ischemia time. Also, any injuries to the pedicle can be identified well in advance of revascularization, an advantage that is perhaps most important when rigid fixation and skin paddle inset are performed prior to the microvascular anastomosis. Other surgeons prefer to perform osteotomies after the pedicle is divided due to increased freedom of movement, potentially avoiding traction injury to the pedicle blood vessels.

We prefer to use a locking titanium reconstruction plate to secure the osteotomized fibula to the remaining native mandibular segments. In recent years, lower-profile hardware has resulted in decreased rates of plate exposure. Some surgeons have had success using smaller, very-low-profile miniplates. Such plates have the advantage of permitting fine adjustments to the final shape of the reconstructed mandible, while locking reconstruction plates are considered to possess superior stability and are able to tolerate higher loads.

In certain cases, a double-barrel approach to mandibular reconstruction is used to increase bony height. In this technique, reconstruction proceeds in the usual manner but the distal portion of the fibula is turned back 180 degrees onto the proximal fibula to add height to the reconstructed mandible so that it more closely approximates the height of the normal dentulous mandible.[6] We reserve use of the double-barrel technique for anterior mandibular defects, as the normal height of the mandible is greater in this region. Laterally, the width of a single fibular segment closely approximates the height of the native mandible. When a single width of fibula is used, we prefer to align the fibula with the lower border of the mandible, rather than the alveolus, to achieve the best possible external contour.

Malocclusion may also occur frequently following mandibular reconstruction. Whenever possible, the mandible is pre-plated prior to mandibular resection so that the reconstruction can be designed to maintain the spatial orientation of the native mandible. When pre-plating is not feasible due to an expansile tumor, pathologic fracture, or prior resection, use of an external fixator can be considered. More recently, use of computer planning and rapid prototype modeling, which are discussed in a separate chapter, has helped improve outcomes, particularly when pre-plating is not feasible.[7]

## Iliac Crest Free Flap

The iliac crest free flap provides a generous amount of cortical and cancellous bone for mandibular reconstruction. The deep circumflex iliac vessels comprise the vascular pedicle of the iliac crest free flap and demonstrate consistent anatomy, reasonable length (an average of 8 to 10 cm), and appropriate vessel diameter (an average of 2 to 3 mm) for microsurgical application. The blood supply of the iliac crest bone flap is robust, incorporating both nutrient perforators and periosteal vessels, which allows the flap to tolerate multiple osteotomies.

The iliac crest bone may be harvested as a full-thickness bicortical or as a partial-thickness unicortical (inner cortex) bone flap. Unicortical bone flaps are associated with a superior donor-site appearance and theoretically less donor-site morbidity, but less bone stock. The natural curved contour of the bone is often considered ideal for lateral mandibular reconstruction. Reconstruction of anterior defects usually requires an osteotomy. The bone stock, particularly when harvested as a full-thickness flap, reliably accommodates osseointegrated dental implants.

The flap may be harvested as a bone-only flap or with an associated skin and/or muscle paddle for reconstruction of composite defects. The skin paddle, which is nourished by several perforators arising from the deep circumflex iliac vessels, may be as wide as 9 to 12 cm in some patients and still allow the donor site to be closed primarily. Previously, osteocutaneous iliac crest free flaps included harvesting a cuff of external oblique muscle, internal oblique muscle, and transversalis fascia with the skin paddle, but in recent years perforator dissection has been more commonly performed, resulting in a less bulky soft tissue component **(Fig. 3.2)**.[8] Even when the skin island is dissected as a perforator flap without a muscular component, iliac crest osteocutaneous free flaps may be excessively bulky in some patients and can require substantial primary or later revisionary thinning, or use of a second, thinner flap for soft tissue reconstruction. Alternatively, a separate internal oblique muscle paddle, based on the ascending branch of the deep circumflex iliac artery, which arises within 1 cm of the anterior superior iliac spine, can also be harvested for reconstruction of composite defects requiring a thin layer of soft tissue coverage.

The donor site, while hidden in clothing, may result in a contour deformity and/or hernia, a complication that may be ameliorated by careful closure techniques and harvest as a split flap. Gait abnormalities have also been reported not infrequently. Harvesting the bone flap as a split-cortical flap decreases the morbidity of the flap by preserving hip contour, minimizing gait disturbances, and providing better support for the abdominal viscera, resulting in a decreased risk of hernia. Meticulous hemostasis and closed suction drainage of the donor site are recommended, because there is significant potential for donor-site hematomas and seromas. Due to the difficulty of flap dissection and the risk of postoperative donor-site hernias, this flap is relatively contraindicated in obese patients.

## Scapular Free Flap

Another alternative for mandibular reconstruction is the scapular free flap. The scapula flap has traditionally been based on the circumflex scapular artery. The length of the pedicle can be increased 4 to 5 cm by including the more proximal subscapular vessels, although this necessarily entails ligation and division of the thoracodorsal vessels that supply, in part, the latissimus dorsi and serratus anterior muscles. The subscapular vessels are also of larger caliber than the circumflex scapular vessels, which may be an advantage in performing the microvascular anastomosis.

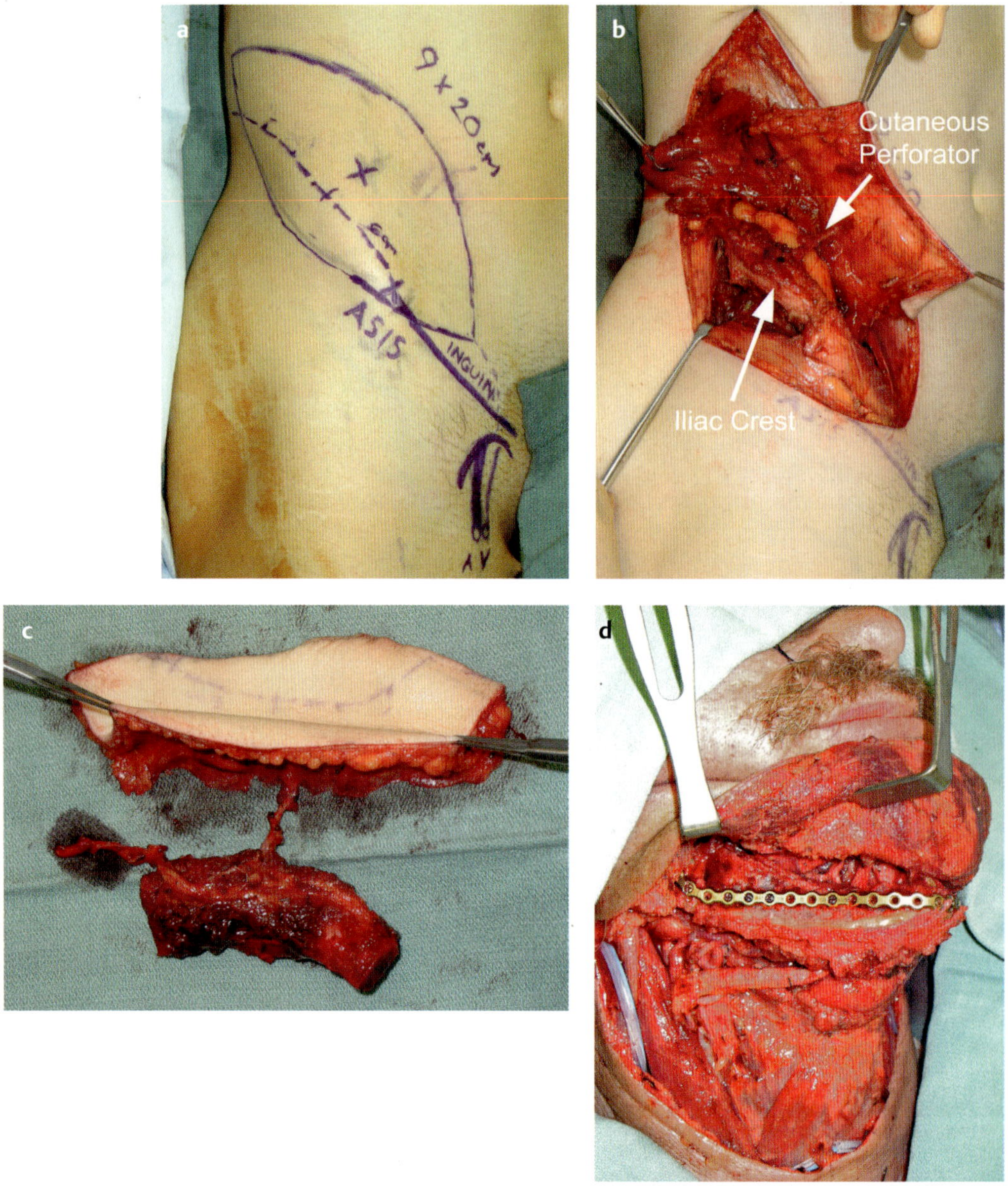


**Fig. 3.2** **(a)** Right hip skin marking for an iliac crest osteocutaneous free flap. The blood supply is the deep circumflex iliac artery. A cutaneous perforator was localized 6 cm from the anterior superior iliac spine (ASIS) and marked with an "X." **(b)** The skin paddle has been elevated and the iliac crest is visible. **(c)** Completed free flap harvest. **(d)** The curved shape of the iliac crest makes it well suited to hemimandibular reconstruction.

The bone may be harvested from either the lateral or the medial edge of the scapula. The lateral scapular bone flap, based on the vertically oriented parascapular branch of the circumflex scapular artery, has the shorter vascular pedicle but is thicker, which is particularly important if osseointegrated implant placement is to be attempted. The medial scapular bone flap, based on the horizontally oriented cutaneous scapular branch of the circumflex scapular artery, is thinner but is associated with a longer pedicle and minimal disturbance of the teres major and minor muscles and the glenohumeral joint, resulting in less postoperative shoulder stiffness. Approximately 10 to 14 cm of linear bone may be harvested from either the lateral or the medial aspect of the scapula.

If needed, a skin paddle, based on a cutaneous branch of the circumflex scapular artery, can be harvested with the osseous portion of the flap. For larger defects, a chimeric flap utilizing the subscapular regional blood supply can be harvested to include a scapular or parascapular skin paddle and the latissimus dorsi (with or without an overlying skin paddle) and serratus anterior muscles. The serratus anterior can be harvested with a rib to allow for a second bony reconstruction. Furthermore, a thoracodorsal artery perforator skin flap can also be harvested, rather than a latissimus dorsi muscle or myocutaneous flap along, with other flaps arising from the subscapular axis. The potential configurations are numerous.

Another variation of the scapular osseous flap involves utilizing the angular branch of the thoracodorsal artery.[9] This branch arises most commonly from the latissimus dorsi branch of the thoracodorsal artery and lies within the submuscular fat pad beneath the superior edge of the latissimus dorsi and teres major muscles. It enters the scapular bone near the inferior angle or tip of the scapula. We prefer to base our scapular flaps on this branch because it allows for a longer pedicle, up to 17 cm if dissected proximally to the axillary artery, and reliably supplies the medial, lateral, and angular portions of the scapular bone. We have used it in anterior mandibular reconstructions in patients who are not candidates for fibular free flap reconstruction (**Fig. 3.3**). In this case, the curved shape of the scapular tip nicely restores the shape of the anterior mandible without the need for osteotomies for shaping. However, a major disadvantage of the scapular bone, regard-

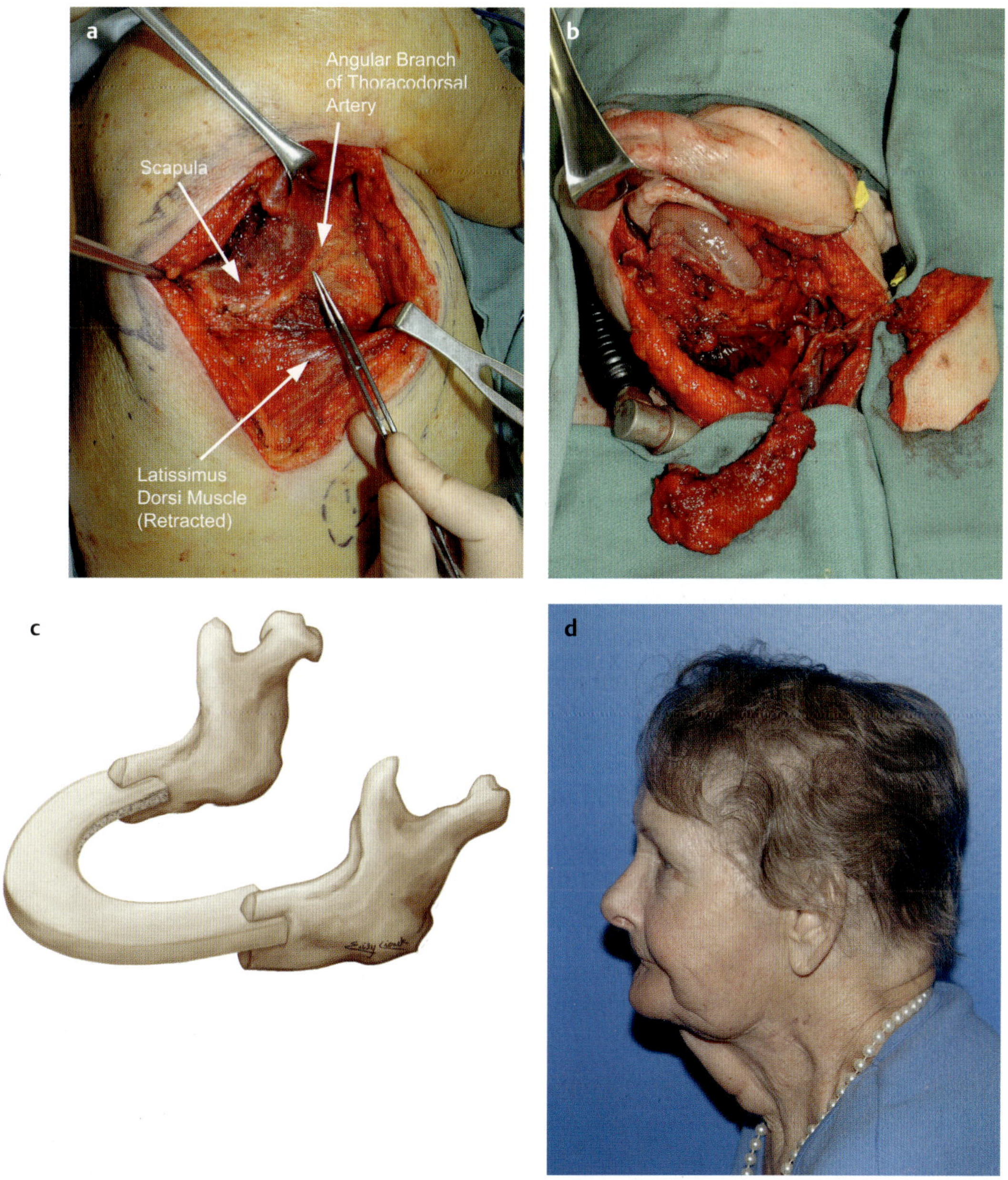


**Fig. 3.3** **(a)** Harvest of a chimeric "scapular tip" osseous free flap based on the angular branch of the thoracodorsal artery. The angular branch travels within a fat pad deep to the latissimus dorsi muscle and enters the scapula near its inferior angle (indicated by the forceps). **(b)** Insetting of a chimeric scapular tip and parascapular cutaneous free flap based on the subscapular artery. **(c)** Schematic explaining the inset of the scapular tip transversely to restore the anterior mandibular shape without the need for osteotomies. **(d)** Postoperative appearance showing good lower facial projection.

less of its pedicle blood supply, is that it is often quite thin and does not consistently provide enough bone stock for osseointegrated implant placement.

Although a potentially reliable donor site, the scapular flap requires careful planning for positioning of the patient during flap harvest, preparation of recipient vessels, microvascular anastomosis, and flap inset. The location of the scapula makes it very difficult to employ a two-team approach for harvesting the flap and preparation of the recipient site. Patients may note a degree of shoulder stiffness and limited abduction following the harvest of the scapula flap. Because of this, physiotherapy should routinely be part of the postoperative course.

### Radial Forearm Free Flap

For soft tissue reconstruction of the head and neck, the radial forearm fasciocutaneous free flap has a reliable, long (up to 20 cm) vascular pedicle. The flap is thin and pliable and can be made sensate by neurorrhaphy of the lateral antebrachial cutaneous nerve to the inferior alveolar nerve. This flap can also be designed as an osteocutaneous flap by inclusion of the anterior (volar) cortex of the radial bone. Up to 14 cm of unicortical radius nourished by periosteal branches from the radial artery may be harvested for selected osseous defects. However, the use of the osteocutaneous radial forearm free flap is typically not a first-line option due to the limited thickness of the bone that may be harvested without disturbing the structural mechanics of the hand and the risk for radial bone fracture in the forearm after harvest.

Patients should be selected based on physical exam of the upper extremity that includes palpation of the distal pulses and the Allen test. Radial artery dominance or equivocal examination of the dual perfusion of the hand should alert the reconstructive surgeon to proceed with caution in the radial forearm. Angiography may be considered to assess the patency of the palmar arch. If ulnar arterial perfusion appears adequate, the nondominant forearm is usually selected as the donor side.

From a third to a half of the radius may be harvested for limited bony defects. Care must be taken not to detach the flexor pollicis longus muscle attachment to the radius, although a portion of the muscle is included in the flap as a muscle cuff that contains the radial artery perforators nourishing the bone. The distal limit of the bony flap is the insertion of the brachioradialis tendon, and the proximal limit is the pronator teres muscle insertion. Osteotomies can be performed on the radial bone flap. Osseointegrated implant placement in the radial bone flap has been accomplished, but it is generally accepted that they are less reliable than those performed in the other bone flaps described in this chapter.

Donor-site morbidity after harvest of an osteocutaneous radial forearm free flap can be significant. Tendon rupture, carpal tunnel syndrome, and a significantly weak extremity have been reported.[10] Radial bone fracture is estimated to occur ~ 15% of the time. Some surgeons suggest prophylactic plating of the radius in the same setting as harvesting the flap. Nonetheless, the potential for chronic hand weakness or pain, coupled with the thinner donor bone stock of the radial forearm osteocutaneous flap, decreases enthusiasm for using this flap as a primary choice in reconstruction of load-bearing segmental mandibular defects, particularly in the anterior mandible.

## Reconstructive Algorithm

In choosing the appropriate reconstructive method, multiple factors must be taken into account, including the length and location of mandibular bone to be replaced, the amount of intraoral lining and type of soft tissue structures that have been resected, and whether or not there is an external skin defect present. Recipient vessel availability also needs to be taken into account. Medical comorbidities, a history of tobacco use, and prior irradiation may influence the type of reconstruction that is most appropriate. The availability and appropriateness of the various pedicled and free flaps described above must also be taken into account. Eliciting a history of prior surgery or trauma as well as preoperatively verifying the vascular status of the donor region are of paramount importance in avoiding donor-site complications.

Concerning the various types of flap choices for osseous mandibular reconstruction, each flap varies in terms of pedicle length, skin paddle, flap length, ability to accept osseointegrated implants, and patient morbidity. The iliac crest and fibular free flaps most reliably accept osseointegrated implants consistently due to their thickness.[11] The scapular free flap offers numerous soft tissue reconstruction options when harvested as part of a chimeric free flap with other skin and muscle components supplied by the subscapular arterial axis, and it may provide adequate bone stock for osseointegrated implants in select patients. The skin paddle of the radial forearm free flap is highly reliable and thin, making inset easier. In terms of vascular pedicle length, the radial osteocutaneous free flap has the longest available potential vascular pedicle. This option may be appealing in the patient with an absence of satisfactory local recipient vessels. However, this flap is limited by the very thin bone stock it provides and the risk for radial bone fracture at the donor site, as mentioned. The fibular free flap provides the longest amount of bone, has a good pedicle length and caliber, and, when dissected appropriately, has a reliable skin paddle. Based on its versatility, as well as acceptable donor-site morbidity, the fibular free flap is generally our preferred method of mandibular reconstruction for defects in which a vascularized bone flap is indicated, with other free flap choices being secondary and based on soft tissue needs, donor-site availability, risk for complications, and patient positioning.

The specific reconstructive technique chosen should also depend on the location of the mandibular defect. Although several defect classification systems have been described, we prefer to simplify the decision-making process by considering whether the mandibular defect is anterior, lateral, or posterior. Anterior defects involve the region of the parasymphysis and symphysis, anterior to the first bicuspid. Lateral defects occur posterior to the canine, encompassing some or all of the mandibular body, and extend to the angle of the mandible or the midramus but spare enough of the ramus and condyle to preserve joint movement and to allow for titanium plate fixation. Posterior defects involve the condyle and can be limited to the ramus or extend anteriorly to encompass the body up to the parasymphysis. Therefore, the presence of the condyle and upper ramus of the mandible differentiate lateral defects from posterior defects.

## ■ Reconstruction of the Anterior Mandible

The anterior mandible is frequently involved with floor of mouth and anterior tongue cancers, as well as occasionally with lower lip cancers by direct extension. As with all cancers possibly involving the mandible, a preoperative computed tomography (CT) scan is requisite, and evidence of cortical invasion is an indication that a segmental mandibulectomy will be required. Note that tumors that abut the mandible but do not invade the cortex are often treated with a marginal mandibulectomy (removal of the upper or lingual bony cortex of the mandible) and can usually be covered with a soft tissue pedicled or free flap alone.

Any defect that includes the anterior mandible should be reconstructed with vascularized bone whenever possible **(Fig. 3.4)**. Failure to reconstruct

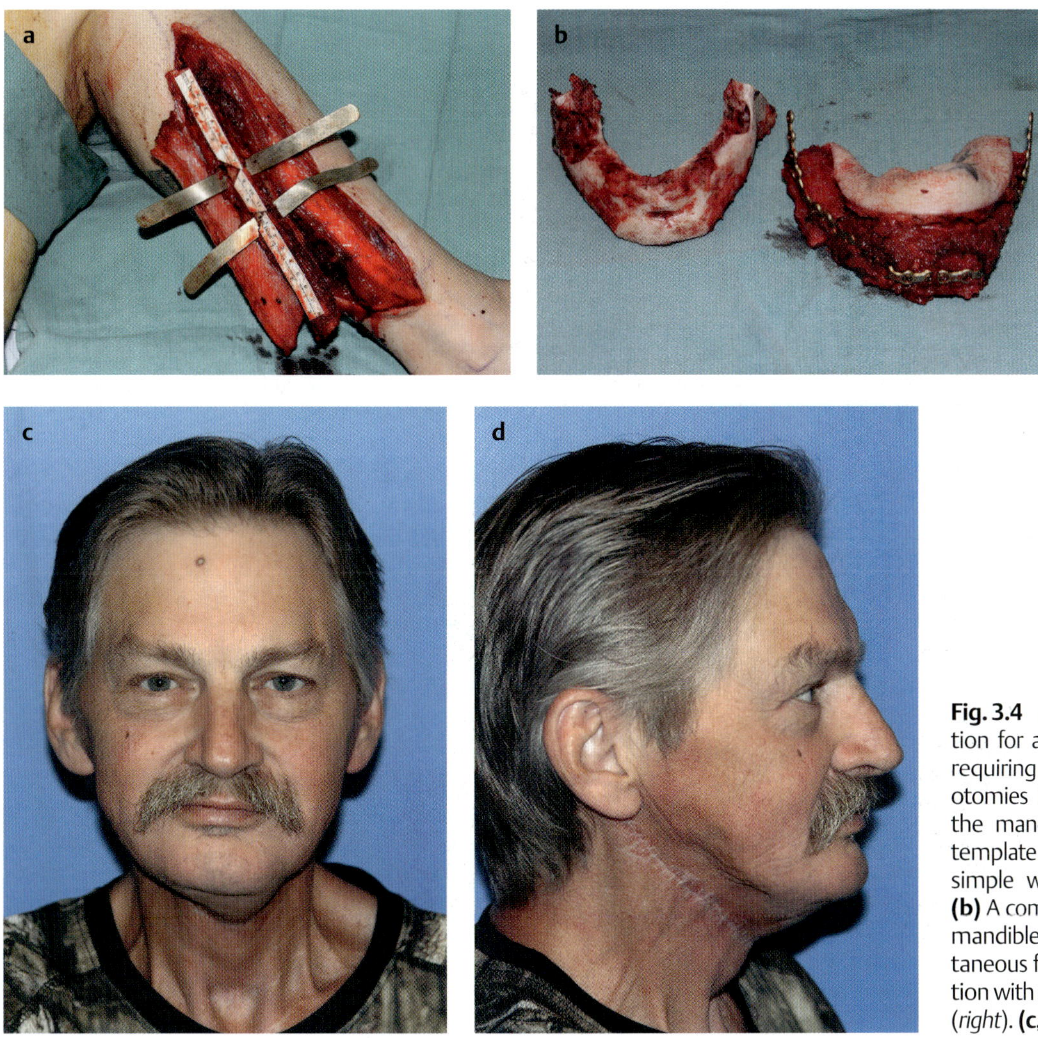

**Fig. 3.4** **(a)** Fibular free flap reconstruction for an anterior mandibular defect, requiring multiple wedge-shaped osteotomies to recreate the curvature of the mandible in this region. A paper template made from a sterile ruler is a simple way of planning osteotomies. **(b)** A comparison between the resected mandible (*left*) and the fibular osteocutaneous free flap after shaping and fixation with a titanium reconstruction plate (*right*). **(c,d)** Postoperative appearance.

the anterior mandible results in the so-called *Andy Gump deformity*, a condition that is disfiguring and may be functionally problematic in terms of mastication, pooling of saliva, and loss of oral competence and even airway support. It is the anterior mandible that forms a curve and provides projection to the lower face, and, therefore, bony reconstruction is required to maintain facial symmetry.

The linear bone of the fibula will require one or more wedge-shaped osteotomies to restore the curvature of the mandible. Whenever possible, we bend a 2.0 mm titanium reconstruction plate to the native mandible prior to the resection. We use the reconstruction plate as a guide for shaping the fibular free flap (or other bone flap). The simplest technique for planning the osteotomies is by cutting a paper or plastic template, such as a sterile paper ruler, to fit the shape of the titanium plate. More recently, computer-generated cutting guides have become available that facilitate making precise osteotomies at the angles dictated by the preoperative plan created using computer-aided design software (see Chapter 16, Robotic Reconstructive Surgery).

In the dentulous patient, mandibular height is greater in the anterior region than in the lateral mandible, averaging 33.5 mm in males and 31.1 mm in females.[12] By comparison, the width of the lateral surface of the fibula averages 17.9 mm in men and 13.1 mm in women, suggesting that a double-barrel configuration may be desirable in this region. In such cases, the lower "barrel" of the fibula should ideally project anteriorly several millimeters further than the upper "barrel" to maintain both chin projection and occlusion. If a single-barrel configuration is used, the fibula is inset so that it matches the occlusion of the maxilla. In edentulous patients, the mandible will tend to over-rotate and anterior projection can be substantially increased. In such cases, if there are no plans for dental restoration, the fibula will need to be set back considerably (1 to 2 cm or more) to limit mandibular excursion and to avoid the appearance of a severe underbite.

## ■ Reconstruction of the Posterior Mandible

Posterior mandibular resections may be required for the surgical treatment of many different types of cancer, including retromolar trigone cancers, tonsillar and lateral pharyngeal wall cancers, and base of tongue cancers. Several primary bone tumors that develop from impacted third molars can require resection of this part of the mandible as well. In some cases, large maxillary and soft palate cancers can extend inferiorly and involve the posterior mandible. Finally, deeply invasive skin cancers, parotid cancers, and temporal bone cancers can require removal of the posterior portion of the mandible, although, in such cases, there will not necessarily be a mucosal defect.

It is established that reconstruction with vascularized bone flaps is preferred for defects that include the anterior mandible, to minimize complications and to maximize oral function. Reconstruction of the posterior mandible, specifically in a mandible lacking sufficient condyle and subcondylar ramus to accommodate secure fixation with titanium hardware, is more controversial. Use of soft tissue alone, with reasonable results, has been reported.[13,14] In these reports, soft tissue free flaps, such as the anterolateral thigh (ALT) free flap and the rectus abdominis myocutaneous (RAM) free flap, were found to allow single-flap closure with adequate tissue bulk to replace the missing mandible and associated soft tissues as well as to provide a skin paddle to resurface the oral mucosal defect **(Fig. 3.5)**. Soft tissue reconstruction can result in acceptable cosmetic appearance and speech and swallowing function. Other advantages include potentially reduced operative time compared with bony flap harvest and shaping, faster recovery, and a low complication rate. Furthermore, in cases where the posterior mandible has been resected, bony reconstruction may not have significant advantages, because the ipsilateral masticatory musculature is generally not reconstructable, nor is there perfect replacement for the condylar joint (see below).

When soft tissue is used, the flap must be adequately bulky to prevent substantial deviation of the mandible toward the resected side. Anticipating soft tissue atrophy, greater in muscle than in fat and much greater when postoperative radiation is administered, some volume overcorrection is desirable. A pectoralis major myocutaneous pedicled flap may also give satisfactory results in posterior mandibular reconstruction. However, the pectoralis major myocutaneous pedicled flap can be limited in reach and arc of rotation for very high or posterior defects. Because later contracture of the pedicle may also cause a descent of the bulk of the flap toward the neck or result in contracture that limits neck mobility, we consider pectoralis major myocutaneous flaps a second choice to a bulky soft tissue free flap, such as the ALT or RAM free flaps. Whether bony or soft tissue reconstruction is utilized, there will be some risk for malocclusion due to loss of the condyle and temporomandibular joint disruption. Dentulous patients tend to experience fewer problems with malocclusion since they can use their remaining teeth to guide their jaws into the proper relationship.

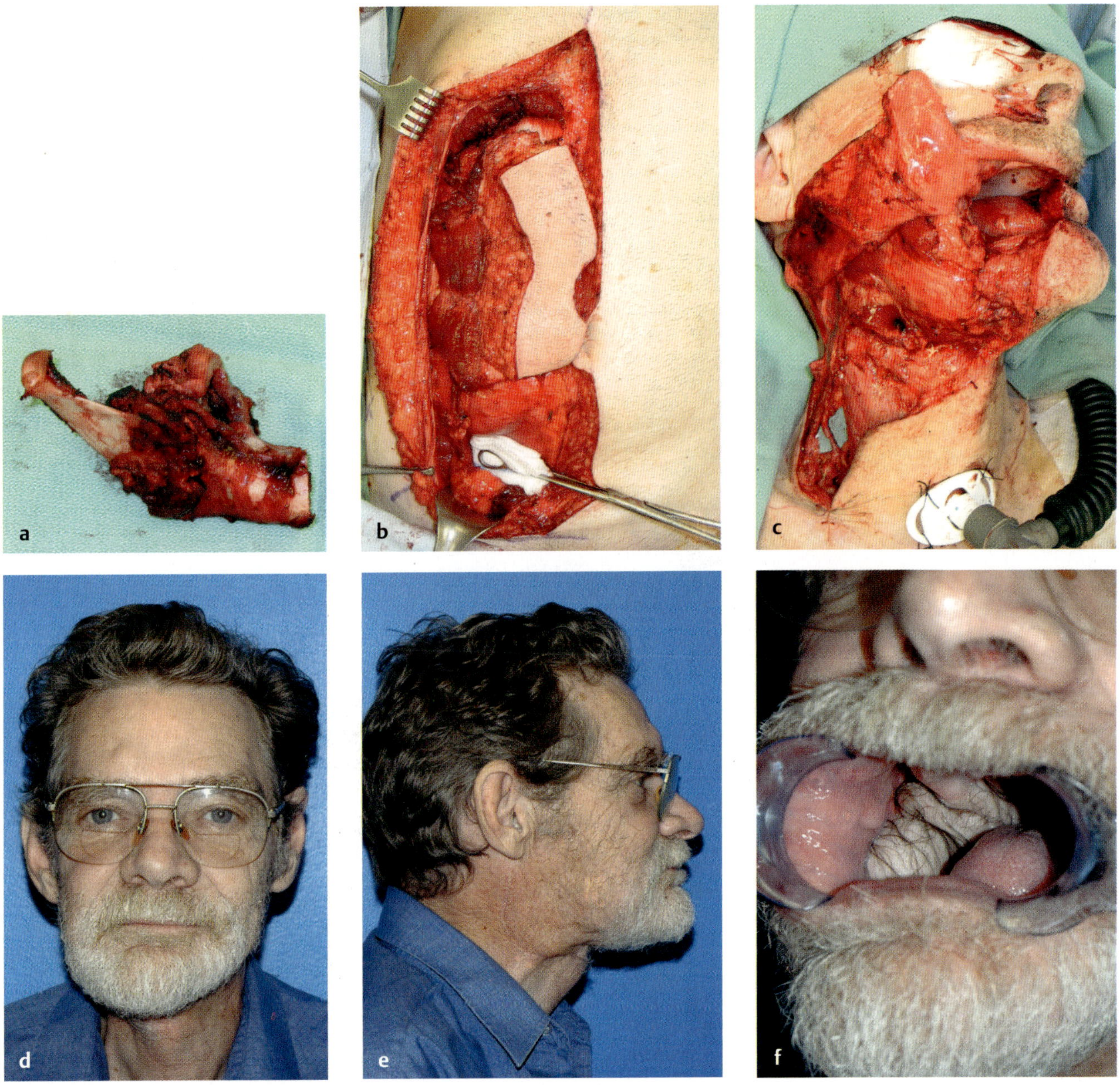


**Fig. 3.5** **(a)** Specimen from a posterior mandibular resection, including the mandibular condyle, ramus, and posterior body. **(b)** Harvest of a right vertical rectus abdominis myocutaneous (VRAM) free flap. **(c)** Inset of the VRAM free flap for reconstruction of the right posterior mandibular composite defect. The anastomoses have been performed to the transverse cervical artery and vein. **(d,e)** Postoperative appearance. The patient has some blunting of the mandibular angle but still has good facial symmetry. **(f)** Intraoral view showing a viable skin paddle and good mouth opening.

Although functional and cosmetic results for posterior mandibular reconstruction with soft tissue free flap can be achieved, we still prefer bony reconstruction for highly functional patients who are able to tolerate more extensive operations and bony free flap harvest (**Fig. 3.6**). In our experience, occlusion is usually, although not always, superior with bony reconstruction. As the defect extends more anteriorly, both the improved occlusion and cosmetic appearance (owing to maintaining a more well-defined jawline) favor bony reconstruction.

## ■ Condylar Reconstruction

The temporomandibular joint is a diarthrodial joint in which the condyle of the mandible is separated from the glenoid fossa of the temporal bone by a cartilaginous disk. Derangement of the joint or removal of the disk or condyle can lead to pain, instability, or trismus. Movement of the temporomandibular joint is complex and comprises both a rotational and a gliding process. Numerous methods of condylar

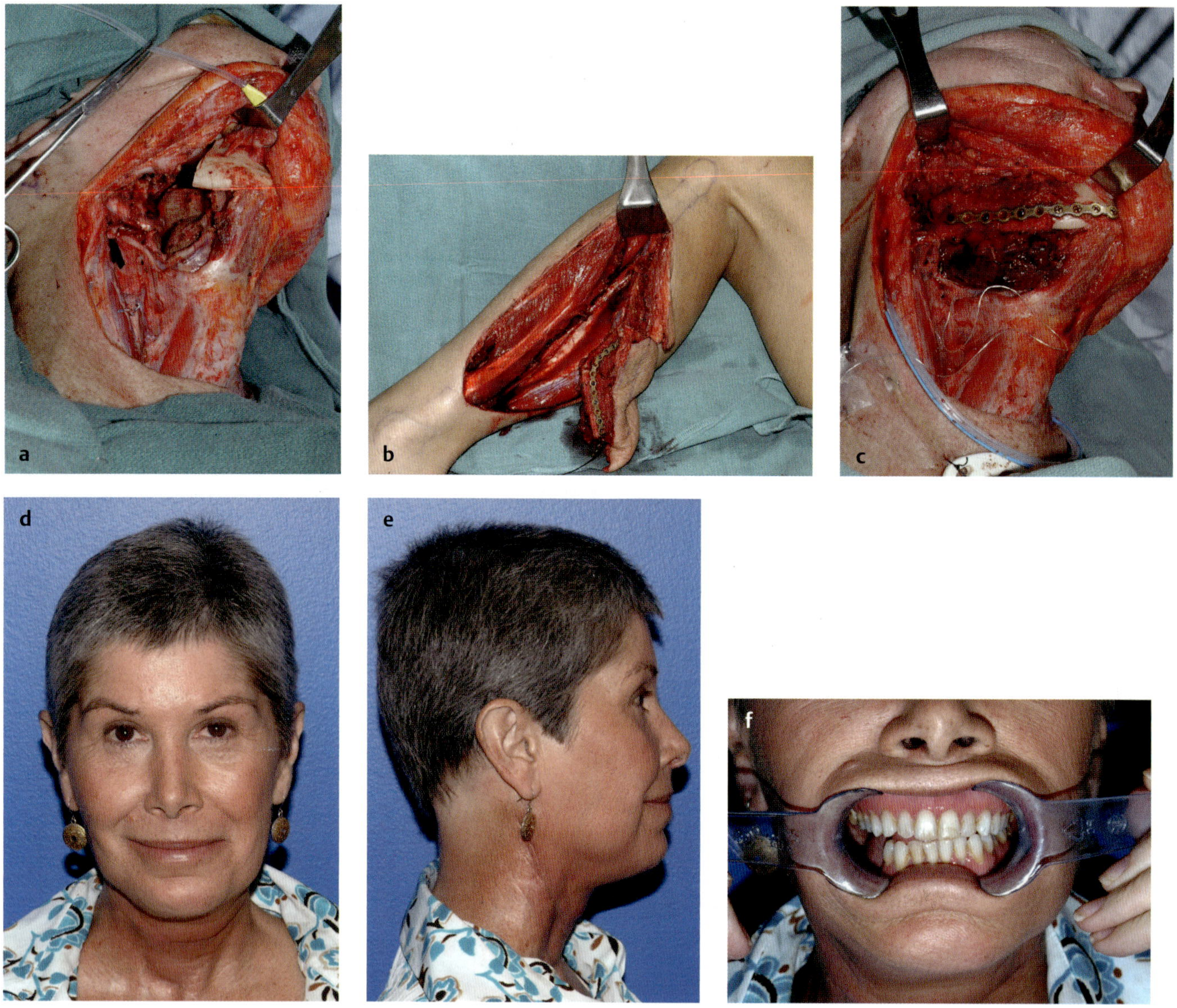

**Fig. 3.6** **(a)** A posterior mandibular defect similar to the one shown in **Fig. 3.5**. The condyle has been removed with the rest of the mandibular specimen and the muscles of mastication have been resected or detached. **(b)** This defect was reconstructed with a fibular osteocutaneous free flap harvested from the contralateral leg. **(c)** Flap inset. The rounded end of the fibular flap was suspended with nonabsorbable sutures to the remnants of the pterygoid muscle tendons. **(d,e)** Postoperative appearance. **(f)** Closed mouth view showing good occlusion.

and temporomandibular joint reconstruction have been described. Because of its complexity, no uniformly satisfactory technique has been found, and reconstruction of this region remains a subject of controversy.

Reconstruction of the rest of the mandible is addressed whenever appropriate with osseous or osteocutaneous free flap reconstruction, as described above. Tumors of the superior ramus rarely invade the temporomandibular joint, and if enough of the upper ramus can be spared, the optimal reconstruction is to fixate the bony free flap to the mandibular remnant. However, the superior cut in posterior segmental mandibulectomies often results in minimal subcondylar bone being left behind, making stable fixation with rigid titanium plates difficult or impossible. In many cases, the condyle is, therefore, completely removed. In addition, all masticatory muscles are detached from the mandible and the ligamentous support of the joint is disrupted.

Reconstruction of the condyle with titanium prostheses has been described. While some success has been noted, complications, including infection, plate fracture, extrusion, and erosion into the middle cranial fossa, are not uncommon. For this reason, such prostheses, even those with a silicone cap, have largely been abandoned in most centers. We avoid this technique in cancer patients, who are at elevated risk for complications, particularly because of the frequent need for radiation therapy.

Reconstruction with costal cartilage grafts has also been described. The costochondral graft appears to be most useful in isolated condylar defects, providing a soft articulating surface with the glenoid fossa. With a larger defect, as is the case in most oncologic resections, a nonvascularized cartilaginous graft lacks adequate length and stability and is prone to resorption, particularly in cases where postoperative radiation therapy is given.

Temporomandibular joint reconstruction with plating of the native condyle onto a vascularized bone flap as a graft has been described by Hidalgo.[15] In a series of 14 patients who underwent hemimandibular resection, the resected condyle was mounted on a free vascular bone flap as a nonvascularized graft. Some condylar resorption was noted in a few patients, but it did not correlate with a decrease in function. It was felt that use of the native condyle aided in accurate free bone flap placement. No tumor recurrences stemming from the transplanted condyle were observed. Wax et al[16] attempted this technique in two patients: one patient experienced displacement of the condyle out of the glenoid fossa and the second had poor cosmetic and functional outcomes. Experience with this procedure has not otherwise been described in the literature.

Replacement of the condyle with the fibular head or a contoured, rounded fibular end has also been used by several centers, including our own. A pseudoarthrosis is thought to form. The end of the bony flap can be anchored by a suture that extends from a hole drilled in the bone or the periosteum to the cut end of the pterygoid tendon or a second hole drilled into the lip of the glenoid fossa to minimize drift of the end of the bony flap out of the temporomandibular joint. The end of the fibular bone flap is rounded with a cutting bur and fits into the glenoid fossa, or the fibular head can be used, although harvesting the fibular head puts the common peroneal nerve at risk for inadvertent injury. The use of a rounded cut end of the fibula to replace the condyle has been our preferred technique for many years and functional results have been good, while avoiding erosion of the bone into the middle cranial fossa.

Whenever possible, it is recommended that the condylar region be addressed immediately rather than in a delayed secondary fashion. The facial nerve is at risk for injury in this region, particularly after scar tissue formation and contracture of the condylar space. Even when the nerve can be identified and protected, it can be compressed and compromised by insertion of a bone graft or flap secondarily.

## Reconstruction of Lateral Defects

Lateral mandibular defects usually arise from extension of lateral tongue and floor of mouth cancers, buccal cancers, and submandibular gland cancers. Osteoradionecrosis may also be an indication for lateral mandibular resection, since this region of the mandible frequently receives substantial radiation during the treatment of oropharyngeal cancers, while the condyle, ramus, and parasymphyseal regions are relative spared.

Missing lateral segments are usually bridged with bone **(Fig. 3.7)**. Bony reconstruction allows for very accurate results, including restoration of preoperative occlusion. Here, too, vascularized bone flaps are usually preferred, but nonvascularized bone grafts may be considered for very small defects in healthy wound beds that neither have been radiated nor are expected to be radiated postoperatively. Some surgeons feel that reconstruction plates can be used to bridge lateral defects, however, because there is a significant risk of plate fracture over time with this technique, as mentioned above, we avoid this method if at all possible. In general, reconstruction of such defects with bony free flaps is usually straightforward, as few if any osteotomies are required. Also, the height of the midpoint of the mandibular body averages only 25.7 mm in males and 24.5 mm in females, so double-barrel fibular reconstruction, which can be more time-consuming and complicated, is usually unnecessary.

In combined lateral and posterior defects (i.e., defects resulting from resection in which the condyle and subcondylar region cannot be spared and

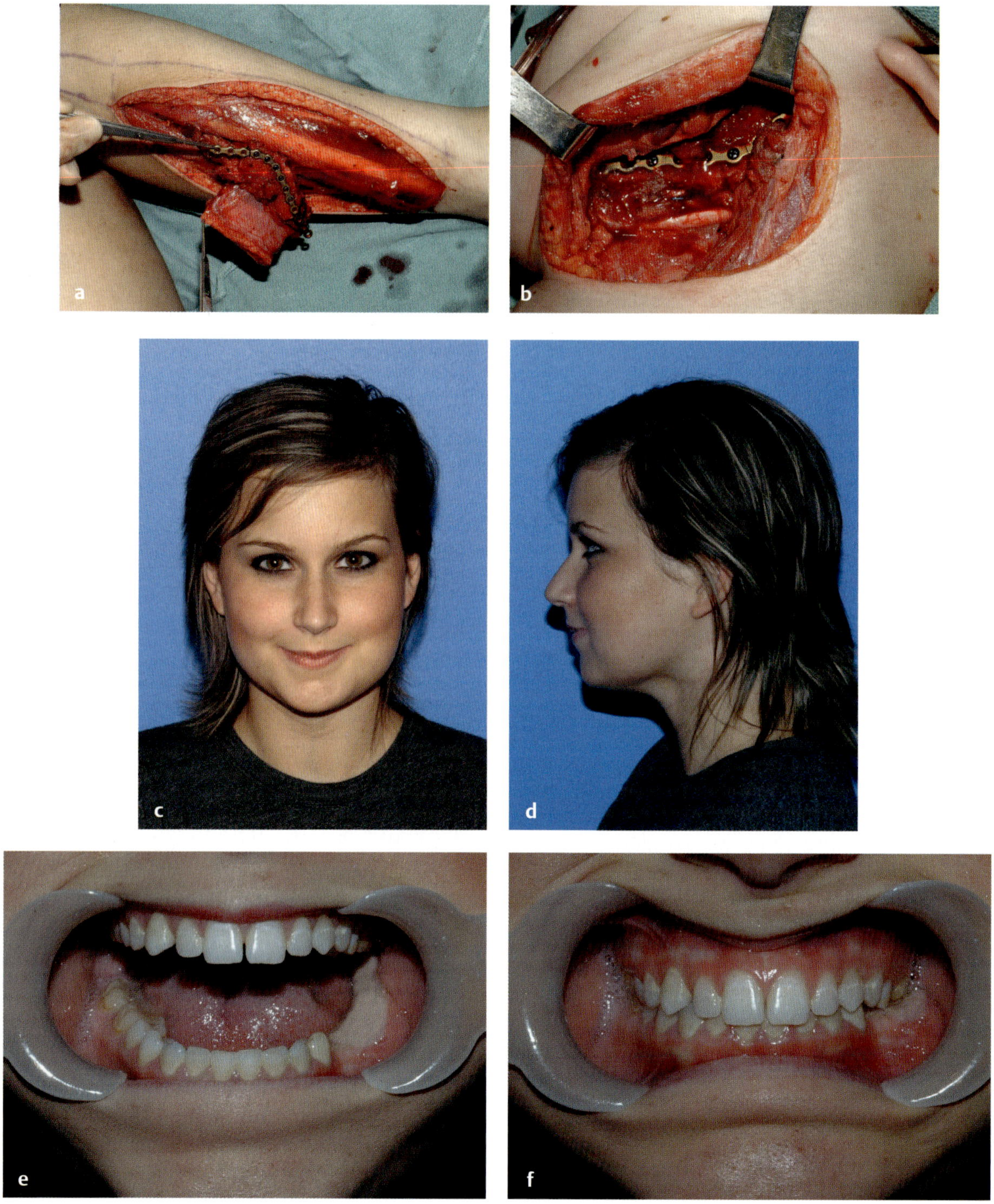

**Fig. 3.7** **(a)** Harvest of a right fibular osteocutaneous free flap for a left lateral mandibular defect, extending from the midramus to the midbody of the mandible. **(b)** The bony defect is "bridged" by the fibula. **(c,d)** Postoperative appearance. **(e,f)** Open and closed mouth views demonstrating excellent occlusion.

that also extend anteriorly to involve the mandibular body), as well as in patients who are not good candidates for bony free flap reconstruction, soft tissue reconstruction can be performed. If lateral segments are not reconstructed with bone, we recommend removing the posterior mandibular segment bearing the condyle to prevent eventual erosion of the bone medially into the oral cavity. In many cases, satisfactory functional and aesthetic results can be achieved with a pedicled or free soft tissue flap for lateral and posterolateral defects, just as in purely posterior defects as described above. The more anteriorly the defect extends, however, the more noticeable a contour deformity will be due to the absence of the lower mandibular bony margin and, often, a visible "step-off" where the native mandible ends. Additionally, the more anterior the defect extends, the greater the potential for malocclusion as the mandible rotates toward the side of the defect due to the pull of the contralateral pterygoid muscles. Our reconstructive algorithm is summarized in **Fig. 3.8**.

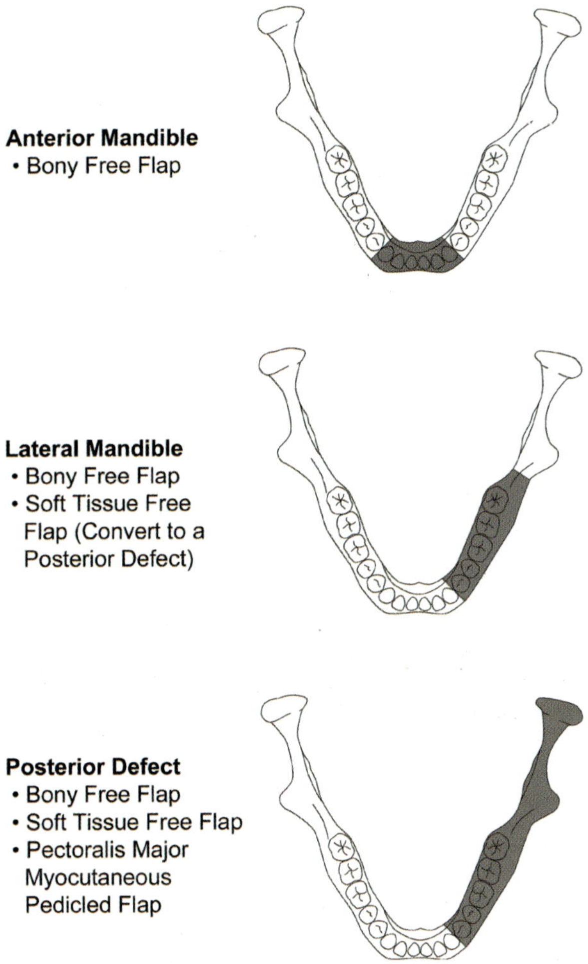


**Fig. 3.8** Algorithm for mandibular reconstruction with pedicled and free flaps. Flap options are listed from most to least favorable in terms of typical functional and aesthetic outcome, but flap selection must also take into account the patient's medical condition, oncologic prognosis, functional prognosis, and donor-site morbidity.

## Defects Requiring More Than One Free Flap

In cases of very large defects involving intraoral, osseous, and external components, reconstruction may not be achievable with a single free flap. In other cases, wound closure may be possible but functionally and aesthetically suboptimal.[17,18] In selected cases, head and neck reconstruction may require a second microvascular free flap or regional pedicled flap. Such reconstructions may be limited by the availability of recipient blood vessels. Strategies like the use of chimeric flaps (e.g., the scapular bone/latissimus dorsi muscle/serratus anterior muscle flap), vein grafting to more distant recipient vessels, such as the transverse cervical or contralateral neck vessels, and the piggy-backing technique, where one flap is anastomosed to the pedicle of another flap, may be required (see chapter on recipient blood vessel dissection and selection).

One commonly used combination is the use of a soft tissue skin or myocutaneous flap for intraoral reconstruction, such as when there is a substantial glossectomy defect, and a bony flap, such as the fibula, to restore the mandible. A thin, pliable flap, such as the radial forearm flap, is recommended for reconstruction of a hemiglossectomy defect, while a bulkier ALT or RAM free flap is recommended for near-total or total glossectomy defects. While the use of a large skin paddle from a single fibular osteocutaneous free flap may close the oral wound, to optimize the functional outcome, a two-flap procedure is advocated to maintain tongue mobility in patients who can tolerate an extended surgery and have a reasonable oncologic prognosis.

When there is a through-and-through defect, an osteocutaneous bone flap is usually used, with its skin paddle providing the intraoral lining and a soft tissue free flap providing the external coverage. Another option is the use of a chimeric osteocutaneous scapular–latissimus dorsi (or thoracodorsal artery perforator) free flap or two-skin-paddle fibular osteocutaneous free flap (when more than one set of cutaneous perforating blood vessels is present). The pectoralis major myocutaneous pedicled flap may also be used to reconstruct the external cheek defect, although we generally reserve this flap as a "lifeboat" in case of complications, such as a flap loss or fistula.

Occasionally, a maxillary and mandibular defect is encountered and may be another indication for a two-free-flap reconstruction **(Fig. 3.9)**. In such cases,

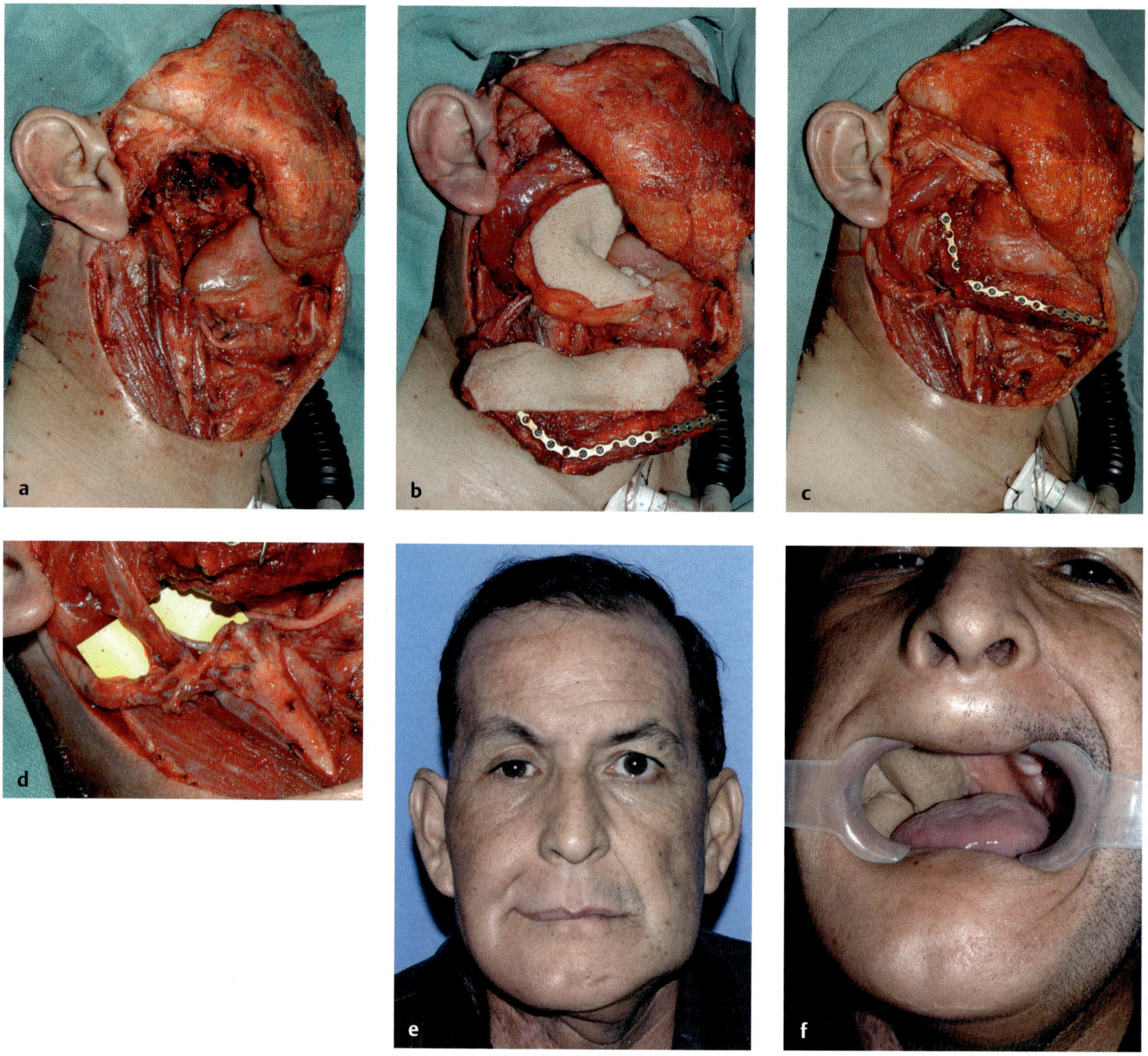


**Fig. 3.9** **(a)** Intraoperative photograph showing reconstruction of a large surgical defect encompassing the right mandible, buccal mucosa, and right maxilla, including half of the hard palate. **(b,c)** A left fibular osseocutaneous free flap was used to reconstruct a right hemimandibular defect that begins at the symphysis and includes the right condyle. An anterolateral thigh myocutaneous free flap has been used to reconstruct the buccal mucosa and right palate. Vastus lateralis muscle is included to provide additional bulk for this reconstruction. Note that the right facial nerve was also sacrificed and tensor fasciae lata static sling is also visible. **(d)** Multiple microvascular anastomoses involving the facial artery, external carotid artery, facial vein, and internal jugular vein on the right side of the neck. **(e)** Postoperative appearance following free flap reconstruction, fascial sling for static facial support, upper eyelid gold weight placement, direct browlift, and lateral canthoplasty. **(f)** Intraoral view showing a viable skin flap and good mouth opening.

a myocutaneous ALT or rectus abdominis flap is used for unilateral maxillary and buccal reconstruction, and a fibular osteocutaneous free flap is used for mandibular reconstruction. However, limited mandibular defects combined with palatomaxillary defects can often be addressed with a single large ALT or RAM free flap when the mandibular defect does not involve the anterior mandible, such as might arise from resection of a retromolar trigone tumor that extends superiorly or a posterior palatal tumor that extends inferiorly.

## Osseointegrated Implants

Dental rehabilitation may be achieved by the use of fixed or removable prostheses that are retained or supported by osseointegrated dental implants. The safety and efficacy of this technique have been demonstrated in the noncancer edentulous population. Use of osseointegrated dental implants is predicated on having adequate bone stock and a well-vascularized recipient tissue bed with stable soft tissue coverage. Insertion of osseointegrated implants into the remaining edentulous native mandible or free vascularized bone flaps has been very successful in carefully selected patients.[19,20] The implants must be surrounded by a minimum of 1 mm of healthy bone. The fibula and iliac crest most reliably offer sufficient bone stock for successful osseointegration, while the scapula and radial forearm do so less reliably. Implant failure is also typically associated with patients who smoke, have had radiation therapy, or who have poor oral hygiene with dental infections.

The choice of timing for placement of osseointegrated implants, either primarily at the time of microvascular free bone flap reconstruction or secondarily after initial healing has been completed, depends on several factors, including whether the resected lesion was benign or malignant, status of adjacent skin and soft tissues, plans for postoperative radiation, and patient motivation. Some authors regard radiotherapy to the host bone as a contraindication to implant placement. Urken et al[20] reported a 92% success rate of endosteal dental implants in vascularized mandibular reconstructions. The rate of implant success when implants were irradiated postoperatively was 86%; implants placed into previously irradiated bone had a 64% success rate. Others have placed implants in irradiated tissues after treatment with hyperbaric oxygen therapy. Still others have had acceptable results without hyperbaric oxygen; however, implant placement in the radiated patient population is regarded as controversial, particularly since there are risks of implant loss, pathological fracture, and osteoradionecrosis. Other issues that are debated include whether implants should be placed prior to or after radiation therapy, the maximum radiation dose associated with acceptable risk for implant placement, and the length of time that should elapse after radiation treatment prior to implant placement in delayed cases.

It should be noted that dental restoration without adequate tongue and oropharyngeal mobility and muscular function needed for deglutition can result in a costly and time-consuming procedure and a disappointing outcome. In addition, the presence of trismus may limit implant placement or may render the patient unable to proceed to abutment and denture installation and therefore to mastication, thus making the implants nonfunctional. As mentioned previously, titanium screws used to secure reconstruction plate hardware may be a problem depending on their location and may need to be removed to accommodate placement of osseointegrated implants. Obviously this would be done only after satisfactory union of the bone flap to the native mandible and any associated osteotomies. One way of avoiding this problem is to place implants immediately at the time of reconstruction so that the plates and screws can be positioned in a way that allows placement of the implants. Immediate implant placement does, however, increase the time and complexity of what is usually already a long and complicated surgery.

## Complications

Specific to bony free flap mandibular reconstruction, malunions and nonunions are rare. If they occur, they can usually be treated with débridement of the bone edges and rigid fixation, provided the free flap remains viable. Fistulas can occur and should be treated promptly with irrigation and débridement if there is purulent fluid in the vicinity of the pedicle, anastomosis, or cervical recipient vessels to prevent thrombosis or vascular rupture.

## Postoperative Care

Patients routinely receive tracheostomy and nasogastric feeding tube placement at the time of surgery. They then receive tube feeds for 2 weeks, while intraoral incisions are allowed to heal. For uncomplicated intraoral defects, a pureed diet is allowed after 2 weeks if all incisions appear to have healed without a fistula. For more complex defects, including combined glossectomy and mandibulectomy defects, a modified barium swallow study is obtained to assess swallowing and to rule out a leak in areas that are not easily visualized by physical exam. Tracheostomy decannulation can usually be performed early, around postoperative day 5, when the immediate postoperative swelling has subsided.

We allow patients who undergo fibular free flap reconstruction to ambulate as early as postoperative day 2, even in a splint, with weight bearing as tolerated on the affected limb. When not ambulating, the patient is required to keep the donor limb elevated, whether in bed or in a chair, to facilitate skin graft healing. Further details involving fibular donor-site care are provided in a separate chapter.

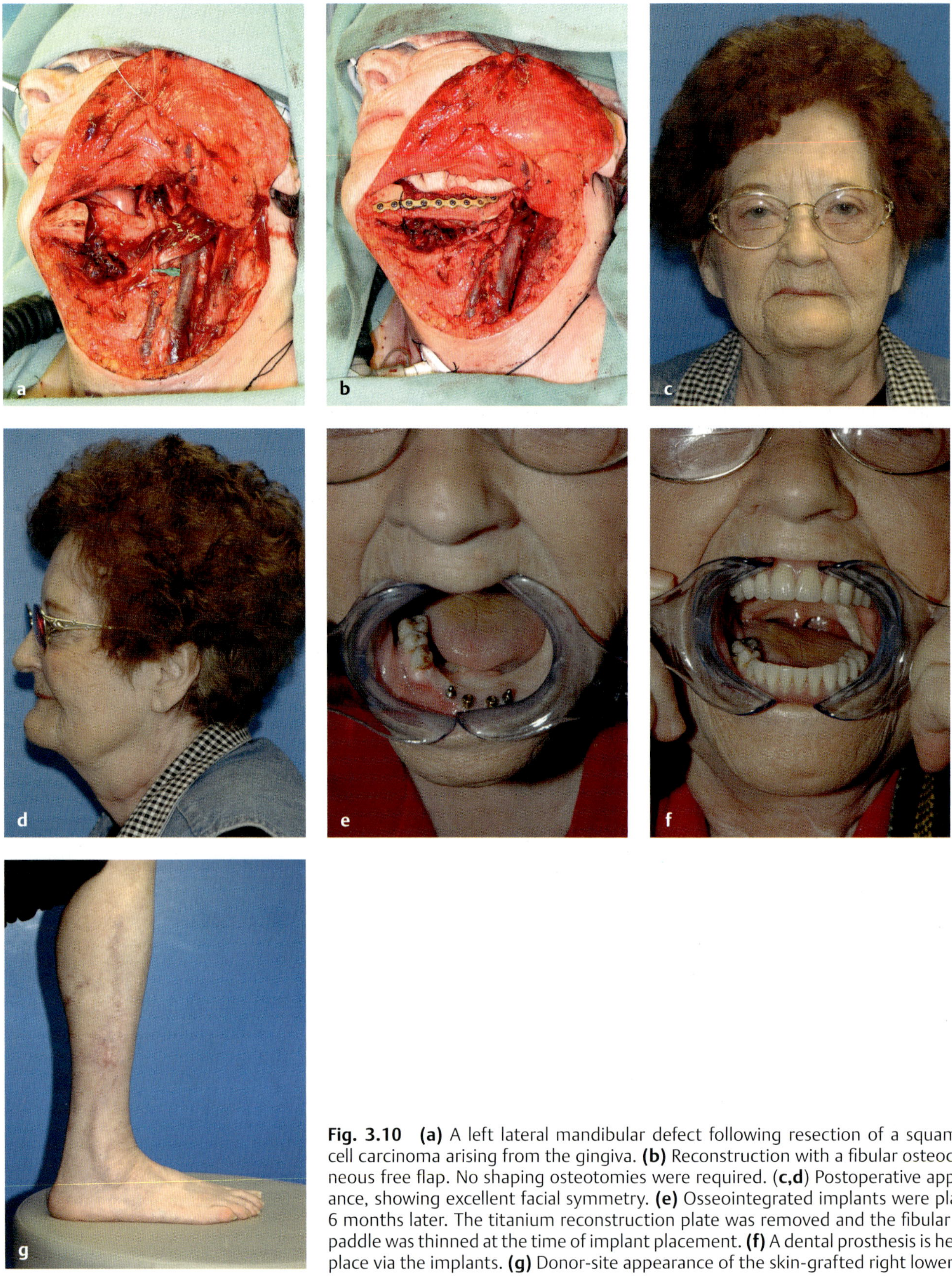


**Fig. 3.10** **(a)** A left lateral mandibular defect following resection of a squamous cell carcinoma arising from the gingiva. **(b)** Reconstruction with a fibular osteocutaneous free flap. No shaping osteotomies were required. **(c,d)** Postoperative appearance, showing excellent facial symmetry. **(e)** Osseointegrated implants were placed 6 months later. The titanium reconstruction plate was removed and the fibular skin paddle was thinned at the time of implant placement. **(f)** A dental prosthesis is held in place via the implants. **(g)** Donor-site appearance of the skin-grafted right lower leg.

## Case Example

A 71-year-old woman presented with a squamous cell carcinoma arising from the left lateral mandibular gingiva (**Fig. 3.10**). She underwent a segmental mandibulectomy of the lateral mandible. A fibular osteocutaneous free flap from the right leg was used to reconstruct the composite defect. The microvascular anastomoses were performed to the facial artery and facial vein. The skin paddle measured 5 cm wide and the donor site required a split-thickness skin graft for closure. Postoperative radiation therapy was not administered. Six months after her initial surgery, she underwent titanium plate and screw removal and thinning of her fibular skin paddle, with placement of titanium osseointegrated implants. Three months after implant placement, the implants were uncovered, and abutments were inserted into the implants after removal of cover screws. Within a week, a dental prosthesis was delivered, allowing her to achieve stable dental restoration. She has normal speech and is able to tolerate an unrestricted diet.

## Pearls and Pitfalls

- Single-stage microvascular free bone flap reconstruction is performed for segmental losses of the anterior mandible whenever possible.
- For anterior defects, the fibular osseous or osteocutaneous free flap is frequently the method of choice. The iliac crest and scapular free flaps are also reasonable secondary options.
- The choice of reconstructive technique for the posterior mandible and condylar region is controversial, and soft tissue reconstruction may be reasonable in many patients, reserving bony reconstruction for highly functional patients, because of the tendency for improved occlusal outcomes.
- Lateral defects should ideally be reconstructed with a vascularized bone flap, to maintain optimal occlusion and to allow the patient to tolerate high functional loads during mastication.
- Mandibular restoration with reconstruction plates alone or with soft tissue flaps, such as the pectoralis major myocutaneous pedicled flap, is associated with high rates of complications, particularly when used in anterior defects and in radiated tissues. Such reconstruction should be reserved for patients deemed to be unsuitable for microvascular free bone flap reconstruction.
- Consideration should be given to dental rehabilitation with dentures or osseointegrated implants, with early involvement of prosthodontists.
- Mandibulectomy-glossectomy defects, mandibulectomy with through-and-through cheek defects, and mandibulectomy-maxillectomy defects may all be indications for multiple free flap surgery.

## Expert Commentary *by Evan Matros and Joseph J. Disa*

The current chapter describes all of the important aspects of mandibular reconstruction to consider prior to proceeding with surgery. This commentary provides additional insights for the reader to contemplate.

The most commonly employed classification system for mandibular defects, the *HCL system*, was described by Boyd et al in 1992[21]: mandibular defects were divided into hemimandible (H), central (C), and lateral (L). Hemimandible defects did not significantly cross the dental midline and were distinguished from lateral defects by the inclusion of the condyle on the surgical specimen. Central defects included the central incisors and the canines. Combinations of defects could also be easily described with this nomenclature. For example, an angle-to-angle defect would be described as LCL. The epithelial status of the defect was also classified using lower-case letters, such as skin (s), mucosa (m), composite (sm), and other (o). While no classification system is perfect, a balance must be achieved between the simplicity of effective communication and permitting sufficient detail to describe the nature of the problem. The system described by Boyd is still relevant and widely used after over 30 years.

The balance between bone and soft tissue described in the current chapter should be underscored. Young surgeons may incorrectly assume that all mandibular resection needs to be reconstructed with osseous flaps. However, the method of reconstruction must be evaluated on an individual basis, depending upon the extent of bone versus soft tissue resection. When the soft tissue defect increases, the fibular skin island is increasingly unlikely to resurface large areas, simultaneously eliminate dead space, and prevent fistula formation. For anterior or central defects, rigidity provided by bone is essential. However, for more posterior defects, more consideration needs to be given to soft tissue flaps, including the pectoralis flaps.[13,14] Disadvantages associated with soft tissue reconstruction are highlighted in the current chapter and often include absence of bone for placement of dental implants, development of crossbite with malocclusion, and minor cosmetic changes. Soft tissue flaps should also be considered for patients who have advanced disease and a limited lifespan, for those with multiple medical comorbidities, and for the very elderly.

While the fibular flap has become the gold standard for osseous mandibular reconstruction, and is employed in the vast majority of cases, there is considerable variation in more subtle aspects of the operation. This includes which leg to use for the fibular flap, the method of bony fixation, and reconstruction of the temporomandibular joint.

Although either the ipsilateral or contralateral leg can reliably be used for reconstruction, we prefer to use the ipsilateral leg.[22] The principal benefit is that the septum, which is based at the posterior border of the bone, is rotated up and over the buccal surface plates used for rigid fixation. This enables all of the hardware to be covered by the vascularized soft tissue of the septum, with the intent of reducing plate exposure and infection. When the contralateral leg is used, the septum emanates from the lingual aspect of the construct, with exposed hardware immediately beneath the final cheek flap and skin island closure. Negative aspects of the ipsilateral leg approach include the unpredictable length and excursion of the septum about the fibula bone, creating potential problems for the soft tissue island to reach the retromolar region. For large defects that approach the maxillary tuberosity, the contralateral leg is often chosen since in the theory there is greater arc of rotation by the septum because of its lingual positioning. Other indications for using the contralateral leg include when recipient vessels are intended to be used in the contralateral neck for patients who have had prior ipsilateral neck surgery or radiation. In such instances, the contralateral leg is used with the pedicle emanating from the mesial aspect of the flap, instead of distally toward the mandibular angle. In this scenario, the septum is still oriented on the posterior aspect of the bone to cover the hardware.

Rigid fixation of the neomandible construct can be reliably achieved with either titanium mini-plates or reconstruction plates. Each approach has advantages. Mini-plates are often less obvious below the overlying skin envelope, especially in attenuated radiated skin **(Fig. 3.11)**. Other advantages include the ease of individual plate removal for infection, loose hardware, or placement of osseointegrated dental implants.[23] With large reconstruction plates, the entire neck needs to be re-explored to accomplish removal. Another advantage of mini-plates is the superior adaptation between the hardware and bone flap, with minimal intervening dead space. The thinness of mini-plates allows for more precise contouring to the parabolic shape of the neomandible construct. Mini-plates have locking screw holes as well. The main advantage of reconstruction bars is their large size, which can tolerate greater loads.

The chapter outlines a variety of methods for condylar reconstruction. As described by Hidalgo, replacement of the native condyle is the preferred method at our center.[24] Marrow from the cut edge of the mandible is sent for frozen evaluation intraoperatively by pathology. In absence of abnormality, it is plated to the neomandible construct. Although there are limited publications describing experience with auto-condyle transplantation, it has been used for many years without notable complication rates. For patients with osteoradionecrosis, consideration has to be given to potential radiation effects in the condyle replacement as well. When the condyle cannot be replaced, the fibula can be wrapped with soft tissue and secured with a suture to the condylar fossa to minimize risk of dislocation. Alternatively, the fibula can be left short, approximately at the level of the sigmoid notch, to allow unimpeded excursion.

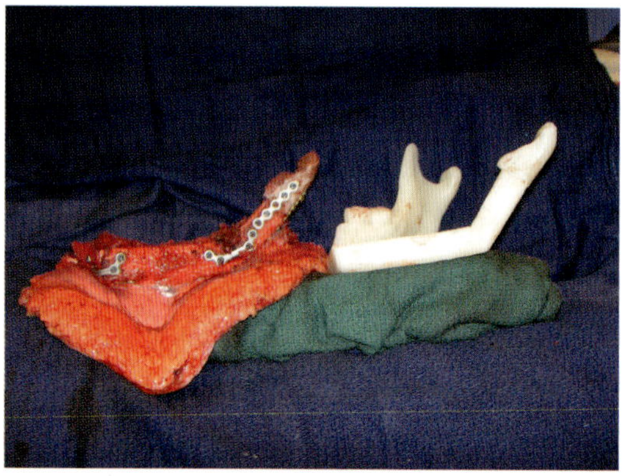

**Fig. 3.11** Hemimandibular reconstruction performed using CAD CAM and three-dimensional (3D) printing. When mini-plate fixation is performed, plates are placed on both the buccal surface and inferior border of the neomandible construct. Auto condyle transplant is completed after frozen-section pathologic evaluation.

## References


1. Wei FC, Celik N, Yang WG, Chen IH, Chang YM, Chen HC. Complications after reconstruction by plate and soft-tissue free flap in composite mandibular defects and secondary salvage reconstruction with osteocutaneous flap. Plast Reconstr Surg 2003;112(1):37–42
2. Mariani PB, Kowalski LP, Magrin J. Reconstruction of large defects postmandibulectomy for oral cancer using plates and myocutaneous flaps: a long-term follow-up. Int J Oral Maxillofac Surg 2006;35(5):427–432
3. Robertson GA. A comparison between sternum and rib in osteomyocutaneous reconstruction of major mandibular defects. Ann Plast Surg 1986;17(5):421–433
4. Hidalgo DA. Fibula free flap: a new method of mandible reconstruction. Plast Reconstr Surg 1989;84(1):71–79
5. Cordeiro PG, Disa JJ, Hidalgo DA, Hu QY. Reconstruction of the mandible with osseous free flaps: a 10-year experience with 150 consecutive patients. Plast Reconstr Surg 1999;104(5):1314–1320
6. Chang YM, Wallace CG, Tsai CY, Shen YF, Hsu YM, Wei FC. Dental implant outcome after primary implantation into double-barreled fibula osteoseptocutaneous free flap-reconstructed mandible. Plast Reconstr Surg 2011;128(6):1220–1228
7. Hanasono MM, Skoracki RJ. Computer-assisted design and rapid prototype modeling in microvascular mandible reconstruction. Laryngoscope 2013;123(3):597–604
8. Safak T, Klebuc MJ, Mavili E, Shenaq SM. A new design of the iliac crest microsurgical free flap without including the "obligatory" muscle cuff. Plast Reconstr Surg 1997;100(7):1703–1709
9. Hanasono MM, Skoracki RJ. The scapular tip osseous free flap as an alternative for anterior mandibular reconstruction. Plast Reconstr Surg 2010;125(4):164e–166e
10. Thoma A, Khadaroo R, Grigenas O, et al. Oromandibular reconstruction with the radial-forearm osteocutaneous flap: experience with 60 consecutive cases. Plast Reconstr Surg 1999;104(2):368–378, discussion 379–380
11. Disa JJ, Hidalgo DA, Cordeiro PG, Winters RM, Thaler H. Evaluation of bone height in osseous free flap mandible reconstruction: an indirect measure of bone mass. Plast Reconstr Surg 1999;103(5):1371–1377
12. Chang EI, Clemens MW, Garvey PB, Skoracki RJ, Hanasono MM. Cephalometric analysis for microvascular head and neck reconstruction. Head Neck 2012;34(11):1607–1614
13. Mosahebi A, Chaudhry A, McCarthy CM, et al. Reconstruction of extensive composite posterolateral mandibular defects using nonosseous free tissue transfer. Plast Reconstr Surg 2009;124(5):1571–1577
14. Hanasono MM, Zevallos JP, Skoracki RJ, Yu P. A prospective analysis of bony versus soft-tissue reconstruction for posterior mandibular defects. Plast Reconstr Surg 2010;125(5):1413–1421
15. Hidalgo DA. Condyle transplantation in free flap mandible reconstruction. Plast Reconstr Surg 1994;93(4):770–781, discussion 782–783
16. Wax MK, Winslow CP, Hansen J, et al. A retrospective analysis of temporomandibular joint reconstruction with free fibula microvascular flap. Laryngoscope 2000;110(6):977–981
17. Wei FC, Demirkan F, Chen HC, Chen IH. Double free flaps in reconstruction of extensive composite mandibular defects in head and neck cancer. Plast Reconstr Surg 1999; 107(1):39–47
18. Hanasono MM, Weinstock YE, Yu P. Reconstruction of extensive head and neck defects with multiple simultaneous free flaps. Plast Reconstr Surg 2008;122(6):1739–1746
19. Chang YM, Santamaria E, Wei FC, et al. Primary insertion of osseointegrated dental implants into fibula osteoseptocutaneous free flap for mandible reconstruction. Plast Reconstr Surg 1998;102(3):680–688
20. Urken ML, Buchbinder D, Weinberg H, Vickery C, Sheiner A, Biller HF. Primary placement of osseointegrated implants in microvascular mandibular reconstruction. Otolaryngol Head Neck Surg 1989;101(1):56–73
21. Boyd JB, Gullane PJ, Rotstein LE, Brown DH, Irish JC. Classification of mandibular defects. Plast Reconstr Surg 1993;92(7):1266–1275
22. Matros E, Schwarz GS, Mehrara BJ, Hu QY, Cordeiro PG, Disa JJ. Indications and outcomes for mandibular reconstruction using sequential bilateral fibula flaps. Plast Reconstr Surg 2010;126(5):1539–1547
23. Cordeiro PG, Hidalgo DA. Conceptual considerations in mandibular reconstruction. Clin Plast Surg 1995;22(1):61–69
24. Hidalgo DA. Condyle transplantation in free flap mandible reconstruction. Plast Reconstr Surg 1994;93(4):770–781, discussion 782–783

# 4 Pharyngoesophageal Reconstruction

*Peirong Yu*

## Introduction

Pharyngoesophageal defects are most commonly the result of a total laryngopharyngectomy for squamous cell carcinoma in the laryngeal region or hypopharynx. Other etiologies include benign strictures, pharyngocutaneous fistulas, and thyroid cancer involving the esophagus. Since radiotherapy has become the primary treatment for early stages of squamous cell carcinoma in these regions, many pharyngoesophageal defects are the results of salvage laryngopharyngectomy after radiation failure, making reconstruction more challenging. Therefore, great care should be taken to carefully plan the surgery with more than one feasible option. One important aspect of surgical planning is to convert a complicated case into a more conventional or simple one to minimize surgical risks and to maximize functional outcomes. Pharyngoesophageal reconstruction requires great attention to detail, and there is no room for error. The ultimate goals of reconstruction are to provide alimentary continuity, to protect important structures, such as the carotid artery, and to restore functions like speech and swallowing. Providing coverage alone is not adequate.

Early attempts at reconstruction using local and regional flaps, such as the Wookey flap and its variations[1,2,3] and the deltopectoral flap,[4] were largely unsuccessful because of the high incidence of partial flap necrosis, high fistula rates, and the need for multistage reconstruction. The gastric pull-up procedure was introduced in the mid-1900s for reconstruction of thoracic esophagectomy defects and was later used for pharyngoesophageal defects.[5,6,7,8,9,10,11,12,13] Subsequently, the pedicled colon and jejunum also became popular flaps for such reconstructions.[14,15,16] Although one-stage reconstruction could be accomplished with these techniques, removing the normal thoracic esophagus and using this technique only to reconstruct a pharyngeal and cervical esophageal defect are rather "inefficient" techniques with high surgical risks. Since the development of myocutaneous flaps and subsequently free flaps, these techniques have been largely abandoned for pharyngeal and cervical esophageal reconstruction.

## Regional Anatomy

The pharynx is anatomically divided into the oropharynx, nasopharynx, and hypopharynx **(Fig. 4.1)**. The nasopharynx essentially consists of the structures around the nasal cavity above the soft palate. The oropharynx is bounded by the nasopharynx superiorly, the oral cavity anteriorly, and the hypopharynx and larynx inferiorly. The superior border of the oropharynx is at the plane of the soft palate, and the inferior border is the level of the hyoid bone. The main structures in the oropharynx are the base of tongue, tonsillar pillars, lateral and posterior oropharyngeal walls, and soft palate. The hypopharynx extends from the level of the hyoid bone to the lower border of the cricoid cartilage, which is congruous with the cervical esophagus below. This is a critical area that is responsible for airway protection and swallowing and speech functions. Common defects of the hypopharynx and cervical esophagus are the result of surgical resection of cancers in the hypopharynx and larynx, advanced thyroid cancers, radiation strictures, and chemical injuries. Isolated tumors in the cervical esophagus, although rare, may also require segmental esophagectomy and reconstruction **(Table 4.1)**. Pharyngoesophageal defects can be circumferential or partial.

## Reconstructive Options

With advances in microsurgery, free flap reconstruction has largely replaced pedicled flaps for large head and neck oncologic defects, especially those

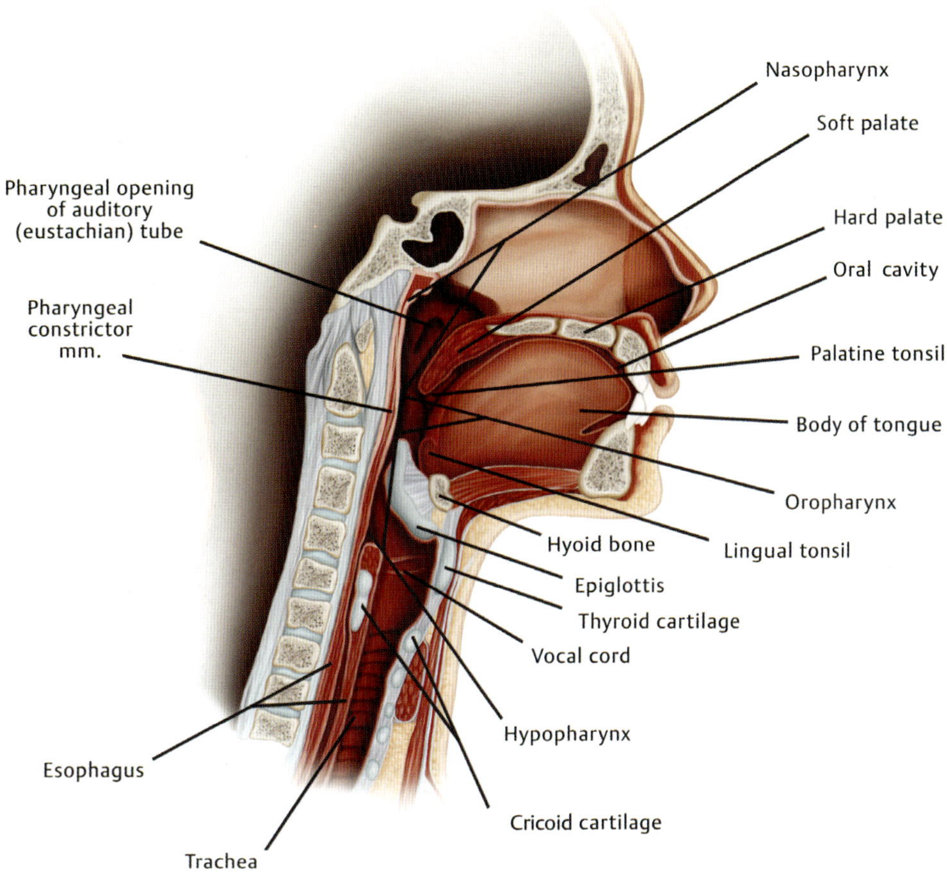


**Fig. 4.1** The hypopharynx is located behind the larynx and in continuity with the oral pharynx superiorly and the cervical esophagus inferiorly. Due to its proximity to the larynx, a total laryngectomy for cancers in this region often results in a partial or circumferential pharyngoesophageal defect requiring reconstruction.

**Table 4.1** Common pathologies causing pharyngoesophageal defects

| Pathology | Defect location | Type of defect |
|---|---|---|
| Primary SCC, advanced stage | Hypopharynx and cervical esophagus | Most commonly partial |
| Recurrent SCC after radiation failure | Hypopharynx and cervical esophagus | Most commonly circumferential |
| Advanced or recurrent thyroid cancer | Hypopharynx and cervical esophagus | Most commonly circumferential |
| Isolated esophageal tumors | Cervical esophagus with an intact larynx | Most commonly partial |
| Pharyngoesophageal or tracheoesophageal fistulas | Cervical esophagus or hypopharynx | Most commonly partial |
| Anastomotic strictures | Cervical esophagus | Most commonly circumferential |
| Radiation-induced strictures | Hypopharynx or cervical esophagus | Partial or circumferential, depending on the degree of stricture |

SCC, squamous cell carcinoma.

with prior radiotherapy, which renders pedicled flaps unreliable. Common free flap options include the anterolateral thigh (ALT) flap, the radial forearm flap, and the jejunal flap. Although reliable and easy to harvest, the radial forearm flap has a reputation for having high fistula rates, especially delayed fistulas. The forearm donor site, which requires a large area of skin grafting, can be conspicuous and incurs risks of partial skin graft loss, tendon exposure, tendon adhesions, and cold intolerance.[17,18,19,20] The jejunal flap proved reliable and became the flap of choice for circumferential pharyngoesophageal defects in the early 1990s.[21,22,23,24,25,26,27] It heals well, with low fistula rates. The major disadvantages are the added abdominal surgery and poor speech rehabilitation. The ALT flap has now been our flap of choice for pharyngoesophageal reconstruction for over a decade[28,29,30,31,32,33] due to its many advantages (**Table 4.2**). However, the ALT flap can be bulky in obese patients. The radial forearm flap is our second choice. The jejunal flap is also a good choice for circumferential defects in otherwise healthy patients with low surgical risks. In patients who have failed free flap reconstruction or are not free flap candidates, the supraclavicular flap, the pectoralis major flap, or the latissimus dorsi flap can be used for selected patients. An algorithm for pharyngoesophageal reconstruction is outlined in **Fig. 4.2**.

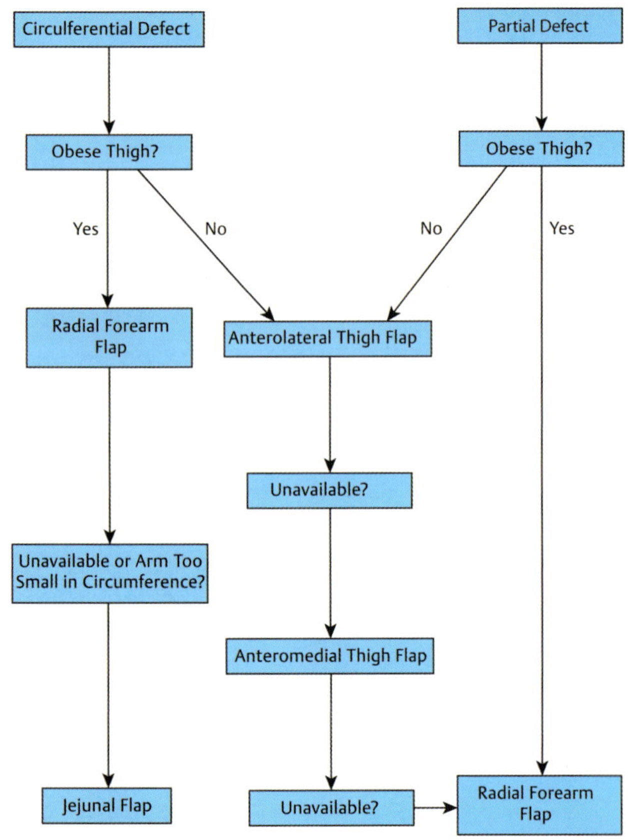


**Fig. 4.2** An algorithm for flap selection in pharyngoesophageal reconstruction.

**Table 4.2** Advantages and disadvantages of flaps commonly used for pharyngoesophageal reconstruction

| | ALT flap | Radial forearm flap | Jejunal flap |
|---|---|---|---|
| Flap elevation | Moderately difficult | Easy | Moderately difficult |
| Flap thickness | Can be too thick | Good | Good |
| Second fascial layer coverage | Yes | No | No |
| Inclusion of muscle | Yes | No | No |
| Primary healing | Good | Good | Best |
| Donor-site morbidity | Low | Moderate | High |
| Recovery time | Quick | Quick | Can be slow |
| Fistula rates | Low | Moderate | Low |
| Stricture rates | Low | Moderate | High |
| TEP voice | Good | Good | Poor |
| Swallowing | Good | Good | Good |
| Use for circumferential defects | Yes | Second choice | Yes |
| Use for partial defects | Yes | Yes | No |
| Contraindications | Obesity, with a very thick thigh | Thin patient with a small arm, radial dominance | Severe comorbidity, prior abdominal surgery |

ALT, anterolateral thigh; TEP, tracheoesophageal puncture.

## The Anterolateral Thigh or Anteromedial Thigh Flap

### Flap Design and Harvesting

There are usually one to three usable cutaneous perforators in the ALT flap territory. The goal of flap design is to capture two or more perforators so that the flap can be divided into two independent skin paddles, one for pharyngoesophageal reconstruction and the other for external neck resurfacing or for flap monitoring. For circumferential defects, a flap width of 9.4 cm is designed to form a tubed neopharynx with a 3 cm diameter (3 x p) **(Fig. 4.3)**.[28] For partial defects, the width of the flap is calculated by subtracting the width of the remaining pharyngeal mucosa from 9.4 cm. For example, if the remaining mucosa is 2 cm wide, the needed flap width would be 7.4 cm.

The perforators are located using the author's "ABC system."[34,35] It is important to keep the leg in a neutral position, with the patella facing the ceiling. The "AP line" is drawn to connect the anterior superior iliac spine (ASIS) and the superolateral corner of the patella (P), and the midpoint of the AP line is marked. Perforator B is marked at the midpoint of the AP line but 1.5 cm lateral to the line. Perforator A is marked ~ 5 cm proximal to perforator B, and perforator C is 5 cm distal to perforator B. Doppler examination can be used to help locate the cutaneous perforators in thin patients. However, the accuracy decreases significantly with increasing thickness of the thigh.[35] Computed tomography angiography (CTA) may be useful to detect unusual perforator anatomy and to help surgeons choose the thigh with favorable perforator anatomy.[36]

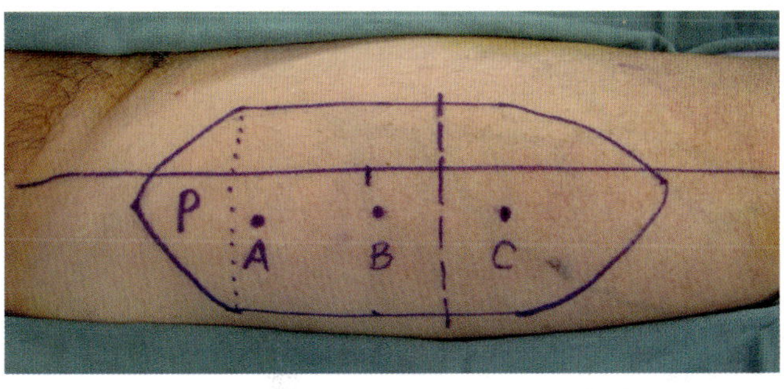


**Fig. 4.3** Design of the ALT flap for pharyngoesophageal reconstruction. The midpoint of the line connecting the anterior superior iliac spine and the superolateral corner of the patella (AP line) is marked. Perforator B is usually located 1.5 cm lateral to the midpoint. Perforators A and C are located 5 cm proximal and distal to perforator B, respectively. The flap is designed to include two or three potential perforators so that a second skin paddle, usually based on perforator C, can be used for neck resurfacing or monitoring. A lip of the flap is extended proximally (P) to form an elongated oblique opening of the tube flap to accommodate the wider opening in the floor of the mouth.

A straight anterior incision ~ 15 cm long is made first across all three cutaneous perforators. This incision is usually placed 1.5 to 2.0 cm medial to the AP line. It also corresponds to the anterior midline of the thigh in most cases. A wider fascia is included to cover the suture lines during flap insetting. Therefore, the fascial incision is made 1 to 2 cm more medially than the anterior skin incision **(Fig. 4.4)**. Subfascial dissection proceeds laterally until the cutaneous perforators are identified. The exact locations of the perforators are marked on the skin surface with a fine permanent suture. The flap is then re-centered, if necessary, based on the actual perforator locations. To accommodate the wide opening in the pharyngeal inlet for the proximal anastomosis, an extended lip of skin is designed at the proximal end of the flap so that an elongated oblique opening can be created when the flap is tubed **(Fig. 4.3)**. Dissection of the perforators and the main pedicle can be performed through the anterior incision only. The remaining flap is incised only after the cutaneous perforators and the main vascular pedicle are located or dissected out.

If no usable perforators are found in the ALT flap territory, the anteromedial thigh (AMT) flap should be explored through the same incision **(Fig. 4.5)**. Overall, the AMT perforators are present in only ~ 50% of patients. However, we have found an inverse relationship between the ALT and AMT perforators.[37,38] When there are no perforators in the ALT flap, the chances of having an AMT perforator are much greater, approaching 100%. Similar to ALT flap dissection, subfascial dissection is performed toward the medial thigh until the intermuscular space between the rectus femoris and the sartorius muscles is identified. The AMT perforators, ranging from one to two in number, originate from the rectus femoris branch of the descending branch artery and enter the skin through the intermuscular space or pierce the medial edge of the rectus femoris muscle **(Fig. 4.5b)**, but never the sartorius muscle. Once the perforators are identified, the medial border of the AMT flap is incised

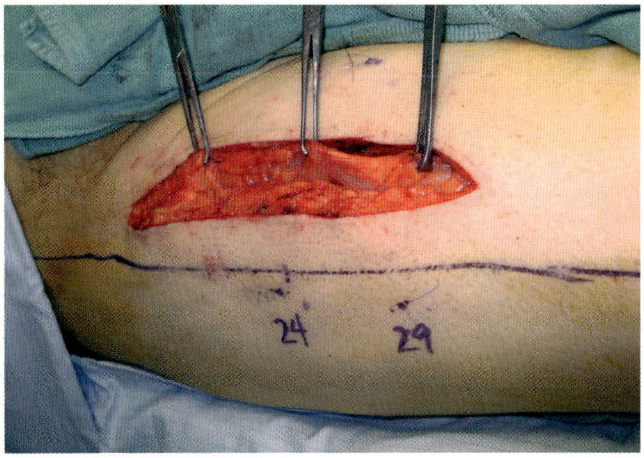


**Fig. 4.4** In the ALT flap, the fascia is wider than the skin so that the fascia can be used to cover the suture line.

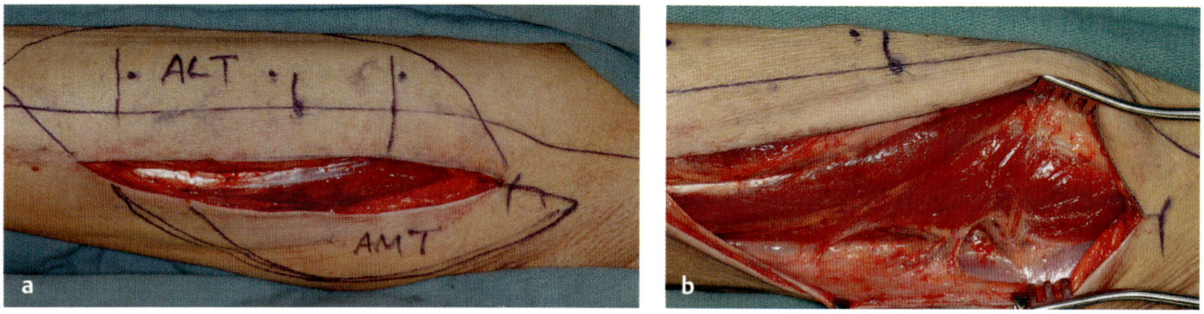


**Fig. 4.5** **(a)** If no suitable ALT flap perforators are found, the AMT flap can be easily explored through the same incision. Subfascial dissection proceeds medially until the intermuscular space between the sartorius and medial edge of the rectus femoris muscles is seen. **(b)** The vascular pedicle of the AMT flap, the rectus femoris branch off the descending branch, travels on the medial edge of the rectus femoris muscle and sends out perforators to the skin.

and the flap can be harvested in the usual fashion. The main vascular pedicle, the rectus femoris branch, can be traced along the medial border of the rectus femoris muscle back to the descending branch. The AMT flap can also be used as a second skin flap when two skin flaps are needed and there is only one ALT perforator. Transecting the descending branch above the origin of the rectus femoris branch allows the descending branch to carry both the ALT and AMT flaps **(Fig. 4.6)**.

## Flap Insetting

Partial flap insetting is performed before vascular anastomoses are completed. The proximal anastomosis of the flap to the base of tongue and posterior pharyngeal mucosa is performed first **(Fig. 4.7)**. If the flap is longer than the defect, the perforator of the flap should be placed near the center of the defect and the extra flap trimmed accordingly. It is easier to perform the proximal anastomosis without tubing the flap first.

Usually, a 3–0 polyglactin suture is used in a simple, interrupted fashion. The longitudinal seam is oriented posterolaterally at 3 to 4 or 8 to 9 o'clock **(Fig. 4.7)**. The proximal anastomosis begins from the corner of the flap, along the posterior wall, followed by the anterior wall. With this "walk around" technique, one should always be aware of the length discrepancy between the pharyngeal inlet and the flap. The other option is to anchor the two corner sutures first, then complete the posterior wall and the anterior wall. Large bites are recommended, with inversion of the skin and mucosal edges into the lumen. Care should be taken to avoid catching the hypoglossal nerve when suturing the flap to the base of the tongue. Next, the longitudinal seam is completed toward the distal end of the flap, also with simple, interrupted sutures. For partial defects, the proximal end of the flap is sewn to the base of the tongue and the lateral edges to the remaining posterior pharyngeal wall mucosa **(Fig. 4.8)**. Vascular anastomo-

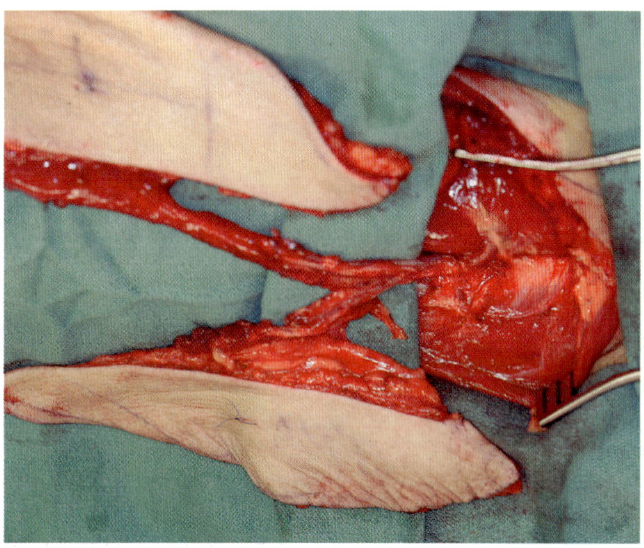

**Fig. 4.6** Since the vascular pedicle of the ALT flap usually comes off the descending branch, the anterolateral thigh flap pedicle, both flaps can be harvested with a single vascular pedicle.

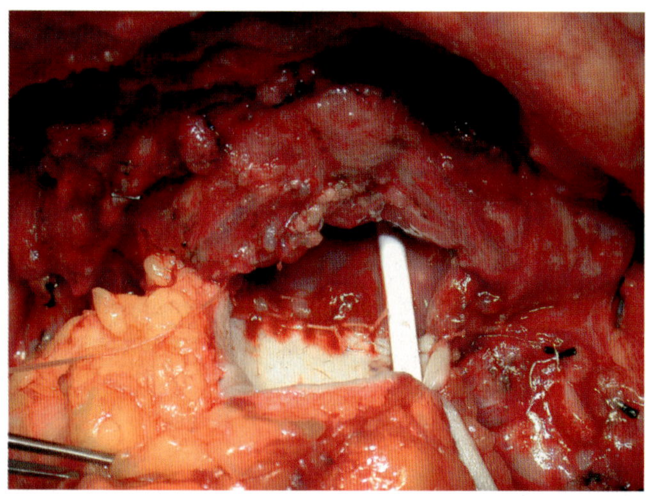

**Fig. 4.7** The proximal anastomosis with the base of tongue and posterior pharyngeal mucosa is performed first. The longitudinal seam of the tubed flap is positioned on the sides.

ses are then performed before completing the distal anastomosis of the flap to the cervical esophagus.

If the thickness of the flap is greater than 10 mm, some degree of flap thinning is necessary. The safest way to thin the ALT flap is to thin the periphery of the flap, to facilitate the suturing of the flap to the remaining pharynx and esophagus. When aggressive thinning is needed, the branches of the perforator within the subcutaneous tissue should be carefully visualized under loupe or microscope magnification and the adipose tissue trimmed away in a radial fashion to avoid injury to the perforators.

For circumferential defects, use of the Montgomery salivary bypass tube (Boston Medical Products, Westborough, Massachusetts) can be considered, which may potentially decrease the incidence of leak and stricture. The value of the bypass tube, however, is unclear. The indications for use of the tube include: a thick flap (narrow lumen), small cervical esophagus, difficult flap insetting due to very low location of the transected cervical esophageal end, and/or poor tissue quality due to radiation injury. A 14 mm diameter tube is used. The tube is inserted through the mouth before the longitudinal seam of the flap is completed (**Fig. 4.9**). The proximal flange of the bypass tube is placed above the proximal anastomosis and the distal end in the esophagus below the distal anastomosis. A 1-0 polypropylene suture is attached to the flange of the tube, brought out through the mouth, and taped to the cheek to prevent distal migration and to facilitate easy removal of the tube. A 10 Fr red rubber catheter is placed over the suture to protect the oral commissure. If a feeding tube has not yet been placed, it is placed through the nose, the tubed flap, or inside the Montgomery salivary bypass tube.

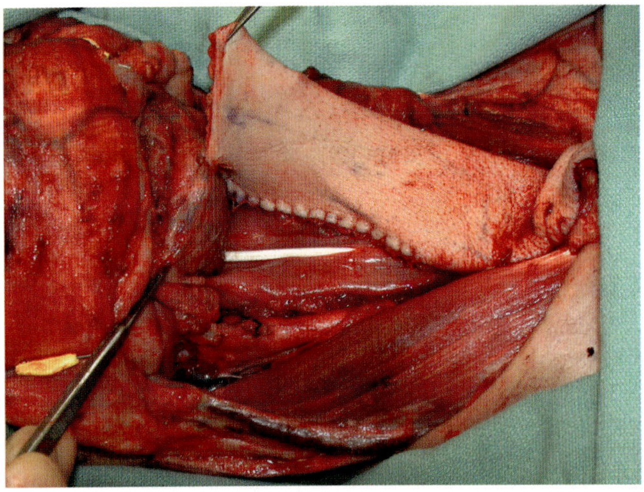

**Fig. 4.8** For partial pharyngoesophageal defects, the flap is sewn to the lateral edges of the posterior pharyngeal mucosa.

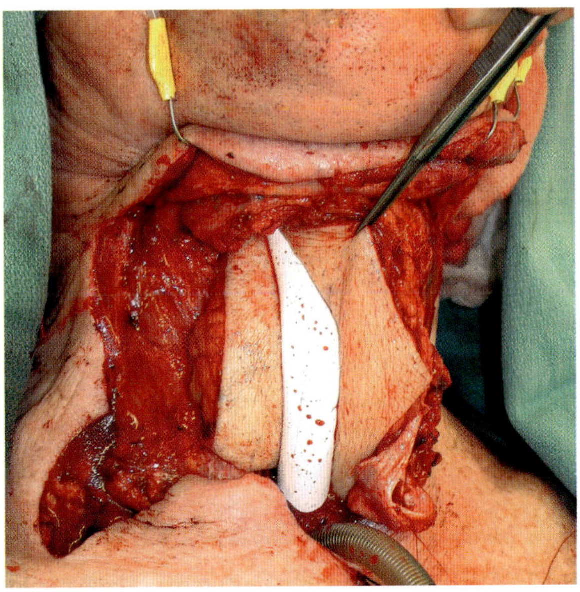

**Fig. 4.9** A Montgomery salivary bypass tube with a diameter of 14 mm can be used to temporarily stent the neopharynx for 2 to 6 weeks. A 1-0 polypropylene suture is placed on the flange of the tube at the proximal end and is brought out through the mouth and taped on the cheek.

Next, the neck is returned to a neutral position from the hyperextended position by removing the shoulder roll. It is not necessary to flex the neck. The anterior wall of the cervical esophagus is split longitudinally for ~ 1.5 cm to spatulate the distal anastomosis (**Fig. 4.10**). This is important to enlarge the distal anastomosis and to minimize the risk of circumferential stricture. On the flap, a triangular lip is created and inserted into the longitudinal split of the esophagus to complete the spatulation (**Fig. 4.11**). The tubed flap is slightly twisted so that the longitudinal seam at the distal anastomosis is facing posteriorly at 6 o'clock. Such positioning of

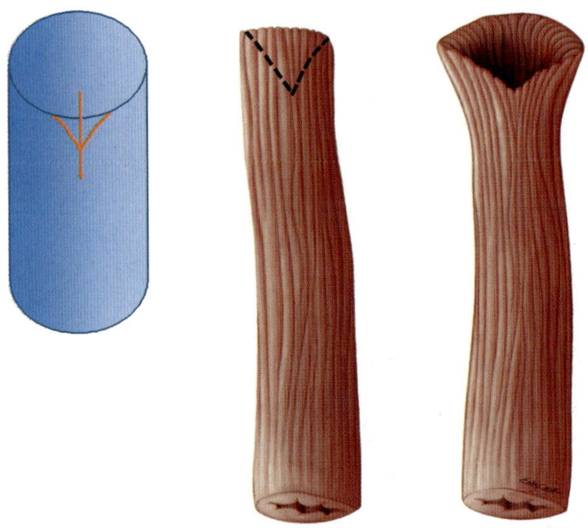

**Fig. 4.10** The cervical esophageal end is incised longitudinally for ~ 1.5 cm to spatulate the anastomosis.

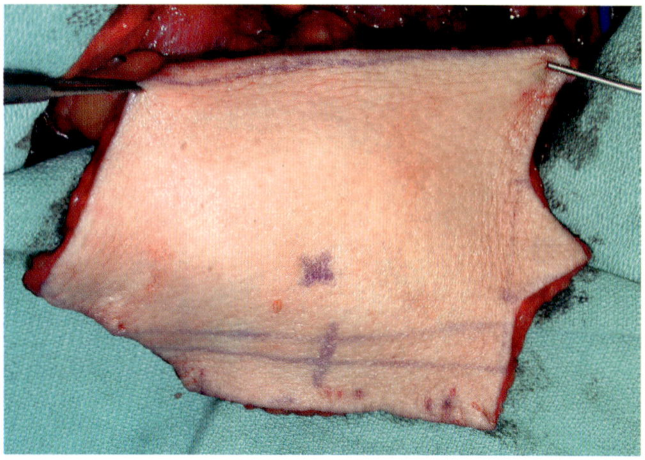

**Fig. 4.11** A triangular lip of flap is created so that it can be sutured to the spatulated cervical esophageal end. This may minimize the risk of stricture formation at the distal anastomosis.

the tubed flap places the perforator vessels anteriorly between 11 and 1 o'clock to avoid compression of the perforators against the prevertebral fascia (**Fig. 4.12**). After completion of the distal anastomosis, the fascia of the flap is used to cover the suture lines. The medial edges of the sternocleidomastoid muscles are detached from the clavicular head insertion for easy fitting of a tracheostoma button for speech rehabilitation later on.

The neck wound is then irrigated with an ample amount of warm normal saline (2 or 3 L), taking care not to squirt the saline directly on the vascular pedicle to avoid vessel spasm. Meticulous hemostasis is essential to avoiding a postoperative hematoma, which can compress the vascular pedicle. A 15 Fr Blake drain is placed on each side of the neck, lateral to the internal jugular vein. Before closing the neck skin, the vascular pedicle is examined again to avoid kinking or compression. The second skin paddle, usually based on perforator C, is externalized to repair any neck skin defects (**Fig. 4.13**) or posterior tracheal defects. It can also be simply used for flap monitoring (**Fig. 4.14a**). If only one perforator is present, a small segment of the vastus lateralis muscle based on a muscular branch is included in the ALT flap and is externalized for monitoring purposes (**Fig. 4.14b**).[39] A 2–0 silk tie is placed around the perforator of the monitoring segment. The monitoring segment can be removed 5 to 7 days later, before the patient is discharged from the hospital, by simply tying the pre-placed tie and cutting the tissue away. Flap monitoring based on a handheld Doppler over the neck skin is not accurate. In addition, it usually detects the arterial signal only, resulting in delayed exploration in the event of the more common venous obstruction. Externalizing a portion of the distal flap by de-epithelializing a strip of skin around the distal anastomosis is not recommended because it results in a high fistula rate.[28]

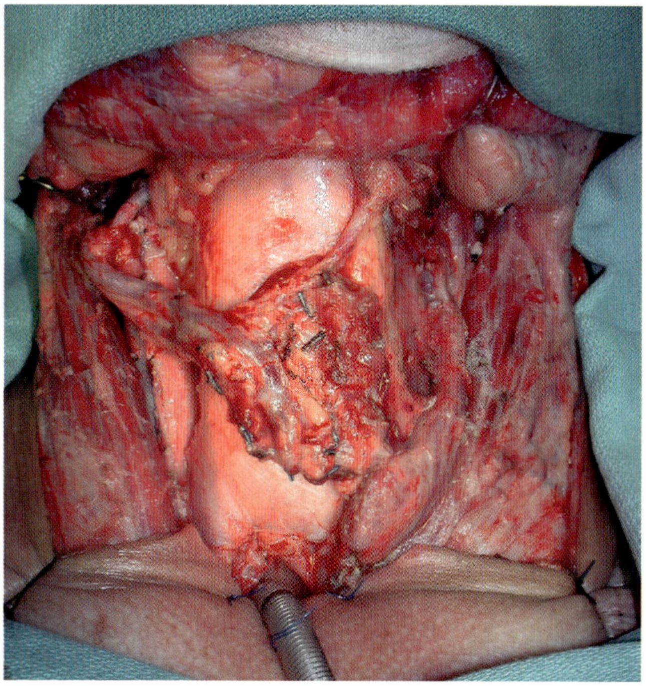

**Fig. 4.12** The perforators are positioned anteriorly to avoid compression of the perforators between the flap and the prevertebral fascia. A wider fascia is designed to cover the suture lines as a second layer after flap insetting.

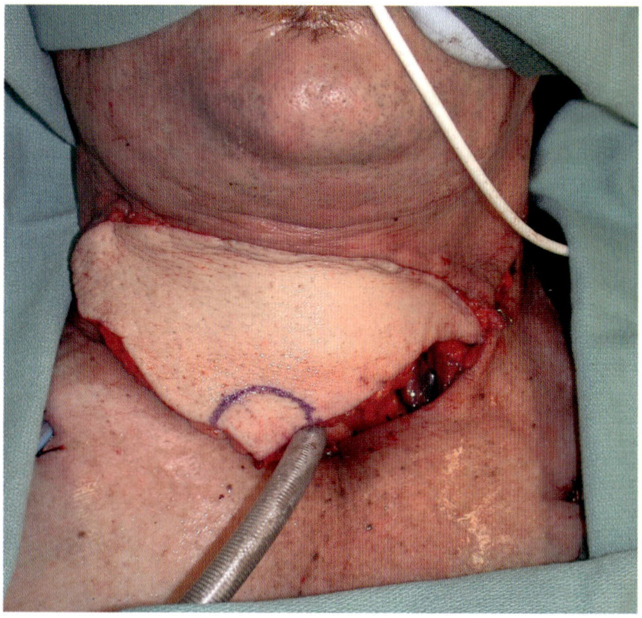

**Fig. 4.13** Including two perforators means the flap can be divided into two skin paddles based on separate cutaneous perforators. The second skin paddle, usually based on perforator C, can be used for neck resurfacing. This avoids the use of a second flap.

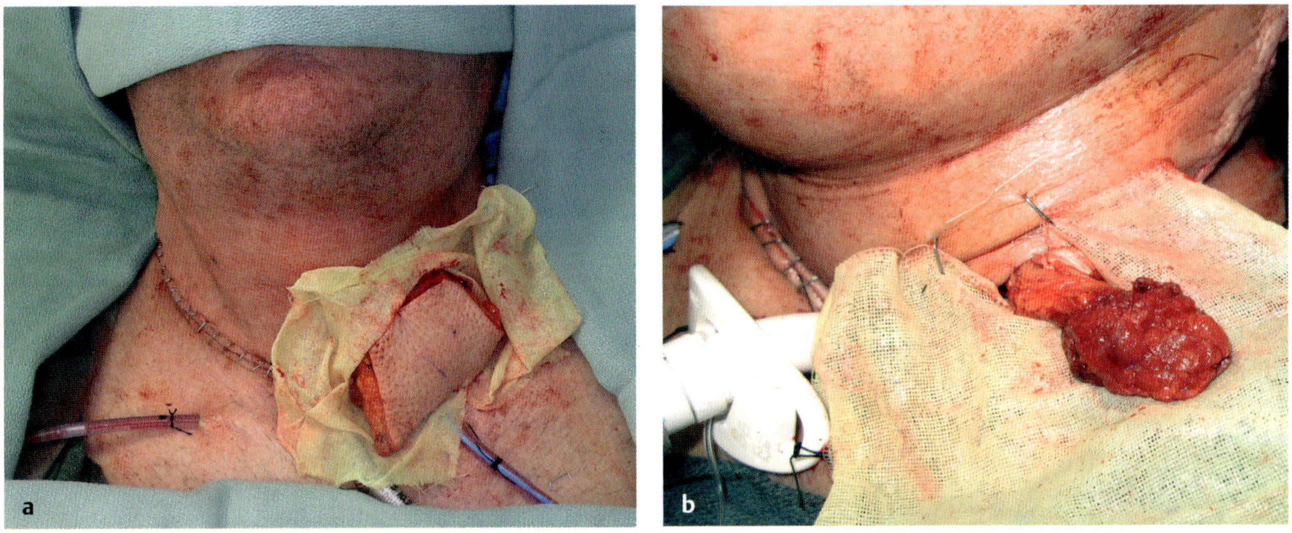

**Fig. 4.14** **(a)** The second skin paddle can also be used solely for monitoring. **(b)** When there is only one perforator present, a segment of the vastus lateralis muscle is used as a monitor.

At the time of neck closure, the tracheostoma is sutured to the surrounding neck and anterior chest skin, and a #8 tracheostomy tube is placed in the tracheostoma and secured to the chest skin. In patients with a short and thick neck, the superior flange of the tracheostomy tube is trimmed to avoid compressing the neck skin and the underlying flap **(Fig. 4.15)**. Skin necrosis and even fistulas can develop owing to such compression.

## The Radial Forearm Flap or Ulnar Artery Perforator Flap

The design of the radial forearm or ulnar artery perforator (UAP) flap is similar to that of the ALT flap. The flap can be designed with an extended lip in the proximal forearm to accommodate the larger opening in the base of the tongue, as with the ALT flap. The circumference of the distal forearm at the wrist crease is 15 to 16 cm in average patients. For circumferential defects, the required flap width of 9.4 cm would require removal of nearly two-thirds of the forearm skin, creating an unsightly donor-site scar. Pharyngoesophageal defects are usually no longer than 10 cm. With shorter defects, the flap can be rotated 90 degrees from the conventional design orientation on the forearm to minimize donor-site morbidity. For instance, for a circumferential defect 6 cm long, the flap width (lateral to medial) is designed as 6 cm and the length (proximal to distal), 9.4 cm. When the flap is tubed, it is rolled from distal to proximal instead of from lateral to medial **(Fig. 4.16)**.

A second skin island can be easily designed with the UAP flap, because all patients have two or more perforators in our experience **(Fig. 4.17)**.[40] As with the

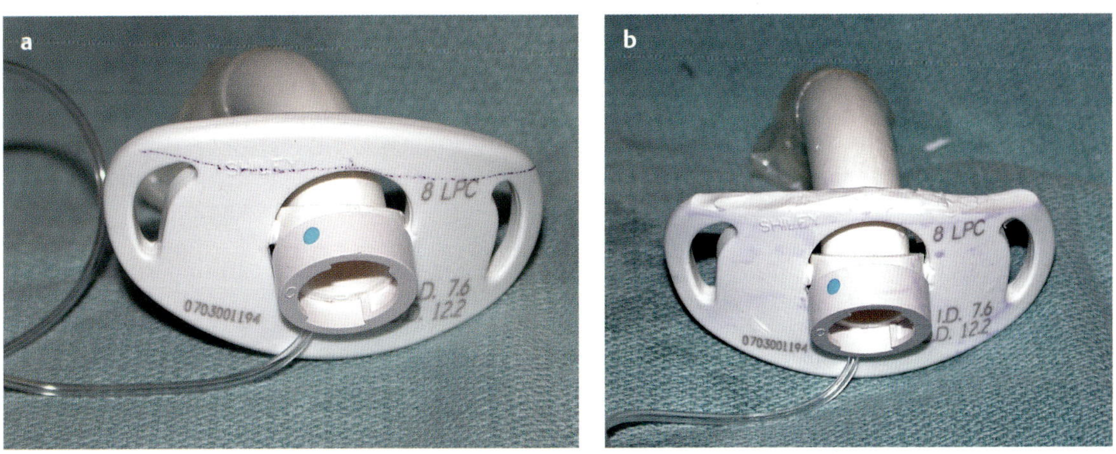

**Fig. 4.15** **(a)** The upper edge of the flange of the tracheostomy tube **(b)** is trimmed to avoid compression of the flange against the flap.

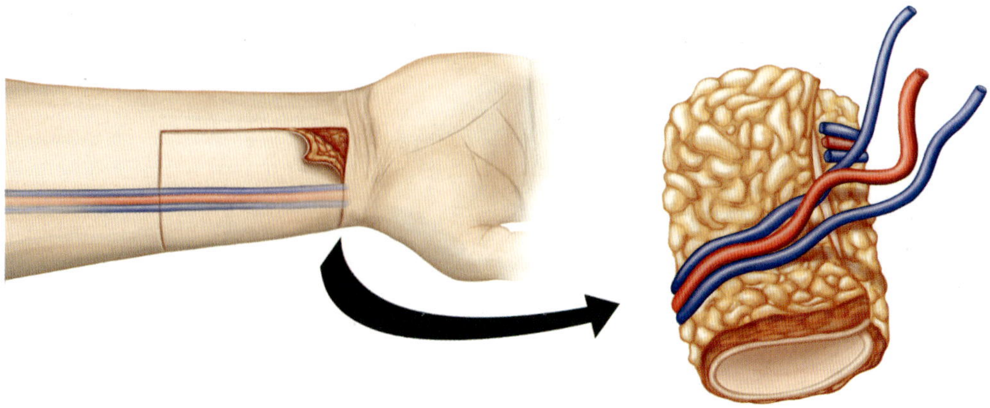

**Fig. 4.16** For short circumferential pharyngoesophageal defects, the radial forearm flap is designed with the width of the flap as the length of the tubed neoesophagus to reduce donor-site morbidity.

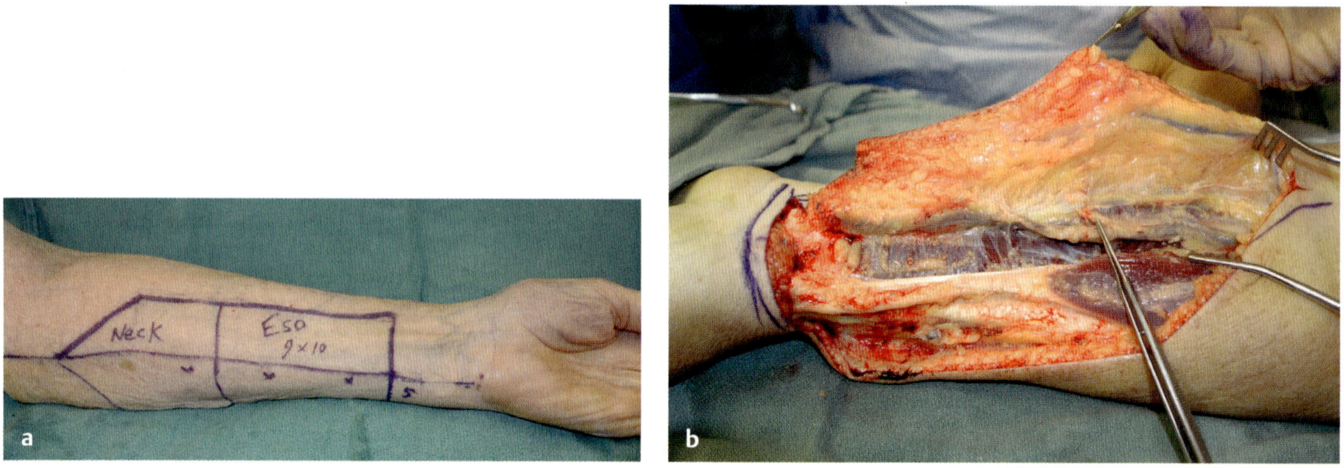


**Fig. 4.17** A second skin island can be created with either the radial forearm flap or the ulnar artery perforator flap. **(a)** The latter consistently has two or more perforators. **(b)** A perforator can also frequently be found in the proximal forearm of the radial forearm flap. The second skin island is externalized to repair a small neck skin defect or as a monitor.

ALT flap, the second skin island can be used to resurface the neck or as a monitor. With the radial forearm flap, a second skin paddle is also possible by including a proximal perforator. Alternatively, a small skin island can be created at the distal end of the flap.

Elevation of the radial forearm flap is well described in the literature, with the following modifications. In most cases, the venae comitantes of the radial forearm flap are adequate for venous drainage without including the cephalic vein. However, the venae comitantes can be extremely small and inadequate in some patients. Therefore, the author's approach is to tentatively outline the flap centered on the radial vessels and to make a small transverse incision at the wrist crease to explore the venae comitantes first. If one of the veins is at least 1 mm in diameter, the proximal end(s) of the venae comitantes are presumed to be of reasonable caliber for straightforward microvascular anastomosis and there is no need to use the cephalic vein. Otherwise, the flap design is shifted laterally to capture the cephalic vein. Suprafascial dissection is preferred,[41] and flap elevation is performed under tourniquet control. The venae comitantes are usually no bigger than 1.5 mm before they converge; therefore, the vein is usually taken above the convergence of the venae comitantes, where the diameter is greater than 2.5 mm in most cases. Once the flap and the vascular pedicle are completely dissected, the tourniquet is released to perfuse the flap and the hand for several minutes before dividing the pedicle. (Harvesting of the UAP flap is described in a separate chapter.) The vascular pedicle is at least 5 cm shorter than that of the radial forearm flap. This should be taken into consideration when choosing recipient vessels. If the recipient vessels are away from the defect, a longer pedicle may be more desirable to avoid vein grafting. Flap insetting is similar to that with the ALT flap.

# The Jejunal Flap

## Flap Harvesting

The vascular pedicle of the jejunal flap is usually the second or third jejunal branch of the superior mesenteric artery and vein. Through an upper midline abdominal incision, the mesentery arcade of the proximal jejunum is examined with fiberoptic backlighting to transilluminate the mesentery **(Fig. 4.18)**. Surgical dissection begins with isolation of the mesentery vessels to their origins at the superior mesenteric artery and vein. The mesentery between the adjacent arcade vessels is divided to the serosal border. The desired jejunal segment, ~ 15 cm long, is divided using a linear cutting stapler. The proximal end of the jejunal segment is marked with a serosal suture to maintain an isoperistaltic orientation during flap insetting. Once the recipient site is ready, the mesentery vessels are ligated and divided. The jejunum flap is removed and the lumen is flushed with cold normal saline until clear.

## Flap Insetting

The diameter of the jejunum is much smaller than the pharyngeal inlet. Therefore, a 2 to 3 cm incision is made in the proximal end of the jejunum along the antimesenteric border to widen the jejunal end, creating a near end-to-side anastomosis **(Fig. 4.19)**. The proximal anastomosis is performed using interrupted 3–0 polyglactin sutures prior to revascularizing the flap. Whether a second-layer Lempert serosal closure is performed usually depends on the surgeon's preference. Care should be taken to avoid the hypoglossal nerve at the base of the tongue during the second-layer closure. The jejunal flap tends to elongate over time, causing redundancy and dysphagia. For the distal anastomosis, the neck is returned to a neutral position and the jejunal flap is slightly stretched in a caudal direction to minimize such redundancy.[42,43] The cervical esophagus is opened longitudinally to spatulate the distal anastomosis, as described above with the ALT flap. The distal anastomosis is performed using a single layer of interrupted 3–0 absorbable sutures.

A monitor segment 3 to 4 cm long is created from the remaining jejunum based on one or two terminal branches of the mesentery arcade **(Fig. 4.20)**. The monitor segment is brought out through the lateral neck incision to avoid obstruction of the tracheostoma and is covered with petroleum jelly-impregnated gauze to prevent desiccation. Both ends of the bowel segment are left open to avoid distention. The monitor segment can also be completely opened longitudinally. A 2–0 silk tie is placed around the segment's small vascular pedicle at the skin level so that the pedicle can be easily tied off when it is time to remove the monitor segment. In the meantime,

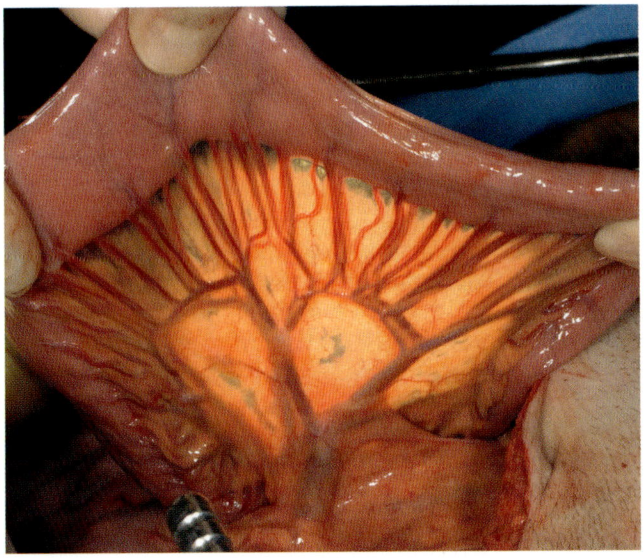

**Fig. 4.18** During jejunal flap harvesting, the mesentery arcades of the jejunal flap are transilluminated with fiberoptic backlighting to facilitate vessel dissection.

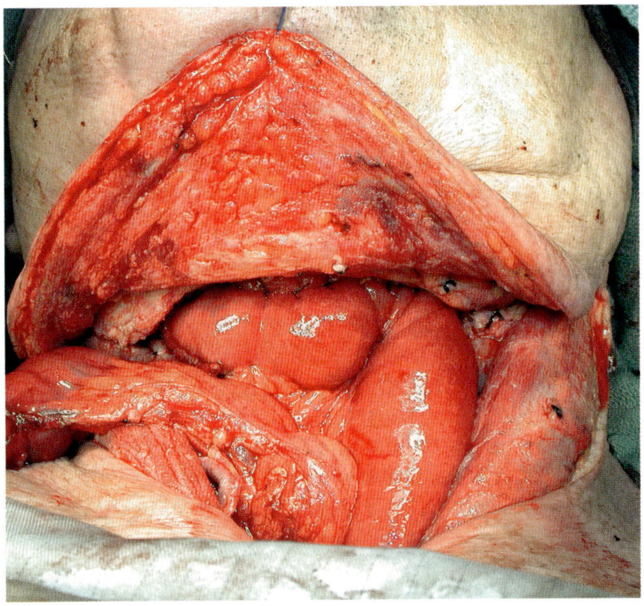

**Fig. 4.19** During jejunal flap insetting, the proximal end of the jejunum was opened longitudinally to accommodate a wider opening at the base of tongue. The flap is slightly stretched in a caudal direction to reduce redundancy.

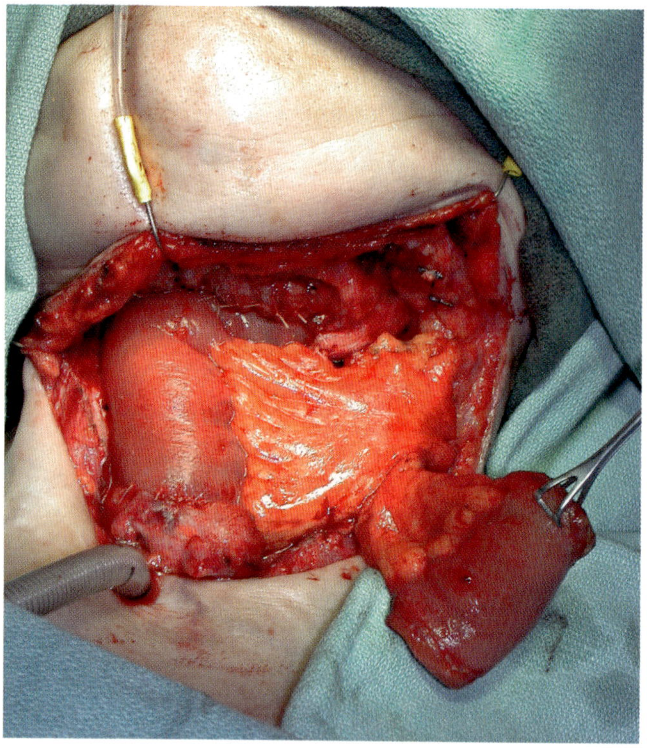

**Fig. 4.20** A short bowel segment is created and externalized as a monitoring segment, which is removed before the patient is discharged from the hospital.

jejunal continuity in the abdomen is re-established, a feeding jejunostomy tube and a gastrostomy tube are inserted, and the abdomen is closed.

## Reconstruction of Isolated Cervical Esophageal Defects with an Intact Larynx

The vast majority of tumors arising in the cervical esophagus are malignant, and laryngectomy is required to achieve tumor-free margins and to prevent aspiration when the cricopharyngeus muscle is resected.[44] For benign tumors, such as schwannomas and granular cell tumors, smaller margins are acceptable to preserve the larynx. However, reconstruction of isolated cervical esophageal defects can be challenging because the resection of a portion of the cricopharyngeus muscle increases the risk of reflux and aspiration. In addition, with an intact larynx and trachea, exposure of the cervical esophagus is limited, making reconstruction technically difficult. Given the small space around the esophagus, a free tissue transfer offers the best flexibility for insetting the flap; a thin flap is required for the same reason. The radial forearm flap is, therefore, the author's flap of choice for both partial and circumferential defects. These defects are usually only a few centimeters long, so the radial forearm flap can be oriented 90 degrees to the conventional flap design so that the width of the flap becomes the length of the neoesophagus. The longitudinal length of the flap is rolled along the vascular pedicle to form a tube **(Fig. 4.16)**. The jejunal flap is also a good choice, with a good size match and excellent healing. However, the need for laparotomy and bowel surgery increases surgical risks, and therefore, it is our second choice.

Because defects of the cervical esophagus are usually located lower in the neck, the external carotid artery is often not exposed. Either the transverse cervical artery or the superior thyroid artery can be used as the recipient artery. The transverse cervical vein and the internal jugular vein are the common recipient veins. The vascular pedicle is often longer than needed and should be carefully looped to avoid kinking or twisting.

### Reconstruction of Postlaryngectomy Pharyngocutaneous Fistulas

Radiotherapy has become the primary treatment for early stages of laryngeal and hypopharyngeal cancers.[45] However, local and regional recurrence rates following radiotherapy for laryngeal and hypopharyngeal cancers can exceed 30%, depending on tumor location and initial tumor stage,[46,47] requiring a salvage total laryngectomy. Although the overall incidence of postlaryngectomy pharyngocutaneous fistulas has decreased significantly in the past decade, it remains very high in previously irradiated patients.[48,49,50,51,52] McCombe et al[49] reported that the incidence increased from 4% to 39% when radiation was included in multimodal therapy. Recent studies have shown that the mean overall survival of patients after salvage total laryngectomy was 7.2 years.[53] The mean 2-, 5-, and 10-year overall survival rates were around 70%, 55%, and 40%, respectively.[45,54,55] These data demonstrate that this patient population still has a reasonable survival expectation. Therefore, reconstruction of these defects may restore function and improve quality of life.

Once fistulas develop, the radiation effects are compounded by salivary contamination of the neck, leading to chronic inflammation and hypoxia of the neck skin and vasculature, which puts the patient at risk for loss of neck skin and the remaining pharynx, tracheostoma compromise, and even carotid artery rupture. Long-standing fistulas will inevitably promote scar formation, leading to pharyngeal stricture and a frozen neck. Pharyngocutaneous fistulas, unlike intraoral fistulas, do not respond to conservative management. Therefore, many such patients were left unreconstructed in the past due to the difficulties of reconstruction. To avoid the development of a frozen neck, early surgical intervention to reconstruct these defects is essential.[56] Reconstructive surgery should be performed within 4 weeks, even within days, after the development of the fistula, before severe fibrosis sets in. Surgical dissection in the neck is therefore much easier than in patients with a long-standing fistula. Thorough débridement of infected and necrotic tissues is mandatory to reconstruct the pharyngeosophageal defect. As with other pharyngeosophageal reconstructions, the two-skin-island ALT flap is our flap of choice. The use of various amounts of the well-vascularized vastus lateralis muscle to cover the neck may help to achieve primary healing. Although the tissues may still be edematous during early surgical intervention, anastomoses can be safely and reliably completed with proper tissue-handling techniques.

Patients with long-standing pharyngocutaneous fistulas often present the worst "frozen neck" **(Fig. 4.21)**. The strategies for reconstruction are the same as those for managing a frozen neck. During surgery, the fistula track and scar tissues are excised, without exposing the great vessels in the neck if they are cancer free **(Fig. 4.22)**. The hypopharynx is opened superiorly to the base of the tongue, where the pharyngeal inlet is incised laterally and widened to approximately two to three finger-widths. This is important because primary closure of the pharynx following a total laryngectomy inevitably narrows the pharyngeal inlet. In patients with a relatively normal pharynx and cervical esophagus, a small degree of narrowing may not cause dysphagia. After pharyngoesophageal reconstruction, however, food transit through the reconstructed conduit is compromised no matter what type of flap is used. Any narrowing in the pharyngeal inlet or weakness of the base of the tongue thus further compounds the problem and causes dysphagia. Inferiorly, the posterior wall of the tracheostoma is carefully separated from the cervical esophagus just far enough, usually 1 cm, for the flap–esophageal anastomosis. Minimal dissection should be performed to avoid ischemia to the remaining cervical esophagus and tracheal stoma. Meticulous tissue-handling techniques must be exercised in these difficult cases because there is no room for error. Once the pharyngoesophageal defect is recreated, the transverse cervical vessels are explored and a multi-island ALT flap is employed to reconstruct the defects as described earlier.

## Managing a Frozen Neck During Pharyngoesophageal Reconstruction

A frozen neck is defined as severe fibrosis in the neck without tissue planes, usually as the result of neck surgery (such as neck dissection) combined with

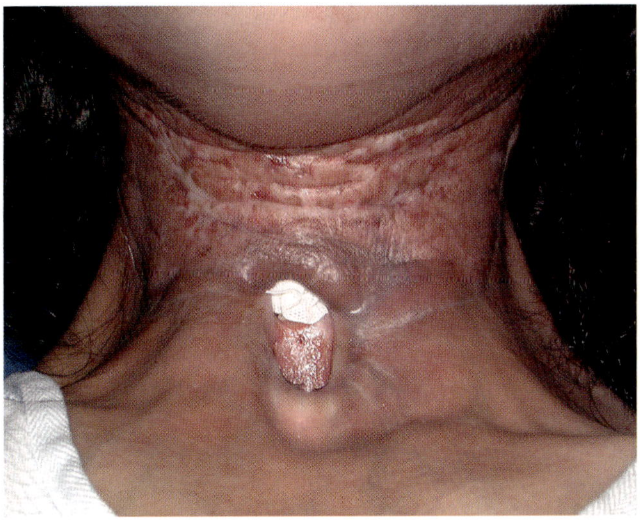

**Fig. 4.21** A long-standing pharyngocutaneous fistula following a total laryngectomy and radiation therapy results in the worst "frozen neck" with severe scarring.

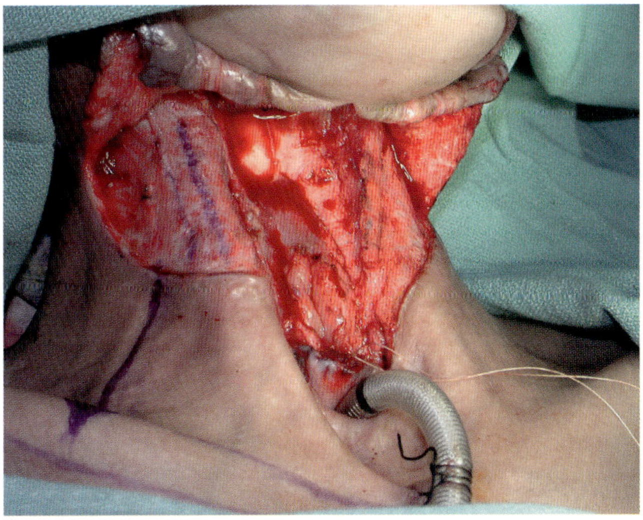

**Fig. 4.22** In patients with pharyngocutaneous fistula following previous total laryngectomy and radiation therapy without tumor recurrence, simply removing the scar tissue in the central neck without exposing the major vessels significantly reduces surgical risks.

radiotherapy. Long-standing pharyngocutaneous fistulas result in the worst cases of frozen neck. There are three major problems associated with managing a frozen neck during reconstruction: (1) risk of carotid artery rupture, (2) lack of recipient vessels, and (3) concomitant defects of the neck skin or trachea. In a frozen neck, the carotid artery and internal jugular vein are usually encased in fibrotic tissue. Surgical dissection around these great vessels during fistula and scar tissue excision and preparation for recipient vessels can easily cause the vessels, which are already damaged by chemoradiation, to rupture, resulting in high rates of morbidity and mortality. The best approach to avoiding carotid artery rupture is to simply stay away from them. Because these patients have already undergone neck dissection, exposing the carotid artery and internal jugular vein is not oncologically indicated. The author's preference is to use the transverse cervical vessels as recipient vessels.

In most cases, the transverse cervical artery arises from the thyrocervical trunk, which originates from the subclavian artery **(Fig. 4.23)**. The transverse cervical artery may arise directly from the subclavian artery in 21% of the sides and from the internal mammary artery in 2% of the sides.[57] The transverse cervical artery crosses anterior to the brachial plexus and middle scalene muscle on its way to the lateral border of the levator scapulae muscle. It travels behind the omohyoid and anterior scalene muscles. The omohyoid muscle immediately above the clavicle is a good landmark to locate the transverse cervical artery, which is deep to it. The transverse cervical artery has an external diameter between 2 and 3 mm after its takeoff from the thyrocervical trunk. When the artery is less than 1.5 mm, it tends to have a vertical course down behind the clavicle rather than a transverse course, suggesting that it may arise from the subclavian or the internal mammary artery rather than the thyrocervical trunk.

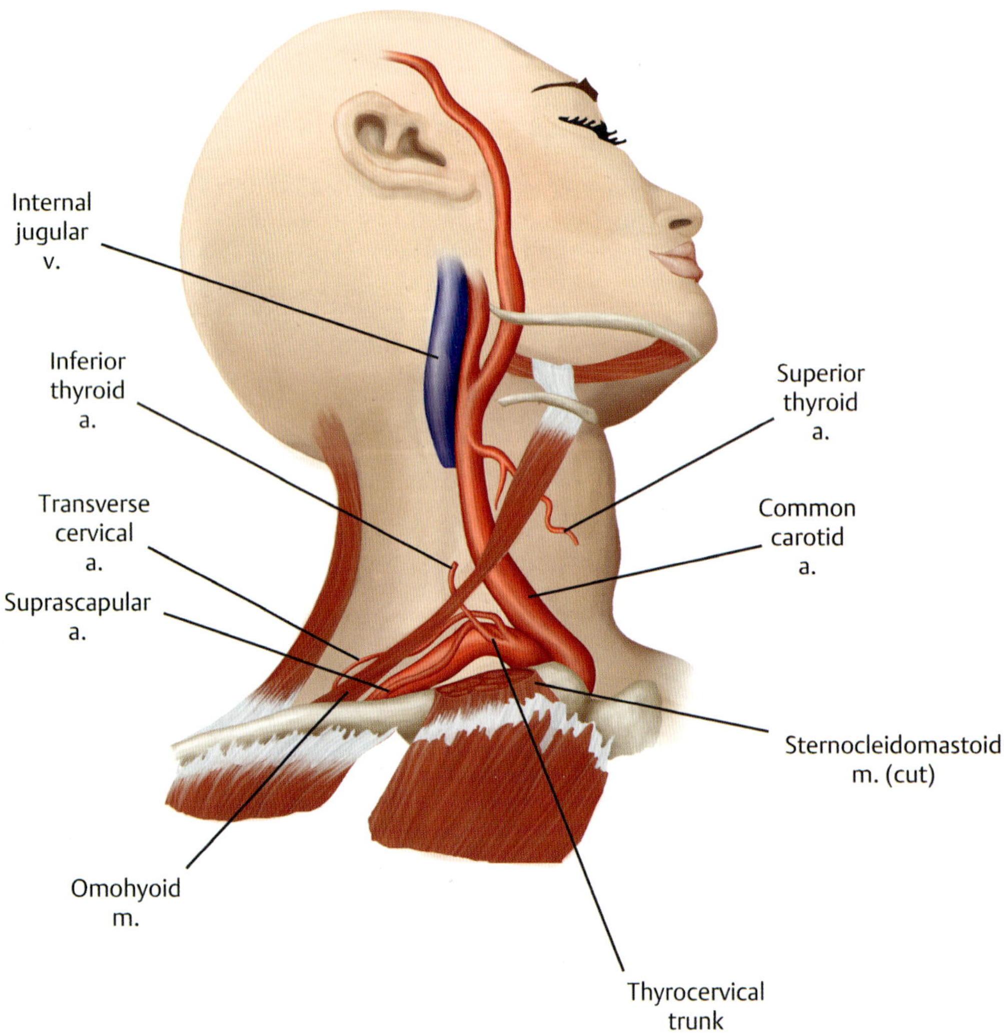


**Fig. 4.23** Anatomy of the transverse cervical vessels. The transverse cervical artery is usually a branch of the thyrocervical trunk, which arises from the subclavian artery.

The transverse cervical vein may run deep (75%) or superficial (25%) relative to the omohyoid muscle.[58] The transverse cervical vein may drain into the external jugular vein or the subclavian vein. In the author's experience, the transverse cervical vein is usually available above the clavicle and has an adequate size regardless of where it drains **(Table 4.3)**. Overall, the transverse cervical vessels are available in 92% of patients and are very similar in size to those of the flap vascular pedicle.[57] In 23% of cases, absence or inadequacy of transverse cervical vessels on one side incurs the need to explore the contralateral transverse cervical vessels. With the visor neck incision typically performed by the tumor ablation team, the supraclavicular region (level V) is usually unexposed and surgical dissection of the transverse cervical vessels is straightforward for most cases. The right side of the neck is preferred to avoid injury to the thoracic duct. The transverse cervical vessels are usually found in the supraclavicular area lateral to the sternocleidomastoid muscle. On the left side of the neck, particular attention should be paid to avoiding injury to the thoracic duct. Dissection should start high, above the supraclavicular fat pad, and proceed deep to it. If the transverse cervical artery is deemed too small, the thyrocervical trunk is explored with dissection under the sternocleidomastoid muscle **(Fig. 4.24)**. The thyrocervical trunk is significantly larger than the transverse cervical artery, usually in the range of 2.5 mm to 3.5 mm. The external jugular vein usually joins the transverse cervical vein before entering the subclavian vein. This part of the external jugular vein is more deeply located and of good quality. If both veins are unavailable, such as in patients who have undergone a radical neck dissection, the internal jugular vein stump immediately above the subclavian vein is usually long enough for an end-to-side anastomosis.

The use of the transverse cervical vessels solves the first two problems associated with a frozen neck. Successful management of the third problem, concomitant neck skin or tracheal defects, is also possible. Elevating an anterior neck skin flap from an area

**Table 4.3** The presence and sizes of the transverse cervical vessels

| Neck | Right side (22) | | Left side (11) | |
|---|---|---|---|---|
| | Artery | Vein | Artery | Vein |
| Absent | 0 | 1 | 0 | 1 |
| Removed | 2 | 2 | 0 | 0 |
| < 2 mm | 4 | 1 | 4 | 1 |
| 2 to 3 mm | 16 | 12 | 7 | 6 |
| > 3 mm | 0 | 6 | 0 | 3 |

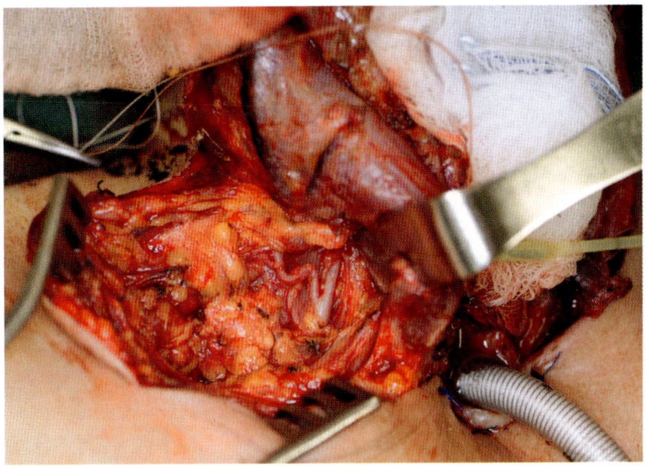

**Fig. 4.24** If the transverse cervical artery is too small, the thyrocervical trunk can be found more medially behind the sternocleidomastoid muscle. The thyrocervical trunk is much larger and can be a good recipient artery.

that has been previously irradiated and operated on often causes skin necrosis. Releasing the contracted neck and removing the scar tissue further creates a large defect in the neck skin. Therefore, a second flap is usually required to reconstruct the external defect when the jejunal flap or radial forearm flap is used for pharyngoesophageal reconstruction,[42,43,59] further complicating an already difficult case. The pedicled pectoralis major myocutaneous flap is probably the most frequently used flap for this purpose.[42,43] The main disadvantage of this flap is its bulk; even when the muscle alone is used, it often produces contour deformity in the neck and sometimes causes obstruction of the tracheostoma. Donor-site morbidity with the pectoralis major flap is particularly undesirable in women. Although the deltopectoral flap is thinner, its use is limited by the need for skin grafting to the donor site, the unreliability of the distal portion of the flap, and sometimes, the need for flap delay. Our choice of flap is the two-skin-island ALT flap, which provides simultaneous pharyngoesophageal reconstruction, neck resurfacing, and tracheostoma reconstruction.[60] In cases where only one cutaneous perforator is present, various amounts of vastus lateralis muscle can be included in the flap to support skin grafting to resurface the neck **(Fig. 4.25)**. The muscle portion of the ALT flap can be separated from the fasciocutaneous portion with only the cutaneous perforator attached, providing more flexibility in flap insetting. Alternatively, the AMT flap can be included with the ALT flap to create two fasciocutaneous flaps based on a single vascular pedicle.

In summary, the use of the transverse cervical vessels and multi-island ALT flap can convert an extremely difficult case with a frozen neck into a relatively straightforward one, reducing surgical risks and donor-site morbidities and improving quality of life.

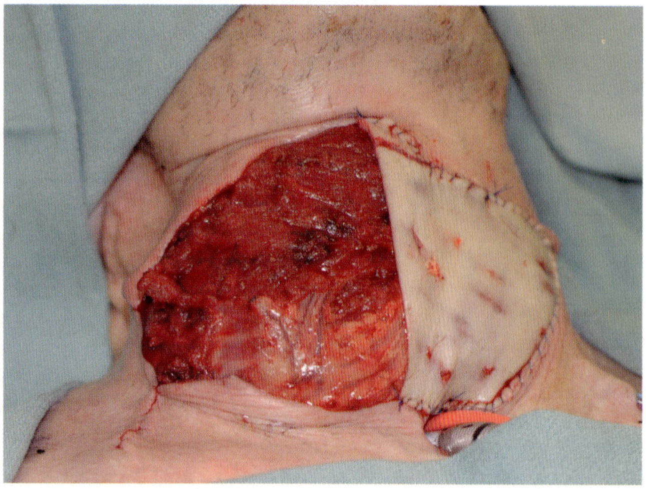

**Fig. 4.25** A through-and-through defect in the neck is inevitable after fistula resection. A multi-island ALT flap can simultaneously reconstruct both defects. When there is only one perforator, various amounts of the vastus lateralis muscle can be included to resurface the neck.

# Complications

## Pharyngocutaneous Fistula

In our experience,[33] pharyngocutaneous fistulas occurred in 9% of patients with ALT flap reconstruction. Fistula rates are similar in partial and circumferential reconstructions. Proximal fistulas are rare with the ALT flap. It has been speculated that the longitudinal seam of a tubed fasciocutaneous flap or two longitudinal suture lines in a partial defect might have contributed to a higher incidence of fistula formation with the radial forearm flap. However, in the author's experience, the fistula rate with the ALT flap is no higher than with the jejunal flap, and no fistulas have occurred through the longitudinal suture lines. Fistulas usually develop between 1 and 4 weeks postoperatively and manifest as leakage of saliva or liquids or, in some patients, as a neck infection. Therefore, any neck infection or abscess that occurs after a pharyngoesophageal reconstruction should raise suspicion for anastomotic leakage. Risk factors for fistula formation include improper suturing techniques, poor tissue quality at the anastomosis site, previous radiotherapy, and turbulent postoperative course. At the time of surgery, any questionable tissue in the proximal pharynx and cervical esophagus should be trimmed until only well-vascularized tissue is seen. The author uses single-layer, simple interrupted 3–0 polyglactin sutures for flap insetting, taking relatively big bites, inverting the skin/mucosa edges into the lumen, spacing each suture 5 to 7 mm apart, and avoiding tight knots.

Once a fistula is identified, oral intake is withheld and local wound care is initiated. Small fistulas, in the absence of tumor recurrence or distal obstruction, usually heal spontaneously within 2 weeks with conservative management. Therefore, a modified barium swallow (MBS) study is repeated 2 weeks later if the leakage has stopped. Larger fistulas or those with infection should be evaluated with computed tomography (CT) to rule out abscess and to assess the proximity of the fistula/abscess to the carotid artery. Any dead space or abscess around the carotid artery, especially in patients who have undergone previous radiotherapy or chemoradiation, should be thoroughly but carefully débrided without jeopardizing the carotid artery. The pectoralis major muscle flap is often used in such cases to protect the carotid artery. This should be done as soon as possible to prevent rupture of the carotid artery. Attempting to repair the leak or dehiscence at this stage will not be successful and may cause more tissue damage. The muscle flap is adequate to obliterate the fistula track and will remucosalize quickly. It is extremely important not to delay the débridement when infection/abscess is identified. Early intervention may achieve rapid healing and prevent life-threatening complications.

With proper management, persistent fistulas are rare. However, if a fistula does persist, the patient should be evaluated for possible tumor recurrence and distal obstruction/stricture. Long-standing fistulas will eventually cause stricture due to scar tissue formation, which in return results in a nonhealing fistula. In these cases, reconstruction with a radial forearm flap may be indicated in motivated patients who are in good general health and have a good prognosis.

## Anastomotic Strictures

Anastomotic strictures usually occur at the distal anastomosis several months or years following reconstruction. Spatulation and the use of the Montgomery bypass tube may reduce the risk of stricture formation. In the author's experience, strictures are most commonly seen in circumferential defect repair. Therefore, removal of the remaining posterior pharyngeal mucosa, thus converting a noncircumferential defect into a circumferential one, as is frequently done when the jejunal flap is used, should be avoided. The preservation of the posterior pharyngeal wall, if it is at least 10 mm wide, may help with the swallowing mechanism as well as prevent stricture.

If a patient develops dysphagia several months after reconstruction, anastomotic strictures should be suspected and an MBS study should be performed to confirm the diagnosis. In the past, surgical dilatation under general anesthesia was used to dilate anastomotic strictures, and serious complications, such as esophageal perforation, occurred. Endoscopic balloon dilatation has become the preferred treatment. This is usually done by a gastroenterologist. Repeated dilatations may be required in some patients. In refractory cases, surgical repair can be achieved with a radial forearm free flap.

## Neck Wound Infection

Neck wound infection is the result of (1) prolonged wound exposure and oral contamination during surgery or (2) an anastomotic leakage. Many patients with head and neck cancer have poor oral hygiene. Prior chemoradiation therapy can also increase the risk of infection. Copious irrigation and obliteration of dead space are important for preventing postoperative wound infection, which often occurs 5 to 7 days after surgery. Once infection occurs, early drainage and thorough débridement and irrigation may enable primary wound closure over a drain. However, part of the wound should be left open for dressing changes if the wound is deemed compromised. Additional flaps are usually not needed to manage infection. Early recognition of wound infection and intervention are crucial to avoiding delays in adjuvant therapy, as postoperative radiotherapy usually starts 4 to 6 weeks after surgery. In patients with diabetes, manifestations of wound infection may be very subtle, because they may not present with fevers or erythema of the neck. Rather, wound infection is indicated by an increase in the white blood cell count and in the blood sugar level. A CT scan can be performed to evaluate the neck when infection is suspected.

# ■ Postoperative Care

## General Postoperative Care

Traditionally, patients undergoing free flap reconstruction for pharyngoesophageal defects are kept in the surgical intensive care unit (ICU) overnight, are sedated, and are placed on a ventilator, with ventilator weaning the next morning. Patients are transferred to a flap monitoring floor by the afternoon. A potential problem with this approach is that sedation often causes hypotension, requiring fluid resuscitation, since pressors are generally considered contraindicated immediately after free flap surgery. This is not a problem for young and otherwise healthy patients. Elderly patients and those with limited cardiopulmonary reserve, however, may suffer fluid overload, congestive heart failure, and respiratory failure. Our recent approach is to extubate patients or to let them breathe spontaneously through the tracheostomy at the conclusion of surgery, thereby avoiding overnight sedation and ventilator support. Patients may go to regular recovery and then to our head and neck surgery/plastic surgery floor with adequate specialized nursing staff to manage the airway and to monitor flaps. Patients can also be admitted to the ICU for cardiac monitoring if indicated. We have found that the rapid awakening protocol significantly reduced medical complications and length of stay.

## Oral Diet

Oral feeding is withheld until an MBS study is performed by the speech pathologists to evaluate the swallowing function and healing process. Scheduling of the MBS study is from 1 to 6 weeks after reconstruction, depending on the type of flap used and prior radiotherapy (**Table 4.4**). MBS study is delayed for fasciocutaneous flaps due to the incidence of delayed fistula formation associated with the use of a fasciocutaneous flap.[20,28] If used, the Montgomery salivary bypass tube is removed before the MBS study. In patients with no evidence of leaks or fistula, a liquid diet is started and then advanced to a soft diet 3 days later if no complications occur. Diet can then be advanced to regular diet as tolerated. In patients with a leak or fistula, oral intake is withheld and an MBS study is repeated in 2 weeks or longer, as clinically indicated. Most leaks heal spontaneously within 2 weeks.

**Table 4.4** Timing of postoperative modified barium swallowing study

| Timing | ALT flap | Forearm flap | Jejunal flap |
|---|---|---|---|
| Prior radiation | 6 weeks | 6 weeks | 2 weeks |
| No radiation | 2 weeks | 2 weeks | 1 week |

ALT, anterolateral thigh.

### Voice Rehabilitation

Tracheoesophageal puncture (TEP) is the preferred method of voice rehabilitation. TEP is commonly used following a total laryngectomy without flap reconstruction. However, an increasing number of patients who undergo a flap reconstruction are being rehabilitated with TEP. TEP can be performed at the time of surgery (primary TEP) or several months after surgery with use of endoscopy (secondary TEP). Because of the higher failure rate of primary TEP with both the ALT and jejunal flaps,[33] secondary TEP, which is usually performed 4 or 5 months after reconstruction in patients without complications, is now preferred by the author. The reasons for the higher success rate of secondary TEP are most likely that these patients are free from surgical complications, are motivated, and are compliant. Patient selection for primary TEP can be difficult in some cases.

## Outcomes

In our early experience with 114 consecutive ALT flaps used for pharyngoesophageal reconstruction,[33] mean ICU stay was 1.9 ± 2.2 days, and mean hospital stay was 9.0 ± 4.7 days. Two patients experienced total flap loss and one patient had partial flap necrosis. Pharyngocutaneous fistulas and strictures occurred in 9% and 6% of patients, respectively. Ninety-one percent of patients tolerated an oral diet without the need for tube feeding. Tracheoesophageal puncture was performed for speech rehabilitation in 51 patients. Eighty-one percent of patients with a secondary TEP achieved fluent speech, versus 41% of patients with a primary TEP.

With jejunal flap reconstruction, average hospital stay was 13 days and average ICU stay was 3 days. The incidence of ileus and bowel obstruction was 9%, abdominal hernia, 6%, and anastomotic stricture, 19%. The fistula rate was lower (only 3%) when the "inexperienced surgeons" were excluded,[30] suggesting the importance of meticulous attention to technical details in such complex reconstructions. In contrast to fistulas with the ALT flap, approximately half of the fistulas with the jejunal flap occur at the proximal anastomosis,[24,26] possibly owing to slight stretching of the thin walls of the jejunal flap during flap insetting. Overall, 65% of patients tolerated an oral diet without supplemental tube feeding, 23% were partially tube-feeding dependent, and 12% were totally tube-feeding dependent. Fluent tracheoesophageal speech was achieved in 22% of patients who received a TEP. The quality of tracheoesophageal speech following jejunal flap reconstruction is usually characterized as "wet" compared with that following a fasciocutaneous flap reconstruction or a total laryngectomy without reconstruction.

Reported fistula rates with the radial forearm flap ranged from 17% to 40%, and stricture rates ranged from 17% to 50%.[18,19,20] Functional outcomes also varied considerably.

### Pearls and Pitfalls

- Although the jejunal flap has several advantages, such as rapid healing, low fistula rate, and no need to form a tube at the time of surgery, its abdominal morbidity and poor speech reproduction with TEP techniques make it less than ideal for pharyngoesophageal reconstruction. The ALT flap is now our flap of choice due to its many advantages. The only contraindication for using the ALT flap is obesity.
- A noncircumferential esophageal defect should not be converted to a circumferential one, because the former rarely results in anastomotic strictures.
- The distal flap–esophageal anastomosis should be spatulated to minimize stricture formation in circumferential defects.
- A layer of well-vascularized fascia of the ALT flap can be used to cover the suture lines, especially the distal anastomosis, to minimize the risk of anastomotic leakage and pharyngocutaneous fistula formation.
- Fasciocutaneous flaps provide better speech function than intestinal flaps.
- High-risk patients with significant comorbid diseases are relative contraindications for jejunal flap reconstruction. Fasciocutaneous flaps have much lower systemic morbidity.
- While bowel heals quickly when used for esophageal reconstruction, fasciocutaneous flaps may experience delayed healing when being soaked with saliva 24 hours a day, which may explain some delayed fistulas. Therefore, delayed oral intake is recommended, particularly in irradiated patients.
- Proper management of postoperative complications is important to prevent life-threatening sequelae and to maximize function.

## Expert Commentary *by Peter C. Neligan*

The chapter is a very complete description of techniques used in pharyngoesophageal reconstruction. As mentioned, free flaps have largely replaced the regional flaps that were once used to reconstruct these defects. While gastric pull-up was frequently used for this indication, and still is in some hands, it is fraught with potential problems and has been associated with a greater than 10% mortality rate.[61,62] One of the biggest problems is that the most distal part of the stomach flap, and therefore the least vascularized, is the very part of that flap that is used to reconstruct the proximal part of the resection, so that breakdown at this site is relatively common.[63] This can be mitigated by adding an extra anastomosis to improve the vascularity of the most distal part of the stomach repair.[64] Similar problems were seen with the older regional flaps and are one of the main reasons why they have largely been abandoned. The progression to free flaps, including the radial forearm, jejunum, and anterolateral thigh (ALT) flaps, is associated with much less morbidity. However, as Dr. Yu points out, the radial forearm flap has a terrible donor site as well as a significant stricture rate and in my practice is used only when the alternative flaps are not available. The jejunum was the go-to flap for this defect in the 1990s but has the disadvantage that the patient requires a laparotomy. This particular problem can be mitigated by endoscopic harvest of the jejunum that minimizes the morbidity traditionally associated with open harvest of the flap.[65] Besides restoring pharyngoesophageal continuity, there remains the problem of speech reproduction. Most pharyngoesophagectomy patients are rehabilitated using a tracheoesophageal puncture (TEP) technique with a voice prosthesis. The consensus is that because of the amount of mucus associated with the jejunum, jejunal speech is very throaty and moist, making it difficult to understand. For that reason, many surgeons, including the author, have switched to the more rigid skin flap that gives better, "drier" speech reproduction. Furthermore, laparotomy, even though it may be endoscopic, is avoided and the potential morbidity is less. One advantage of the ALT flap, which Dr. Yu points out, is that one can achieve a two-layered closure of the defect (the skin and the thigh fascia). One potential area of leakage is the vertical closure that is used to tube the flap. It has been my practice to place this line of repair against the prevertebral fascia and then to seal the repair laterally with sutures from the thigh fascia to the prevertebral fascia on either side. One other area where our approaches may differ slightly is that, in my practice, closure is routinely achieved over a Montgomery salivary tube, whereas in Dr. Yu's practice this is reserved for specific cases and is not used routinely. Instead of relying on specific measurements, the flap is designed to be three times the diameter of the tube being used. The tube, which is left in place for several weeks during healing, has been found to minimize the risk of fistula formation and is thought also to help with reducing the risk of stricture formation.[31] Our current practice is to suture the tube to a feeding tube. This makes removal easy and ensures that the salivary tube doesn't migrate distally, something that happened in the first few patients we used it in.

I fully agree with Dr. Yu that, when possible, the ALT can be split into two separate skin paddles. This is particularly important in cases where the pharyngoesophagus needs reconstruction in patients who also need external skin cover. In patients with only one perforator available, a second free flap might be required for the latter purpose. As Dr. Yu rightly points out, preoperative CT angiography is useful for showing the location and number of the perforators so that the case can be planned properly and in advance. However, if CTA has not been done or is not available, the fallback of the anteromedial thigh (AMT) flap is invariably available. Making the medial incision first allows the surgeon to evaluate the perforators and to go to the medial thigh if there are no suitable ALT perforators.

It has been our practice to avoid a second free flap if possible. This is achieved by utilizing the IMAP flap, based on the internal mammary perforators, if neck skin reconstruction is needed and a two-paddle ALT free flap is not possible. The IMAP flap can easily be pedicled up to replace the neck skin while the secondary defect can be closed directly on the chest.[66] This flap can also be used in cases of incomplete resection of the pharyngoesophagus as a pedicled flap to reconstruct the defect **(Fig. 4.26)**, again with direct closure of the donor defect.

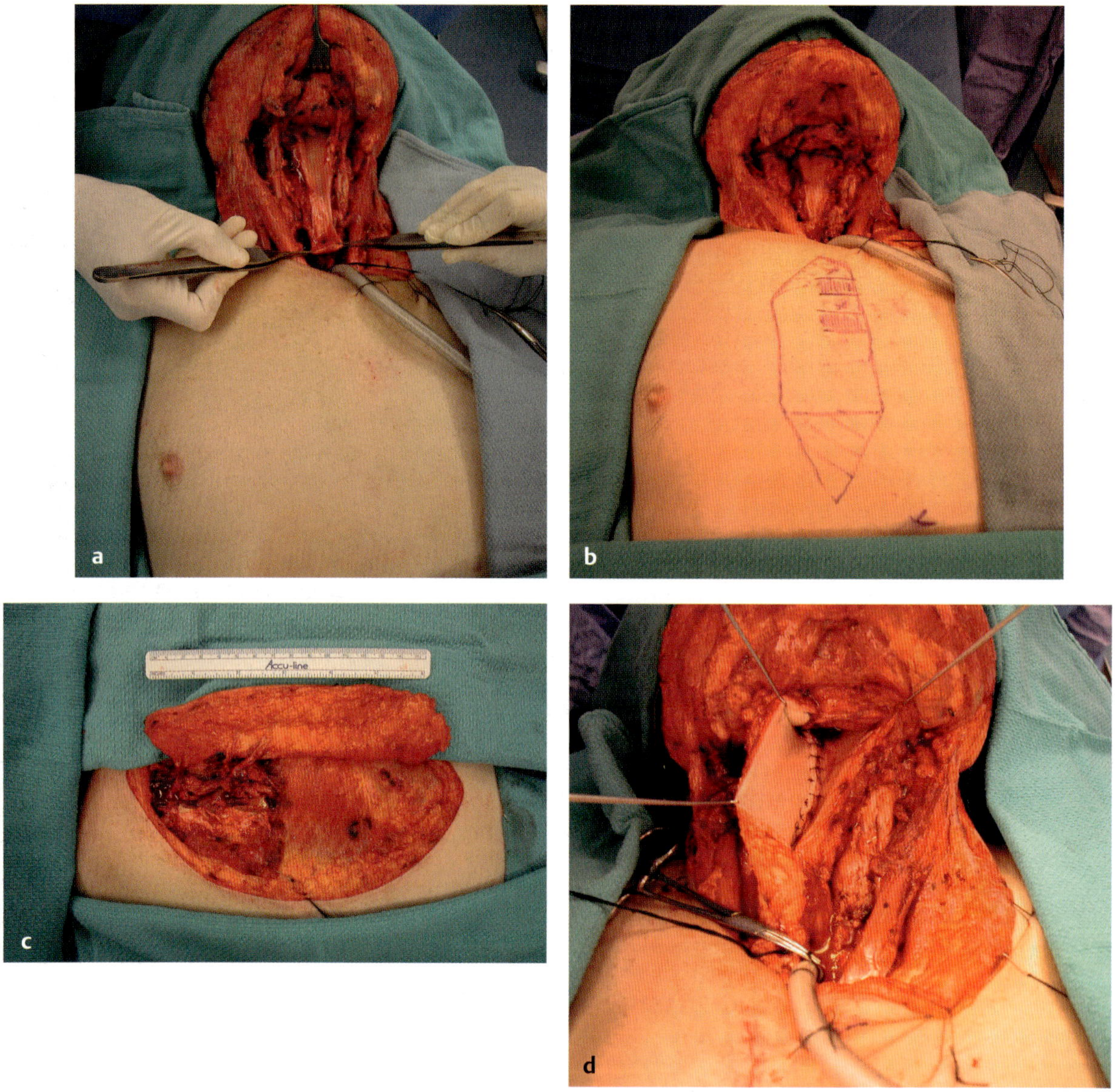


**Fig. 4.26** **(a)** Partial circumference hypopharyngeal defect following laryngopharyngectomy. **(b)** Design for internal mammary artery perforator (IMAP) flap to be used for pharyngeal reconstruction. **(c)** Elevation of IMAP flap. **(d)** Tubed inset of the pedicled IMAP flap into the neck to repair the subtotal pharyngectomy defect.

In terms of flap monitoring, we have moved away from using an external skin paddle and now routinely use a Synovis Flow Coupler (Synovis Micro Companies Alliance, Birmingham, AL) to monitor our flaps. It is placed on the draining vein and, in our hands, is very reliable.

In summary, then, Dr. Yu has provided a comprehensive overview of reconstruction of the pharyngoesophageal defect. He supplies great technical detail on how he completes the repair and imparts extremely useful information for anyone undertaking this surgery.

## References

1. Wookey H. The surgical treatment of carcinoma of the pharynx and upper esophagus. Surg Gynecol Obstet 1941;75:449
2. Moore FT, Faulkner T. Repair following pharyngo-oesophago-laryngectomy. Br J Plast Surg 1953;6(2): 102–113
3. Conley JJ. Management of pharyngostome, esophagostome and associated fistulae. Ann Otol Rhinol Laryngol 1956;65(1):76–91
4. Bakamjian VY. A two-stage method for pharyngoesophageal reconstruction with a primary pectoral skin flap. Plast Reconstr Surg 1965;36:173–184

5. Shefts LM, Fischer A. Carcinoma of the cervical esophagus with one-stage total esophageal resection and pharyngogastrostomy. Surgery 1949;25(6):849–861
6. Jack GD. Carcinoma of the hypopharynx and upper oesophagus. Br J Surg 1955;42(175):530–532
7. Ong GB, Lee TC. Pharyngogastric anastomosis after oesophago-pharyngectomy for carcinoma of the hypopharynx and cervical oesophagus. Br J Surg 1960;48:193–200
8. Le Quesne LP, Ranger D. Pharyngolaryngectomy, with immediate pharyngogastric anastomosis. Br J Surg 1966;53(2):105–109
9. Leonard JR, Maran AGD. Reconstruction of the cervical esophagus via gastric anastomosis. Laryngoscope 1970;80(6):849–862
10. Harrison DFN, Thompson AE, Buchanan G. Radical resection for cancer of the hypopharynx and cervical oesophagus with repair by stomach transposition. Br J Surg 1981;68(11):781–783
11. Lam KH, Wong J, Lim ST, Ong GB. Pharyngogastric anastomosis following pharyngolaryngoesophagectomy. Analysis of 157 cases. World J Surg 1981;5(4):509–516
12. Fredrickson JM, Wagenfeld DJ, Pearson G. Gastric pull-up vs deltopectoral flap for reconstruction of the cervical esophagus. Arch Otolaryngol 1981;107(10):613–616
13. Spiro RH, Shah JP, Strong EW, Gerold FP, Bains MS. Gastric transposition in head and neck surgery. Indications, complications, and expectations. Am J Surg 1983;146(4):483–487
14. Harrison AW. Transthoracic small bowel substitution in high stricture of the esophagus. J Thorac Surg 1949;18(3):316–326
15. Goligher JC, Robin IG. Use of left colon for reconstruction of pharynx and oesophagus after pharyngectomy. Br J Surg 1954;42(173):283–290
16. Slaney G, Dalton GA. Problems of viscus replacement following pharyngo-laryngectomy. J Laryngol Otol 1973;87(6):539–546
17. Anthony JP, Singer MI, Mathes SJ. Pharyngoesophageal reconstruction using the tubed free radial forearm flap. Clin Plast Surg 1994;21(1):137–147
18. Cho BC, Kim M, Lee JH, Byun JS, Park JS, Baik BS. Pharyngoesophageal reconstruction with a tubed free radial forearm flap. J Reconstr Microsurg 1998;14(8):535–540
19. Azizzadeh B, Yafai S, Rawnsley JD, et al. Radial forearm free flap pharyngoesophageal reconstruction. Laryngoscope 2001;111(5):807–810
20. Scharpf J, Esclamado RM. Reconstruction with radial forearm flaps after ablative surgery for hypopharyngeal cancer. Head Neck 2003;25(4):261–266
21. Coleman JJ III, Searles JM Jr, Hester TR, et al. Ten years experience with the free jejunal autograft. Am J Surg 1987;154(4):394–398
22. Coleman JJ III, Tan KC, Searles JM, Hester TR, Nahai F. Jejunal free autograft: analysis of complications and their resolution. Plast Reconstr Surg 1989;84(4):589–595, discussion 596–598
23. Schusterman MA, Shestak K, de Vries EJ, et al. Reconstruction of the cervical esophagus: free jejunal transfer versus gastric pull-up. Plast Reconstr Surg 1990;85(1): 16–21
24. Reece GP, Schusterman MA, Miller MJ, et al. Morbidity and functional outcome of free jejunal transfer reconstruction for circumferential defects of the pharynx and cervical esophagus. Plast Reconstr Surg 1995; 96(6):1307–1316
25. Cordeiro PG, Shah K, Santamaria E, Gollub MJ, Singh B, Shah JP. Barium swallows after free jejunal transfer: should they be performed routinely? Plast Reconstr Surg 1999;103(4):1167–1175
26. Chang DW, Hussussian C, Lewin JS, Youssef AA, Robb GL, Reece GP. Analysis of pharyngocutaneous fistula following free jejunal transfer for total laryngopharyngectomy. Plast Reconstr Surg 2002;109(5): 1522–1527
27. Disa JJ, Pusic AL, Hidalgo DA, Cordeiro PG. Microvascular reconstruction of the hypopharynx: defect classification, treatment algorithm, and functional outcome based on 165 consecutive cases. Plast Reconstr Surg 2003; 111(2):652–660, discussion 661–663
28. Yu P, Robb GL. Pharyngoesophageal reconstruction with the anterolateral thigh flap: a clinical and functional outcomes study. Plast Reconstr Surg 2005;116(7): 1845–1855
29. Genden EM, Jacobson AS. The role of the anterolateral thigh flap for pharyngoesophageal reconstruction. Arch Otolaryngol Head Neck Surg 2005;131(9):796–799
30. Yu P, Lewin JS, Reece GP, Robb GL. Comparison of clinical and functional outcomes and hospital costs following pharyngoesophageal reconstruction with the anterolateral thigh free flap versus the jejunal flap. Plast Reconstr Surg 2006;117(3):968–974
31. Murray DJ, Gilbert RW, Vesely MJ, et al. Functional outcomes and donor site morbidity following circumferential pharyngoesophageal reconstruction using an anterolateral thigh flap and salivary bypass tube. Head Neck 2007;29(2):147–154
32. Spyropoulou GA, Kuo YR, Chien CY, Yang JC, Jeng SF. Buried anterolateral thigh flap for pharyngoesophageal reconstruction: our method for monitoring. Head Neck 2009;31(7):882–887
33. Yu P, Hanasono MM, Skoracki RJ, et al. Pharyngoesophageal reconstruction with the anterolateral thigh flap after total laryngopharyngectomy. Cancer 2010;116(7): 1718–1724
34. Yu P. Characteristics of the anterolateral thigh flap in a Western population and its application in head and neck reconstruction. Head Neck 2004;26(9):759–769
35. Yu P, Youssef A. Efficacy of the handheld Doppler in preoperative identification of the cutaneous perforators in the anterolateral thigh flap. Plast Reconstr Surg 2006;118(4):928–933, discussion 934–935
36. Garvey PB, Selber JC, Madewell JE, Bidaut L, Feng L, Yu P. A prospective study of preoperative computed tomographic angiography for head and neck reconstruction with anterolateral thigh flaps. Plast Reconstr Surg 2011;127(4):1505–1514
37. Yu P, Selber J. Perforator patterns of the anteromedial thigh flap. Plast Reconstr Surg 2011;128(3):151e–157e

38. Yu P, Selber J, Liu J. Reciprocal dominance of the anterolateral and anteromedial thigh flap perforator anatomy. Ann Plast Surg 2013;70(6):714–716
39. Ferguson RE Jr, Yu P. Techniques of monitoring buried fasciocutaneous free flaps. Plast Reconstr Surg 2009;123(2):525–532
40. Yu P, Chang EI, Selber JC, Hanasono MM. Perforator patterns of the ulnar artery perforator flap. Plast Reconstr Surg 2012;129(1):213–220
41. Chang SC, Miller G, Halbert CF, Yang KH, Chao WC, Wei FC. Limiting donor site morbidity by suprafascial dissection of the radial forearm flap. Microsurgery 1996;17(3):136–140
42. Reece GP, Bengtson BP, Schusterman MA. Reconstruction of the pharynx and cervical esophagus using free jejunal transfer. Clin Plast Surg 1994;21(1):125–136
43. Disa JJ, Cordeiro PG. Reconstruction of the hypopharynx and cervical esophagus. Clin Plast Surg 2001;28(2):349–360
44. Marin VP, Yu P, Weber RS. Isolated cervical esophageal reconstruction for rare esophageal tumors. Head Neck 2006;28(9):856–860
45. Wolf GT, Hong WK, Fisher SG, et al; The Department of Veterans Affairs Laryngeal Cancer Study Group. Induction chemotherapy plus radiation compared with surgery plus radiation in patients with advanced laryngeal cancer. N Engl J Med 1991;324(24):1685–1690
46. León X, Quer M, Orús C, López M, Gras JR, Vega M. Results of salvage surgery for local or regional recurrence after larynx preservation with induction chemotherapy and radiotherapy. Head Neck 2001;23(9):733–738
47. Moore BA, Holsinger FC, Diaz EM Jr, Weber RS. Organ-preservation laryngeal surgery in the era of chemoradiation. Curr Probl Cancer 2005;29(4):169–179
48. Genden EM, Rinaldo A, Shaha AR, Bradley PJ, Rhys-Evans PH, Ferlito A. Pharyngocutaneous fistula following laryngectomy. Acta Otolaryngol 2004;124(2):117–120
49. McCombe AW, Jones AS. Radiotherapy and complications of laryngectomy. J Laryngol Otol 1993;107(2):130–132
50. Hier M, Black MJ, Lafond G. Pharyngo-cutaneous fistulas after total laryngectomy: incidence, etiology and outcome analysis. J Otolaryngol 1993;22(3):164–166
51. Natvig K, Boysen M, Tausjø J. Fistulae following laryngectomy in patients treated with irradiation. J Laryngol Otol 1993;107(12):1136–1139
52. Weber RS, Berkey BA, Forastiere A, et al. Outcome of salvage total laryngectomy following organ preservation therapy: the Radiation Therapy Oncology Group trial 91-11. Arch Otolaryngol Head Neck Surg 2003;129(1):44–49
53. Fowler BZ, Muller S, Chen AY, Johnstone PAS. Factors influencing long-term survival following salvage total laryngectomy after initial radiotherapy or conservative surgery. Head Neck 2006;28(2):99–106
54. Forastiere AA, Goepfert H, Maor M, et al. Concurrent chemotherapy and radiotherapy for organ preservation in advanced laryngeal cancer. N Engl J Med 2003;349(22):2091–2098
55. Goodwin WJ Jr. Salvage surgery for patients with recurrent squamous cell carcinoma of the upper aerodigestive tract: when do the ends justify the means? Laryngoscope 2000;110(3 Pt 2, Suppl 93):1–18
56. Iteld L, Yu P. Pharyngocutaneous fistula repair after radiotherapy and salvage total laryngectomy. J Reconstr Microsurg 2007;23(6):339–345
57. Yu P. The transverse cervical vessels as recipient vessels for previously treated head and neck cancer patients. Plast Reconstr Surg 2005;115(5):1253–1258
58. Goodwin WJ Jr, Rosenberg GJ. Venous drainage of the lateral trapezius musculocutaneous island flap. Arch Otolaryngol 1982;108(7):411–413
59. McCarthy CM, Kraus DH, Cordeiro PG. Tracheostomal and cervical esophageal reconstruction with combined deltopectoral flap and microvascular free jejunal transfer after central neck exenteration. Plast Reconstr Surg 2005;115(5):1304–1310, discussion 1311–1313
60. Yu P. One-stage reconstruction of complex pharyngoesophageal, tracheal, and anterior neck defects. Plast Reconstr Surg 2005;116(4):949–956
61. Collin CF, Spiro RH. Carcinoma of the cervical esophagus: changing therapeutic trends. Am J Surg 1984;148(4):460–466
62. Joshi P, Nair S, D'Cruz AK. Hypopharyngeal cancers requiring reconstruction. Otolaryngol Head Neck Surg 2012;147:161
63. Joshi P, Nair S, Chaturvedi P, et al. Hypopharyngeal cancers requiring reconstruction: a single institute experience. Indian J Otolaryngol Head Neck Surg 2013;65(Suppl 1):135–139
64. Kawai KI, Kakibuchi M, Sakagami M, Fujimoto J, Toyosaka A, Nakai K. Supercharged gastric tube pull-up procedure for total esophageal reconstruction. Ann Plast Surg 2001;47(4):390–393
65. Kim WW, Gagner M, Fukuyama S, et al. Laparoscopic harvesting of small bowel graft for small bowel transplantation. Surg Endosc 2002;16(12):1786–1789
66. Vesely MJ, Murray DJ, Novak CB, Gullane PJ, Neligan PC. The internal mammary artery perforator flap: an anatomical study and a case report. Ann Plast Surg 2007;58(2):156–161

# 5 Reconstruction of Tracheal Defects

*Peirong Yu*

## Introduction

Tracheal reconstruction after surgical resection is difficult because of several tracheal characteristics, including the rigidity needed to maintain an open lumen, the need for an intact luminal lining, the required ability to clear secretions, and the trachea's proximity to major blood vessels. Reconstruction of long tracheal defects has not been possible until recently.[1] Therefore, patients with extensive tracheal involvement are typically not considered surgical candidates, or they may require total laryngectomy and possibly a mediastinal tracheostomy, which has high mortality rates. Successful tracheal reconstruction may extend surgical indications, preserve laryngeal function, avoid the high-risk mediastinal tracheostomy, and improve quality of life. The ultimate goal of tracheal reconstruction is to provide a noncollapsible airway, with a stable epithelial lining and reliable, well-vascularized tissue coverage.

Tracheal reconstruction requires careful planning and expert team effort from many disciplines, including head and neck surgery, thoracic surgery, reconstructive surgery, critical care, and anesthesiology, as well as extensive nursing care to avoid life-threatening complications. Anesthesiologists must have experience in airway surgery and a good basic understanding of the sequence of tracheal reconstruction, and they must be prepared to frequently change the endotracheal tube during surgery. Many patients have unilateral vocal cord paralysis, which further complicates surgery by increasing the risk for aspiration and airway compromise. A history of external-beam radiation therapy also greatly increases the degree of difficulty in surgical dissection and the surgical risks. Major tracheal surgery and reconstruction thus should be performed in specialized centers with expertise from multiple disciplines.

## Regional Anatomy

The adult human trachea has an average length of 11.8 cm, with a range of 10 to 13 cm from the lower border of the cricoid cartilage to the top of the carina. There are usually 18 to 22 cartilaginous rings in the trachea, thus ~ 2 rings per centimeter of length. Three-fifths of the trachea is above the sternal notch in juveniles; the proportion changes to about one-half of the trachea in young adults, and only one-third or less in older adults. However, with the neck flexed, the trachea is almost entirely mediastinal and the cricoid cartilage drops to the thoracic inlet. There is ~ 1.5 cm of subglottic larynx present between the vocal cords and the lower margin of the cricoid. The tracheal wall is ~ 3 mm thick. The trachea has an average inner diameter of 2.3 cm across and 1.8 cm in the anterior-posterior dimension in adult males, and 2.0 cm and 1.4 cm, respectively, in females. The trachea is smaller and more circular in children. The cartilaginous rings that surround the anterior two-thirds of the trachea provide tracheal rigidity. In youth, the tracheal wall is elastic laterally. The elasticity decreases significantly with age, particularly when calcification occurs in cartilages. The posterior wall is membranous-muscular and contracts during coughing and spasm, with the trachealis muscle pulling the lateral cartilaginous walls of the trachea medially. The intercartilaginous muscles between the rings and muscles in the membranous wall contract simultaneously.

Histologically, the trachea is lined with respiratory mucosa. The epithelial cells are columnar cells and are ciliated. The cilia function to clear particulate matters and secretions. There are numerous submucosal mucous glands, which are connected to the surface by ducts. In smokers and patients with chronic irritation, squamous metaplasia may occur, and the cilia are destroyed. Secretions may still be successfully cleared by cough despite metaplasia.

The blood supply to the trachea is segmental and shared with the esophagus. The upper half of the trachea is mainly supplied by three tracheoesophageal branches of the inferior thyroid artery, which is a branch of the thyrocervical trunk arising from the subclavian artery. The posterior membranous wall of the trachea is also supplied by secondary small branches from the primary esophageal vessels branching from the tracheoesophageal arteries. The tracheal cartilages receive nourishment from the submucosal plexus only. The superior thyroid artery does not give direct branches to the trachea, but it does anastomose with the inferior thyroid artery. The arteries approach the trachea and esophagus laterally. Therefore, extensive dissection laterally may devascularize the trachea and/or esophagus. Circumferential dissection of the trachea should not exceed 1 or 2 cm. The lower half of the trachea is supplied by bronchial arteries.

The main surgical diseases of the trachea are tumor, trauma, and congenital anomalies, such as tracheal atresia. Most trauma-related diseases of the trachea are strictures from prolonged intubation. Tumors of the trachea can be primary or secondary. Primary tracheal tumors are uncommon, but most are malignant and are diagnosed long after the onset of symptoms.[2] The two most common tracheal tumors are adenoid cystic carcinoma and squamous cell carcinoma. Secondary tracheal neoplasms are more common and usually result from direct invasion by carcinomas of the esophagus, larynx, thyroid, or lung. Most patients with lung cancer present with locally advanced (T3 or T4 lesions) or metastatic disease. Patients with T4 tumors of the lung (e.g., invasion of the trachea or carina) can still benefit from extended surgical resections.[3,4,5,6] In our practice, the most common tracheal lesions are the result of advanced thyroid cancer involving the trachea.

## ■ Historical Perspective on Tracheal Reconstruction

Small windows in the trachea can be patched or closed primarily. Short tracheal defects (up to 2 cm) may be closed primarily.[1] With the neck in 15 to 35 degrees of flexion, 1,000 to 1,200 g of tension applied to the divided tracheal ends may permit a reapproximation of a 4.5 cm gap.[5,6] Mobilizing the right hilum with the pleura open may allow an additional 1.4 cm of resection but with increased anastomotic complications and mortality.[4,5] A longer gap cannot be closed primarily; therefore, reconstruction with a tracheal conduit will be required. In elderly patients, a radiated trachea, or a previously operated neck, even a 4 or 5 cm defect may not be able to be closed primarily due to tracheal calcification, fibrosis, and reduced elasticity and blood supply.

Early methods in experimental studies were limited to rigid prosthetic replacement, such as with metal tubes, polypropylene mesh, and polytetrafluoroethylene (PTFE) graft. Without viable lining and tissue integration of the prosthetic materials, such primitive replacements were doomed to fail.[7,8,9,10,11] Simple prosthetic replacement resulted in nonhealing tracheal ends, occlusion by granulation tissue, infection, strictures, and erosion of major blood vessels.

A soft tissue flap alone will collapse immediately. Intraluminal stenting with a prosthesis causes irritation and inflammatory responses that result in problematic secretions and will eventually fail.[12] Therefore, the supporting material needs to be placed outside the flap lining to support it and prevent collapse. Many prosthetic materials have been tested, but few are suitable for clinical use. Cartilage has been shown to resorb, causing airway collapse.[13] Processed cadaveric tracheal allografts are highly subject to infection and rejection when exposed. A short allograft may survive initially if wrapped with vascularized tissue, such as the omentum, but such reconstructions are prone to resorption and loss of rigidity, leading to stricture, airway collapse, and death.[14,15,16,17] These materials are particularly unsuitable for cancer patients because of the need for radiotherapy. Recent advances in tissue engineering show some promise,[18,19,20] but use of engineered tissue in cancer patients, who often require chemotherapy and radiation, can be very limited. In addition, tissue engineering needs time. Cancer patients may not have the luxury of time to wait for the creation of a tissue-engineered trachea. Reconstruction of oncologic tracheal defects needs to be immediate and well vascularized, such as with microvascular free tissue transfer.

## ■ Methods of Reconstruction

Methods of reconstruction depend on the size of the defects. To guide surgical planning, a defect classification system is proposed **(Table 5.1)**. Patients with types I and II defects have an intact larynx, whereas those with type III defects do not.[21,22,23,24,25,26,27,28,29,30,31,32,33]

### Type I Defects

Type I defects are small defects that can be closed primarily with or without additional maneuvers. Defects less than 2 cm in length (type Ia) in

**Table 5.1** Classification of tracheal defects

| Type | Description | Defect size | Larynx | Reconstruction technique |
|---|---|---|---|---|
| I | Small defects | Ia: < 2 cm in length<br>Ib: 2–5 cm in length | Intact | Ia: Simple primary closure.<br>Ib: Primary closure with laryngeal release ± hilar mobilization |
| II | Large defects | Length > 5 cm | Intact | Free flap with rigid support, tissue-engineered trachea, tracheal transplantation |
| III | Tracheostoma defects | IIIa: part of laryngopharyngectomy<br>IIIb: tracheostoma defect | Absent or nonfunctional | Local flap or free flap without rigid support |

the longitudinal dimension can be closed primarily by direct approximation with interrupted 2–0 polydioxanone sulfate (PDS) sutures. Larger defects with a length less than 4 or 5 cm (type Ib) can still be closed primarily in an end-to-end fashion with suprahyoid laryngeal release **(Fig. 5.1)**. Suprahyoid release can typically provide an additional 1.5 to 2 cm for closure, depending on the elasticity of the trachea, which further depends on the patient's age and history of prior surgery and radiation therapy. Mobilization of the right hilum may provide an additional 1.4 cm of length. Thus, a 5.5 cm long defect can potentially be closed primarily with suprahyoid release and hilar mobilization, with the neck flexed at 15 to 35 degrees by suturing the chin to the chest skin. Such maneuvers, however, do not provide adequate length for primary closure in patients who have had multiple operations or radiation therapy in the past or in older patients. Serious airway complications and mortality increase significantly with increasing length of the defect beyond 4 cm. Coverage of the tracheal anastomosis with a muscle flap, such as a pectoralis major, is strongly recommended in all patients who undergo aggressive paratracheal dissection resulting in a significant dead space in the neck, have had prior radiotherapy, or plan to have postoperative radiotherapy. Suprahyoid laryngeal release should be performed judiciously in patients with vocal cord paralysis, especially in those with compromised pulmonary function, as it increases the risk for dysphagia and aspiration.

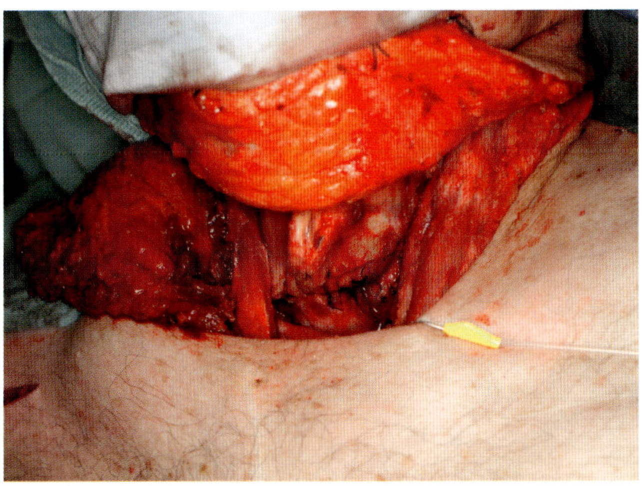

**Fig. 5.1** Small defects can be closed primarily with or without laryngeal release. A pectoralis major muscle flap is often used to cover the suture line and to obliterate dead space.

## Type II Defects

The ultimate goals of tracheal reconstruction of type II defects are to provide a noncollapsible airway with a functional epithelial lining and reliable, well-vascularized tissue coverage. This requires microsurgical reconstruction.

### Supporting Material

The first priority in tracheal reconstruction is to maintain a rigid airway that does not collapse. Supporting materials for tracheal reconstruction are not readily available. We have tested several materials in animal studies, including polytetrafluoroethylene (PTFE) ring vascular grafts, Medpor porous polyethylene sheets (Stryker, Kalamazoo, MI), Hemashield vascular grafts (Boston Scientific, Natick, MA), and PolyMax poly-L-lactide resorbable mesh (Synthes, West Chester, PA). We have found that both PTFE and Medpor materials have poor tissue integration and are prone to exposure and extrusion. The Hemashield graft has good tissue integration but lacks rigidity. The PolyMax mesh is rigid but resorbable. Therefore, we combined the Hemashield and PolyMax mesh to create a noncollapsible airway.

To maintain an adequate airway and to accommodate a soft tissue flap lining, the diameter of the rigid construct needs to be ~ 30 mm. The thickness of the lining flap with a certain degree of swelling will account for at least 10 mm. Therefore, a 30 mm diameter prosthetic construct will leave a 20 mm diameter final airway lumen. The Hemashield vascular graft has a diameter of 26 mm. The Hemashield graft is longitudinally opened and reinforced with a sheet of 0.5 mm thick Synthes PolyMax resorbable mesh.[34,35] The PolyMax mesh with the desired width and length is placed in hot water (> 70°C) in a sterile water bath. Once it becomes soft in hot water, the sheet of mesh is placed on a large sterile syringe with a diameter of 30 mm to form a semicircular tube. The mesh hardens at room temperature. Additional trimming can be easily done with a pair of Mayo suture scissors. The mesh is then placed inside the Hemashield graft. Depending on the circumference involved in the tracheal defect, this construct can be fashioned as a small patch, a half circle, or up to three-quarters of the circumference.

## Soft Tissue Flap

The lining flap of the neotrachea needs to have a reliable blood supply and an epithelial surface, and it must be thin. The radial forearm flap meets these criteria. The dimensions of the flap are outlined according to the size of the defect, with the distal border of the flap near the wrist crease. The flap is elevated with suprafascial dissection. A cutaneous perforator can usually be found in the proximal forearm to create a monitoring skin island **(Fig. 5.2)**. Before its

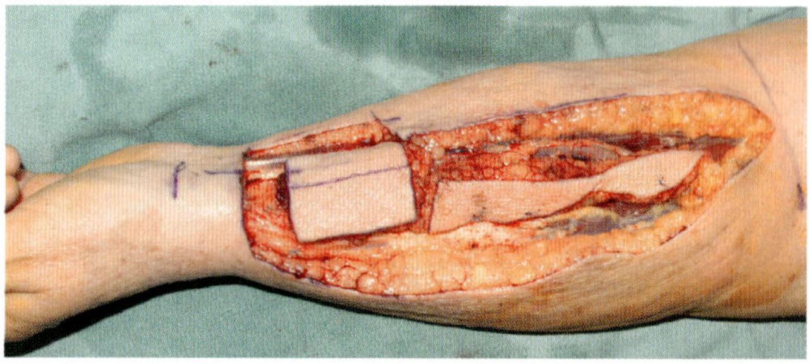

**Fig. 5.2** When raising the radial forearm flap, a small monitoring flap can be designed in the proximal forearm based on a separate perforator.

vascular pedicle is divided, the radial forearm flap is placed inside the construct, with the skin side facing the lumen. The flap is suspended to the construct with multiple 3–0 polypropylene sutures through the dermis of the flap to prevent collapse. These suspension sutures should be placed away from the vascular pedicle and are loosely tied to avoid vascular compromise of the flap **(Fig. 5.3)**. A small window is created at the end of the prosthesis where the vascular pedicle will be brought out. The final neotrachea is now ready for transfer.

## Flap Insetting

For most tracheal defects, reconstruction can be performed through the neck incision with or without removing the clavicular head and manubrium.

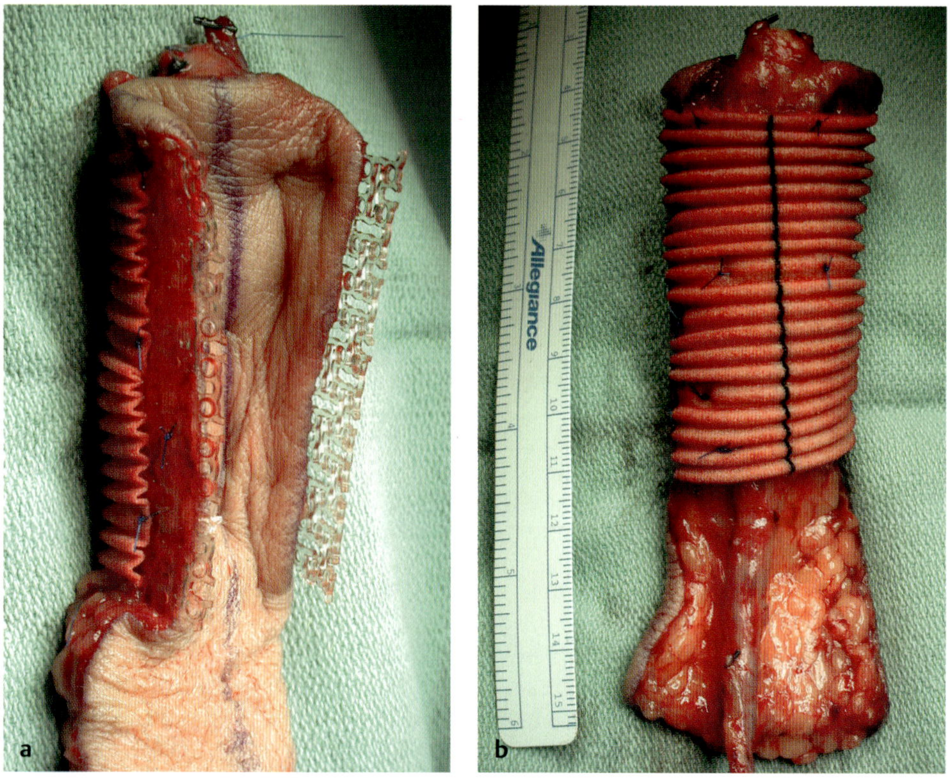



**Fig. 5.3** Fabrication of the neotrachea. **(a)** A Hemashield aortic graft is longitudinally opened and stented with PolyMax mesh. **(b)** A radial forearm flap is placed inside the lumen and is suspended to the construct with polypropylene sutures.

Recipient vessels for microvascular anastomosis are usually readily available in the neck. If the upper neck is not exposed, the transverse cervical artery and vein lower in the neck are good recipient vessels with good size match with the flap vascular pedicle. The superior thyroid artery and a branch of the common facial vein stump that drains into the internal jugular vein are also good recipient vessel choices. Alternatively, the internal mammary artery and vein can be used if the clavicular head and manubrium are removed.

The neotrachea is placed over the tracheal defect with the vascular pedicle coming out on the laryngeal end. The radial forearm flap is sewn to the remaining tracheal wall on the recipient vessel side first using 3–0 polyglactin sutures **(Fig. 5.4)**. Vascular anastomoses are then performed under an operating microscope. Once the neotrachea is revascularized, the remaining flap insetting is completed **(Fig. 5.5)**. The patient is allowed to breath spontaneously at this point. The endotracheal tube is withdrawn above the tracheal defect. A Montgomery T-tube (Boston Medical Products, Westborough, MA) tracheal stent is inserted into the neotracheal lumen between the distal end of the flap and the native trachea. The prosthetic material around the T-tube is trimmed back for a few millimeters so that it is not exposed to the tracheostomy site. The endotracheal tube is completely withdrawn. Bronchoscopy is performed through the T-tube to evaluate the reconstruction and airway patency. The T-tube is an important temporary measure to "stent" the lumen to prevent occlusion from flap swelling and to avoid high airway pressure during coughing, which may cause air leak or even anastomosis disruption.

The neotrachea is then covered externally with well-vascularized tissue. This can be accomplished with either a sternocleidomastoid or a pectoralis major muscle flap. The latter is preferred in patients with a big neck and extensive lymph node dissection that leaves some dead space around the trachea or in a previously irradiated neck. The muscle flap covers the entire tracheal reconstruction and wraps around the T-tube **(Fig. 5.6)**. A 15 Fr Blake drain is placed on each side of the neck. A small monitoring skin flap, based on a perforator vessel in the proximal forearm, is brought outside the neck through the neck incision for flap monitoring purposes **(Fig. 5.7)**.

The neck is irrigated with an ample amount of normal saline and is returned to a neutral position.

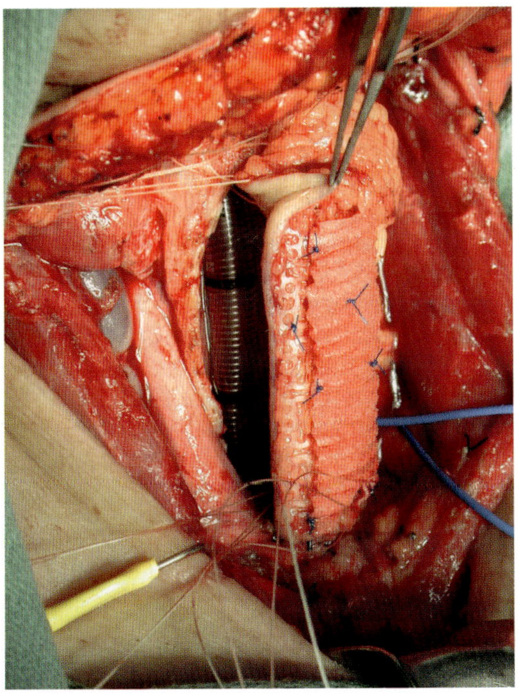

**Fig. 5.4** The neotrachea is placed over the tracheal defect with the vascular pedicle coming out on the laryngeal end. The radial forearm flap is sewn to the remaining tracheal wall on the recipient vessel side first, before revascularization, using 3–0 polyglactin sutures.

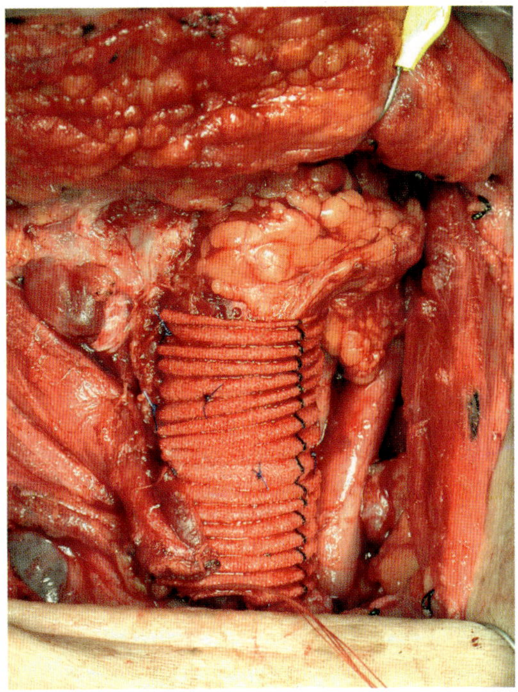

**Fig. 5.5** The remaining flap insetting is completed after vascular anastomoses are completed.

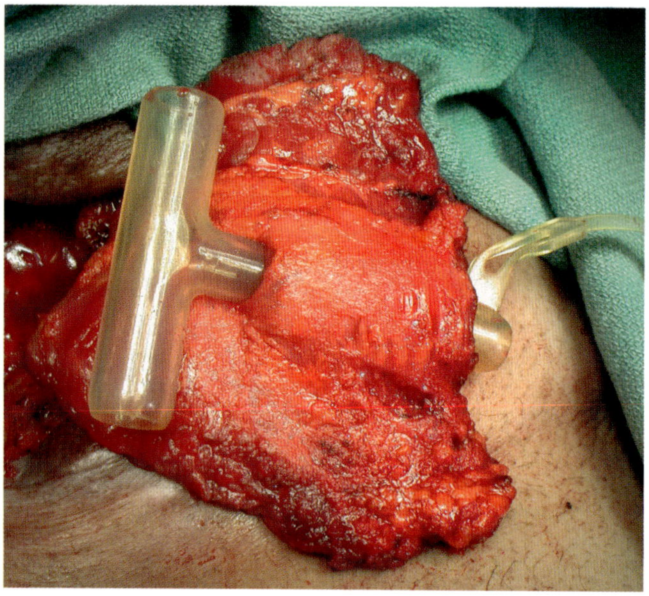

**Fig. 5.6** A pectoralis muscle flap covers the entire tracheal reconstruction and wraps around the T-tube tracheostomy tube.

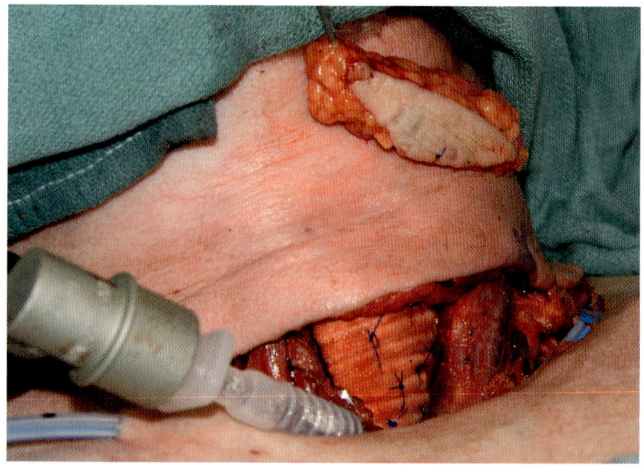

**Fig. 5.7** A 15 Fr Blake drain is placed on each side of the neck. The small monitoring skin flap, based on a perforator vessel in the proximal forearm, is brought outside the neck through the neck incision for flap monitoring purposes and is removed at bedside before discharge.

The vascular pedicle and anastomoses are inspected to ensure that there is no kinking, twisting, or compression on the vascular pedicle before closure of the neck incision. A Dobhoff nasogastric feeding tube is placed for temporary feeding during the acute postoperative period.[36]

## Postoperative Care

Meticulous perioperative care is given as part of a combined team effort. Patients are placed in a surgical intensive care unit (ICU) after surgery for close monitoring of their airway. Since there is no cuff on the T-tube to provide positive ventilation, patients are awake and breathing spontaneously at the time of T-tube placement, and they are kept awake throughout the postoperative period. Bronchoscopy through the T-tube is performed daily for 3 days to assess flap viability and airway patency and to clear secretions. Because many patients have unilateral vocal cord paralysis, a bedside swallowing test is given to all patients by a speech pathologist before feeding is attempted during recovery. Once the patient is tolerating an oral diet, the Dobhoff feeding tube is removed. Neck drains are removed once drainage is less than 30 mL in a 24-hr period for 2 consecutive days with no air leak. The monitoring skin flap outside the neck is removed at the bedside 5 to 7 days after surgery.

Patients are followed up in the clinic at regular intervals after discharge. Bronchoscopy is performed before discharge and at 6-month follow-up or as clinically indicated. Postoperative radiation therapy can be started 5 to 6 weeks after surgery. The T-tube can usually be removed 4 to 6 weeks after surgery when the reconstructed airway has healed and airway patency is confirmed with bronchoscopy. Follow-up imaging studies are performed for tumor surveillance and to assess the reconstructed trachea.

## Type III Defects

Type III defects involve the tracheal wall below the tracheostoma in patients with a total laryngectomy. Because of the absence of a larynx, the goal of tracheal reconstruction is to repair the tracheostoma or to extend the tracheostoma from the mediastinal trachea to the neck above the sternal notch with a soft tissue flap. The tracheostoma can be easily stented with a silicon tube (Larry tube), so rigid reconstruction is not required. Tracheal resection can be part of an extensive total laryngopharyngectomy that involves simultaneous reconstruction of the cervical esophagus and trachea (IIIa). An isolated tracheostoma/tracheal defect (IIIb) is usually the result of tracheostomal recurrence.

A type IIIa defect associated with a total laryngopharyngectomy usually involves only the posterior wall of the cervical trachea. Simultaneous reconstruction of the tracheostoma and pharyngoesophageal defect is best served with a two-skin-island anterolateral thigh (ALT) flap, which provides reliable reconstruction with a single flap, superior functional outcome, and minimal donor-site morbidity.[37,38,39,40] The main flap is used for pharyngoesophageal reconstruction. A second skin paddle based on an independent perforator is used for tracheostoma reconstruction.

When a total laryngectomy and total esophagectomy with extensive tracheal resection are performed, the remaining trachea above the carina is usually only 3 to 4 cm long. Therefore, double free flap reconstruction for the esophagus and trachea is indicated. The total esophagectomy defect requires a supercharged jejunal flap to reach all the way to the base of the tongue.[41] The tracheal defect is reconstructed with a tubed ALT free flap. The reconstructive sequence requires careful planning. If the jejunal flap is pulled up to the neck first before tracheal reconstruction, it would be nearly impossible to inset the ALT flap to the mediastinal tracheal end due to limited exposure. If tracheal reconstruction is performed first, pulling up the jejunal flap through the mediastinum may risk disrupting the ALT-tracheal anastomosis. The author's approach is to harvest the ALT flap first. Sutures are then placed between the ALT flap and the mediastinal trachea as parachuting sutures. These sutures are not tied, and the flap is placed outside the mediastinum. The ALT flap is then revascularized. At this point, the jejunal flap is prepared. The second mesentery vessels are usually used for supercharging in the neck to either the transverse cervical vessels or the internal mammary vessels. The third mesentery vessels are divided and are ligated to increase the reach. The fourth mesentery vessels serve as the vascular pedicle for the pedicled portion of the flap **(Fig. 5.8)**. The mesentery between the second and third mesentery vessels is divided to the bowel wall to unfurl the small bowel, while the mesentery arcade vessels between the third and fourth mesentery vessels are kept intact so that the small bowel that is normally supplied by the third mesentery vessel can be supplied by the fourth mesentery vessel through arcade connections. The jejunal flap is placed in a long plastic bag and is pulled through the mediastinum to the neck **(Fig. 5.9)**. Vascular anastomoses are then performed. A small segment of jejunum based on one or two terminal mesentery vessels is separated and later externalized for monitoring purpose. The main jejunal flap is then sewn to the base of the tongue and posterior pharynx. Once the esophageal reconstruction is completed, the ALT flap is inset by tying the previously placed parachuting sutures. The other end of the ALT flap is sewn to the neck skin above the sternal notch to create a "tracheostoma" **(Fig. 5.10)**.

For isolated tracheostomal defects (type IIIb) **(Fig. 5.11)**, the internal mammary artery perforator

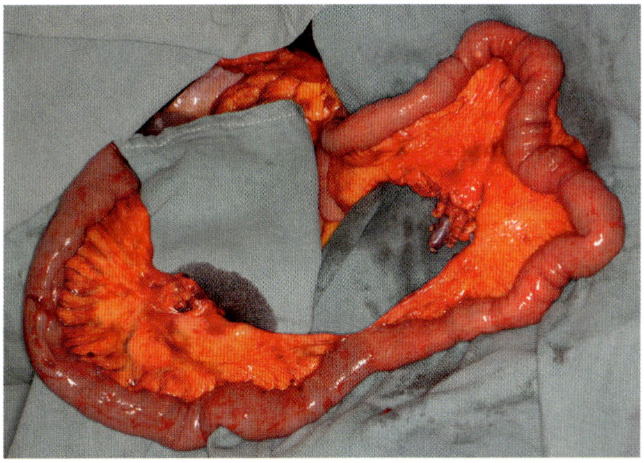

**Fig. 5.8** The supercharged jejunal flap. The second mesentery vessels are usually used for supercharging in the neck either to the transverse cervical vessels or internal mammary vessels. The third mesentery vessels are divided and ligated to increase the reach. The fourth mesentery vessels serve as the vascular pedicle for the pedicled portion of the flap.

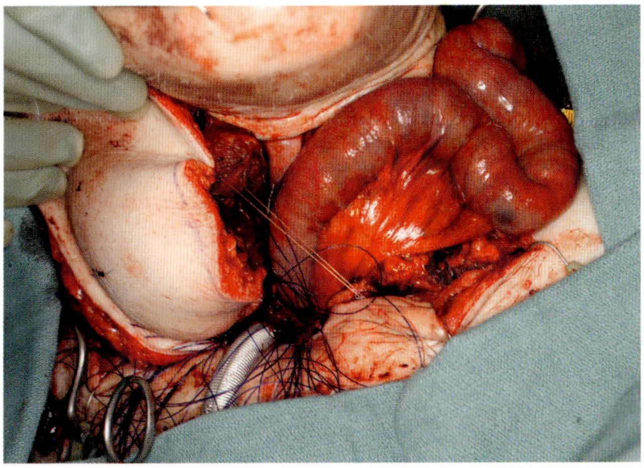

**Fig. 5.9** The ALT flap is tubed and sutured to the remaining trachea with parachuting sutures. The jejunal flap is placed in a long plastic bag and pulled through the mediastinum to the neck.

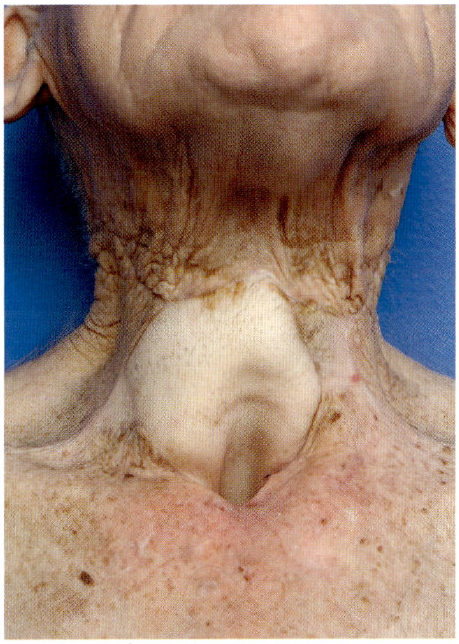

**Fig. 5.10** The other end of the ALT flap is sewn to the neck skin above the sternal notch to create a "tracheostoma" and to resurface the neck.

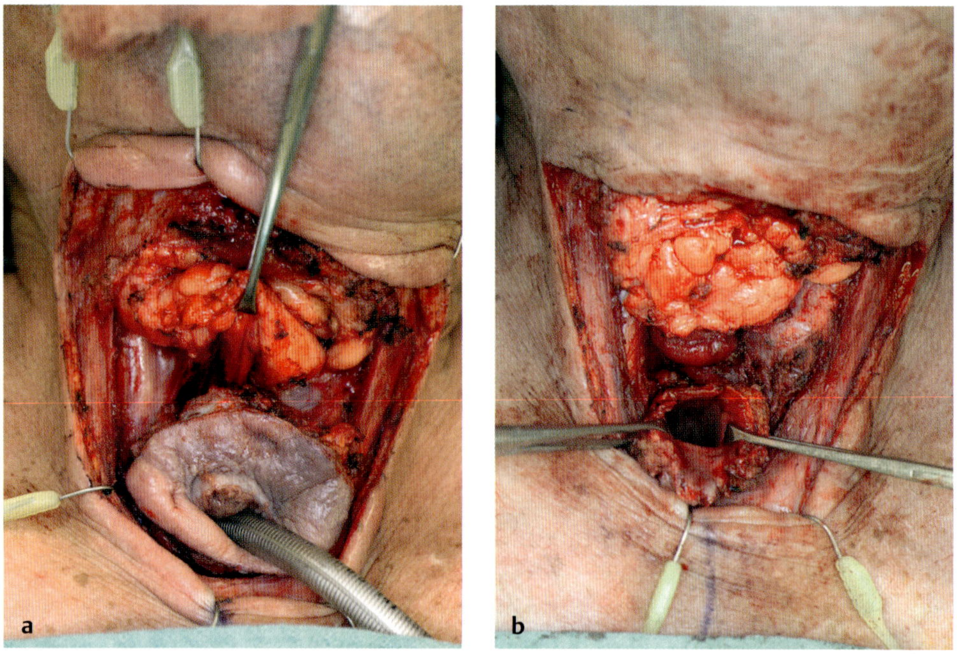

**Fig. 5.11 (a)** An isolated tracheostomal defect (type IIIb) **(b)** after resection for stomal recurrence.

(IMAP) flap provides quick and simple reconstruction with predictable results.[42] The flap is islanded on the internal mammary artery perforators at the second intercostal space and is designed parallel to the ribs **(Fig. 5.12)**. The distal end of the flap can be reliably extended beyond the anterior axillary fold for a width of 5 to 6 cm and length of 13 to 15 cm. Such a long and narrow island flap is still well perfused and is suitable for tracheostoma and anterior neck reconstruction. A width of 5 to 6 cm can usually be closed primarily to avoid donor-site deformity. For circumferential tracheostoma defects, bilateral IMAP flaps are required **(Fig. 5.13)**. For longer tracheal defects, a tubed ALT or radial forearm free flap works well. These patients usually require the removal of the manubrium and unilateral clavicular head to get access to the mediastinal trachea for tumor resection. The neck and upper mediastinum are often previously radiated. Therefore, muscle flap coverage of the great vessels is essential to prevent catastrophic complications. The vastus lateralis muscle can be included with the ALT flap for this purpose. If a radial forearm flap is planned, the pectoralis major muscle flaps can be used. Care should also be taken

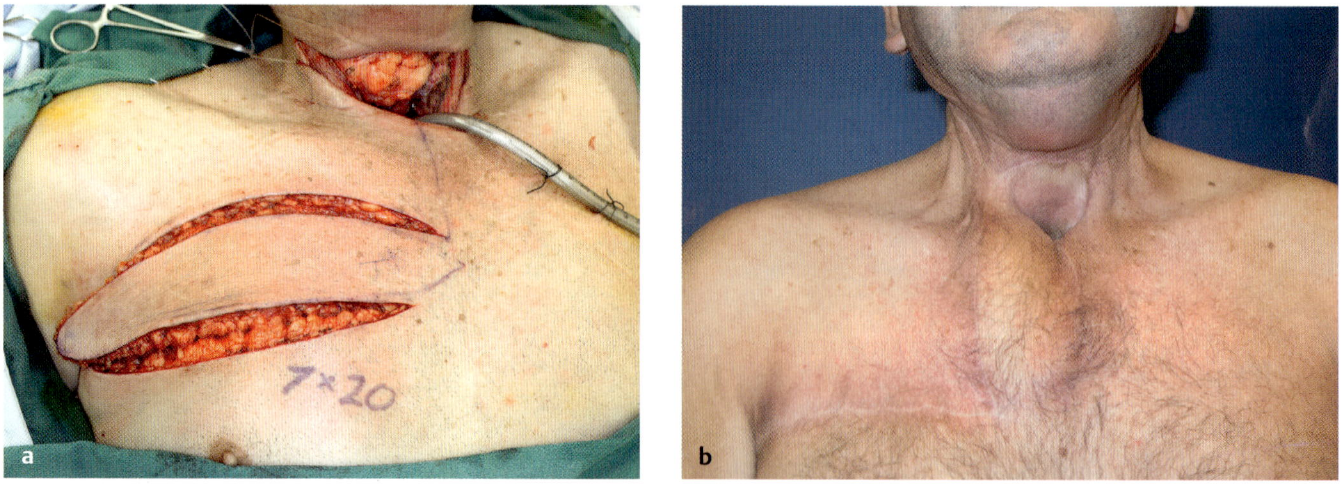

**Fig. 5.12 (a)** The internal mammary artery perforator (IMAP) flap is islanded on the internal mammary artery perforators at the second intercostal space and is designed parallel to the ribs. The distal end of the flap can be reliably extended beyond the anterior axillary fold for a width of 5 to 6 cm and a length of 13 to 15 cm. **(b)** Such a long and narrow island flap is still well perfused and is suitable for tracheostoma and anterior neck reconstruction.

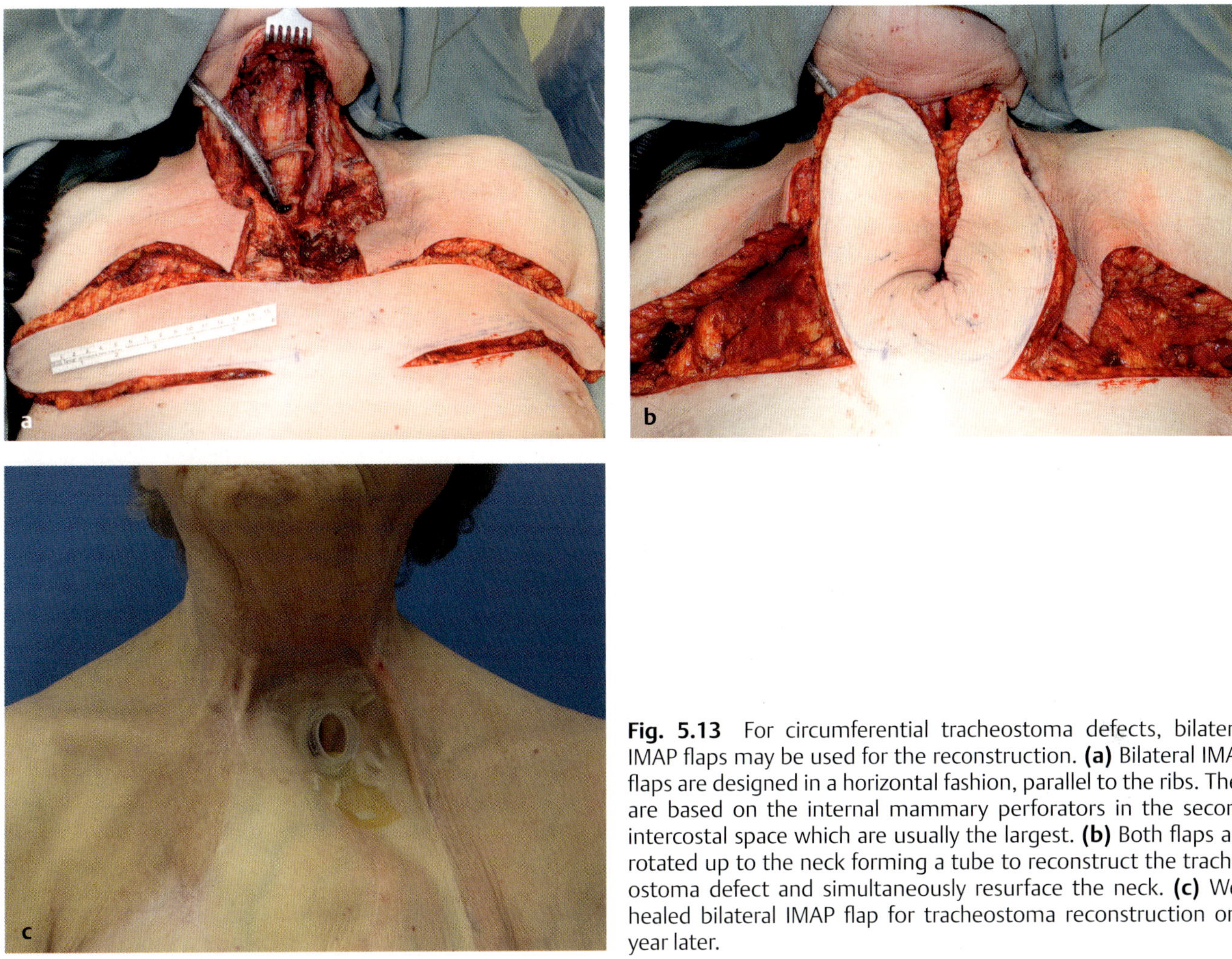

**Fig. 5.13** For circumferential tracheostoma defects, bilateral IMAP flaps may be used for the reconstruction. **(a)** Bilateral IMAP flaps are designed in a horizontal fashion, parallel to the ribs. They are based on the internal mammary perforators in the second intercostal space which are usually the largest. **(b)** Both flaps are rotated up to the neck forming a tube to reconstruct the tracheostoma defect and simultaneously resurface the neck. **(c)** Well healed bilateral IMAP flap for tracheostoma reconstruction one year later.

to smooth the bony edges of the clavicle and sternum to minimize the risk of delayed traumatic injury to the vessels.

## Complications

### Issues with Skin Flap for Lining

Although respiratory epithelial lining is preferred, we have demonstrated that skin flap lining is not as problematic as once thought. The concern regarding using skin for the tracheal lining stems from the possibility that the shedding of keratin debris into the bronchial system can cause airway irritation and infection. Long-term follow-up of our patients suggests that they tolerate skin lining well, with no respiratory symptoms. Bronchoscopy also revealed clean airways, free of debris or secretions. It is likely that a small amount of keratin shedding can be easily cleared by coughing. Our animal study showed that a buried 6 cm long, 3 cm diameter skin tube produced 1 g of keratin and sebaceous debris in 4 weeks. Thus, the hourly production was merely 1.5 mg, which is negligible.

### Air Leak through the Anastomosis

Air leakage is the most common surgical complication after tracheal reconstruction and usually occurs during coughing. Air leakage can come from two sources. Most patients have their cricoid cartilage resected, and the flap is sewn to the thyroid cartilage. The thyroid cartilage is severely calcified in most patients, with a very thin mucosal lining. Healing between the skin flap and calcified thyroid cartilage can be delayed, a source of leakage. Needle holes through calcified cartilage could be another source of air leak. Small leaks produce minimal symptoms and are usually detected by subcutaneous emphysema or imaging studies. A catheter placed percutaneously under computed tomographic guidance is adequate for managing minor leaks. The catheter can be connected to a PleuroVac in a manner similar to the management of pneumothorax. Large air leaks may require surgical repair and additional muscle coverage. Coverage of the anastomosis with a muscle flap at initial surgery may reduce the risk of air leak. Placement of a T-tube at the time of reconstruction is also important to prevent high airway pressure during coughing in order to minimize air leakage.

## Issues with Supporting Materials

The supporting material is the key to successful tracheal reconstruction. PTFE grafts are more prone to exposure and infection, and therefore should be avoided. Exposure of the supporting material either to the lumen or to the outside skin may require removal of the prosthesis and insertion of a T-tube tracheostomy tube to support the airway. We have not experienced exposure of the Hemashield graft and PolyMax mesh. PolyMax mesh is widely used for craniofacial surgery. Although the mesh loses strength over time and is resorbed in 12 to 18 months, our experience shows that scarring around the Hemashield graft apparently can prevent airway collapse by the time the mesh is resorbed. This has been confirmed in our patients both clinically and with imaging studies during long-term follow-up of up to 4 years.

## Medical Complications

As with other major surgical procedures, cardiopulmonary and other systemic comorbidities remain major risk factors for postoperative morbidity and mortality after tracheal reconstruction. Therefore, patient selection is of paramount importance for such complex reconstructive endeavors. Severe systemic comorbidities should be considered contraindications for microsurgical tracheal reconstruction. Obese patients with a thick radial forearm flap also may not be good candidates for reconstruction because excessive flap thickness incurs an inability to maintain a patent lumen.

### References


1. Grillo HC. Primary tracheal neoplasms. In: Grillo HC, ed. Surgery of the Trachea and Bronchi. Hamilton, Ontario: BC Decker Inc., 2004
2. Grillo HC, Mathisen DJ. Primary tracheal tumors: treatment and results. Ann Thorac Surg 1990;49(1):69–77
3. American Cancer Society. Cancer Facts and Figures 2002. Atlanta, GA: American Cancer Society, 2002
4. Gandhi S, Walsh GL, Komaki R, et al. A multidisciplinary surgical approach to superior sulcus tumors with vertebral invasion. Ann Thorac Surg 1999;68(5):1778–1784, discussion 1784–1785
5. Mitchell JD, Mathisen DJ, Wright CD, et al. Clinical experience with carinal resection. J Thorac Cardiovasc Surg 1999;117(1):39–52, discussion 52–53
6. Mitchell JD, Mathisen DJ, Wright CD, et al. Resection for bronchogenic carcinoma involving the carina: long-term results and effect of nodal status on outcome. J Thorac Cardiovasc Surg 2001;121(3):465–471
7. Rendina EA, Venuta F, De Giacomo T, et al. Sleeve resection and prosthetic reconstruction of the pulmonary artery for lung cancer. Ann Thorac Surg 1999;68(3):995–1001, discussion 1001–1002
8. Belsey R. Resection and reconstruction of the intrathoracic trachea. Br J Surg 1950;38(150):200–205
9. Daniel RA Jr. The regeneration of defects of the trachea and bronchi; an experimental study. J Thorac Surg 1948;17(3):335–349
10. Teramachi M, Okumura N, Nakamura T, et al. Intrathoracic tracheal reconstruction with a collagen-conjugated prosthesis: evaluation of the efficacy of omental wrapping. J Thorac Cardiovasc Surg 1997;113(4):701–711
11. Cull DL, Lally KP, Mair EA, Daidone M, Parsons DS. Tracheal reconstruction with polytetrafluoroethylene graft in dogs. Ann Thorac Surg 1990;50(6):899–901
12. Moghissi K. Tracheal reconstruction with a prosthesis of Marlex mesh and pericardium. J Thorac Cardiovasc Surg 1975;69(4):499–506
13. Beldholm BR, Wilson MK, Gallagher RM, Caminer D, King MJ, Glanville A. Reconstruction of the trachea with a tubed radial forearm free flap. J Thorac Cardiovasc Surg 2003;126(2):545–550
14. Anderl H, Haid B. Total reconstruction of the trachea: a 22-year follow-up. Plast Reconstr Surg 2005;115(2): 548–552
15. Letang E, Sánchez-Lloret J, Gimferrer JM, Ramírez J, Vicens A. Experimental reconstruction of the canine trachea with a free revascularized small bowel graft. Ann Thorac Surg 1990;49(6):955–958
16. Cavadas PC. Tracheal reconstruction using a free jejunal flap with cartilage skeleton: experimental study. Plast Reconstr Surg 1998;101(4):937–942
17. Genden EM, Gannon PJ, Smith S, Keck N, Deftereos M, Urken ML. Microvascular transfer of long tracheal autograft segments in the canine model. Laryngoscope 2002;112(3):439–444
18. Delaere P, Vranckx J, Verleden G, De Leyn P, Van Raemdonck D; Leuven Tracheal Transplant Group. Tracheal allotransplantation after withdrawal of immunosuppressive therapy. N Engl J Med 2010;362(2):138–145
19. Zalzal GH, Barber CS, Chandra R. Tracheal reconstruction using irradiated homologous grafts in rabbits. Otolaryngol Head Neck Surg 1989;100(2):119–125
20. Kunachak S, Kulapaditharom B, Vajaradul Y, Rochanawutanon M. Cryopreserved, irradiated tracheal homograft transplantation for laryngotracheal reconstruction in human beings. Otolaryngol Head Neck Surg 2000;122(6):911–916
21. Bjork VO, Rodriguez LE. Reconstruction of the trachea and its bifurcation; an experimental study. J Thorac Surg 1958;35(5):596–603

22. Mukaida T, Shimizu N, Aoe M, et al. Experimental study of tracheal allotransplantation with cryopreserved grafts. J Thorac Cardiovasc Surg 1998;116(2):262–266
23. Jacobs JP, Elliott MJ, Haw MP, Bailey CM, Herberhold C. Pediatric tracheal homograft reconstruction: a novel approach to complex tracheal stenoses in children. J Thorac Cardiovasc Surg 1996;112(6):1549–1558, discussion 1559–1560
24. Macchiarini P, Walles T, Biancosino C, Mertsching H. First human transplantation of a bioengineered airway tissue. J Thorac Cardiovasc Surg 2004;128(4):638–641
25. Walles T, Giere B, Hofmann M, et al. Experimental generation of a tissue-engineered functional and vascularized trachea. J Thorac Cardiovasc Surg 2004;128(6):900–906
26. Grimmer JF, Gunnlaugsson CB, Alsberg E, et al. Tracheal reconstruction using tissue-engineered cartilage. Arch Otolaryngol Head Neck Surg 2004;130(10):1191–1196
27. Kojima K, Ignotz RA, Kushibiki T, Tinsley KW, Tabata Y, Vacanti CA. Tissue-engineered trachea from sheep marrow stromal cells with transforming growth factor beta2 released from biodegradable microspheres in a nude rat recipient. J Thorac Cardiovasc Surg 2004;128(1):147–153
28. Macchiarini P, Jungebluth P, Go T, et al. Clinical transplantation of a tissue-engineered airway. Lancet 2008;372(9655):2023–2030
29. Pribaz JJ, Weiss DD, Mulliken JB, Eriksson E. Prelaminated free flap reconstruction of complex central facial defects. Plast Reconstr Surg 1999;104(2):357–365, discussion 366–367
30. Pribaz JJ, Fine N, Orgill DP. Flap prefabrication in the head and neck: a 10-year experience. Plast Reconstr Surg 1999;103(3):808–820
31. Fändrich F, Schröder DW. Experimental tracheal replacement using a revascularized ileal segment for transplantation in rats. J Surg Res 1995;59(5):560–568
32. Matloub HS, Yu P. Engineering a composite neotrachea in a rat model. Plast Reconstr Surg 2006;117(1):123–128
33. Zang M, Chen K, Yu P. Reconstruction of large tracheal defects in a canine model: lessons learned. J Reconstr Microsurg 2010;26(6):391–399
34. Yu P, Clayman GL, Walsh GL. Human tracheal reconstruction with a composite radial forearm free flap and prosthesis. Ann Thorac Surg 2006;81(2):714–716
35. Yu P, Clayman GL, Walsh GL. Long-term outcomes of microsurgical reconstruction for large tracheal defects. Cancer 2011;117(4):802–808
36. Ferguson REH Jr, Yu P. Techniques of monitoring buried fasciocutaneous free flaps. Plast Reconstr Surg 2009;123(2):525–532
37. Yu P. One-stage reconstruction of complex pharyngoesophageal, tracheal, and anterior neck defects. Plast Reconstr Surg 2005;116(4):949–956
38. Yu P. Characteristics of the anterolateral thigh flap in a Western population and its application in head and neck reconstruction. Head Neck 2004;26(9):759–769
39. Yu P, Robb GL. Pharyngoesophageal reconstruction with the anterolateral thigh flap: a clinical and functional outcomes study. Plast Reconstr Surg 2005;116(7):1845–1855
40. Yu P, Hanasono MM, Skoracki RJ, et al. Pharyngoesophageal reconstruction with the anterolateral thigh flap after total laryngopharyngectomy. Cancer 2010;116(7):1718–1724
41. Poh M, Selber JC, Skoracki R, Walsh GL, Yu P. Technical challenges of total esophageal reconstruction using a supercharged jejunal flap. Ann Surg 2011;253(6):1122–1129
42. Yu P, Roblin P, Chevray P. Internal mammary artery perforator (IMAP) flap for tracheostoma reconstruction. Head Neck 2006;28(8):723–729

# 6 Laryngotracheal Reconstruction with Prefabricated Free Flaps and Tracheal Allotransplantation

*Jan Jeroen Vranckx*

## Reconstruction of Hemilarynx after Hemilaryngectomy

Despite the popularity of organ-sparing combined radiation and chemotherapy protocols, laryngectomy continues to be indicated for patients with recurrent laryngeal cancers and some locally advanced cancers. For cancers that obviously cross the midline, a total laryngectomy is often performed, which results in loss of both of the vocal cords and thus loss of natural speech. In many cases, a unilateral advanced tumor on one vocal fold is also treated surgically by total laryngectomy since the reconstruction of a hemilarynx with the aim of sparing one vocal cord is often considered too complex.[1] However, since the loss of speech and the need for a permanent tracheostoma dramatically change the patients' quality of life, we make every attempt to avoid a total laryngectomy when oncologically feasible.

The goal of the reconstruction is to restore the extended hemilaryngectomy defect and to obtain a morphology after reconstruction that is comparable to that seen in unilateral vocal fold paralysis with the affected vocal cord in the paramedian position. Indications are a unilateral lateralized glottic cancer with subglottic extension and lateralized chondrosarcomas of the cricoid cartilage **(Fig. 6.1)**.

To restore the cartilaginous framework after extended hemilaryngectomy, donor tissues should be used that mimic the resected tissues. The trachea is nearby and represents the ideal donor tissue, with a similar cartilaginous structure and an internal lining consisting of respiratory mucosa. A four-ring horseshoe-shaped configuration that mimics the hemilaryngeal convex shape can be obtained when the trachea is opened at the posterior membrane.

Because of the proximity of the cervical trachea to the larynx, a one-stage reconstruction of the hemilarynx is possible, with preservation of the tracheal continuity if a segment of four rings can be transposed up to the hemilaryngeal defect. However, to allow upward mobilization, the trachea has to be dissected from the surrounding tissues over a length of 8 cm. This interrupts the extrinsic blood supply of this segment and can result in necrosis of the central part of the trachea. Tracheal vascularity is further diminished after remodeling the upper 4 cm of membranous tra-

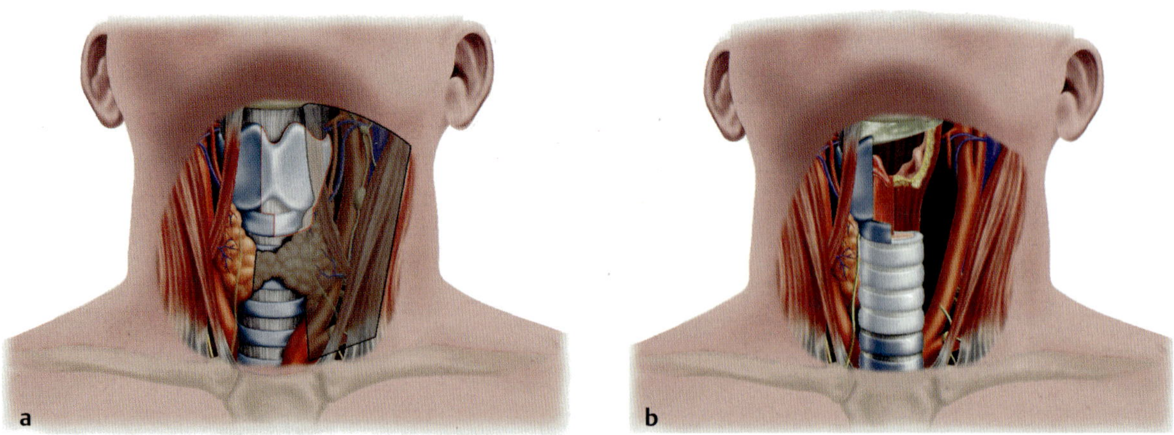


**Fig. 6.1** **(a)** Diagram representing unilateral laryngeal cancer. The shaded area is to be resected. **(b)** Defect shown after hemilaryngectomy. Mark the contralateral half of the larynx. Note the donor tracheal rings under the defect (in white).

chea to create the convex patch and by placement of a temporary tracheostomy at the anterior wall.[2,3]

Zur and Urken[4] used a single-stage procedure to transfer the trachea to the laryngeal defect, with the trachea pedicled on the thyroid artery and vein along with the adjacent thyroid gland. However, there is an inherent risk of occult metastases to the thyroid gland and the paratracheal lymph nodes, which are commonly seen when there is significant subglottic extension of the cancer. We, therefore, modified our operative sequence to reduce the oncologic risk. In our initial series of patients, we performed the prefabrication of a four-ring trachea segment by wrapping it with a radial forearm fascia flap and a microvascular anastomosis to head and neck blood vessels.[5] Neovascularization of the tracheal segment following this step takes ~ 2 weeks. In a second stage, the tumor was resected and the hemilarynx was restored with the prefabricated tracheal segment.

Although we were successfully able to perform reconstruction in this manner, the concern with this protocol was that the first-stage prefabrication step, before the resection of the tumor in the second stage, has the theoretic risk of manipulating tumor cells and eliciting their spread. However, changing the sequence of surgery is problematic. When the tumor is resected primarily in the first stage, a hemilaryngeal defect is created before the prefabrication of the trachea has been started.[5,6] The hemilaryngeal defect needs to be temporarily closed to allow for breathing and swallowing while the prefabrication step takes place.

We, therefore, defined a novel reconstructive design for extended hemilaryngectomy repair leading to optimal functional results without diminishing oncologic safety. In the first stage, an extended hemilaryngectomy is performed. Only patients who have tumors without extension to the supraglottic area are considered candidates for this reconstructive protocol. For a T3 glottic cancer, the tumor is resected along with the anterior commissure and half of the cricoid cartilage. The ipsilateral thyroid lobe and tracheoesophageal lymph nodes are also removed, as well as the lymph nodes in levels II, III, and IV. During the same surgery, we harvest a radial forearm flap, consisting of a proximal fasciocutaneous segment and a distal fascial component, from the nondominant arm. The fascial paddle is wrapped around the upper 4 cm of the cervical trachea and the fasciocutaneous paddle is used to temporarily close the extended hemilaryngectomy defect (**Fig. 6.2**).

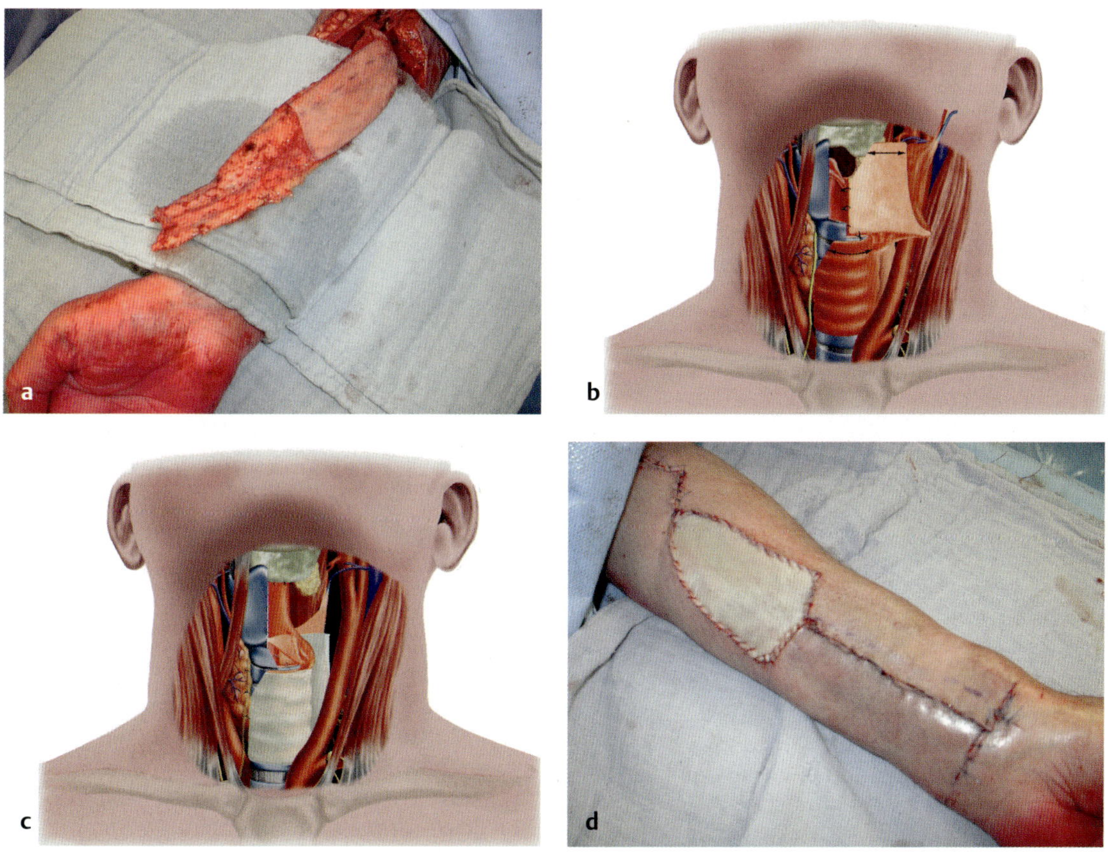

**Fig. 6.2** **(a)** Harvest of the fasciocutaneous (FC) and fascia (F) radial forearm free flap. **(b)** The FC segment is used to temporarily close the hemilarynx defect and the F segment to wrap and prefabricate the trachea. **(c)** A microvascular anastomosis is performed on the neck vessels. Appearance at the end of the first stage. There is a monitoring skin flap at the inferolateral FC border. An ePTFE sheet covers the fascia flap and the vascular pedicle to avoid adhesions in preparation for the second stage. **(d)** Donor site after flap harvest.

After microsurgical anastomosis of the radial vascular pedicle to the neck vessels, the flap and the pedicle are covered with an expanded polytetrafluoroethylene (ePTFE) membrane to prevent adhesion formation. We suture the inferolateral corner of the fasciocutaneous segment in the skin of the neck for monitoring the perfusion of the buried tissues after microsurgical anastomosis. The monitor skin paddle also serves as the roof of the temporary tracheostoma and can be used in the second stage to close the skin defect after removal of the tracheostoma.

After 4 months, we perform a second look at the section margins. If histology confirms absence of tumor recurrence, definitive reconstruction is initiated **(Fig. 6.3)**. The ePTFE membrane is removed and the skin paddle is de-epithelialized to serve as posterior bulk at the end of reconstruction. The fascia-wrapped revascularized tracheal segment is isolated, opened, and transferred upward into the laryngeal defect. Next, the mediastinal tracheal stump is mobilized and is sutured to the reconstructed larynx. During the second stage, the microvascular pedicle of the radial forearm flap in which the trachea segment was wrapped is left intact. A tracheostomy is maintained in the suture line between the reconstructed larynx and the mediastinal trachea. The tracheostomy is closed after restoration of all laryngeal functions, 1 to 2 months after the second stage. The tracheostomy is closed by inverting the skin around the tracheostomy, a small procedure performed under local anesthesia.

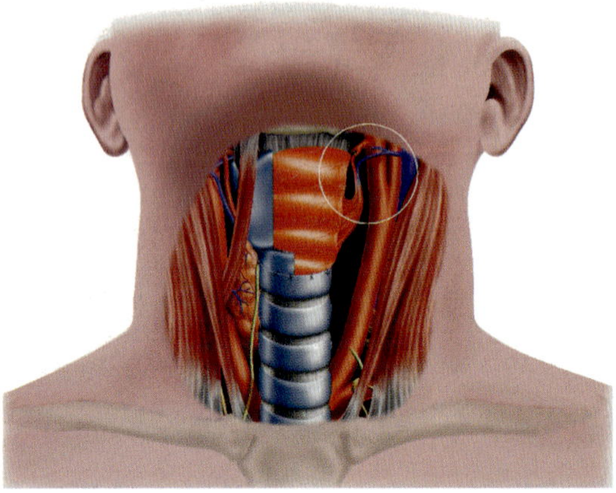

**Fig. 6.3** Diagram showing the end result after the second stage of hemilaryngeal reconstruction. The prefabricated trachea is opened so that it is horseshoe-shaped and is trimmed to match the hemilaryngeal defect. The initial fasciocutaneous segment is de-epithelialized and serves as posterior bulk. The hemilarynx defect is restored with the prefabricated tracheal segment. In all these steps, the microvascular anastomosis performed during the first stage remains intact.

This tracheal "autotransplantation" protocol leads to an efficient reconstruction of the extended hemilaryngectomy defect. Swallowing of solids and liquids is possible after 1 week and speaking is possible during finger occlusion of the temporary tracheostomy.[5,6] After the second operation, the tracheal patch and the vascularized forearm flap restore the sphincteric and respiratory function of the larynx. Hand-free speech is possible after closure of the tracheostoma ~ 6 weeks after the second stage of reconstruction. The voice sounds natural although moderately hoarse. Some aspiration of saliva is seen during the first days after surgery; however, most patients resume oral feeding after 1 week. The tracheostomy closure may be delayed because of swallowing problems caused by postirradiation pharyngeal hypocontractility.

The revascularized tracheal patch restores the subglottic luminal concavity required to preserve function.[1,6] Two sutures at the lateral site of the defect between the epiglottis and the aryepiglottic fold bring the aryepiglottic fold into a midline position posteriorly. Complete posterior closure is important to obtain good voice and swallowing function, so the reconstruction has to be placed in the posterior midline. Complete glottic closure is less critical anteriorly; therefore, a paramedian position of the graft will permit good respiratory function.

The most challenging part of the reconstruction is repair of the airway lumen at the subglottic level. Tracheal autografts have the combined characteristics of a respiratory mucosal lining and cartilaginous support, tissue characteristics that are necessary for restoration of a luminal convexity. Hirano et al[7] showed that, in the normal larynx, the anterior glottis plays the most important role for phonation, while the posterior glottis plays an equally important role in respiration. Closure of the posterior larynx is important for swallowing without aspiration. After extended hemilaryngectomy, the posterior larynx becomes the sphincteric larynx. After reconstruction, the phonatory glottis is moved from anterior to posterior, while the respiratory glottis is moved from posterior to anterior. With the tracheal patch in a paramedian position, the amount of airway lumen that is lost in the posterior larynx will be gained anteriorly.

The 4-month prefabrication period allows for laryngeal repair with a well-vascularized tracheal patch. The delay between the tumor resection and the definitive reconstruction allows for a second look to verify that there is no recurrent tumor at the resection margins. In cases of local recurrence, total laryngectomy can be performed during the second procedure.

# Reconstruction of Tracheal Stenosis

## Reconstruction of Recurrent Short-Segment Stenosis of the Trachea

For a stenosis of less than 50% of the tracheal length, segmental tracheal resection with end-to-end anastomosis is the treatment of choice.[8] However, traction or tension on the proximal and distal tracheal segment may lead to local necrosis, leakage, and fistulization. Scarring due to previous interventions may limit a tensionless suture.[9,10] In that situation, augmentation of the tracheal lumen by inserting local, regional, or distant tissue is necessary.[11]

To restore the trachea, tissues should be used that resemble the mucosa-lined elastic cartilaginous framework of the trachea and preserve its functions under respiratory forces, deglutition, speech, and flexion and extension of the neck.[12] However, spare tissues are not available from an autologous donor site. Therefore, tracheal reconstruction using other tissues has been utilized. The most frequently used reconstructive tissues consist of cartilage grafts, pericardium, and muscle flaps that are used as a carrier for skin, periosteum, or bone.[13] Since these donor tissues all lack one or more features for optimal tracheal repair, the outcome is unpredictable. Composite tissues flaps consisting of vascularized fascia for blood supply, buccal mucosa for internal lining, and elastic cartilage for support can be a reasonable option for reconstructing composite tracheal defects **(Fig. 6.4)**. Bare cartilage undergoes necrosis when directly exposed to the airway lumen. Cartilage exposure can be avoided by using a prefabrication procedure, as described above for hemilaryngeal reconstruction.[13,14] The cartilage is sutured to a vascularized fascia layer, such as the radial forearm fascia and its intrinsic blood supply from the radial artery and comitant veins. After 2 weeks, orthotopic transfer can be performed.

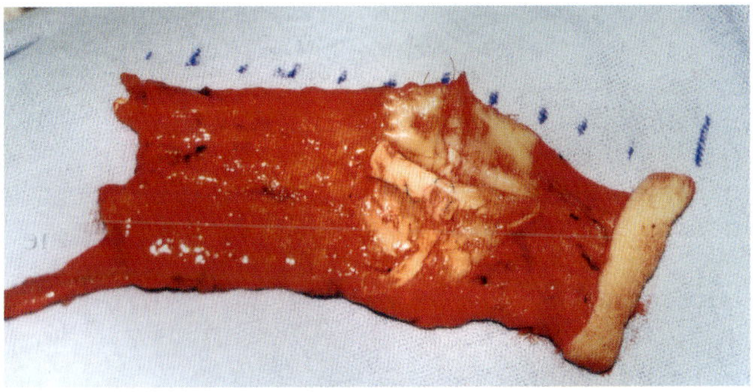

**Fig. 6.4** Two-stage prefabrication–prelamination procedure for short-segment tracheal stenosis. Auricular cartilage is sutured on the radial forearm fascia. The skin is closed on top. After the 2-week prefabrication step to vascularize the cartilage grafts, orthotopic transfer to the tracheal defect is performed.

Since buccal mucosa is thinner than cartilage, a buccal mucosa–vascularized fascial free flap composite can be created in a one-stage procedure without a prefabrication step to reconstruct partial-circumference tracheal defects. Vascularized mucosa can repair airway defects with primary healing of the reconstructed site. When using a mucosa-lined fascia flap to repair an airway defect, it is essential that the mucosal patch and the defect have a similar size. A smaller size may create granulation tissue at the suture line, which may trigger restenosis. The advantage of the mucosa-lined laminated free flap is that it is a single-stage repair. A disadvantage is the absence of supportive tissue and the diminished convexity of the airway lumen because the cartilaginous supportive component is not available. Simultaneous use of the Dumon silicone stent (Novatech SA, La Ciotat Cedex, France) will prevent prolapse of the mucosa-lined fascia and will prevent collapse of the incised and expanded airway. Short-term stenting of 4 to 6 weeks is sufficient to anticipate collapse during healing of the reconstructed airway.

This reconstructive technique is indicated for treating stenoses after segmental tracheal resection. Anastomotic stricture is usually related to excessive tension at the suture line, which occurs in ~ 10% of patients undergoing tracheal resection.[13,14] A mucosa-laminated fascia free flap currently is the preferred strategy for the treatment of an airway stenosis in which segmental resection and primary anastomosis are impossible or deemed risky because of excessive tension. The mucosa-lined reconstruction features fast primary healing with an excellent take of the buccal mucosa on the fascial vascular carrier **(Fig. 6.5)**. No re-epithelialization is necessary during healing, and this may be advantageous in a restenosis where a scarred wound bed is encountered. A mucosal lining is preferable for airway lining. A skin graft or a cutaneous flap may undergo crusting and desquamation. Another advantage of the mucosa-lined fascia is that the donor defect at the forearm site can be closed primarily, resulting in a scar that is less visible than the defect created in dissection of a fasciocutaneous flap.

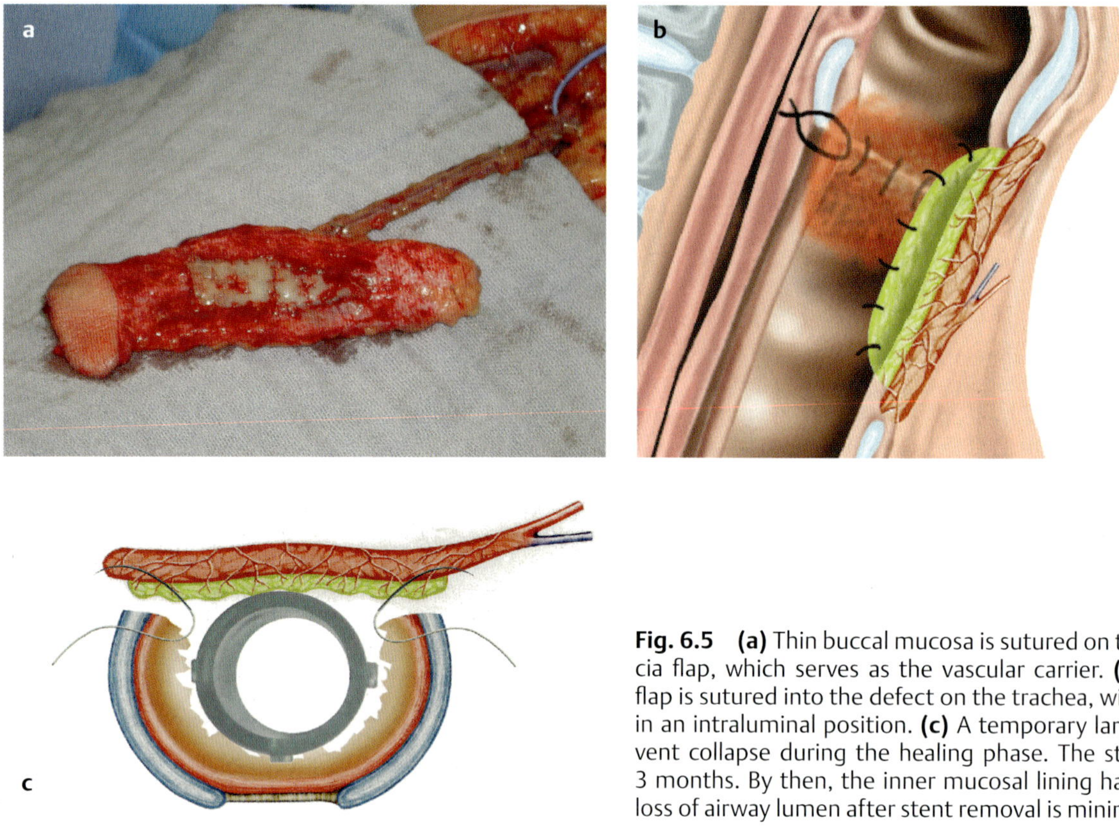

**Fig. 6.5** **(a)** Thin buccal mucosa is sutured on the radial forearm fascia flap, which serves as the vascular carrier. **(b)** The prelaminated flap is sutured into the defect on the trachea, with the mucosal patch in an intraluminal position. **(c)** A temporary laryngeal stent will prevent collapse during the healing phase. The stent is removed after 3 months. By then, the inner mucosal lining has been restored. The loss of airway lumen after stent removal is minimal in limited defects.

## Reconstruction of Long-Segment Stenosis of the Trachea

A one-stage mucosa–prelamination technique or two-stage cartilage–prefabrication procedure cannot be performed for long-segment tracheal defects because there are no sufficient autologous donor tissues available to restore the mucosa-lined elastic cartilaginous framework.

One theoretical option is utilizing tissue engineering to cultivate a three-dimensional vascularized tubular trachea. Recently, successful restoration of a mainstem bronchus was accomplished by means of a tissue-engineered transplant colonized by the recipient's epithelial and chondrogenic mesenchymal cells, which avoided the use of immunosuppressive therapy. However, the main drawback of the procedure was the lack of an intrinsic blood supply. An avascular tissue-engineered trachea would be unsuitable for reconstructing a long tracheal defect, where the graft would be exposed to the airway lumen. Such constructs collapse and ultimately require a stent, which itself can incite formation of hypertrophic granulation tissue that can occlude the tracheal lumen.[15] The highly vascularized inner mucosal lining of the trachea plays an important role in primary defense against airborne molecules. Moreover, continuous movements during respiration, swallowing, and coughing require elasticity and flexibility. Without intrinsic vascularization, scar tissue will be generated, and healing is unpredictable at best. Current tissue-engineering protocols are not able to generate a vascularized hollow tubular trachea that remains stable over time.[16]

The only current option to authentically restore a long tracheal gap is an allogeneic tracheal transplant. The problem is that the trachea does not have its own extrinsic vascular pedicle, so it is not transplantable like a heart, kidney, or facial transplant. A vascular pedicle can be "generated" around an allogeneic donor trachea using prefabrication techniques in a heterotopic position, preventing exposure to air until the tissue is well vascularized. The donor trachea should be fresh: that is, the inner mucosal lining must be intact.

To preserve the mucosal lining of the tracheal transplant, rapid revascularization is mandatory. An allogeneic trachea from the tissue bank could be used instead to bridge the gap, similar to stored bone grafts. However, although the vascular requirements of the cartilaginous framework are limited and cartilage elicits a limited immunologic rejection, the inner mucosal lining needs a significant vascular supply and its immunologic response is as strong as that of regular skin.[14] A cryopreserved or decellularized tracheal tube no longer has a viable mucosal lining, and a new one would need to be created with thin, vascularized skin flaps.[17] However, the functional outcome is unpredictable, since even a very thin skin flap is still much thicker than true mucosal lining and may obliterate the inner lumen. When a wider outer cartilage skeleton is made with cartilage grafts to avoid obstructing the inner lumen with a vascular free skin flap, it is very difficult to predictably create an optimal tubular and flexible shape.

Since the blood supply to the trachea makes it unsuitable for direct revascularization, most previous attempts at tracheal transplantation have been performed after indirect revascularization. Rose et al[18] reported the first allogeneic tracheal transplantation in a human. The donor trachea was implanted heterotopically in the sternocleidomastoid muscle of the recipient and was transferred to the orthotopic position 3 weeks later. However, the recipient was not given immunosuppressive therapy, and the report did not document the long-term outcome or the viability of the allograft. Klepetko et al[19] reported that they preserved the viability of a heterotopically revascularized allograft by wrapping it in the omentum of a patient who received a lung transplant from the same donor. Its viability was documented at 60 days.

Restoration of arterial inflow and venous outflow is essential for the survival of the tracheal allograft. Indirect revascularization of a donor trachea is perfectly feasible, as demonstrated by the successful revascularization of tracheal allografts and autografts using vascularized fascia flaps in both laboratory animals and humans.[8,19,20] When the recipient tissue is perfused by an identifiable vascular pedicle, a microvascular transfer can be performed after the prefabrication step. Proof of concept in immunosuppressed rabbits showed complete revascularization and restoration of mucosal lining in tracheal allografts after 2 to 4 weeks of heterotopic revascularization in the lateral thoracic area.[21]

In 2007, we performed the first tracheal allotransplantation and reconstructed a long-segment tracheal defect by using a blood type-matched donor allograft that was revascularized in a first stage by heterotopic wrapping in vascularized radial forearm fascia.[22] Immunosuppressive therapy was required during the prefabrication step to establish connections between the donor's capillary network around the trachea and the recipient's blood vessels from the surrounding forearm arm fascia flap. This occurred rapidly, preserving the viability of the cartilaginous trachea. Nonetheless, unlike in the rabbit model, where this process occurred efficiently and predictably, the posterior membranous trachea underwent avascular necrosis. After débridement of the necrotic tissue, we replaced the areas with buccal mucosa from the recipient.

The autologous mucosa grew over the lumen of the cartilaginous tracheal transplant, creating a chimeric patchwork of (male) donor epithelium and (female) recipient buccal mucosa. In situ hybridization analysis for the Y chromosome in biopsies showed that endothelial and respiratory cells originating from the male donor disappeared shortly after the withdrawal of immunosuppressive therapy. The immunologic rejection occurred silently because of the repopulation by the recipient's surrounding vascular network and buccal mucosal cells. The cartilaginous framework was not recognized by the immune system because adult cartilage lacks blood vessels. The stealth activity of the highly differentiated chondrocytes may be based on their encasement in dense matrix. This event allowed all immunosuppressive therapy to be tapered and permanently stopped. The viability of the tracheal cartilage was maintained after stopping all immunosuppressive drugs (**Fig. 6.6**).

So far, five patients have been treated with allogeneic tracheal transplants, with variable outcomes.[23] The first patient is doing very well. In two cases, the cartilage framework remained well vascularized, wrapped in the free vascular fascia flap, but the inner mucosal lining was gradually rejected. Unfortunately, the inner mucosal lining determines the outcome. First, the remaining allogeneic respiratory epithelium was rejected, and, subsequently, the autologous mucosal grafts succumbed to secondary thrombosis.

We have modified the procedure to enhance the mucosal healing by making gaps in the intercartilaginous spaces. This seems to limit the barrier function of the intercartilaginous ligaments for angiogenesis.[24] There is a balance between the speed of formation of neovascular connections and the oxygen requirements of the allogeneic trachea. We are currently investigating proangiogenic cell-based strategies to accelerate and enhance the neovascularization processes of the inner mucosal lining using blood-originating endothelial progenitor cells and plasma-based matrix elements.[24,25]

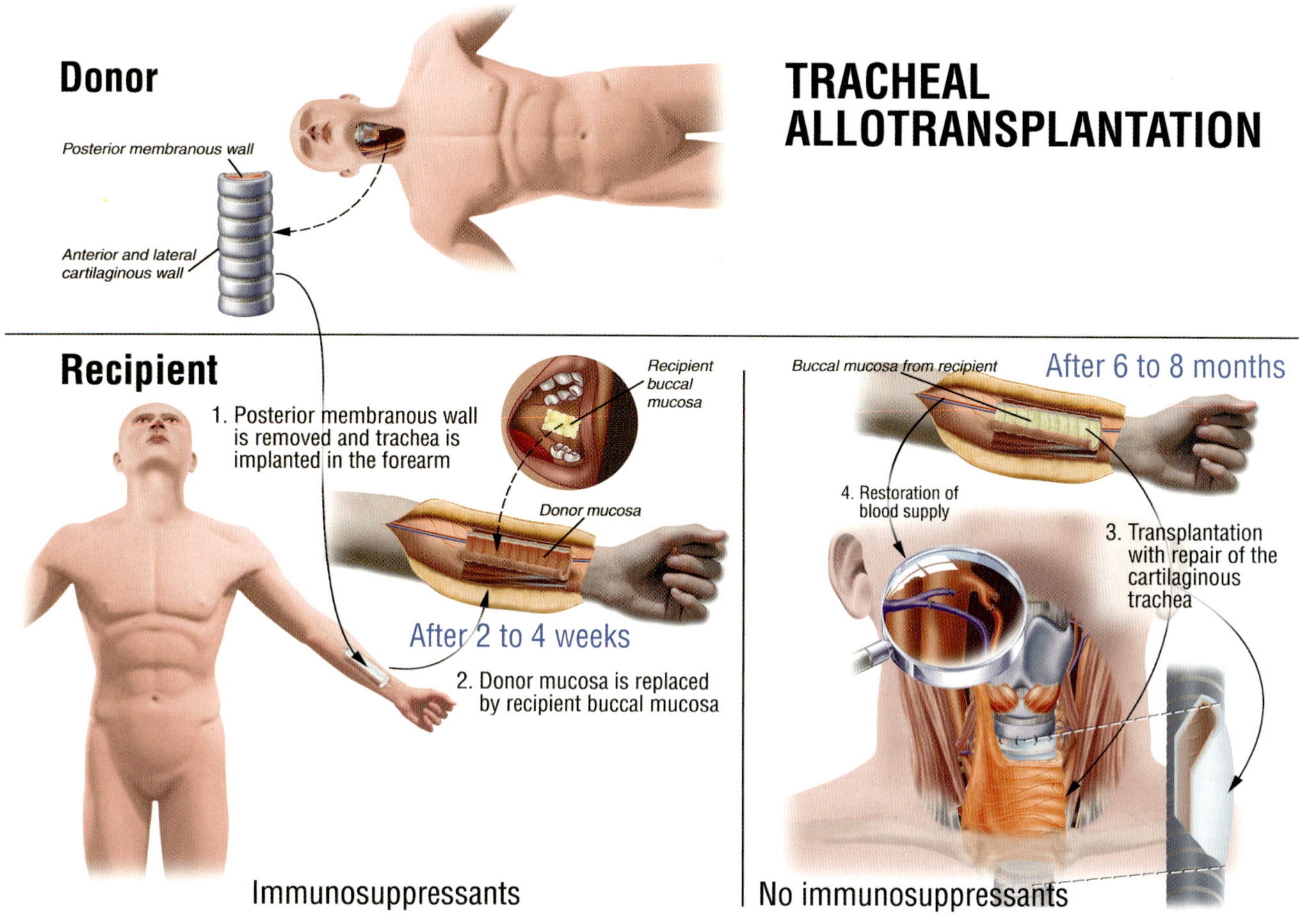


**Fig. 6.6** Overview of the tracheal allotransplantation procedure. A donor trachea is wrapped by radial forearm fascia in the forearm in heterotopic position. Buccal recipient mucosa replaces the posterior membrane and patches of allogeneic respiratory epithelium of the donor trachea. After prefabrication, the vascularized trachea is transferred to the neck in orthotopic position. Immunosuppression is tapered and stopped when the trachea is in place and bronchoscopy shows a well-vascularized inner mucosal lining within the tracheal allogeneic framework.

## References

1. Pearson BW, Keith RL. Near-total laryngectomy. In: Johnson JT, Blitzer A, Ossoff RM, Thomas IR, eds. Instructional Courses: American Academy of Otology-Head Neck Surgery, Vol. 2. St. Louis, MO: Mosby; 1990:309–330
2. Vranckx JJ, Den Hondt M, Delaere P. Prefabrication and prelamination strategies for the reconstruction of complex defects of trachea and larynx. J Reconstr Microsurg 2013;
3. Delaere PR, Poorten VV, Goeleven A, Feron M, Hermans R. Tracheal autotransplantation: a reliable reconstructive technique for extended hemilaryngectomy defects. Laryngoscope 1998;108(6):929–934
4. Zur KB, Urken ML. Vascularized hemitracheal autograft for laryngotracheal reconstruction: a new surgical technique based on the thyroid gland as a vascular carrier. Laryngoscope 2003;113(9):1494–1498
5. Delaere P, Goeleven A, Poorten VV, Hermans R, Hierner R, Vranckx J. Organ preservation surgery for advanced unilateral glottic and subglottic cancer. Laryngoscope 2007;117(10):1764–1769
6. Delaere PR, Vranckx JJ, Dooms C, Meulemans J, Hermans R. Tracheal autotransplantation: guidelines for optimal functional outcome. Laryngoscope 2011;121(8):1708–1714
7. Hirano M, Kurita S, Kiyokawa K, Sato K. Posterior glottis. Morphological study in excised human larynges. Ann Otol Rhinol Laryngol 1986;95(6 Pt 1):576–581
8. Grillo HC. Tracheal replacement. Ann Thorac Surg 1990;49(6):864–865
9. deLorimier AA, Harrison MR, Hardy K, Howell LJ, Adzick NS. Tracheobronchial obstructions in infants and children. Experience with 45 cases. Ann Surg 1990;212(3):277–289
10. Idriss FS, DeLeon SY, Ilbawi MN, Gerson CR, Tucker GF, Holinger L. Tracheoplasty with pericardial patch for extensive tracheal stenosis in infants and children. J Thorac Cardiovasc Surg 1984;88(4):527–536
11. Eliachar I, Roberts JK, Welker KB, Tucker HM. Advantages of the rotary door flap in laryngotracheal reconstruc-

tion: is skeletal support necessary? Ann Otol Rhinol Laryngol 1989;98(1 Pt 1):37–40

12. Wright CD, Grillo HC, Wain JC, et al. Anastomotic complications after tracheal resection: prognostic factors and management. J Thorac Cardiovasc Surg 2004; 128(5):731–739
13. Delaere P, Hierner R, Vranckx J, Hermans R. Tracheal stenosis treated with vascularized mucosa and short-term stenting. Laryngoscope 2005;115(6):1132–1134
14. Vranckx JJ, Den Hondt M, Delaere P. Prefabrication and prelamination strategies for the reconstruction of complex defects of trachea and larynx. J Reconstr Microsurg 2014;30(3):145–152
15. Vogel G. Trachea transplants test the limits. Science 2013;340(6130):266–268
16. Ott LM, Weatherly RA, Detamore MS. Overview of tracheal tissue engineering: clinical need drives the laboratory approach. Ann Biomed Eng 2011;39(8):2091–2113
17. Yu P, Clayman GL, Walsh GL. Long-term outcomes of microsurgical reconstruction for large tracheal defects. Cancer 2011;117(4):802–808
18. Rose KG, Sesterhenn K, Wustrow F. Tracheal allotransplantation in man. Lancet 1979;1(8113):433–434
19. Klepetko W, Marta GM, Wisser W, et al. Heterotopic tracheal transplantation with omentum wrapping in the abdominal position preserves functional and structural integrity of a human tracheal allograft. J Thorac Cardiovasc Surg 2004;127(3):862–867
20. Buckwalter JA, Mankin HJ. Articular cartilage. Part II: degeneration and osteoarthritis, repair, regeneration and transplantation. J Bone Joint Surg Am 1997; 79:612–632
21. Delaere PR, Liu ZY, Hermans R, Sciot R, Feenstra L. Experimental tracheal allograft revascularization and transplantation. J Thorac Cardiovasc Surg 1995; 110(3):728–737
22. Delaere P, Vranckx J, Verleden G, De Leyn P, Van Raemdonck D; Leuven Tracheal Transplant Group. Tracheal allotransplantation after withdrawal of immunosuppressive therapy. N Engl J Med 2010;362(2):138–145
23. Delaere PR, Vranckx JJ, Meulemans J, et al. Learning curve in tracheal allotransplantation. Am J Transplant 2012;12(9):2538–2545
24. Hendrickx B, Vranckx JJ, Luttun A. Cell-based vascularization strategies for skin tissue engineering. Tissue Eng Part B Rev 2011;17(1):13–24
25. Vermeulen P, Dickens S, Degezelle K, Van den Berge S, Hendrickx B, Vranckx JJ. A plasma-based biomatrix mixed with endothelial progenitor cells and keratinocytes promotes matrix formation, angiogenesis, and reepithelialization in full-thickness wounds. Tissue Eng Part A 2009;15(7):1533–1542

# 7 Midfacial Reconstruction

*Matthew M. Hanasono and Roman J. Skoracki*

## Introduction

Management of midfacial defects is among the most complicated and controversial areas of head and neck oncologic reconstruction. Options include use of prosthetic obturators, pedicled flaps, and free flaps, sometimes combined with grafts or alloplasts. While the popularity of pedicled flaps has declined in recent years due to limited reach and volume, prosthetic obturators remain a good solution for select patients with limited palatal defects. However, for extensive defects, obturators may be difficult or impossible to retain, particularly in edentulous patients. Furthermore, obturators are usually inappropriate for defects that involve resection of the skull base, orbital floor, orbital contents, or soft tissues of the face. Finally, some patients may not like the inconvenience of an obturator, which must be removed and cleaned regularly and periodically adjusted or replaced for fit and/or chronic fungal colonization.

Midfacial reconstructions with various bony and soft tissue free flaps have been described, and the best techniques are a subject of debate.[1,2,3,4,5] One of the fundamental problems with reconstructing the midface is that the defects created by oncologic resection are highly variable. Such defects usually not only involve the maxillary bones, but also may include several adjacent facial and cranial bones, as well as soft tissues of the face, palate, and orbit. Successful outcomes in midfacial reconstruction involve a mastery of a broad range of soft tissue and bony flaps and craniofacial plating techniques, as well as an understanding of the requirements for prosthetic rehabilitation, which is used in place of reconstruction in some cases, often in concert with local and distant tissue-transfer procedures. This chapter discusses reconstruction of both orbital and palatomaxillary defects, because the two frequently occur in concert.

## Regional Anatomy and Nomenclature

The pivotal structures of the midface are the paired maxillary bones, which are fused at the intermaxillary suture to form the upper jaw **(Fig. 7.1)**. The maxillae contribute to forming the boundaries for three cavities: the roof of the mouth, the floor and lateral wall of the nasal cavity, and the floor and medial walls of the orbit. The maxillae attach laterally to the zyomatic bones, which comprise part of the orbital floor and the lateral orbital wall, as well as provide shape to the cheek. In addition to the zygomatic bones, the maxillae also articulate with the frontal and ethmoid bones of the cranium, and the nasal, lacrimal, inferior nasal conchal, palatine, and vomer bones of the face.

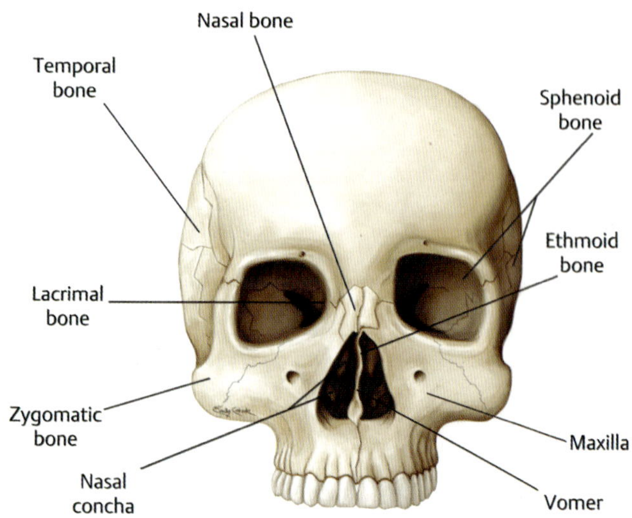


**Fig. 7.1** Bony anatomy of the midface, including the maxilla and orbit.

Many maxillary tumors extend into or arise from the orbit, which is a conical or pyramidal structure ~ 30 mL in volume that contains the eye, extraocular muscles, and extraocular fat, as well as blood vessels and cranial nerves II, III, IV, V, and VI. The superior margin of the orbit is the frontal bone, the inferior margin is the maxilla, palatine, and zygomatic bones, the medial margin is the frontal, lacrimal, and ethmoid bones, and the lateral margin is the zygomatic and sphenoid bones. The orbit lies below the anterior cranial fossa, above the maxillary sinus, lateral to the nasal cavity, and anterior to the middle cranial fossa (medially) and the temporal fossa (laterally). From the orbital rim, the orbit tapers posteriorly to an apex, the entrance of the optic canal. Two large discontinuities, the superior and inferior orbital fissures, converge upon one another in the back of the orbit just lateral to the apex.

Oncologic resections of maxillary tumors can be quite variable. There is no consensus in the literature on the nomenclature of types of maxillectomy. In many publications, the terms *partial* and *subtotal* have been used interchangeably. Spiro et al[6] divided maxillectomies into limited, subtotal, and total, depending on whether the resection involved predominantly one wall, at least two walls including the palate, or the entire maxilla. Others subclassify partial maxillectomy into infrastructure (where only the upper alveolus and hard palate below the level of the nasal floor are removed), medial (where the medial wall of the maxilla, often along with the medial third of the inferior orbital wall and the medial orbital wall, is removed), suprastructure (where all the walls of the maxilla, except the hard palate and upper alveolus, are removed), and subtotal (where all the walls of the maxilla, except the orbital floor and the zygomatic buttress, are removed).

Orbital exenteration involves removal of all the orbital contents, in contrast to enucleation, which involves removal of only the globe. In standard orbital exenteration, both eyelids and at least the anterior part of the orbit are removed. This technique is used for many adnexal cancers involving the eyelid with orbital extension. When the eyelid skin and orbicularis muscles are not involved in the cancerous process, such as in some palpebral conjunctival and orbital cancers, the anterior lamella of the eyelid (skin or musculocutaneous layer) can be spared and used for coverage of the exenterated orbital defect. As a matter of aesthetic preference, the eyelids may still be removed by some surgeons and replaced by skin from the reconstructive flap. In extended orbital exenteration, cancers of the paranasal sinuses, nasal cavity, and periorbital and facial soft tissues extending to the orbit require more radical surgical ablation, in which one or more orbital bony walls and neighboring structures, such as the sinuses and facial skin, may be resected. Both total maxillectomy and suprastructure maxillectomy may be combined with orbital exenteration, technically making each procedure an extended orbital exenteration but more often referred to as an orbitomaxillectomy by most surgeons.

## Reconstructive Approach

Medial maxillectomy involves resection of the medial wall of the maxilla and inferior turbinate. This surgery is usually indicated for benign or low-grade tumors arising from the lateral nasal wall. Formerly performed through a lateral rhinotomy incision, it is now frequently performed endoscopically. If no other structures are removed, reconstruction is unnecessary. For the remainder of maxillary and orbital resections, reconstruction or rehabilitation must be addressed with flaps, grafts, and/or prosthetics.

In terms of reconstruction, there are several key considerations.[7] The palate should be considered first (**Fig. 7.2**). The amount of hard and soft palate resected, as well as the location of the resection and the plans for dental restoration, will dictate whether a prosthetic obturator is indicated or a bony or soft tissue flap should be performed. The status of the orbital floor is important if the orbital contents are to be preserved (**Fig. 7.3**). Accurate reconstruction here, with grafts, implants, or bony flaps, is mandatory for useful eye function. If an extended orbital exenteration or orbitomaxillectomy is performed, a pedicled or free flap may be indicated to separate the orbit from the nasal cavity and sinuses, or occasionally the intracranial cavity. A pedicled or free flap may also be needed to serve as the lining of the remaining orbit for an orbital prosthetic if one is desired by the patient. A final consideration is whether facial skin and soft tissues, such as the lips, eyelids, or nose, will be included in the resection. Facial skin may be reconstructed with local tissues (e.g., cervicofacial rotation flap) or a pedicled or free flap, while other facial structures are usually addressed separately, most commonly with local tissue techniques (e.g., paramedian forehead flap for nasal reconstruction) that are beyond the scope of this chapter.

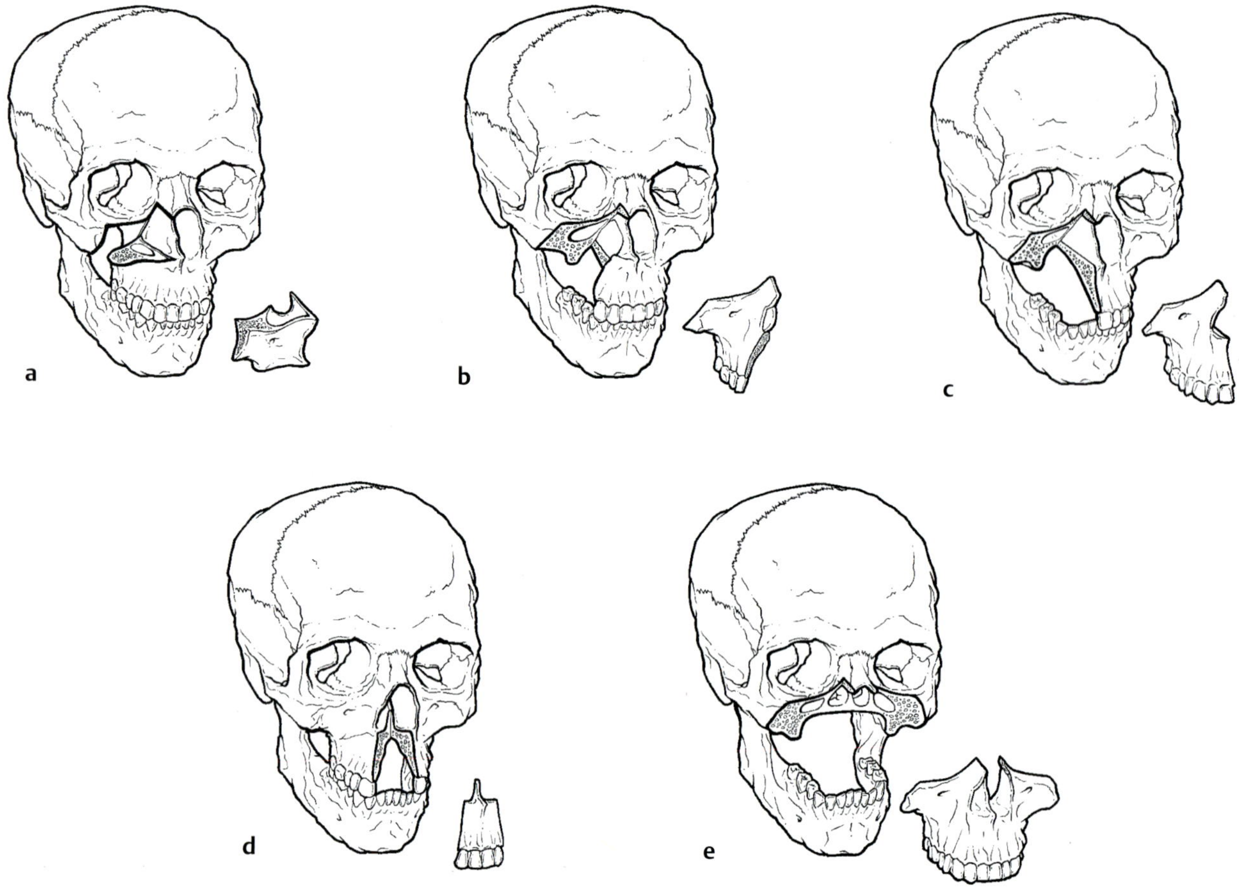

**Fig. 7.2** Reconstructive classification of palatomaxillary defects based on ability to accommodate an obturator and need for bony or soft tissue reconstruction. Maxillectomy types include: **(a)** superstructure maxillectomy, **(b)** posterior palatomaxillectomy, **(c)** hemipalatomaxillectomy, **(d)** premaxillary resection, and (**e**) bilateral palatomaxillectomy.

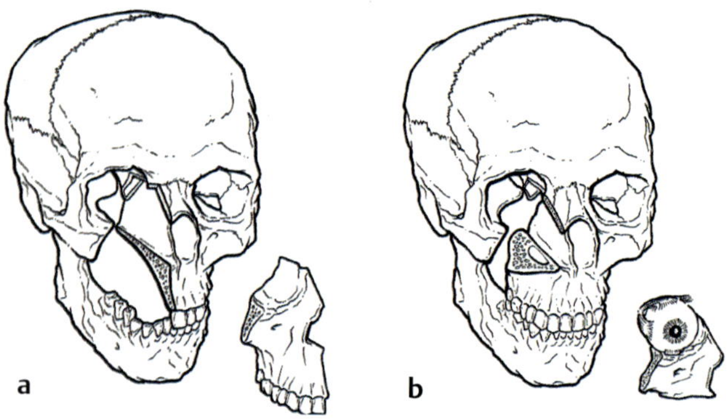

**Fig. 7.3** **(a)** Maxillectomy with orbital floor resection. In this case, a hemipalatomaxillectomy is performed with resection of the orbital floor, which is termed a *total maxillectomy* by some, although others use this term to include defects in which the orbital floor is spared. To avoid confusion, the status of the orbital floor should be mentioned separately. **(b)** Maxillectomy with orbital exenteration. In this case, orbital exenteration is combined with a superstructure maxillectomy, which is termed an *orbitomaxillectomy* by some authors.

## Suprastructure Maxillectomy

Suprastructure maxillectomies result in defects that do not involve the palate. Suprastructure defects that do not violate the bony orbit usually do not need reconstruction. Exceptions include when facial soft tissues are included in the resection and soft tissue cheek reconstruction is needed. Another exception may be when intracranial contents at the skull base have been exposed. In the latter case, a bulky soft tissue free flap that obliterates the maxillary sinus is recommended to isolate the intracranial cavity from the nasal cavity by creating a watertight seal against the dura or brain, thereby preventing cerebrospinal fluid leaks and meningitis, although small defects are often sealed with local or pedicled flaps, such as the temporoparietal fascial flap.

## Unilateral Posterior Palatomaxillectomy

While any number of palatoalveolar defects are possible, Okay et al[2] have recommended distinguishing defects based on whether function can be satisfactorily restored with an obturator or if a free flap is required. Palatoalveolar defects that spare both canine teeth can often be successfully treated with an obturator. In these cases, cantilever forces resulting in unstable prosthetic retention are minimized because of the favorable root morphology of the canine adjacent to the obturator and the generous arch length provided by the remaining alveolus. Thus, defects including unilateral posterior palatomaxillectomy defects or anterior defects limited to the premaxilla, which bears the four incisor teeth, can be obturated and should be considered separately from those that cannot, including those that involve half the palate and those that involve the entire anterior arch or whole palate.

Based on this information, unilateral palatomaxillectomy defects posterior to the canine tooth can usually be treated with an obturator. However, due to inadequate stability of the obturator in some patients, especially edentulous ones, and long-term costs associated with periodic adjustment and replacement of the prosthesis, autologous tissue may still be preferred in some patients. Additionally, exposure of the intracranial contents, loss of the orbital floor or orbital contents, and resection of the facial soft tissues are indications for free flap reconstruction.

We reconstruct posterior palatomaxillary defects with soft tissue rather than bony free flaps. The aesthetic challenge is usually to provide adequate volume to the cheek to support the facial soft tissues and to avoid a hollow appearance. An analogous situation is present in the mandible, where posterior mandibular reconstruction with soft tissue flaps can often achieve good results with regard to both function and appearance, provided the flap has adequate bulk. As with the mandible, restoration of posterior maxillary dentition, which is not easily visible even when smiling, is not a priority to many patients.

The anterolateral thigh (ALT) and rectus abdominis myocutaneous (RAMC) free flaps are usually well suited to providing the appropriate amount of tissue for posterior palatomaxillary reconstruction **(Fig. 7.4)**. These flaps tend to be thicker in Western

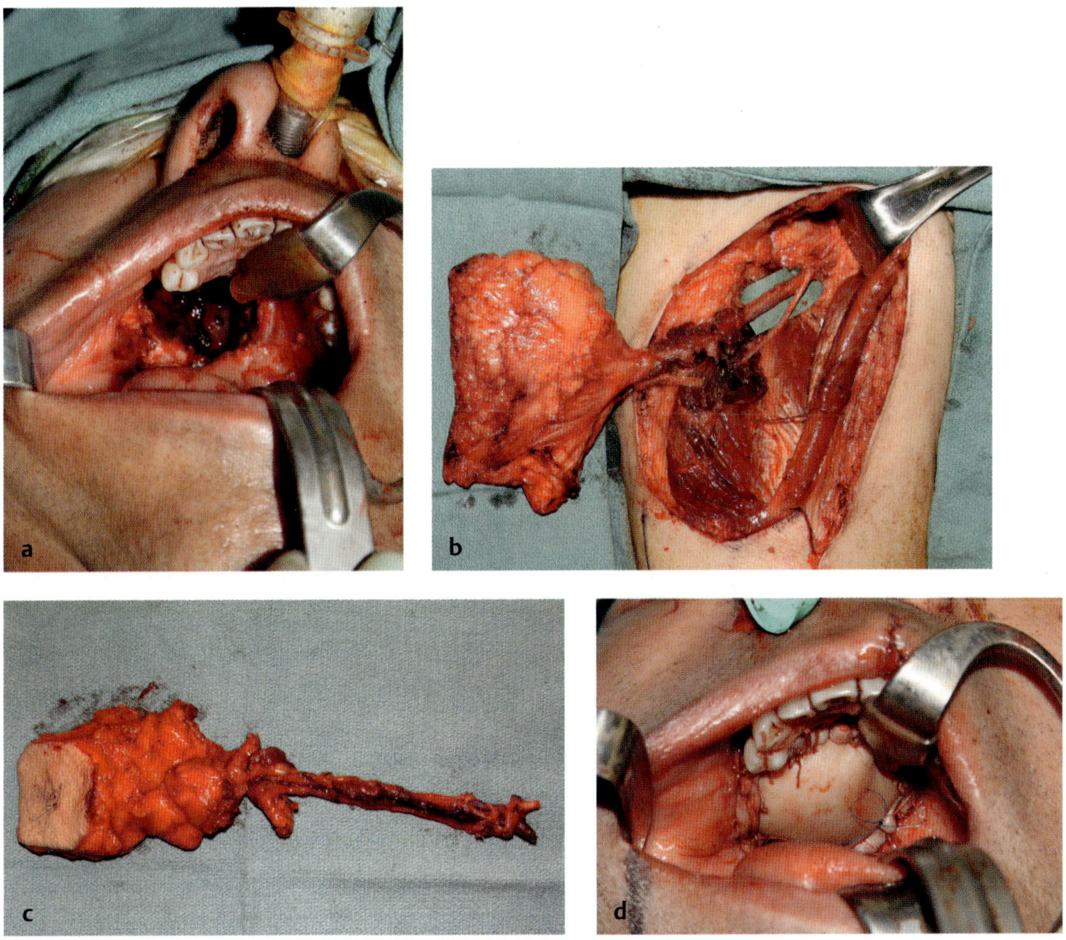

**Fig. 7.4** **(a)** Patient with a posterior palatomaxillectomy defect sparing the orbital floor and orbital contents **(b,c)** undergoing an anterolateral thigh free flap reconstruction. **(d)** The maxillary sinus is obliterated after complete removal of the mucosa with a diamond bur drill. The flap is inset so that it does not hang into the oral cavity. (*Continued on page 104*)

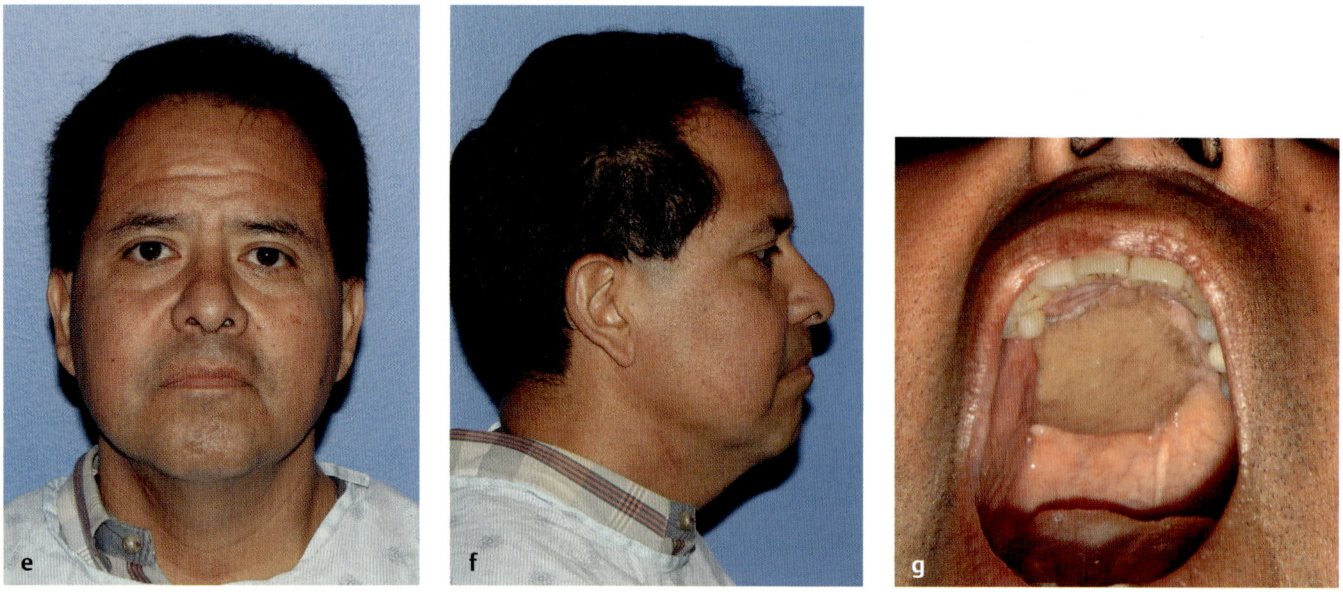


**Fig. 7.4** (*Continued*) **(e–g)** Postoperative external and intraoral appearance.

patients and will partially obliterate the maxillary sinus. Both flaps can be dissected in a way that minimizes their muscular components, and the flaps can be safely defatted in patients who have more subcutaneous adipose tissue than desired. By utilizing distal perforators, pedicle length is usually satisfactory in both flaps to reach the neck blood vessels without need for interposition vein grafting. The radial forearm fasciocutaneous free flap can be used on more obese individuals or for small defects in which bulk is not needed to provide cheek projection. Suturing to the palatal mucosa should ideally take place over the bony palatal remnant to avoid an oronasal fistula, or drill holes can be made in the bony palate and a deep layer of sutures placed through them for an extra degree of wound closure stability.

For all free flap reconstructions in the midface, the facial artery and vein or the superficial temporal artery and vein are the preferred recipient vessels when available. When the facial artery and vein are used as recipient blood vessels, a subcutaneous tunnel is created within the cheek to the neck, which should prevent injury to the distal branches of the facial nerve. Care is taken not to injure the parotid duct during tunnel creation.

## Unilateral Hemipalatomaxillectomy

Unlike unilateral posterior palatomaxillectomy defects, defects where the resection of the palate and alveolus extends anterior to the canine tooth are difficult to obturate because of the greater cantilever forces acting on the prosthesis, which must rely on less dentition for retention. This is consistent with our experience, in which many patients who desire dental restoration are unable to accommodate a conventionally retained prosthesis, in contrast to patients who undergo a posterior palatomaxillectomy. Free flap selection for these defects is somewhat controversial. Soft tissue free flaps are usually more straightforward surgically. However, they do not provide a rigid skeletal framework, which can result in a loss of anterior maxillary projection on the side of the defect, and they cannot accept osseointegrated implants for dental restoration. To accommodate a conventional dental prosthesis, the soft tissue flap must not protrude excessively into the oral cavity. However, achieving a concave palatal reconstruction with soft tissue flaps can be technically challenging, especially if the lateral portion of the defect includes some or all of the buccal mucosa.

We favor the use of osteocutaneous free flaps for hemipalatomaxillectomy defects in highly functional patients with a reasonable oncologic prognosis **(Fig. 7.5)**.[8] Besides providing better anterior projection, osteocutaneous free flaps offer the possibility of osseointegrated implants for dental restoration.[9] A caveat is that postoperative radiation therapy may render placement of osseointegrated implants risky, thus defeating one of the main purposes of bony reconstruction. In such cases, options include initial placement of an obturator, if possible, followed by delayed osteocutaneous free flap reconstruction after the conclusion of radiation, or proceeding with immediate bony reconstruction and simultaneous osseointegrated implant placement. Some centers do perform delayed osseointegrated implant placement even into irradiated bony free flaps after treatment with hyperbaric oxygen therapy, although the efficacy of this strategy still needs to be established.

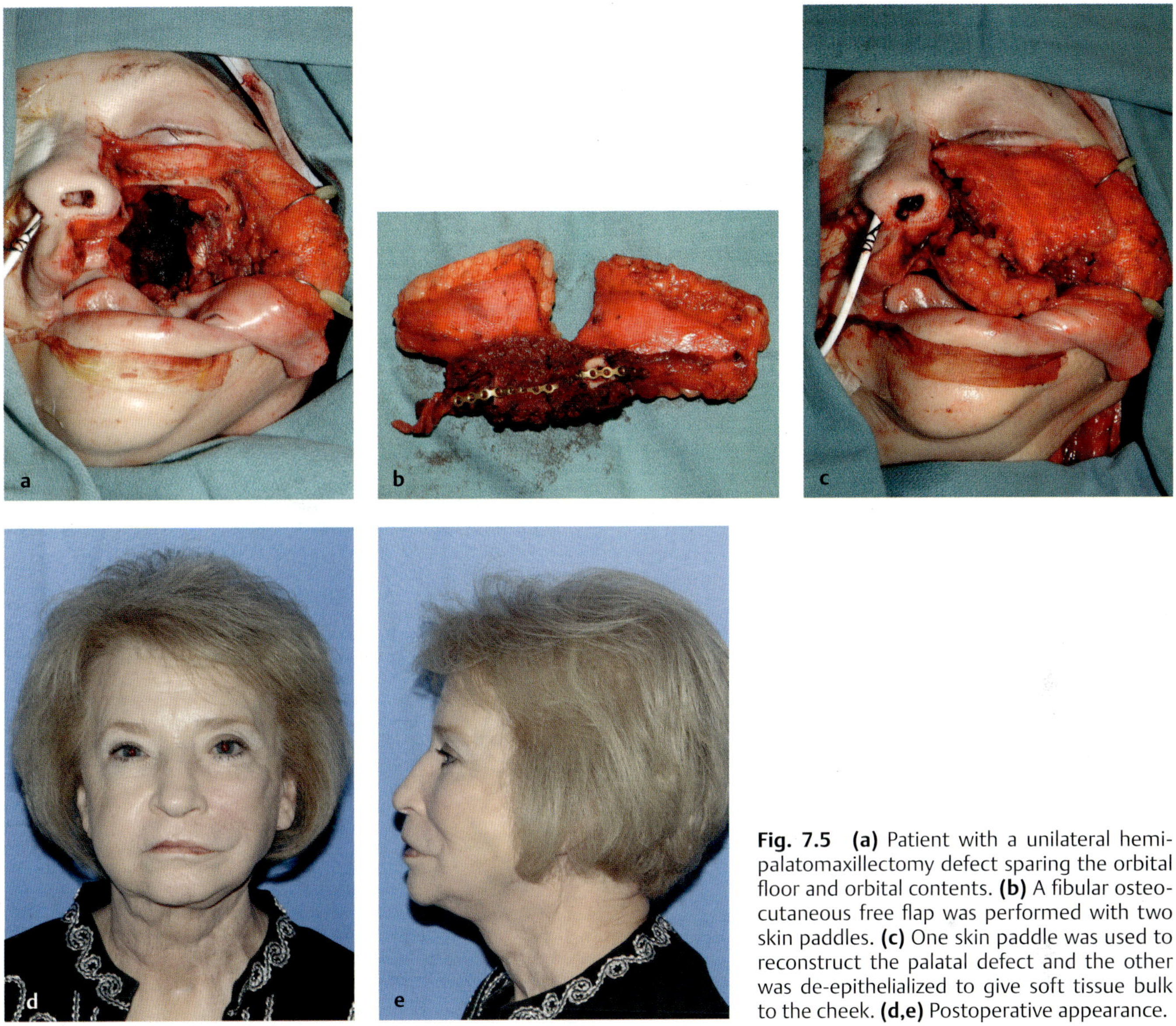

**Fig. 7.5 (a)** Patient with a unilateral hemipalatomaxillectomy defect sparing the orbital floor and orbital contents. **(b)** A fibular osteocutaneous free flap was performed with two skin paddles. **(c)** One skin paddle was used to reconstruct the palatal defect and the other was de-epithelialized to give soft tissue bulk to the cheek. **(d,e)** Postoperative appearance.

In terms of bony free flap selection, many donor sites have been suggested, including the fibula,[10] scapula,[11] radius,[12] rib, and iliac crest.[13,14] We favor the fibula because of its high-quality bone stock, which easily accommodates osseointegrated implants, and thin skin paddle, which is relatively adherent to the bone, as is desirable for palatal reconstruction without ptosis of the soft tissue component of the flap into the mouth. Regardless of which flap is used, we recommend making osteotomies to simulate the complex shape of the native maxilla as closely as possible. While it is tempting to simply place vascularized bone in a nonanatomic position and shape, our experience is that the soft tissues of the cheek will eventually contract and reveal the shape of the underlying bone, especially when postoperative radiation is administered. We discuss fibula shaping more below.

## Anterior Palatomaxillectomy (Premaxillary Resection)

Premaxillary defects usually arise from resection of lip or nasal pathologies. Most such defects are amenable to obturation alone or a soft tissue free flap combined with a dental prosthesis that clasps to the remaining teeth to maintain midfacial projection and to support the lip and nose. Osteocutaneous free flaps, such as the fibular osteocutaneous free flap or the radial forearm osteocutaneous free flap, may also be used to reconstruct the defect. The advantage of an osteocutaneous flap in this area is maintenance of upper lip and nose support without an obturator as well as the possibility of osseointegrated implant dental restoration.

## Bilateral Palatomaxillectomy

Bilateral palatomaxillectomy defects that involve loss of the anterior maxillary alveolar arch, including the canine teeth, require bony reconstruction to maintain midfacial height, width, and projection. They also require bony reconstruction for dental restoration with osseointegrated implants, which are usually necessary to retain a prosthesis. Bilateral palatomaxillectomy defects can rarely, if ever, be stably obturated.[2,8] Although other osteocutaneous free flaps have been advocated, the fibular free flap is our preferred flap for bilateral palatomaxillectomy reconstruction, for the same reasons noted above. In addition, for sizable defects involving both maxillary bones, the fibula offers the longest length of bone of the various flap options.

In our experience, 14 to 16 cm of bone length is typically needed to reconstruct a bilateral maxillectomy defect.[15,16] Therefore, the entire fibular length, sparing only 5 to 7 cm distally and 5 to 7 cm proximally, is initially harvested and the proximal bone is then trimmed to maximize vascular pedicle length. The lateral surface of the fibula is used to restore the vertical maxillary height, measured from the orbital rim to the occlusal plane of the hard palate, by orienting it such that it faces anteriorly on the face. The peroneal vessels, therefore, assume a posterior position facing the maxillary sinus. Some flexor hallucis longus muscle is usually included with the flap to obliterate the maxillary sinus cavity and to provide adequate soft tissue around the vascular pedicle to prevent its desiccation. The skin paddle of the flap is used to reconstruct the palatal defect. The orientation of the skin paddle depends on the location of its perforator blood supply, and it may be longitudinally or transversely oriented in relation to the long axis of the fibula.

When the bony defect extends more laterally or posteriorly on one side than another, that side is usually preferred for the microvascular anastomosis due to closer proximity to the recipient blood vessels. Alternatively, the side with better recipient blood vessels, if any, is selected for the microvascular anastomosis. The leg that is ipsilateral to the side of the planned microvascular anastomosis is selected for fibular osteocutaneous free flap harvest so that the skin paddle can be used to restore the palate. Vein grafts are used when pedicle length is inadequate to reach the recipient vessels. We prefer to use the facial blood vessels as recipients when available, due to their proximity to the defect and their good caliber match to the peroneal blood vessels.

After the resection is complete, a titanium reconstruction plate is fashioned in the approximate shape of the Greek letter omega in the transverse plane (**Fig. 7.6** and **Fig. 7.7**). The configuration of the reconstruction plate is such that it simulates the width and projection of the native maxilla. The lateral portions of the reconstruction plate must be long enough to allow fixation with two or three screws

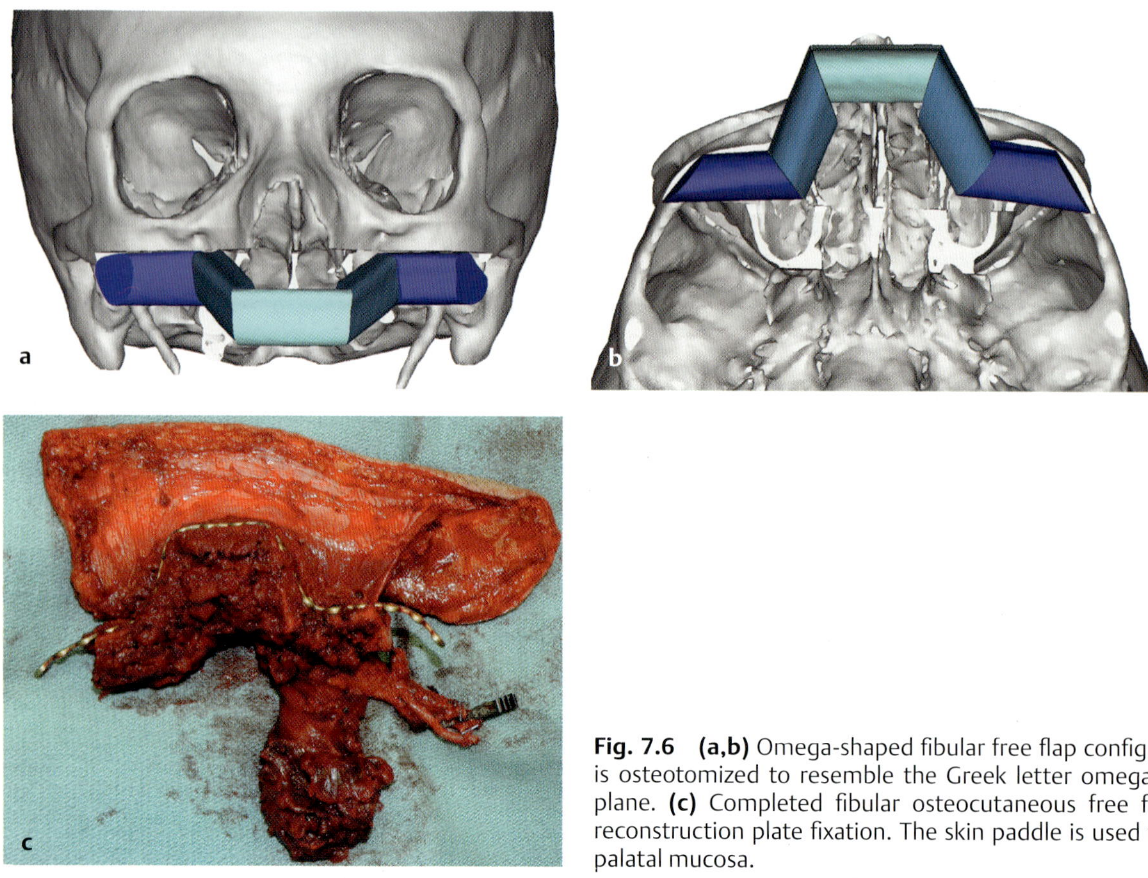

**Fig. 7.6** **(a,b)** Omega-shaped fibular free flap configuration. The fibula is osteotomized to resemble the Greek letter omega in the horizontal plane. **(c)** Completed fibular osteocutaneous free flap with titanium reconstruction plate fixation. The skin paddle is used to reconstruct the palatal mucosa.

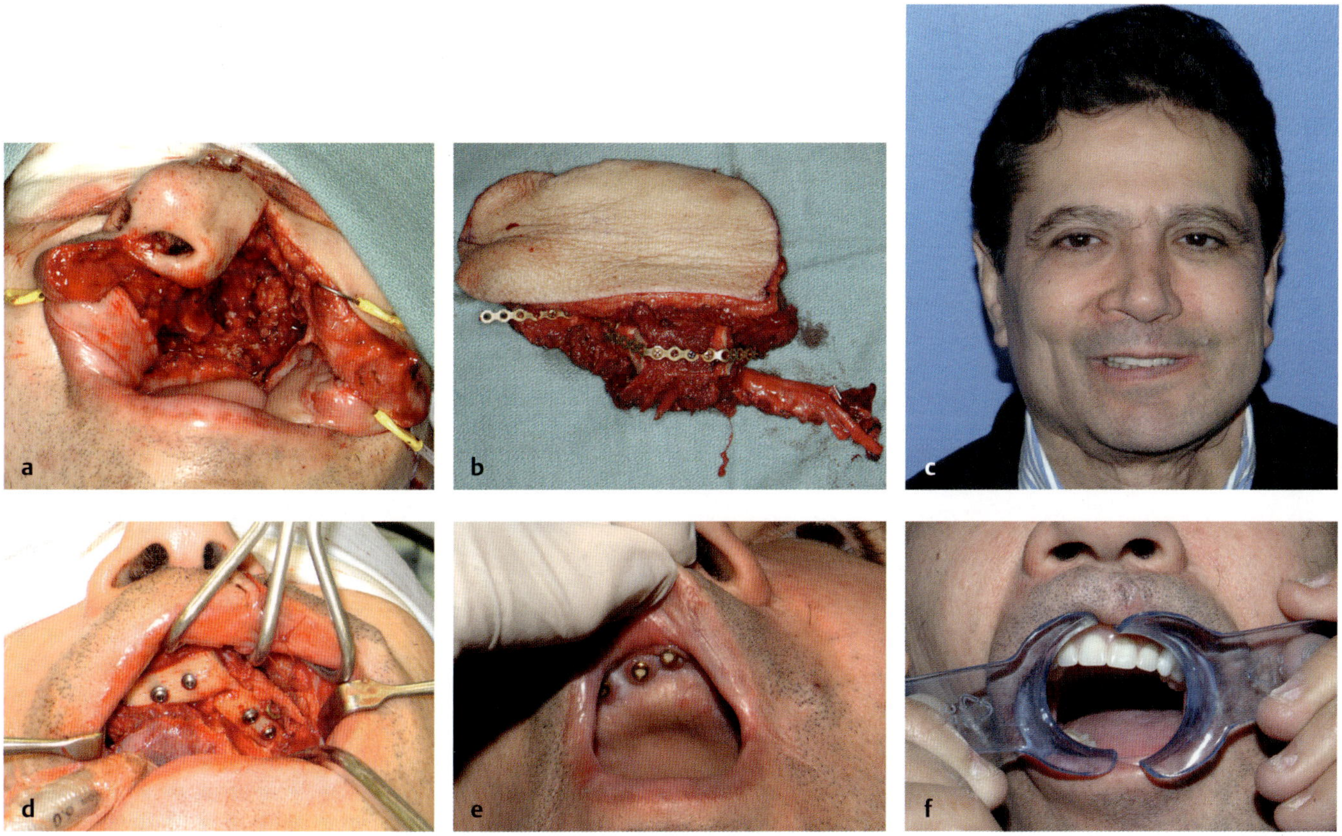

**Fig. 7.7** **(a)** Patient with a bilateral palatomaxillectomy defect sparing the orbital floors and orbital contents undergoing a **(b)** fibular osteocutaneous free flap reconstruction. **(c)** Postoperative appearance. **(d)** Osseointegrated implants were placed 6 months after the initial reconstruction for dental restoration. **(e)** Abutments were then placed through the fibular free flap skin paddle and **(f)** were used to retain a dental prosthesis.

to the remaining zygomatic bones laterally. Separate plates may be used to fix the fibular construct to the remaining facial skeleton, thereby facilitating anterior plate removal at a later date, if needed to allow room for osseointegrated implant placement.

Closing wedge osteotomies are performed on the fibula with a reciprocating saw, taking care not to injure the vascular pedicle. When reconstructing bilateral maxillectomy defects, the lateral portions of the omega recreate the malar regions. The central portion of the fibular free flap restores the maxillary alveolus. For unilateral (see the section on hemipalatomaxillectomy, above) or less than complete bilateral defects, a shorter segment of bone is used and one or more osteotomies can be omitted (i.e., the fibula resembles a half or incomplete omega).

Generally, two to three screw holes are available to secure each fibular segment. The portion of the fibular free flap that replaces the anterior maxillae is inset at the vertical level of the resected alveolus, rather than at the level of the dentition, to provide room for an implant-retained dental prosthesis. A slight downward angulation of the portion of the fibula used to recreate the anterior maxillae is usually desirable to fully restore vertical facial height.

Dental restoration with osseointegrated implants is performed 3 to 6 months after fibular free flap reconstruction. In patients with significant subcutaneous adipose tissue in their fibular free flap skin paddle, thinning of the fat is usually performed simultaneously with placement of the implants. Partial or total hardware removal is sometimes necessary to place the osseointegrated dental implants.

## Orbital Floor Defects

Our experience suggests that, when supported by a soft tissue free flap, the orbital floor can usually be successfully reconstructed with bone grafts or alloplasts, even when postoperative radiation therapy is administered (**Fig. 7.8**). Many surgeons, however, feel that bone grafts are relatively more resistant to radiation-associated complications than alloplasts are.[17] In a recent review of orbital floor reconstruction for trauma, Kirby et al[18] found that autologous bone reconstructions were more likely to be complicated by orbital dystopia and enophthalmos than were titanium mesh and porous polyethylene, possibly due to increased difficulty in shaping the reconstructed

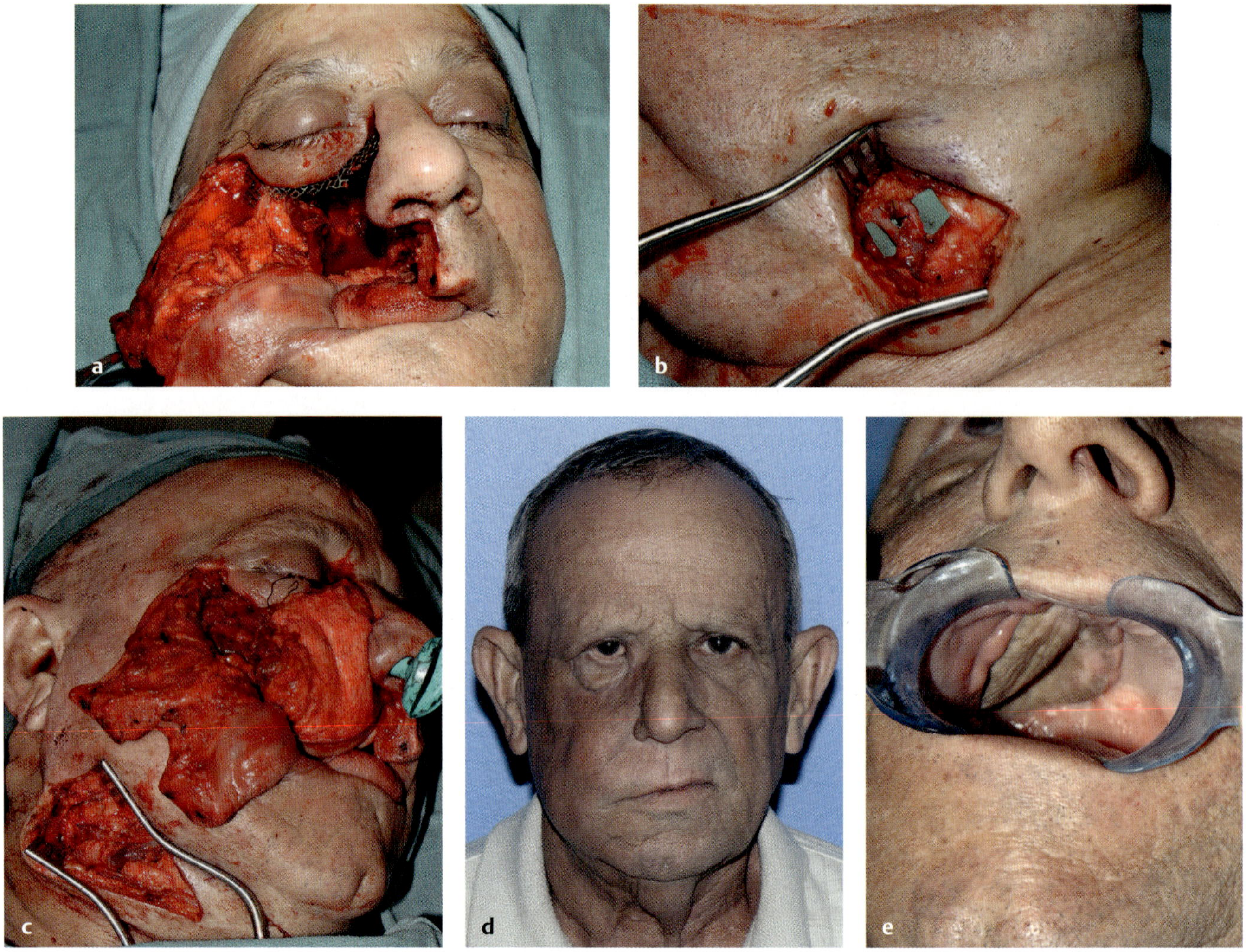


**Fig. 7.8** Patient with a superstructure maxillectomy with orbital floor defect. **(a)** An orbital floor reconstruction with titanium mesh was performed. **(b)** A limited neck incision was used to gain access to the facial artery and vein for use as free flap recipient blood vessels. **(c)** This was followed by an anterolateral thigh free flap to support the hardware as well as to provide shape to the cheek. **(d,e)** Postoperative external and intraoral appearance.

orbital floor, irregular thickness, and unpredictable resorption. Obviously, alloplastic materials have the advantages of being available in virtually unlimited quantities and of incurring no donor-site morbidity.

When using the fibular osteocutaneous free flap for reconstructing hemipalatomaxillectomy and bilateral palatomaxillectomy defects that include resection of the orbital floor, we include some soleus or flexor hallucis longus muscle with the fibular osteocutaneous free flap to support a bone graft or alloplastic orbital floor reconstruction. A double-barreled design to reconstruct both the floor and the hard palate is possible[19] but challenging because of the limited space in the midface. Patients who have had a complication following nonvascularized reconstruction can usually be reconstructed secondarily with a bony free flap, such as the fibula, scapula, or radial forearm osteocutaneous free flaps or even the serratus anterior with rib **(Fig. 7.9)**.

## Orbital Exenteration Defects

The primary goal of reconstruction of orbital exenteration defects is to line the orbital cavity with durable tissue and to exclude the nasal or sinus cavities when the medial or inferior orbital wall has been removed, as well as to protect the brain when the orbital roof has been removed. In addition, the patient's desire for prosthetic rehabilitation should be considered when planning the reconstruction. A deep orbital cavity facilitates prosthetic fit, while a shallow orbital cavity, or an orbital reconstruction that sits flush with the face or is convex, may not securely hold a prosthesis without osseointegrated implants or may cause the prosthesis to protrude unnaturally.

Healing by secondary intention and granulation may be the simplest treatment after tumor resection. The entire process will take 2 to 3 months and

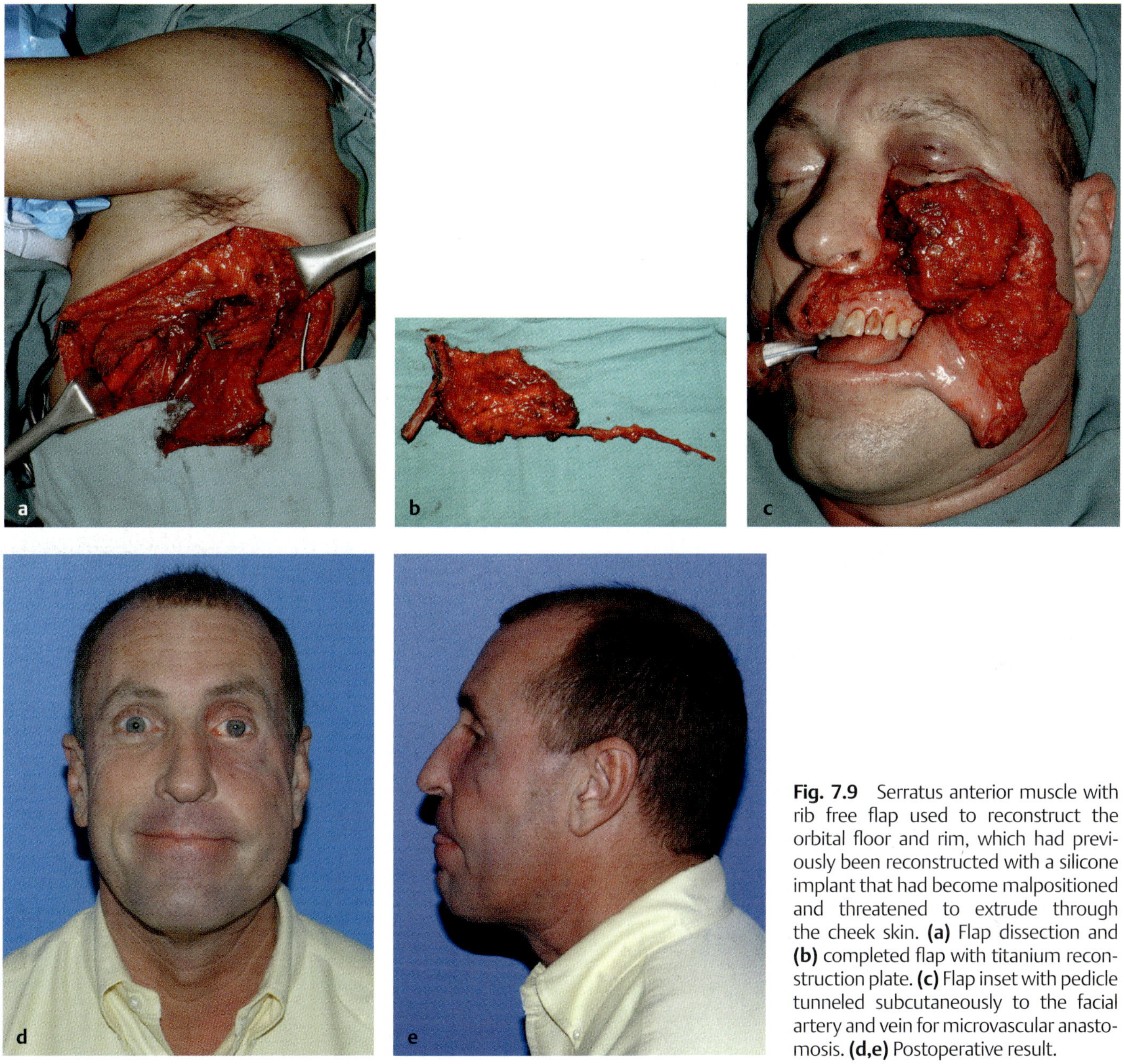


**Fig. 7.9** Serratus anterior muscle with rib free flap used to reconstruct the orbital floor and rim, which had previously been reconstructed with a silicone implant that had become malpositioned and threatened to extrude through the cheek skin. **(a)** Flap dissection and **(b)** completed flap with titanium reconstruction plate. **(c)** Flap inset with pedicle tunneled subcutaneously to the facial artery and vein for microvascular anastomosis. **(d,e)** Postoperative result.

requires daily wound care with wet-to-dry dressings. When completely healed by secondary intention, the orbital cavity is only slightly shallowed by granulation tissue, rendering inspection of local tumor recurrence relatively easy. It is our preference to accelerate wound closure using a meshed or unmeshed split-thickness skin graft, which can be utilized to line the orbital cavity. Similar to healing by secondary intention, split-thickness skin grafting of the orbital defect also results in the ability to perform excellent visualization of the orbital cavity. Due to their thinness, skin graft reconstructions usually result in a deep orbital cavity that provides an excellent fit for an orbital prosthesis if one is desired by the patient. When there is no history of prior radiation and no postoperative radiation is planned, healing by secondary intention or skin grafting, even on bare orbital bone, is usually successful for addressing the standard orbital exenteration wound.

If the orbital cavity is to be irradiated after surgery, more durable, well-vascularized lining of the orbital cavity with soft tissue rather than just spontaneous epithelialization or skin graft coverage is necessary to avoid chronic bone exposure and osteoradionecrosis. Among local pedicled flaps used, the most common ones are the temporalis muscle flap or temporoparietal fascia flap, by virtue of their proximity to the orbit. The temporalis muscle flap, based on the anterior and posterior deep temporal arteries arising from the internal maxillary artery, is thin enough to permit a reasonably secure fit for an orbital prosthesis, even without osseointegrated implants, but results in a depression at the donor site, which may be cosmetically unfavorable in many patients. The temporal parietal fascia flap covered by a split-thickness skin graft may be preferable in that there is no donor-site deformity. In both cases, reach of the flaps may be limited, and it may be necessary to remove the lateral orbital wall to cover the medial orbital cavity and to avoid a bulge caused by the proximal flap soft tissue over the lateral orbital rim. Large scalp or forehead flaps should be avoided when other reconstructive options are available because of their donor-site disfigurement.

In extended orbital exenteration, the size of the cavity usually necessitates soft tissue coverage larger than what local or regional flaps can provide.[19] An exception is the resection of the lateral orbital wall alone, which is usually inconsequential from a reconstructive standpoint. The orbital cavity may still be reconstructed with a skin graft or regional flap. In addition, limited defects of the medial orbital wall can often still be reconstructed with a temporalis flap. For all other defects, we recommend reconstruction with a microvascular free flap. A multitude of soft tissue free flaps are satisfactory for reconstruction of the extended orbital exenteration cavity.

Our preference is to reconstruct the cavity with a radial forearm fasciocutaneous free flap in cases where the bony resection is limited. This flap provides an adequate amount of tissue, with relatively little bulk in nonobese patients, to accommodate an orbital prosthetic without revision surgery. In cases where the bony resection is more extensive, such as in the case of an orbitomaxillectomy, a larger, bulkier flap is preferred. The rectus abdominis myocutaneous and the ALT free flaps are good choices in this situation. Both flaps may be designed so that muscle tissue obliterates the sinuses and creates a tight seal over any exposed dura, preventing infection with sinonasal bacterial flora. Bulkier flaps like these are required to restore midfacial volume and to preserve cheek contour. In these cases, the reconstruction usually results in a convex orbital reconstruction, which will require flap revision at a later date if an orbital prosthesis is desired.

Orbital exenteration performed in concert with a suprastructure maxillectomy (i.e., orbitomaxillectomy) adds another reconstructive priority: closure of the nasal cavity to prevent the escape of air and nasal drainage. Because the formation of a sinonasocutaneous fistula along the suture line between the medial flap (or native cheek skin) and the nose can be difficult to treat, every effort should be made to obtain a secure closure. While thin fasciocutaneous flaps that result in a concave orbital cavity are beneficial for patients with isolated orbital exenteration defects who wish to have an orbital prosthesis, for patients with orbitomaxillectomy defects, we recommend bulkier free flaps that obliterate the orbital cavity to minimize the chance of a fistula as well as to maintain cheek contour. The rectus abdominis free flap, harvested as a myocutaneous flap or as a muscle-sparing variant (i.e., muscle-sparing rectus abdominis free flap, or deep inferior epigastric perforator flap), is suitable and can be tailored to the specifics of the defect in terms of size, volume, and desired pedicle length. The ALT free flap also works well for orbitomaxillectomy reconstruction **(Fig. 7.10)**. A myocutaneous ALT free flap, incorporating some or all of the thickness of the vastus lateralis muscle, can be used when the thigh is thin and has insufficient adipose tissue to restore cheek contour, although muscle atrophy may result in significant volume loss in the future.

Defects resulting from both orbital exenteration and palatomaxillectomy are best reconstructed with flaps that allow for multiple skin paddles to close the three defects (external orbital skin, nasal lining, and palatal coverage) separately, allowing for airtight skin-to-skin and skin-to-mucosa closure. Both the rectus abdominis myocutaneous free flap and ALT free flap are usually good choices here as well, again with the flap design tailored to include more or less muscle based on the extent of the defect. In cases where the pedicle of the ALT free flap gives rise to only a single cutaneous perforator, a portion of the skin paddle can be de-epithelialized to reconstruct two or more surfaces. It is usually the author's preference to leave a "raw" (noncutaneous) flap surface facing the nasal cavity and to allow it to spontaneously remucosalize. A soft silicone nasal trumpet is left in the adjacent nostril for ~ 2 weeks to prevent adhesions from developing between the flap and the nasal septum.

We have never encountered a bilateral/anterior palatomaxillectomy defect that was combined with orbital exenteration, although they are a theoretical possibility. Ideally, in such cases, an osteocutaneous free flap is used to reconstruct the palatoalveolar defect and a soft tissue free flap is used to reconstruct the orbital defect. Such complex reconstruction should obviously be weighed against the patient's medical condition and overall prognosis.

Custom-made orbitofacial prostheses may be used for aesthetic rehabilitation after orbital exenteration. The aesthetic result is pleasing, especially when camouflaged with eyeglasses. Options for retention include the use of adhesive or osseointegrated titanium implants. Such implants are placed into the bony orbital margins. A minimum of 3 or 4 mm of bone thickness must be present to accommodate the

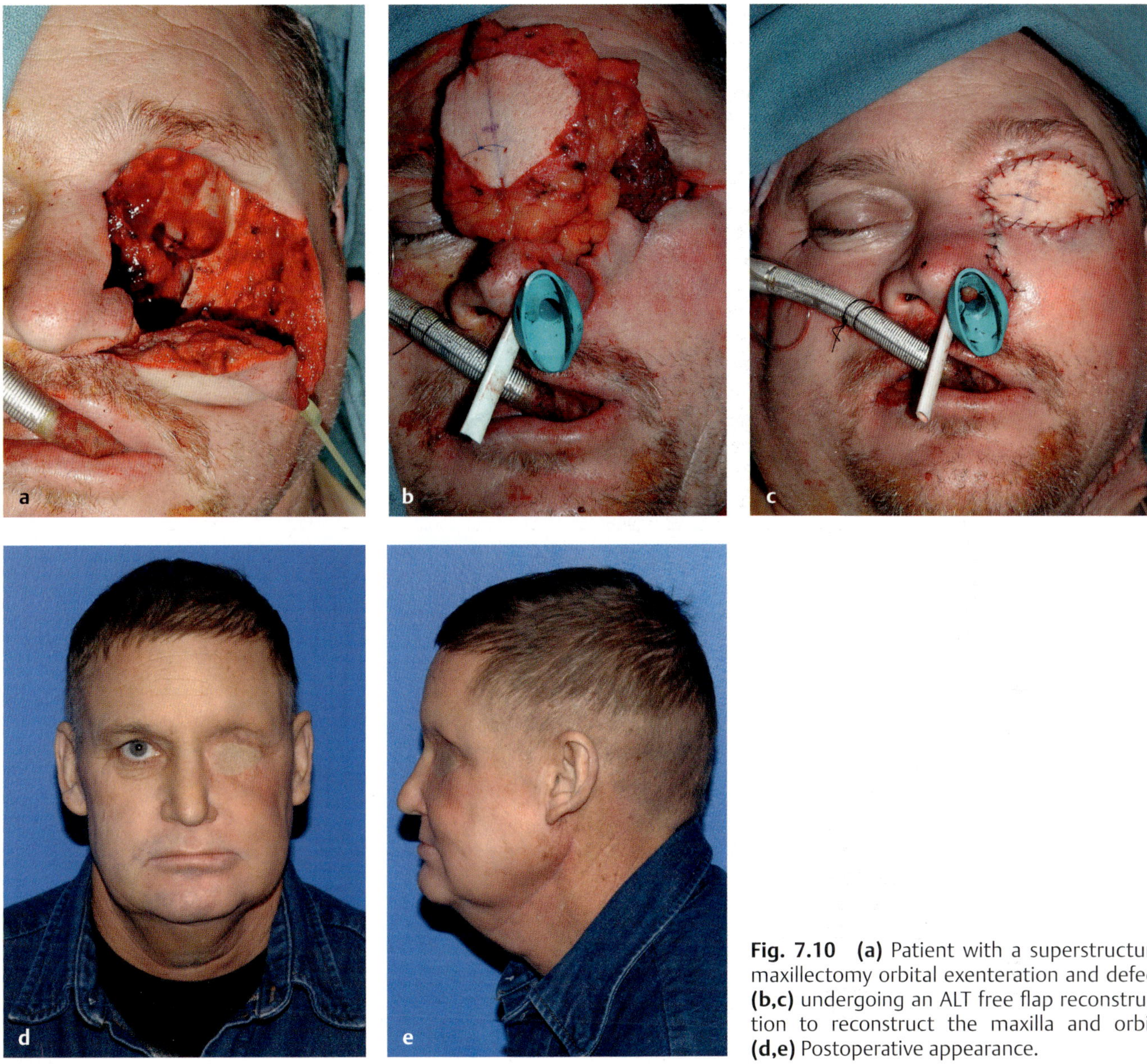


**Fig. 7.10** **(a)** Patient with a superstructure maxillectomy orbital exenteration and defect **(b,c)** undergoing an ALT free flap reconstruction to reconstruct the maxilla and orbit. **(d,e)** Postoperative appearance.

implants, which are then covered with skin and soft tissue. Thin, immobile soft tissue coverage is desirable to minimize excessive abutment lengths and to avoid chronic tissue irritation. Implants may be left buried for several months to allow osseointegration, or they may be exposed immediately and abutments, which protrude above the level of the skin, can be attached to the implants. Finally the prostheses are coupled to the abutments via magnetic or clasp-retained attachments.

Multistage prosthetic rehabilitation demands significant motivation from patients. An eye patch or dark glasses may be satisfactory for some patients. As mentioned, a bulky flap may limit accommodation of an orbital prosthetic or may cause the prosthesis to protrude excessively compared with the contralateral side. In some cases, the fit and appearance of an orbital prosthetic can be improved by debulking or recontouring of the reconstructive flap. Limitations of prosthetics include the inability of the eye to move and the static nature of the eyelids. Several fittings may also be needed, and the prosthetics, which can be costly, need to be replaced periodically due to normal wear and tear.

Our reconstructive algorithm is summarized in **Fig. 7.11**.

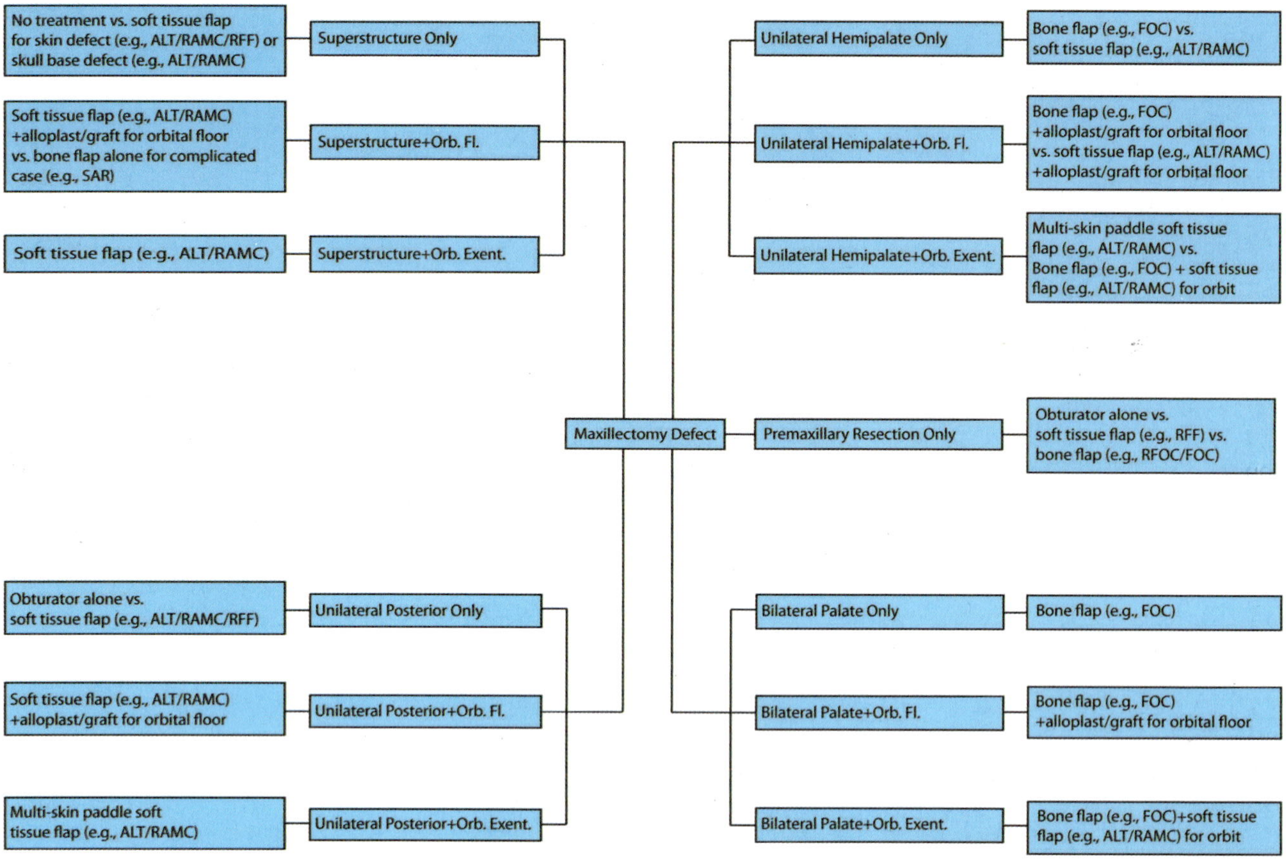


**Fig. 7.11** Reconstructive algorithm. ALT, anterolateral thigh; RAMC, rectus abdominis myocutaneous; FOC, fibular osteocutaneous; RFF, radial forearm fasciocutaneous; RFOC, radial forearm osteocutaneous.

## Postoperative Care

As with most head and neck reconstructions, the head of the bed should be elevated postoperatively. Some nasal drainage is expected. We usually favor placement of a soft silicone nasal trumpet for 1 to 4 weeks to stent the nasal passage open. The nasal trumpet is secured loosely to the membranous septum with a suture. If the reconstruction includes an oral suture line, a feeding tube is placed and the patient is not allowed oral intake for 1 to 2 weeks, depending on the risk for fistulization.

In patients who have had orbital wall reconstruction, periodic light perception and visual acuity checks are necessary to rule out optic nerve injury or globe compression. Any signs of decreased vision should prompt an immediate ophthalmology consult. Extraocular movements should be assessed as well, although a forced duction test at the conclusion of the surgery should have been performed to rule out entrapment.[20]

## Complications

In our experience, the success rate of free flaps used in midfacial reconstruction is as high as that for free flaps used to reconstruct other head and neck defects. Because of the greater distance from the cervical recipient blood vessels, there is the potential for pedicle length to be inadequate. In such instances, interposition vein grafting is preferable to performing anastomoses under tension. Also, care must be taken to make an adequately large subcutaneous tunnel for the pedicle to reach the neck without compression.

Specific to maxillary and orbital reconstruction is the potential for fistula formation, including both oronasal (i.e., palatal) fistulas and sino-nasocutaneous fistulas, usually near the medial canthus. Closure along palatal and facial suture lines must be multilayered and meticulous. Nasal obstruction should be avoided, as air under pressure can cause wound breakdown along lateral rhinotomy incisions and medial orbital incisions. In our experience, late-occurring fistulas in irradiated patients rarely heal spontaneously and usually require another free flap for closure.[7]

With regard to orbital reconstruction, there is a potential for graft or implant exposure along the orbital rim when tissues are thin and poorly vascularized, especially when incisions are placed over bony prominences or titanium hardware. In such cases, consideration should be given to placing flap tissue between bone grafts, implants, or hardware and the cheek or eyelid skin or to replacing the skin with a flap skin. Also, accurate positioning of the reconstructed orbital walls is critical to avoiding orbital content entrapment, enophthalmos or exophthalmos, vertical dystopia (eyes at different levels), or even blindness due to elevated intraocular pressure or impingement of the optic nerve if grafts and implants are placed too far posteriorly in the region of the orbital apex.

Other common sequelae of maxillary reconstruction are lower eyelid ectropion and notching of the lid. Careful closure with care taken to suspend the lower eyelid, but avoiding orbital rim and subciliary incisions if at all possible, is usually the best prevention for avoiding ectropion. Ectropion may also be avoided by using a transconjunctival approach, as described by Cordeiro et al.[17] Secondary corrective procedures, such as canthoplasty or lower eyelid suspension with fascial or cartilage grafts, can also help to correct ectropion but will usually not achieve perfect symmetry in irradiated patients. Lid notching occurs with less predictability, but care should nevertheless be taken to evert the lid closure. Incorporation of a z-plasty on the mucosal side of the lid may be helpful in avoiding notching.

## Pearls and Pitfalls

- When reconstructing the midface, consideration must be given to reconstruction of the palate, the orbital floor, and the orbital cavity.
- Partial palatomaxillary defects posterior to the canine tooth can be obturated or satisfactorily reconstructed with a soft tissue free flap, such as an anterolateral thigh, radial forearm fasciocutaneous, or rectus abdominis myocutaneous free flap.
- Hemipalatomaxillary defects are reconstructed with either a bulky soft tissue free flap or a bony free flap in patients with a good functional and oncologic prognosis, particularly when dental restoration is planned.
- Bilateral anterior palatomaxillary defects are best reconstructed with bony free flaps, such as the fibular osteocutaneous free flap.
- Small anterior premaxillary defects can be obturated or reconstructed with a small osteocutaneous free flap.
- The orbital floor can usually be satisfactorily reconstructed with bone graft or titanium mesh as long as they are both supported by well-vascularized pedicled or free flap tissue.
- Accurate reconstruction of the orbital floor is important to prevent diplopia, visual changes, or even blindness.
- When the orbit has been exenterated, a thin pedicled flap or free flap facilitates prosthetic retention.
- A bulky free flap is indicated for an extended orbital exenteration, including an orbitomaxillectomy, to separate the nasal and sinus cavities from the orbit and to prevent a sinonasocutaneous fistula.

## Expert Commentary *by James S. Brown*

This chapter is a comprehensive description of an approach to maxillary reconstructive surgery, but the central part of the midface (the nasal bones and medial orbital walls) has not been included. The techniques are similar to Cordeiro's,[3] with the addition of the fibular osteocutaneous flap and the serratus anterior with rib. The techniques are clearly described, an algorithm is included to guide selection among the reconstructive options, and the quality of the cases presented is very high.

It is acknowledged early in the chapter that there are many varieties of midface and maxillary defects and a mastery of a broad range of hard and soft tissue free flap options is required. The importance of prosthetic options is also emphasized. The bone flap favored by the authors is the fibular flap, while the soft tissue flaps favored are the anterolateral thigh flap, rectus abdominis flap, and fasciocutaneous radial forearm flap, which are commonly known and used. The lack of appropriate discussion to compare other hard tissue options, including iliac crest with internal oblique or the scapula tip with teres major, latissimus dorsi, or serratus anterior, is an omission. These other bone options offer support of the nasal piriform and paranasal regions, adequate support of facial tissues when orbital floor resection is required, and, most importantly, the advantage of a muscle flap component, which, in my opinion, provides the natural result for restoring the hard palate and the nasal lining after spontaneous remucosalization.

In my own practice, the least frequently utilized bone reconstruction for the midface is the fibular flap. While the fibula will take an implant well and the flap withstands radiotherapy, the bone height is only adequate in low-level (inferior) maxillectomies, in which the nasal piriform is retained. Also, the problem of orbital floor removal is addressed by the author with titanium mesh, but this does not give bony support to the orbital rim, which is needed to prevent ectropion and lid contraction. Bony reconstruction of the orbital rim is required for the periorbital tissues to maintain their proper position in the longer term. Reconstruction of the orbital rim is very challenging with the fibular flap but more straightforward with scapular tip and iliac crest (deep circumflex iliac artery) flaps **(Fig. 7.12)**.

Having contributed to the methods of classification,[4] I wonder why the Class I–VI **(Fig. 7.13)** classification has not been used, because the proposed algorithm is very similar and includes Classes I to V b, c, and d, and would provide appropriate comparison and uniformity rather than further complicating the subject.

Removal of part or all of the nasal bones in midface resection was not addressed in the chapter. This is very important in Class III (maxillectomy including the orbital floor but not the orbit), when the resection involves the lateral nasal bones and loss of support to the medial canthus is easily restored with the iliac crest flap, but is more difficult with fibular and scapular tip flaps. In addition, a defect that requires the complete removal of the nasal bones and the related ethmoid sinuses (Class VI) requires composite reconstruction, which is achieved most effectively with the composite radial forearm flap.

The implication in this chapter is that obturation cannot be considered for bilateral maxillectomy defects; however, obturation is very possible for any Class II a to c defect if implants are used.[21] The best results for patients, especially for those less able to recover from major reconstructive surgery, are achieved by appropriate discussion with a prosthodontist. The prosthodontist will have to look after the dental side of the restoration and rehabilitation; therefore, the prosthodontist must be involved in the discussions with the patient and the surgeon from the start. In our service, virtually all obturated patients receive immediate implants, which can be loaded at the first obturator change. This relationship is the key to the team building and understanding that are so important for this patient group, when there are genuine choices with similar outcomes, and allows a significant de-escalation of surgery where appropriate through patient choice or medical necessity.

I must emphasize that my comments are opinion-based, because building reliable and consistent data for due comparison of outcomes is difficult with the small numbers of patients from most units. Dr. Hanasono continues to make valuable contributions to the literature in head and neck reconstructive surgery, and this chapter is further evidence of the experience and quality of MD Anderson in all its aspects.

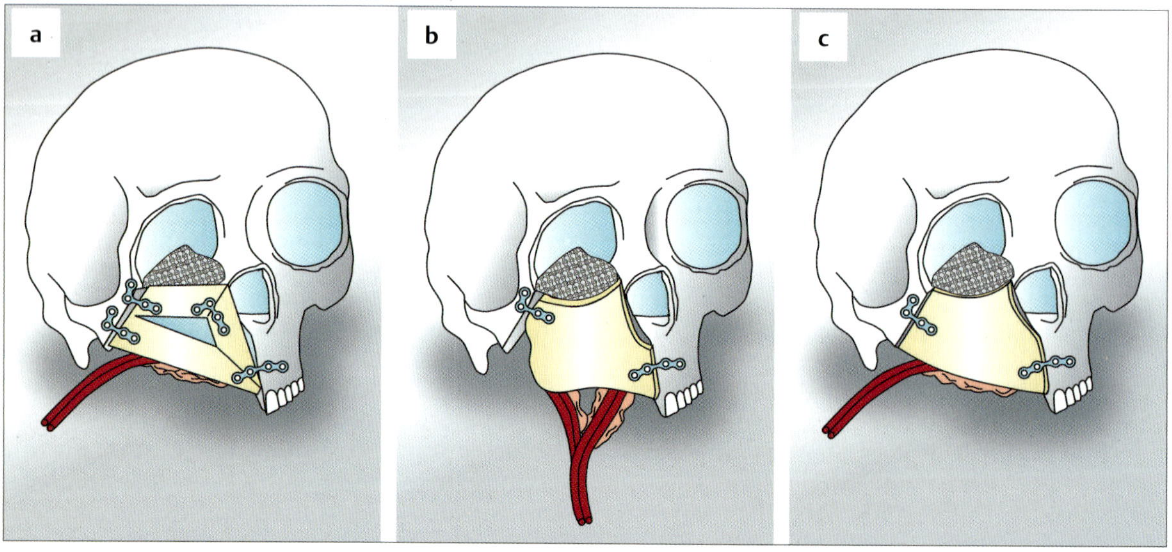


**Fig. 7.12** Possible reconstructions for maxillectomy defects that require orbital rim and floor restoration. **(a)** Fibular flap. This figure shows the acute angles needed and illustrates the difficulty of planning skin islands when utilizing this flap. **(b)** Scapular tip flap, based on the angular branch of the thoracodorsal artery. The flap is oriented so that the thicker lateral bone of the scapula forms the alveolus. **(c)** Iliac crest flap. This flap fills the defect and is the best option with regard to accepting an implant-retained prosthesis. Reprinted with permission from Brown and Shaw.[4]

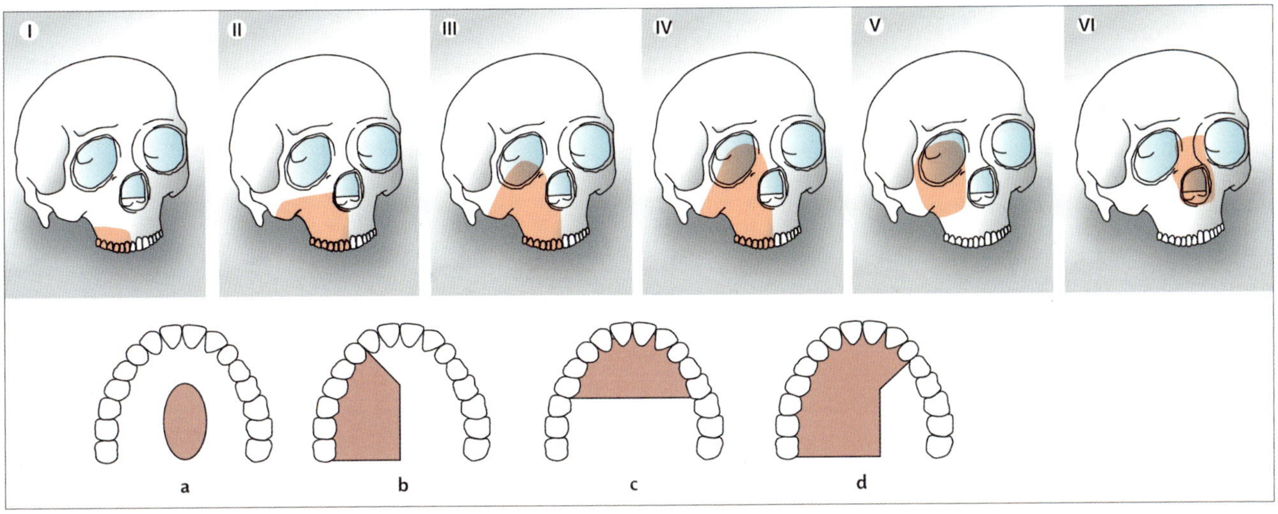


**Fig. 7.13** Classification of vertical and horizontal maxillectomy and midface defects. Vertical classification: I—maxillectomy not causing an oronasal fistula; II—not involving the orbit; III—involving the orbital adnexae with orbital retention; IV—with orbital enucleation or exenteration; V—orbitomaxillary defect; VI—nasomaxillary defect. Horizontal classification: a—palatal defect only, not involving the dental alveolus; b—less than or equal to one-half unilateral; c—less than or equal to one-half bilateral or transverse anterior; d—greater than one-half maxillectomy. Letters refer to the increasing complexity of the dento-alveolar and palatal defect, and qualify the vertical dimension. Reprinted with permission from Brown and Shaw.[4]

## References

1. Brown JS, Rogers SN, McNally DN, Boyle M. A modified classification for the maxillectomy defect. Head Neck 2000;22(1):17–26
2. Okay DJ, Genden E, Buchbinder D, Urken M. Prosthodontic guidelines for surgical reconstruction of the maxilla: a classification system of defects. J Prosthet Dent 2001;86(4):352–363
3. Cordeiro PG, Santamaria E. A classification system and algorithm for reconstruction of maxillectomy and midfacial defects. Plast Reconstr Surg 2000;105(7):2331–2346, discussion 2347–2348
4. Brown JS, Shaw RJ. Reconstruction of the maxilla and midface: introducing a new classification. Lancet Oncol 2010;11(10):1001–1008
5. Archibald S, Jackson S, Thoma A. Paranasal sinus and midfacial reconstruction. Clin Plast Surg 2005;32(3):309–325, v
6. Spiro RH, Strong EW, Shah JP. Maxillectomy and its classification. Head Neck 1997;19(4):309–314
7. Hanasono MM, Silva AK, Yu P, Skoracki RJ. A comprehensive algorithm for oncologic maxillary reconstruction. Plast Reconstr Surg 2013;131(1):47–60
8. Moreno MA, Skoracki RJ, Hanna EY, Hanasono MM. Microvascular free flap reconstruction versus palatal obturation for maxillectomy defects. Head Neck 2010;32(7):860–868
9. Chang YM, Coskunfirat OK, Wei FC, Tsai CY, Lin HN. Maxillary reconstruction with a fibula osteoseptocutaneous free flap and simultaneous insertion of osseointegrated dental implants. Plast Reconstr Surg 2004;113(4):1140–1145
10. Yazar S, Cheng MH, Wei FC, Hao SP, Chang KP. Osteomyocutaneous peroneal artery perforator flap for reconstruction of composite maxillary defects. Head Neck 2006;28(4):297–304
11. Clark JR, Vesely M, Gilbert R. Scapular angle osteomyogenous flap in postmaxillectomy reconstruction: defect, reconstruction, shoulder function, and harvest technique. Head Neck 2008;30(1):10–20
12. Cordeiro PG, Chen CM. A 15-year review of midface reconstruction after total and subtotal maxillectomy: part I. Algorithm and outcomes. Plast Reconstr Surg 2012;129(1):124–136
13. Genden EM, Wallace D, Buchbinder D, Okay D, Urken ML. Iliac crest internal oblique osteomusculocutaneous free flap reconstruction of the postablative palatomaxillary defect. Arch Otolaryngol Head Neck Surg 2001;127(7):854–861
14. Brown JS, Jones DC, Summerwill A, et al. Vascularized iliac crest with internal oblique muscle for immediate reconstruction after maxillectomy. Br J Oral Maxillofac Surg 2002;40(3):183–190
15. Hanasono MM, Skoracki RJ. The omega-shaped fibula osteocutaneous free flap for reconstruction of extensive midfacial defects. Plast Reconstr Surg 2010;125(4):160e–162e
16. Hanasono MM, Jacob RF, Bidaut L, Robb GL, Skoracki RJ. Midfacial reconstruction using virtual planning, rapid prototype modeling, and stereotactic navigation. Plast Reconstr Surg 2010;126(6):2002–2006
17. Cordeiro PG, Chen CM. A 15-year review of midface reconstruction after total and subtotal maxillectomy: part II. Technical modifications to maximize aesthetic and functional outcomes. Plast Reconstr Surg 2012;129(1):139–147

18. Kirby EJ, Turner JB, Davenport DL, Vasconez HC. Orbital floor fractures: outcomes of reconstruction. Ann Plast Surg 2011;66(5):508–512
19. Rodriguez ED, Martin M, Bluebond-Langner R, Khalifeh M, Singh N, Manson PN. Microsurgical reconstruction of posttraumatic high-energy maxillary defects: establishing the effectiveness of early reconstruction. Plast Reconstr Surg 2007; 120(7, Suppl 2):103S–117S
20. Hanasono MM, Lee JC, Yang JS, Skoracki RJ, Reece GP, Esmaeli B. An algorithmic approach to reconstructive surgery and prosthetic rehabilitation after orbital exenteration. Plast Reconstr Surg 2009;123(1):98–105
21. Boyes-Varley JG, Howes DG, Davidge-Pitts KD, Brånemark I, McAlpine JA. A protocol for maxillary reconstruction following oncology resection using zygomatic implants. Int J Prosthodont 2007;20(5):521–531

# 8 Skull Base Reconstruction

*Matthew M. Hanasono*

## Introduction

The skull base is a complex anatomical region, through which the major blood vessels of the head and neck, multiple cranial nerves, and the spinal cord pass. Lesions affecting the skull base include a variety of congenital, vascular, endocrine, and neoplastic entities. Surgical removal of these lesions usually involves a multidisciplinary effort between neurosurgeons, head and neck surgeons, and otologic surgeons. Except for lesions removed via minimally invasive endoscopic techniques, reconstructive surgeons usually play a major role in treatment of skull base lesions because of the substantial anatomical and functional deficits that can result from resection of the various craniofacial structures involved, such as the orbital contents, midface, mandible, and calvarium, as well as the eyes, nose, ears, scalp, and facial soft tissues.

Defects involving the skull base are especially challenging to treat because of the major, life-threatening complications that may occur should the reconstruction fail, such as dural or brain exposure, pneumocephalus, cerebrospinal fluid (CSF) leak, meningitis, and osteomyelitis. Reconstructive techniques that minimize the risks for such complications as well as restore facial appearance and function have become a critical part of most skull base surgeries. Although historically skull base resections were associated with poor outcomes, advances in reconstruction that minimize complications, loss of function, and disfigurement, concomitant with advances in oncologic treatment, have substantially decreased the morbidity and even increased the efficacy of skull base tumor treatment.

Local flaps, such as pericranial flaps, temporalis muscle flaps, and temporoparietal fascia flaps, remain useful for limited defects and specific indications, such as endoscopic resections and for reinforcing dural repairs intracranially. However, microvascular free flaps are now routinely utilized for most major skull base reconstructions.[1,2] Microvascular free flaps typically involve an extracranial or combined resection and supply larger volume and reach than local options can offer. Microvascular free flaps have also demonstrated higher reliability in previously radiated patients, in which local flaps may have compromised vascularity because they are included in the radiation field.[3,4] In addition, local flaps can have compromised vascularity when extensive skull base resections include transection of the blood supply that would be used for local flaps, particularly in reoperative cases.

Adding substantially to the morbidity of skull base surgery is the possibility of cranial nerve (CN) deficits. Many skull base tumors invade and spread intracranially via cranial nerves, while others surround the nerve in such a way that surgical removal necessitates nerve sacrifice. In particular, facial nerve (CN VII) reconstruction, by direct repair or cable nerve graft, as well as dynamic and static facial reanimation, may be indicated in the treatment of many skull base tumors, particularly those that arise from the parotid gland or the temporal bone. Nerve repair or grafting of other cranial nerves may also be indicated as part of the reconstructive treatment.

## Regional Anatomy

Oncologic skull base defects can be broadly defined as defects occurring from resection of tumors arising from or involving the floor of the anterior, middle, or posterior cranial fossae. The resection involves removal of cranial bone, with or without incision of the dura. The classification system described by Irish et al[5] is useful for describing skull base tumors, since it communicates the general location of the defects and predicts the reconstructive challenges associated with a given region of the skull base **(Fig. 8.1)**.

Region I involves defects from tumors arising in and around the orbits, nose, sinuses, and cribriform plate, and they can extend into the anterior cranial fossae, and those originating in the clivus or extending as far

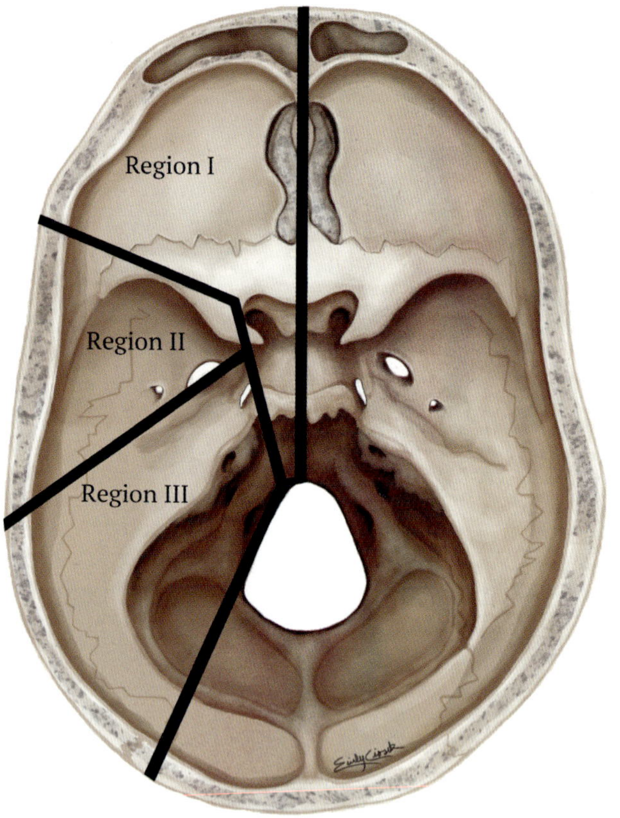


**Fig. 8.1** Skull base regions. Adapted, with permission, from Irish JC, Gullane PJ, Gentili F, et al. Tumors of the skull base: outcome and survival analysis of 77 cases. Head Neck 1994;16:3–10.

posteriorly as the foramen magnum. Region I can be further subdivided into midline and lateral or paramedian regions. Midline Region I tumors often originate from the ethmoid and sphenoid sinuses or the cribriform plate, as is the case with esthesioneuroblastomas. Lateral Region I tumors include those that arise from the orbit or periorbital structures, such as lacrimal gland tumors.

Region II extends from the petrous temporal bone to the posterior orbital wall. Region II defects result from tumors originating from the lateral skull base, primarily the infratemporal and pterygopalatine fossae, and they can extend into the middle cranial fossa. Tumors that originate in this region include juvenile nasopharyngeal angiofibromas, nasopharyngeal carcinomas, glomus jugulare tumors, sphenoid wing meningiomas, and clival chordomas, as well as parotid tumors that grow deeply and maxillary or even cheek neoplasms that spread posteriorly, usually via the maxillary division of the trigeminal nerve ($V_2$).

Region III defects are usually associated with tumors arising from the ear, parotid, or temporal bone, and may extend into the middle or posterior cranial fossae. Region III tumors include cutaneous tumors involving the external auditory canal, such as squamous and basal cell carcinomas, as well as parotid tumors and, occasionally, sarcomas that arise directly from the temporal bone.

## Preoperative Considerations

The location of the tumor, as evidenced by physical exam and preoperative imaging, predicts the reconstructive needs, as outlined below. In addition to an assessment of reconstructive flap choices, including both local or regional flaps and free flaps, the possibility of grafts or implants should be considered. Autologous bone grafts and manmade implants, such as titanium mesh, porous polyethylene, or methylmethacrylate, may be necessary for concurrent calvarial reconstruction, as well as to restore the orbital walls and orbital rim.[6]

Cranial nerve deficits should be anticipated based on the location of the tumor, as well as by a full preoperative physical exam of cranial nerve function, which should be documented in detail in the preoperative note. Various procedures to address facial nerve paralysis should be discussed with the patient preoperatively in any case where transection of the facial nerve is a possibility. Such procedures include direct nerve repair, cable nerve grafting, dynamic reanimation with vascularized muscle transfer, anastomosis to other cranial nerves (e.g., masseteric nerve to facial nerve or hypoglossal nerve to facial nerve transfers), and static reanimation with a fascial graft, and periocular procedures, such as gold eyelid weight placement, canthoplasty, and lateral tarsorrhaphy.

Other functional deficits might include those arising from loss of glossopharyngeal (CN IX), vagus (CN X), spinal accessory (CN XI), and hypoglossal (CN XII) nerve function. Resection of the glossopharyngeal nerve can result in uncoordinated swallowing and aspiration, which may be addressed with temporary or permanent gastrostomy tube placement as well as postoperative speech and swallowing therapy. Unilateral hypoglossal nerve deficits are generally well tolerated but may also require speech and swallowing therapy. Vocal cord paralysis after transection of the vagus nerve can be addressed by an otolaryngologist postoperatively with vocal cord injection of various filler materials and/or medialization thyroplasty. Transection of the spinal accessory nerve results in shoulder drop that is best addressed with physical therapy.

A discussion of the patient's desire for an orbital or ear prosthesis should take place preoperatively, since the planning for a prosthesis may influence the choice of flap or shape of the reconstructive flap, particularly for an orbital prosthesis (discussed below). Both orbital and ear prostheses may require osseointegrated implants for stable fixation, and consideration may be given to immediate placement, particularly when postoperative radiation is anticipated, since many have reported decreased implant reliability when the implant is placed after radiation is given. In many cases, placement of an osseointegrated implant is challenging after substantial resection of bone, since fairly thick bone stock must surround the implant in order for it to be stable, and implant placement usually must be within a small area to be included in the prosthetic part. In such cases, it may be unrealistic to offer an orbital or ear prosthesis, or at least one that is rigidly fixed by attachment to an osseointegrated implant. Implants and prosthetics are discussed more thoroughly in a separate chapter.

## Reconstructive Approach

### Region I

As mentioned above, Region I resections may involve the midline or lateral anterior cranial fossa, or both. Midline Region I tumors are usually resected with an anterior craniofacial approach, resulting in a communication of the nasal cavity with the intracranial space. Skull base defects restricted to the upper nasal cavity can be reconstructed with a pericranial flap or a galea–frontalis flap, transposed to line the floor of the anterior cranial fossa. These flaps derive their blood supply from the paired supratrochlear and supraorbital vessels, which are both branches of the ophthalmic arteries, which, in turn, are branches of the internal carotid arteries. The supratrochlear and supraorbital vessels both have superficial and deep branches, which supply the galea–frontalis flap and the pericranial flap, respectively. Sizable defects that encompass the external nose, forehead, and/or orbit are usually best reconstructed with a free flap. Free flaps may also be required when prior surgery has resulted in the division of the supratrochlear and supraorbital blood supply of the galea–frontalis and pericranial flaps. **(Fig. 8.2)**

Nasal reconstructions are usually addressed separately from the skull base. Such reconstructions are delicate, multistaged procedures utilizing local flaps, such as the paramedian forehead flap, and auricular

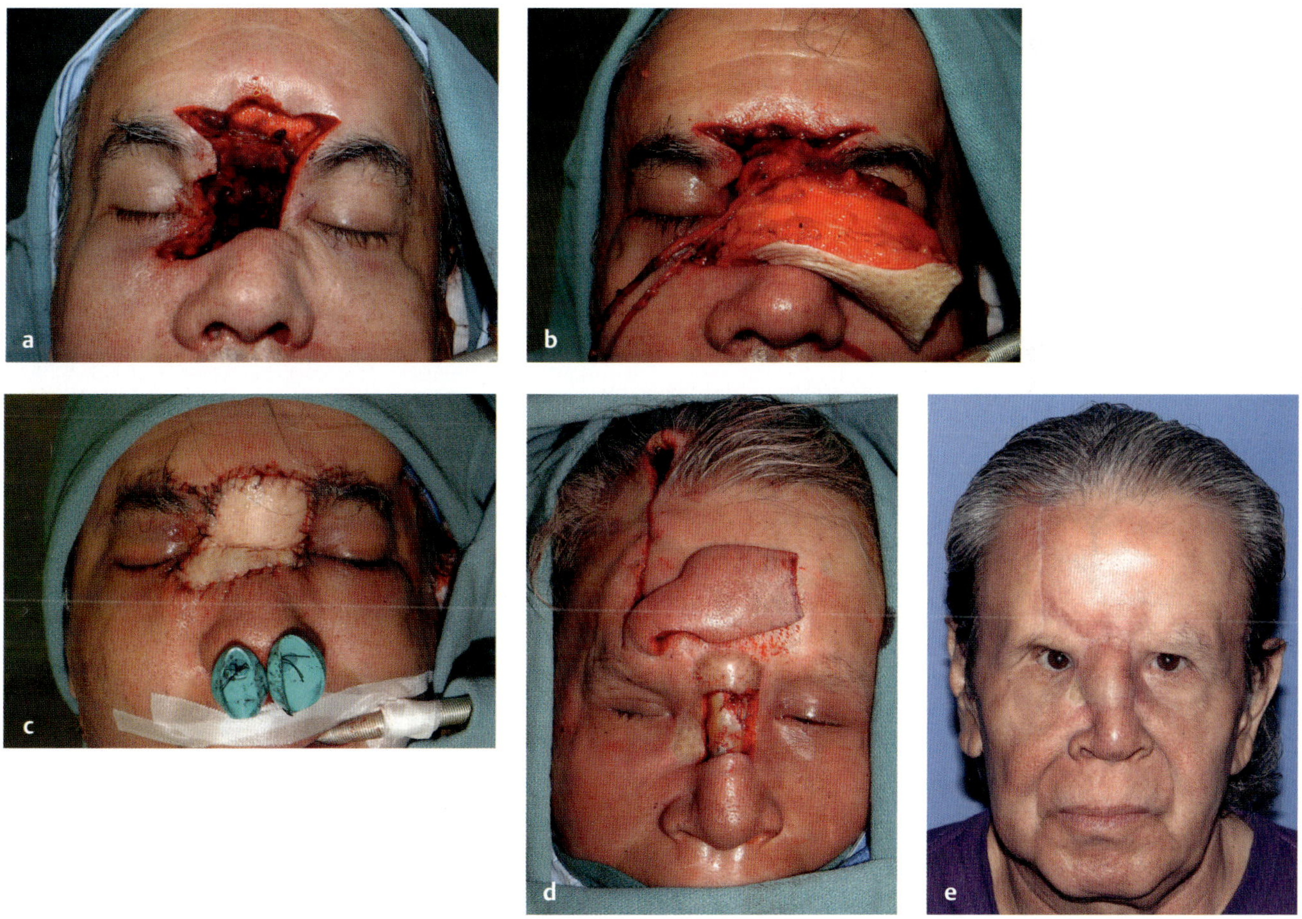

**Fig. 8.2** **(a)** A Region I skull base defect involving an anterior craniofacial resection, frontal sinusectomy, partial rhinectomy, and removal of the medial orbital walls for a nasal squamous cell carcinoma. **(b)** The defect was reconstructed with an ALT free flap, separating the anterior cranial fossa from the nasal cavity. Following radiation therapy, delayed nasal reconstruction with **(c)** autologous cartilage and **(d)** bone grafts as well as a paramedian forehead flap. **(e)** Final postoperative appearance.

or costal cartilage grafts. Reconstruction should be delayed for many months following the conclusion of adjuvant radiation therapy, to avoid fibrosis and contracture of the reconstructed nose. Prostheses are another option for nasal reconstruction that often produce an even better aesthetic result than autologous tissues and do not require multiple operations. If a substantial amount of the forehead has been previously resected or in cases where the forehead has been irradiated, the paramedian forehead flap may not be reliable and prosthetics may be the only aesthetically acceptable option.

Lateral Region I resections frequently involve orbital exenteration or orbitomaxillectomy. In orbital exenterations that spare the medial and inferior orbital walls, a thin fasciocutaneous free flap, such as the radial forearm fasciocutaneous free flap, can resurface the orbit and protect exposed dura and bone. If the patient desires an orbital prosthesis, reconstruction with thin flaps results in a concave orbital cavity that is suited to prosthetic retention.

A temporalis muscle pedicled flap can also be used to resurface the orbital cavity, provided the inferior and medial walls are intact. In such cases, it is usually necessary to remove the lateral wall of the orbit to extend the reach of the flap and to avoid the excess bulk of the muscle over the bone of the lateral orbit. One disadvantage of the temporalis muscle flap is that it usually leaves a noticeable hollowing in the temporal fossa. However, the donor-site hollowing can often be addressed satisfactorily with autologous fat grafting performed as an elective, outpatient, secondary procedure. Temporoparietal fascia flaps (supplied by the superficial temporal artery) and pericranial flaps are probably not durable enough for long-term coverage of dura that is exposed to the external environment, particularly if postoperative radiation is planned.

In orbitomaxillectomies and orbital exenterations that result in communication with the nasal and sinus cavities, bulkier flaps, such as the anterolateral thigh (ALT) free flap or rectus abdominis myocutaneous (RAM) free flap, more reliably close orbital wall dehiscences **(Fig. 8.3)**. Both flaps have the advantage of being highly versatile with respect to including a variable amount of muscle (i.e., the vastus lateralis muscle in the ALT free flap, and the rectus abdominis muscle in the RAM free flap) to achieve the volume needed. Conversely, both flaps can usually be harvested with minimal or no muscle, and even thinned (primarily or during a secondary procedure) when less thickness is desired.

In our experience, it is usually preferable to include enough flap tissue for Region I reconstructions so that all dehiscences are sealed, to minimize the chances of developing a sinonasocutaneous fistula. Such fistulas rarely, if ever, heal spontaneously due to the air pressures generated by nasal breathing and nose blowing. Closure in the region of the medial orbit and lateral nose must be meticulous and multilayered. Where the closure may be tenuous, it is probably safer to resect additional skin, so that the external skin incision overlies healthy bone. One drawback of filling the orbit with flap tissue is that prosthetic retention may be difficult and the prosthesis may protrude unnaturally due to the lack of a concave orbit.

## Region II

Resection of Region II tumors may involve an anterior transmaxillary approach. When the skull base has been resected, leaving the dura exposed, the defect must be reconstructed to isolate the intracranial contents from the nasal cavity, ruling out prosthetic obturation as a potential method of reconstruction. Muscle or myocutaneous flaps are used to obliterate the maxillary cavity **(Fig. 8.4)**.

The temporalis muscle may reach this area, but often it does not provide adequate bulk to restore facial contour when the malar maxillary and zygomatic bones have been resected, especially following radiation, which usually results in substantial muscle flap atrophy over time. In such cases, a myocutaneous free flap, such as the ALT or RAM free flap, again, is usually a better choice. When there is no oral or cheek defect, the skin paddle of the free flap can be de-epithelialized and the entire flap buried. The muscle component usually provides an adequate seal against dural leaks. The adipose component of the flap usually undergoes minimal atrophy, even following radiation; therefore, facial contours are maintained and adequate support of the skull base is achieved to prevent brain herniation.[7,8]

Accurate reconstruction of the orbital floor is mandatory if the orbital floor is included as part of the resection while the globe is spared. Malposition of the orbital floor can result in enophthalmos, exophthalmos, or vertical dystopia (eyes at uneven heights). Most of what is known about orbital floor reconstruction comes from the trauma literature. Both alloplastic materials, such as titanium mesh or porous polyethylene, as well as autogenous grafts, such as calvarial or iliac crest bone grafts, have been successfully used. Autogenous grafts have the theoretical advantage of revascularization by the surrounding tissues, making them potentially more resistant to radiation-associated complications, such as infection or exposure. Our own experience does not strongly support use of one material over another; however, well-vascularized tissue coverage

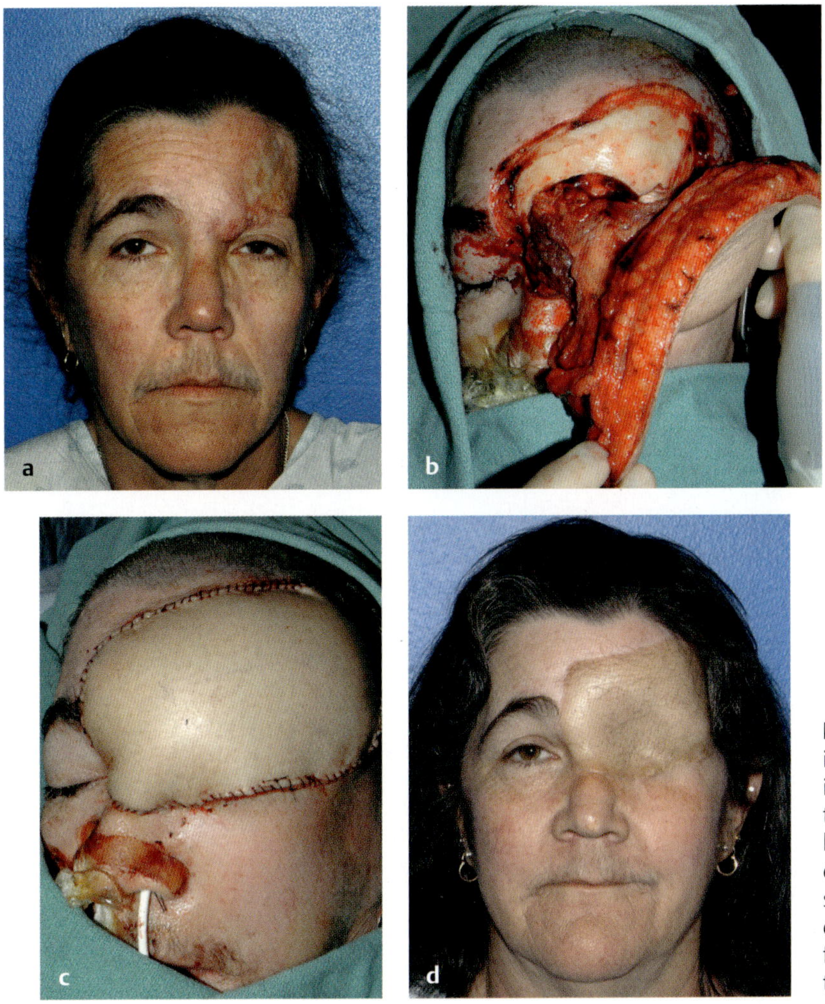

**Fig. 8.3** **(a)** Patient with a basal cell carcinoma invading the right orbit and frontal bone. **(b)** An intraoperative view shows the extent of the resection, including exposure of the frontal dura. **(c)** A lateral Region I skull base defect following frontal craniectomy and orbital exenteration was reconstructed with an ALT myocutaneous free flap, obliterating the orbital cavity and separating the dura from the sinuses and nasal cavity. **(d)** Postoperative appearance.

of the entire implant or graft is mandatory regardless of the material used if postoperative radiation is planned. Care must also be taken not to impinge on the optic nerve during orbital floor reconstruction, or visual impairment, even blindness, can result.

Some resections for tumors in Region II are approached laterally rather than anteriorly. These resections require removal of several structures, including the parotid, posterior mandible, and posterolateral maxilla. For these defects, which may include both a cutaneous component and an intraoral component, we use the ALT and RAM free flaps, which can be designed to include multiple skin paddles based on separate perforators, to reconstruct the oral defect separately from the facial defect. Good results with soft tissue reconstruction alone can be achieved for posterior mandibular defects. Resections that encompass both Regions I and II often involve orbitomaxillectomies and are reconstructed in an identical manner to those orbitomaxillectomies that involve only Region I, with a bulky free flap that fills both the orbit and the sinus cavities.[9,10]

## Region III

In Region III, small defects are often amenable to reconstruction with the temporalis muscle flap, which lies within the operative field, provided that the blood supply, the anterior and posterior deep temporal branches of the internal maxillary artery, remains intact.[11] The radial forearm fasciocutaneous free flap can also be used for small superficial defects, such as those arising from a partial or total auriculectomy.

The ALT and RAM free flaps work well in this region when a larger flap is needed **(Fig. 8.5)**. They are configured so that a muscle component of the flap fills the deep portion of the wound and the skin paddle resurfaces the cutaneous defect, if there is

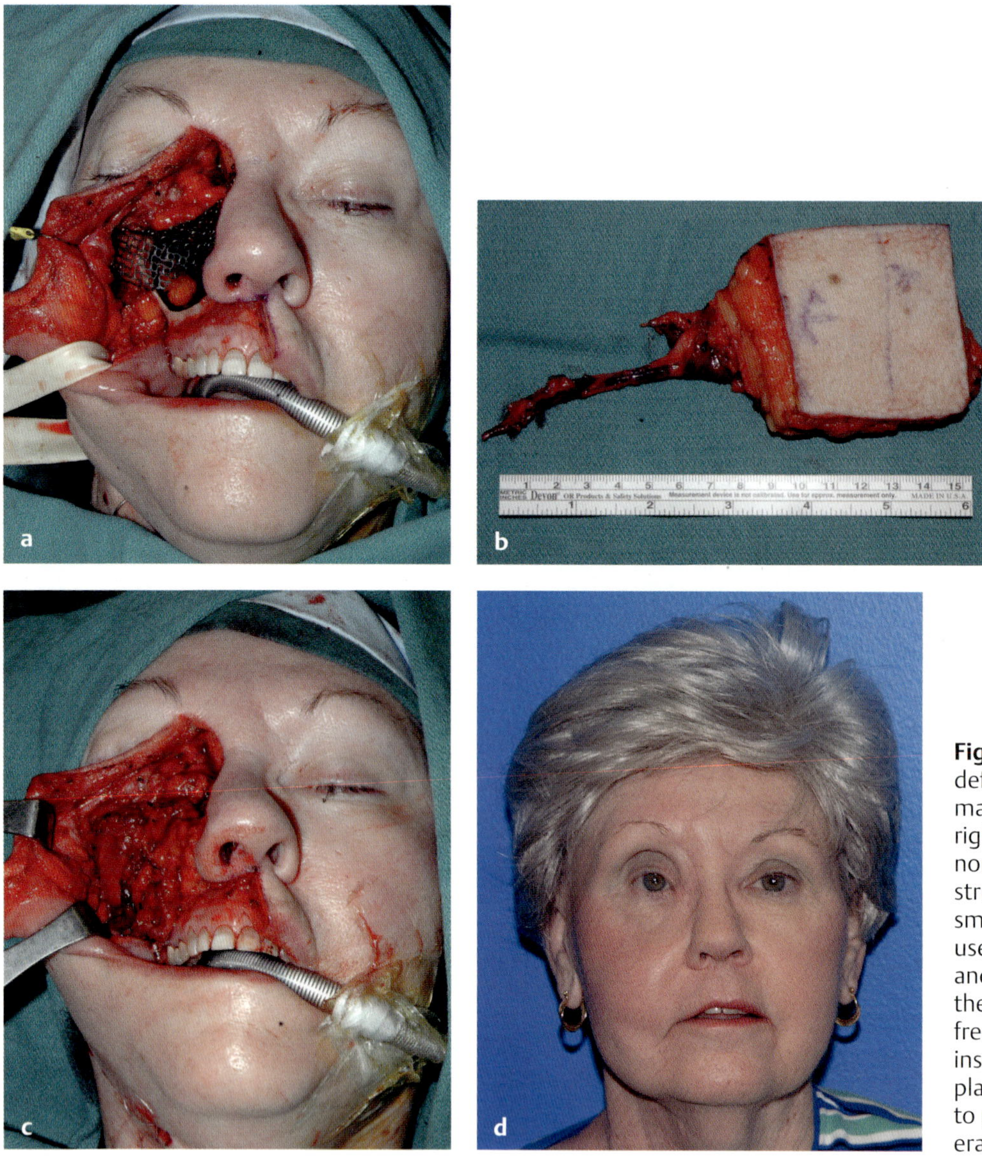

**Fig. 8.4** **(a)** A Region II skull base defect involving an anterior transmaxillary approach for removal of a right maxillary squamous cell carcinoma. The orbital floor was reconstructed with titanium mesh. **(b)** A small (~ 5 × 5 cm) ALT free flap was used to support the titanium mesh and separate the maxillary sinus from the middle cranial fossa. **(c)** The ALT free flap was de-epithelialized and inset so that some of the flap was placed anterior to the titanium mesh, to prevent later exposure. **(d)** Postoperative appearance.

one. If there is no cutaneous defect, the skin paddle can be de-epithelialized and entirely buried, as discussed for Region II defects. Although the latissimus dorsi muscle free flap covered by a split-thickness skin graft is often used to reconstruct very large defects that involve the scalp, ALT free flaps have also been shown to close very large defects reliably. Reconstructions for defects that include both Region II and III also tend to require larger, bulky free flaps, occasionally with two skin paddles if an oral cavity defect exists in addition to an external defect (**Fig. 8.6**).[12,13,14]

The pectoralis major, trapezius, and even the latissimus dorsi myocutaneous pedicled flaps have also been used to reconstruct defects of Region III. We restrict their use to modest defects only, in patients who are not candidates for free flaps and in whom the temporalis muscle flap is unavailable or of inadequate size. Pedicled flaps from the torso often have problems with reaching the most superior portion of the surgical defect. Even when they do reach, the closure is tight, and postoperative contracture of the proximal muscle and pedicle usually restricts neck movement. When neck movement becomes restricted or there is an aesthetically unappealing bulkiness in the neck due to the mass of the muscular pedicle, a revision procedure to debulk the proximal flap can be performed 3 months after the initial surgery or 6 months following the conclusion of postoperative radiation, whichever is later (**Fig. 8.6**).

The external ear, if resected, is usually best reconstructed separately in a delayed manner if postoperative radiation is anticipated, as it is with nasal reconstruction. Prosthetic rehabilitation for total auricular reconstruction is usually the mainstay

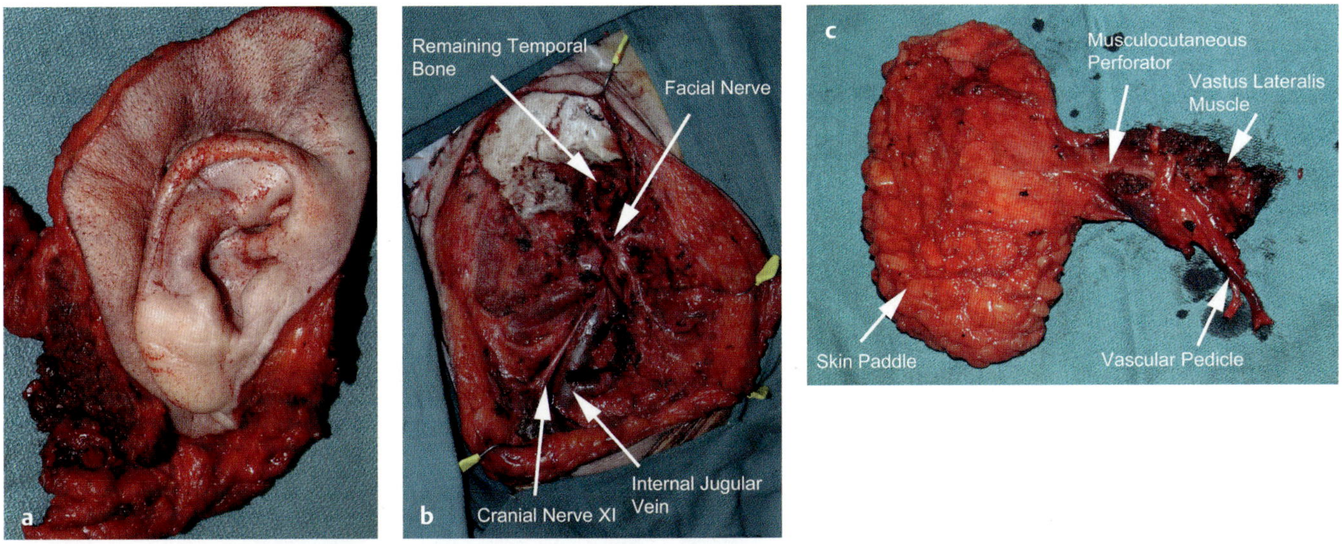


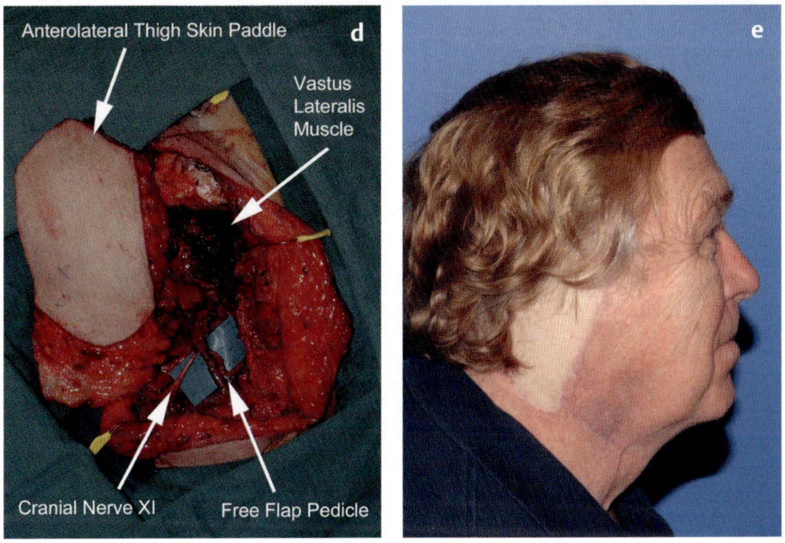


**Fig. 8.5** A Region III defect resulting from **(a)** a total auriculectomy and **(b)** lateral temporal bone resection for a recurrent auricular melanoma. **(c)** The defect was reconstructed with a musculocutaneous ALT free flap, incorporating a skin paddle based on a single perforating blood vessel and a portion of the vastus lateralis muscle. **(d)** The muscular component was placed into the deep part of the temporal bone defect, obliterating the eustachian tube, and the skin paddle was used to close the auriculectomy defect. **(e)** Postoperative appearance.

in oncologic surgery due to the lack of thin, pliable cutaneous tissue to cover a cartilaginous framework carved from costochondral grafts or alloplasts, such as porous polyethylene. Partial defects of the auricle can be reconstructed with local tissue flaps or can be incorporated into the design of a free flap used to close the skull base wound and eliminate dead space.

Our institutional treatment algorithm is summarized in **Fig. 8.7**. Microvascular free flaps are selected over regional flaps whenever vascularized tissue coverage is needed and regional flaps are not suitable due to limitations in size, reach, or reliability. Additionally, microvascular free flaps should be used in medically suitable candidates whenever such reconstruction holds promise for a better quality of life (via improved function or aesthetic appearance) than can be achieved with other techniques. Because placement of either a regional or free flap may inhibit the ability to detect a local recurrence by physical examination, serial imaging is mandatory for disease surveillance.

With regard to recipient artery choice for microvascular free flaps, the facial and superficial temporal arteries are most commonly used in Region I, the facial artery is most commonly used in Region II, and the facial and distal external carotid arteries are most commonly used in Region III, all based on proximity to the defect. Similar to recipient artery choice, the facial and superficial temporal veins are most commonly used in Region I. In Regions II and III, the facial and internal jugular veins are most commonly used. The transverse cervical artery and vein are occasionally useful as recipient vessels in Region III when the external carotid artery and internal jugular vein, or their branches, are not available.

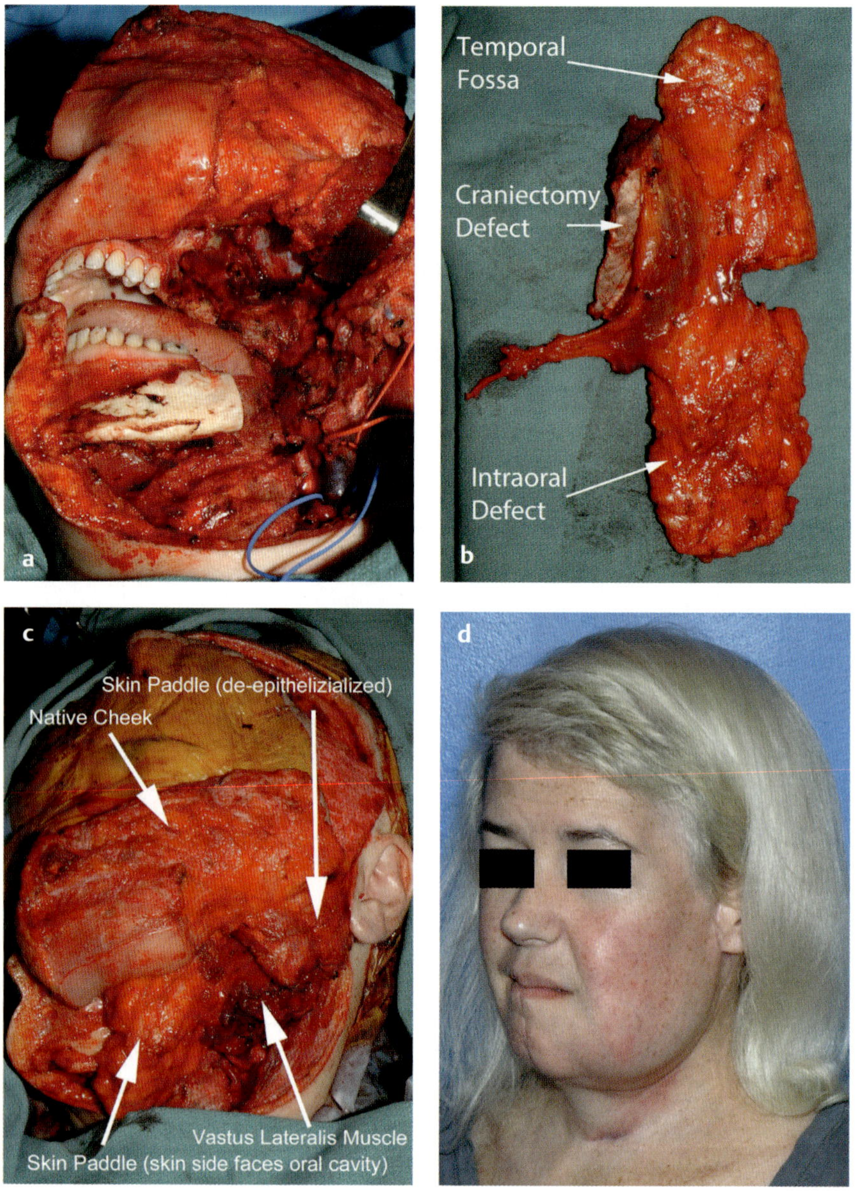


**Fig. 8.6** **(a)** A combined Region II and III defect involving a lateral approach to the infratemporal fossa with resection of the posterior mandible and maxilla, as well as an extradural middle cranial fossa resection, in a patient with recurrent metastatic melanoma. **(b)** A dual skin paddle ALT free flap was used to reconstruct the intraoral and temporal bone defects, and **(c)** a portion of the vastus lateralis muscle was placed against the craniectomy defect and helped provide soft tissue bulk to obliterate the dead space in the infratemporal and pterygopalatine regions. **(d)** Postoperative appearance.

## Complications

Patients undergoing skull base surgery are at risk for neurologic complications, including cerebrovascular accident, meningeal or brain infections, pneumocephalus, and CSF leak. Such complications should be managed with a neurosurgeon. Dural repairs and known CSF leaks should be discussed intraoperatively at the commencement of the reconstruction. Empirically, we have found that soft tissue free and pedicled flaps inset so that they completely cover the dural repair or leak help to seal the leak. A mild amount of volume overcorrection in these areas may be indicated, though not so much as to put pressure on the brain by increasing the intracranial pressure. Similarly, meticulous isolation of the dura and brain from the sinonasal and oral cavities by well-vascularized flap tissues is necessary to prevent meningitis, cerebritis, or brain abscess.

When the orbital walls are reconstructed with flaps, grafts, or implants, there is a risk for orbital entrapment, and a forced duction test should be performed prior to leaving the operating room. Failure to adequately support the orbits can lead to early or late diplopia. Care

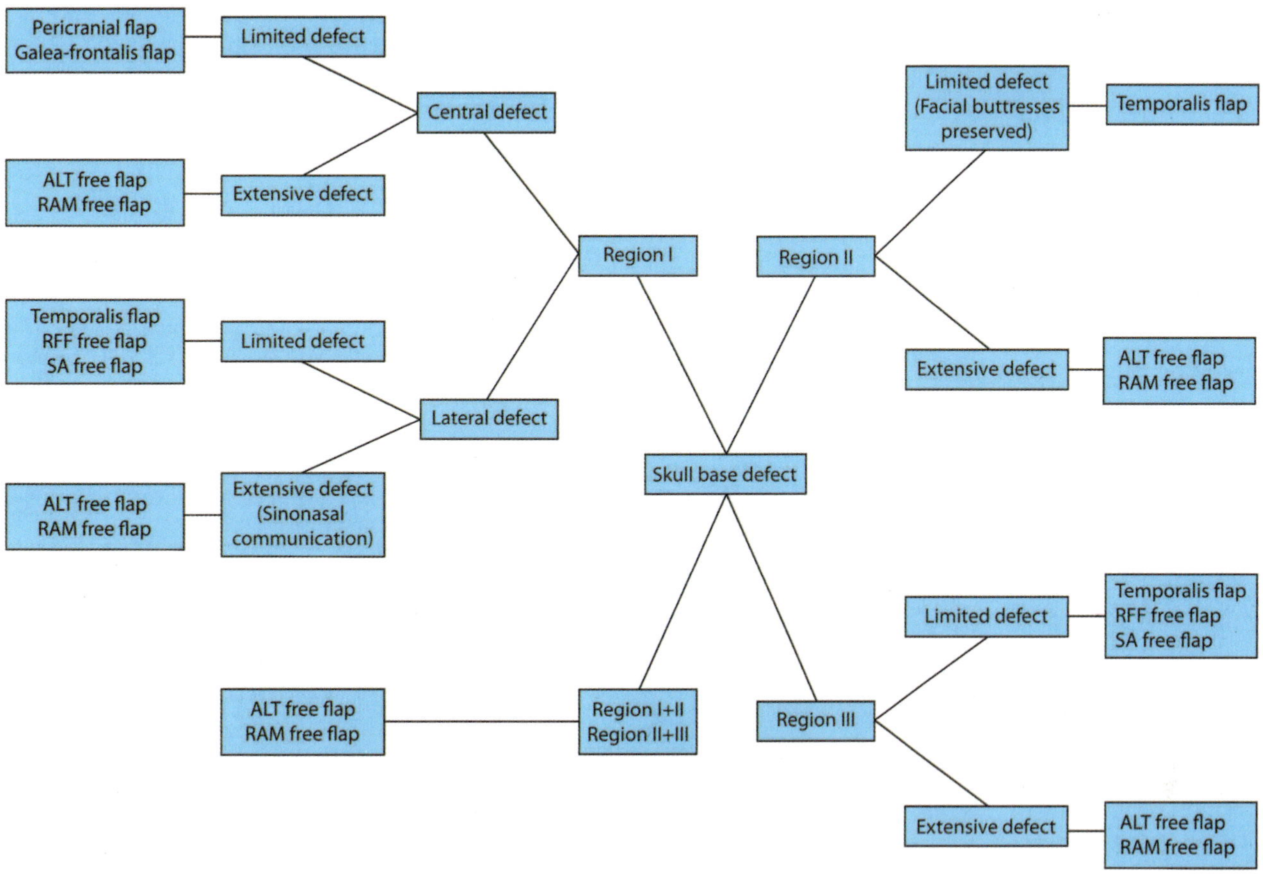


**Fig. 8.7** Reconstructive algorithm for skull base defects. ALT, anterolateral thigh; RAM, rectus abdominis muscle; RFF, radial forearm fasciocutaneous; SA, serratus anterior (muscle).

must be taken when the posterior orbit is reconstructed not to injure the optic and oculomotor nerves at the orbital apex. Typically, 0.5 to 1.0 cm of space is left open in the region of the apex when performing orbital floor reconstruction to avoid impinging on the nerves. Excessive pressure on the globe by the reconstructive flap or orbital wall reconstruction must also be avoided. Prior to the patient's leaving the operating room, gentle palpation for excessive pressure on the operated eye(s) should be performed, and the orbits are checked for symmetry, although this may be difficult to assess when substantial facial swelling occurs during the course of surgery.

Partial or total loss of local pedicled flap, such as from galea–frontalis, pericranial, temporoparietal fascia, and temporalis muscle flaps, can result if the vascular supply has been damaged or ligated as a part of the resection. Such flaps may also be unreliable in previously irradiated patients. The risk for free flap loss in this region does not appear to be increased compared with other head and neck sites, with our recent experience demonstrating a 1.6% free flap loss rate. Exposure of dura or brain is an indication for further surgery, and it can sometimes be addressed with local tissue rearrangement, such as a scalp- or forehead-based flap, but often requires a second free flap.

## Postoperative Care

In addition to flap monitoring, regular neurologic monitoring should be performed. Postoperative computed tomography (CT) or magnetic resonance imaging (MRI) is obtained per the recommendations of the neurosurgeon. While it is not uncommon to see a minor amount of intracranial air on imaging in the early postoperative period, clinical neurologic findings and evidence on serial imaging suggesting increasing pneumocephalus are indications for a prompt return to the operating room. Minor CSF leaks can be observed or treated with a lumbar drain. Recalcitrant or severe CSF drainage may require further surgery. Prophylactic antibiotics with good CSF penetration should be used to prevent perioperative infection. Vision should also be assessed, particularly following Region I or Region II reconstructions, where optic nerve injury or compression from swelling flaps may occur. Any concern about decreased visual acuity should prompt an ophthalmologic consultation, with imaging or a possible return to the operating room. Likewise, diplopia secondary to orbital entrapment must be ruled out, and, if diagnosed, it should be addressed with very early surgical revision. Vigilant flap monitoring is particularly indicated in skull base reconstruction, since loss of a flap in this region can result in dural or brain contamination and exposure.

## ■ Case Example

A 52-year-old man presented with a basal cell carcinoma of his left auricle and external auditory canal invading his temporal bone **(Fig. 8.8)**. He underwent a lateral temporal bone resection and a partial auriculectomy, involving removal of his tragus and conchal bowl. An anterolateral thigh myocutaneous free flap was used for reconstruction. A portion of the vastus lateralis muscle was placed into the deep portion of the wound, against the sigmoid sinus and eustachian tube orifice. Microvascular anastomoses were performed to the facial artery and facial vein. The skin paddle was used to close the auricular defect. The skin paddle was designed so that the perforator supplying it was in the epicenter of the exposed flap, which facilitated postoperative monitoring with handheld Doppler ultrasound in addition to physical examination.

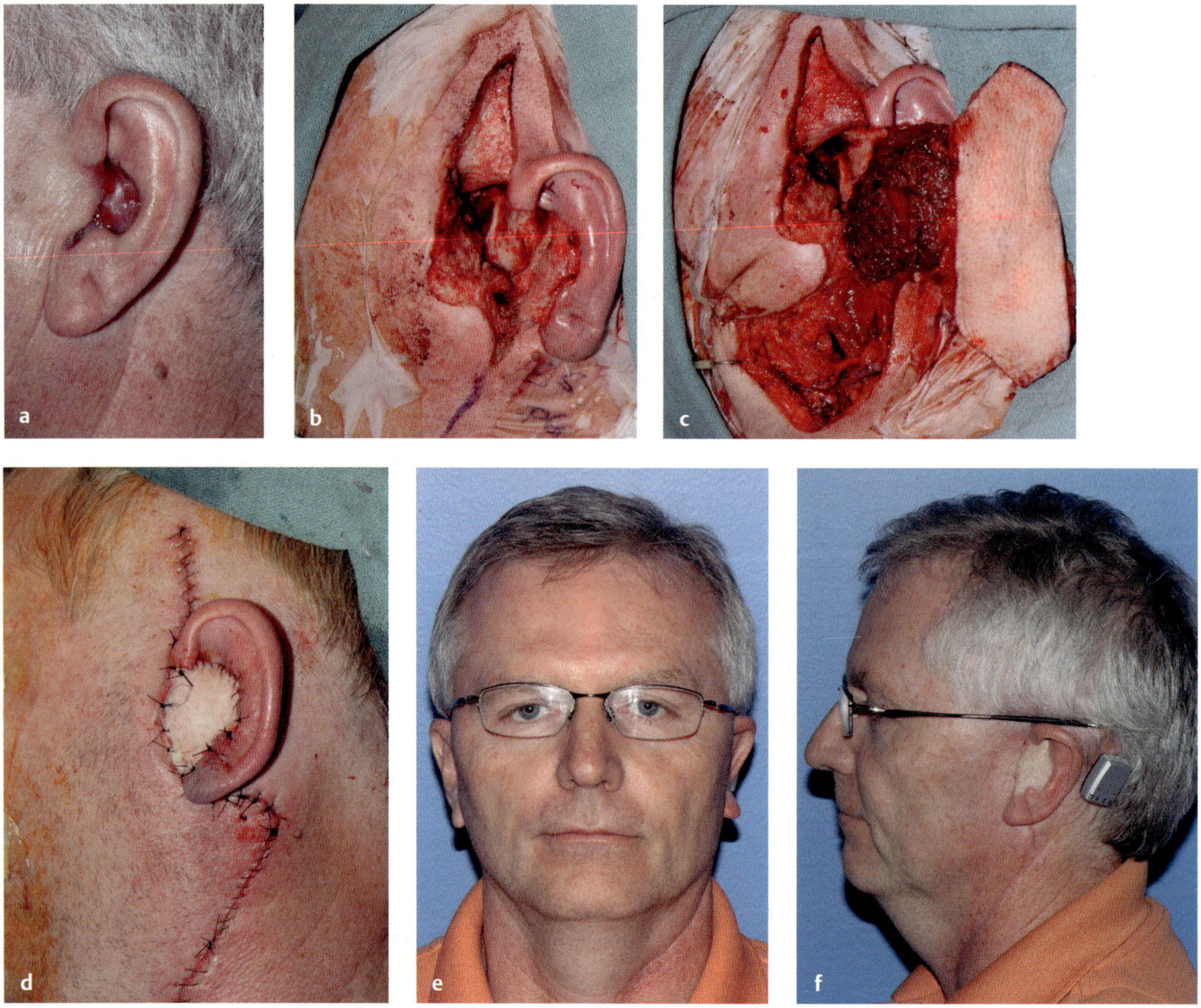

**Fig. 8.8** **(a)** Patient with a recurrent basal cell carcinoma of the left auricle and external auditory canal. **(b)** He underwent a lateral temporal bone resection and partial auriculectomy. **(c)** Reconstruction was performed with an ALT free flap, including a small skin paddle for the conchal-tragal region. **(d)** Postoperative appearance following a second-stage otoplasty to improve symmetry; **(e,f)** a bone-anchored hearing aid was also affixed to an osseointegrated implant that was placed at the time of the initial surgery.

At the time of the resection, an osseointegrated implant was placed into the remaining temporal bone. At a secondary procedure, 4 months later, the implant was uncovered and an abutment was attached to the implant. A bone-anchored hearing aid (BAHA) was then attached to the abutment. At the same time, revisionary surgery was performed to reposition the left auricle, which had become malpositioned in an inferior and lateral location. We have found this to be a common occurrence following temporal bone resection and try to suspend the cartilage of the auricle or auricular remnant to periosteum and deep temporal fascia with sutures. However, lateral migration of the auricle is common, since the external auditory canal is transected at the time of temporal bone resection. Repositioning was performed using skin excision and permanent sutures to resuspend the auricular cartilage.

## Pearls and Pitfalls

- The goals of craniofacial reconstruction after skull base surgery include creating a watertight dural seal, providing a barrier between the dura and the aerodigestive tract, supporting the orbit, and restoring facial function and appearance.
- Classifying skull base lesions into regions based on key anatomical structures helps to predict the reconstructive needs and outcomes.
- Repair and rehabilitation of the facial nerve, if it is resected, must be considered in the reconstructive approach.
- The orbital walls need to be accurately reconstructed to avoid enophthalmos, exophthalmos, or vertical dystopia. Care must be taken to avoid optic and oculomotor nerve injury in the region of the orbital apex, as well as to avoid entrapment of extraocular muscles and soft tissues.
- Local flaps, such as the temporalis muscle flap, are mostly useful in Region I and Region II for limited defects, but they may be rendered unreliable by the surgical resection or prior radiation therapy.
- Most major skull base reconstructions require soft tissue free flaps to isolate the dura from the sinonasal and oral cavities and to provide adequate bulk to eliminate dead space and restore facial contours.
- Prosthetic rehabilitation may be the most appropriate way of replacing resected facial structures like the orbit, nose, or ear, or it may be used while awaiting autologous tissue reconstruction.
- Patients must be vigilantly monitored postoperatively for pneumocephalus, CSF leak, and cerebromeningeal infection, as well as visual impairment.

## References


1. Chang DW, Langstein HN, Gupta A, et al. Reconstructive management of cranial base defects after tumor ablation. Plast Reconstr Surg 2001;107(6):1346–1355, discussion 1356–1357
2. Hanasono MM, Silva A, Skoracki RJ, et al. Skull base reconstruction: an updated approach. Plast Reconstr Surg 2011;128(3):675–686
3. Neligan PC, Mulholland S, Irish J, et al. Flap selection in cranial base reconstruction. Plast Reconstr Surg 1996;98(7):1159–1166, discussion 1167–1168
4. Califano J, Cordeiro PG, Disa JJ, et al. Anterior cranial base reconstruction using free tissue transfer: changing trends. Head Neck 2003;25(2):89–96
5. Irish JC, Gullane PJ, Gentili F, et al. Tumors of the skull base: outcome and survival analysis of 77 cases. Head Neck 1994;16(1):3–10
6. Hanasono MM, Lee JC, Yang JS, Skoracki RJ, Reece GP, Esmaeli B. An algorithmic approach to reconstructive surgery and prosthetic rehabilitation after orbital exenteration. Plast Reconstr Surg 2009;123(1):98–105
7. Chiu ES, Kraus D, Bui DT, et al. Anterior and middle cranial fossa skull base reconstruction using microvascular free tissue techniques: surgical complications and functional outcomes. Ann Plast Surg 2008;60(5):514–520
8. Hanasono MM, Utley DS, Goode RL. The temporalis muscle flap for reconstruction after head and neck oncologic surgery. Laryngoscope 2001;111(10):1719–1725
9. Rosenthal EL, King T, McGrew BM, Carroll W, Magnuson JS, Wax MK. Evolution of a paradigm for free tissue transfer reconstruction of lateral temporal bone defects. Head Neck 2008;30(5):589–594
10. Disa JJ, Rodriguez VM, Cordeiro PG. Reconstruction of lateral skull base oncological defects: the role of free tissue transfer. Ann Plast Surg 1998;41(6):633–639
11. Hanasono MM, Silva AK, Yu P, Skoracki RJ, Sturgis EM, Gidley PW. Comprehensive management of temporal bone defects after oncologic resection. Laryngoscope 2012;122(12):2663–2669
12. Moncrieff MD, Hamilton SA, Lamberty GH, et al. Reconstructive options after temporal bone resection for squamous cell carcinoma. J Plast Reconstr Aesthet Surg 2007;60(6):607–614
13. Malata CM, Tehrani H, Kumiponjera D, Hardy DG, Moffat DA. Use of anterolateral thigh and lateral arm fasciocutaneous free flaps in lateral skull base reconstruction. Ann Plast Surg 2006;57(2):169–175, discussion 176
14. Hanasono MM, Sacks JM, Goel N, Ayad M, Skoracki RJ. The anterolateral thigh free flap for skull base reconstruction. Otolaryngol Head Neck Surg 2009;140(6):855–860

# 9 Scalp and Calvarial Reconstruction

*Albert Chao and Matthew M. Hanasono*

## Introduction

Scalp and calvarial reconstruction can present unique challenges to the reconstructive surgeon, both as a result of the effects of oncologic treatment, such as radiation therapy, and due to the specific anatomical features of this region of the body. Scalp tissue is intrinsically inelastic, limiting the application of primary closure and adjacent tissue rearrangement techniques. The location of the scalp provides few regional flap options other than the temporalis major muscle and the temporoparietal fascia flaps. Due to the close relationship of the scalp and calvarium, oncologic disease affecting the scalp often involves the underlying calvarium, and vice versa, which can complicate reconstruction. The ideal reconstruction should be durable enough to protect skull and/or intracranial contents, should confer a normal contour, and, ideally, should maintain the hairline and hair follicle orientation.

## Regional Anatomy

The scalp is composed of five layers, which can be remembered by the familiar mnemonic SCALP: (1) **s**kin, (2) sub**c**utaneous fat, (3) galea **a**poneurotica, (4) **l**oose areolar tissue, and (5) **p**ericranium. The skin of the scalp is the thickest in the body, measuring 3 to 8 mm, and, in most patients, is hair-bearing. The scalp is inelastic, with the galea aponeurotica being poorly distensible and the pericranium being essentially nondistensible. The galea aponeurotica is continuous with the frontalis muscle anteriorly and occipitalis muscle posteriorly. Laterally, the galea aponeurotica is continuous with the temporoparietal (superficial temporal) fascia. The layer of loose areolar tissue is also known as the subgaleal or innominate fascia. The pericranium, which is the periosteum of the skull, fuses with the deep temporal fascia laterally. A thorough understanding of the anatomical layers is important, particularly when rotation and advancement flaps are planned. In these cases, dissection should be performed within the loose areolar tissue layer to preserve the pericranium, in case skin grafting of the flap donor site is needed.

Blood vessels, lymphatics, and sensory nerves are found within the subcutaneous layer, superficial to the galea aponeurotica. Blood vessels that supply the scalp and forehead include the paired supratrochlear, supraorbital, superficial temporal, posterior auricular, and occipital arteries and their accompanying veins **(Fig. 9.1a)**. The supratrochlear and supraorbital arteries arise from the ophthalmic artery, a branch of the internal carotid artery. The remaining arteries that supply the scalp originate from the external carotid artery. These blood vessels are the basis for axial flaps used in local flap reconstruction of scalp defects. Robust interconnections between vascular territories allow for relatively long and large flaps to be used reliably. Caudal to the nuchal line, blood vessels that perforate the trapezius and splenius capitis muscles supply the skin of the posterior scalp and nape of neck.

Sensory nerves of the scalp are also paired and include the supratrochlear ($V_1$), supraorbital ($V_1$), zygomaticotemporal ($V_2$), auriculotemporal ($V_3$), lesser occipital (C2, C3), and greater occipital (C2) nerves **(Fig. 9.1b)**. The supraorbital and supratrochlear nerves supply the forehead and frontoparietal scalp. The zygomaticotemporal nerve supplies the region lateral to the brow and the temporal scalp up to the temporal crest. The auriculotemporal nerve supplies the lateral scalp, and the greater and lesser occipital nerves supply the occipital region.

Motor nerves in the scalp innervate the muscles of this region, which include the frontalis, temporalis, auricularis (anterior, superior, and posterior), and occipitalis muscles. Of these, the most clinically significant is the temporal branch of the facial nerve, which supplies the frontalis muscle. This branch is located on the deep surface of the temporoparietal fascia and

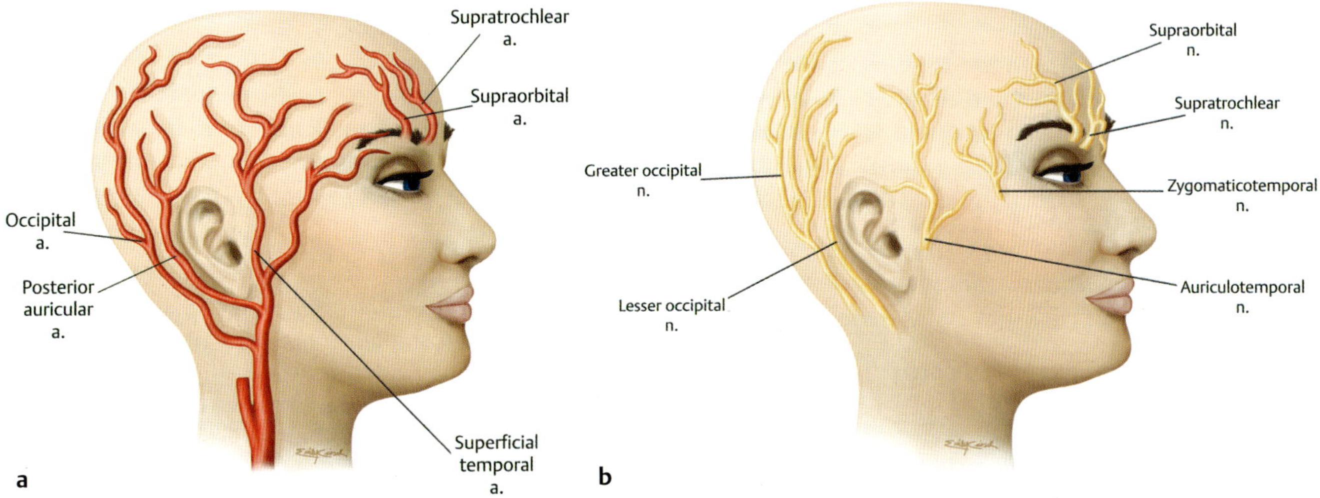


**Fig. 9.1** **(a)** Arterial blood supply of the scalp. **(b)** Sensory nerves of the scalp.

follows a course approximated by a line from 0.5 cm inferior to the external auditory meatus to a point 1.5 cm above the lateral eyebrow (Pitanguy's line). Dissection in this region is usually performed in a plane deep to the superficial layer of the deep temporal fascia in the region of the zygoma to prevent nerve injury. Elevation of the temporal fat pad and dissection in the plane of the zygomatic periosteum is the safest way to avoid injury to the temporal branch of the facial nerve in the zygomatic arch area. The temporalis muscle is innervated by the mandibular branch of the trigeminal nerve, which enters the deep surface of the muscle. The postauricular branch of the facial nerve, which arises from the main trunk near its emergence from the styloid foramen of the temporal bone, innervates the auricularis and occipitalis muscles.

The calvarium includes bones that form by intramembranous ossification (frontal, parietal, and temporal bones) as well as those that form by endochondral ossification (occipital and sphenoid bones). Structurally, the calvarium comprises three layers: an outer table, a diploic (or medullary) space, and an inner table. Burring of the outer table with entry into the vascular diploic space facilitates take of skin grafts on the calvarium in cases where the periosteum has been removed.

## ■ Reconstructive Options

### Preoperative Assessment

Any plan for scalp and calvarial reconstruction should be preceded by a thorough history and physical examination. Medical comorbidities, such as vascular disease, diabetes mellitus, and tobacco use, should be factored into the overall reconstructive strategy. Corticosteroid use should be elicited, particularly in patients with concomitant intracranial pathology. A history of prior radiation therapy may preclude the use of local flaps due to compromised regional vascularity. The details of prior surgical procedures should be reviewed.

On physical examination, mobility of scalp tissue and hair growth patterns should be noted. In patients who have had prior procedures, scars should be carefully assessed, because they may indicate that the axial blood supply to potential local flaps has been interrupted, making them unreliable for use in reconstruction. Evaluation of the superficial temporal blood vessels as potential recipient vessels is advisable in cases where free tissue transfer is being considered, either by palpation or by handheld Doppler ultrasound. A preoperative CT scan of the head and neck provides valuable information about the extent of disease and anticipated defect, including calvarial involvement and the potential need for bony reconstruction.

Prior to embarking on reconstruction, negative margins should be confirmed through the use of frozen and permanent sections. If there are concerns about the margin status, the wound can be temporized with dressing changes while awaiting final pathology results. The reconstructive plan should also take into consideration patient positioning during surgery and postoperatively. In many cases, use of a horseshoe head support with the patient in either supine or prone position can facilitate the wide exposure required to elevate scalp flaps. Postoperatively, use of a halo device may help protect the reconstruction; use of the halo should be arranged preoperatively with the neurosurgeon, although we have rarely found this device necessary.

## Scalp Reconstruction

All rungs of the reconstructive ladder have a place in scalp reconstruction, including both nonmicrosurgical and microsurgical techniques. The choice of reconstructive method depends on the surface area and depth of the scalp defect as well as the quality of remaining scalp tissue. Unlike many other types of head and neck reconstruction, tissue expansion may occasionally play a role in scalp reconstruction.

### Scalp Reconstruction: Nonmicrosurgical Techniques

Nonmicrosurgical techniques include primary closure, local scalp flaps, tissue expansion, skin grafts, and regional flaps.

#### Primary Closure

Primary closure with adjacent hair-bearing tissue is an appropriate first choice for the closure of small scalp defects. However, due to the inelasticity of scalp tissue, this approach is typically limited to defects no greater than 3 cm in diameter **(Fig. 9.2)**. Even in these circumstances, wide undermining of the scalp is usually necessary. Excessive wound tension can result in wound breakdown and/or scar alopecia and should be avoided. Tension can be minimized by designing resections so that the direction of wound closure is perpendicular to relaxed skin tension lines. In the scalp, these lines are generally oriented sagittally, while in the forehead they are oriented transversely.

Galeal scoring is an adjuvant technique that can increase scalp flap length and reduce tension, and it may be used with both primary closure and local scalp flaps. To confer the greatest effect, scoring should occur parallel to the leading edge of a flap and scores should be spaced at least 1 cm apart. Care must be taken to divide only the galea and not the subcutaneous layer directly adjacent to it in which the blood supply to the scalp resides. While it has been found that each galeal incision increases flap length by only 1.67 mm, multiple incisions can substantially minimize wound-closure tension.

#### Local Flaps

Local flaps are used for larger defects where primary closure is not possible. One major advantage of local flaps is adherence to the principle of replacing like tissue with like tissue. Local flaps are typically based on one or more of the axial vessels that supply the scalp, which include the supratrochlear, supraorbital, superficial temporal, postauricular, and occipital arteries **(Fig. 9.3)**.[1]

Local flaps are commonly designed as rotation-advancement flaps, whose diameter may need to measure five times or more the diameter of the defect to avoid excessive tension. For defects where this is not feasible, such as centrally located defects, multiple smaller rotation-advancement flaps may be performed **(Fig. 9.4)**. The parietal region has relatively greater laxity and therefore is a preferable donor site for scalp flaps. Donor sites should be chosen in less aesthetically sensitive areas when possible (i.e., incisions should be planned so that they do not violate the forehead if possible), and flap design should attempt to match hair follicle orientation following flap transposition, ideally with minimal disruption of the hairline. Rotation-advancement flaps invariably result in a standing cone, or "dog-ear," at the flap base closest to the defect, which should not be excised primarily to avoid potentially compromising flap vascularity. In many cases, excision of a Burow's triangle away from a rotation flap on the side opposite the standing cone can redistribute tissue and minimize the deformity.

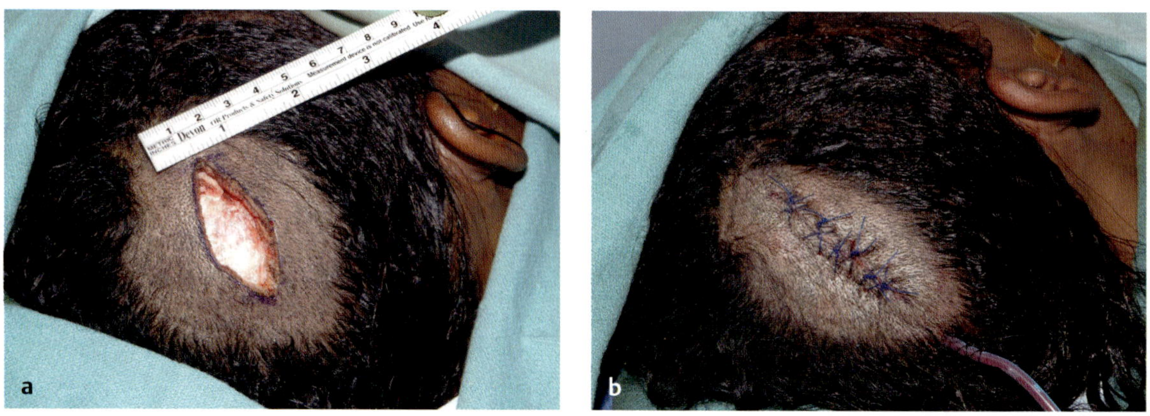


**Fig. 9.2** **(a)** Defects less than 3 cm in width **(b)** can be closed primarily following undermining in the subgaleal plane.

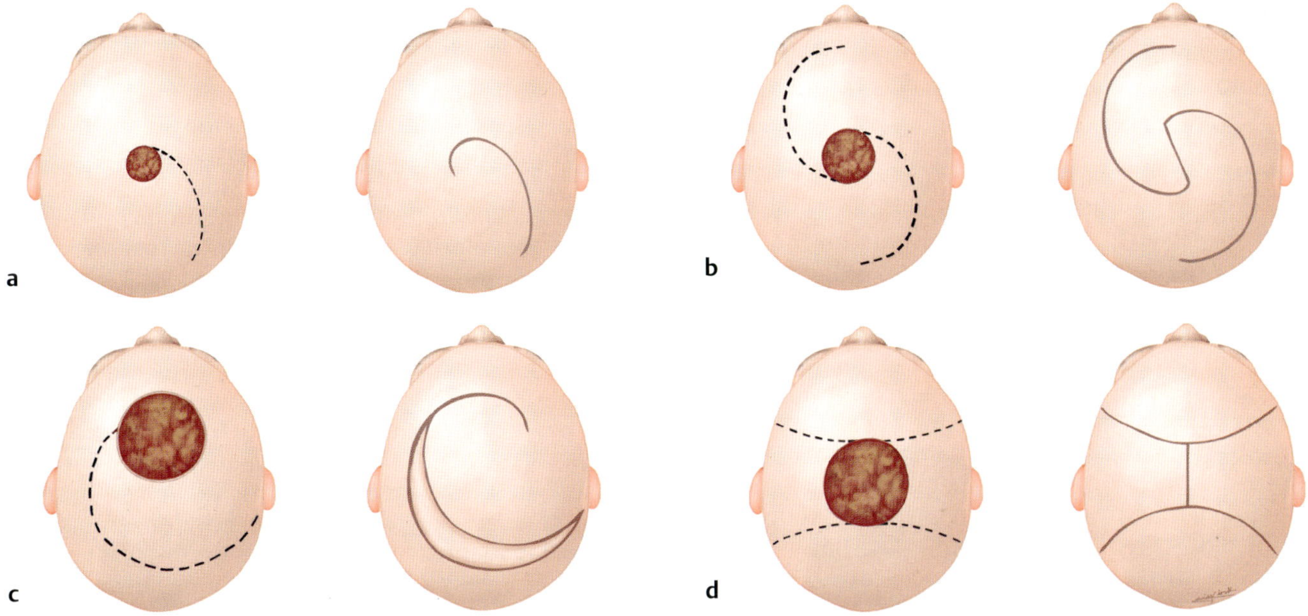


**Fig. 9.3** Local flap designs for reconstructing scalp defects. **(a)** Rotation flap. **(b)** Double opposing rotation flaps ("yin–yang" flaps). **(c)** Large rotation-advancement flap ("scalping" flap) with skin grafting of the flap donor site (shaded region). **(d)** Orticochea tripartite flaps.

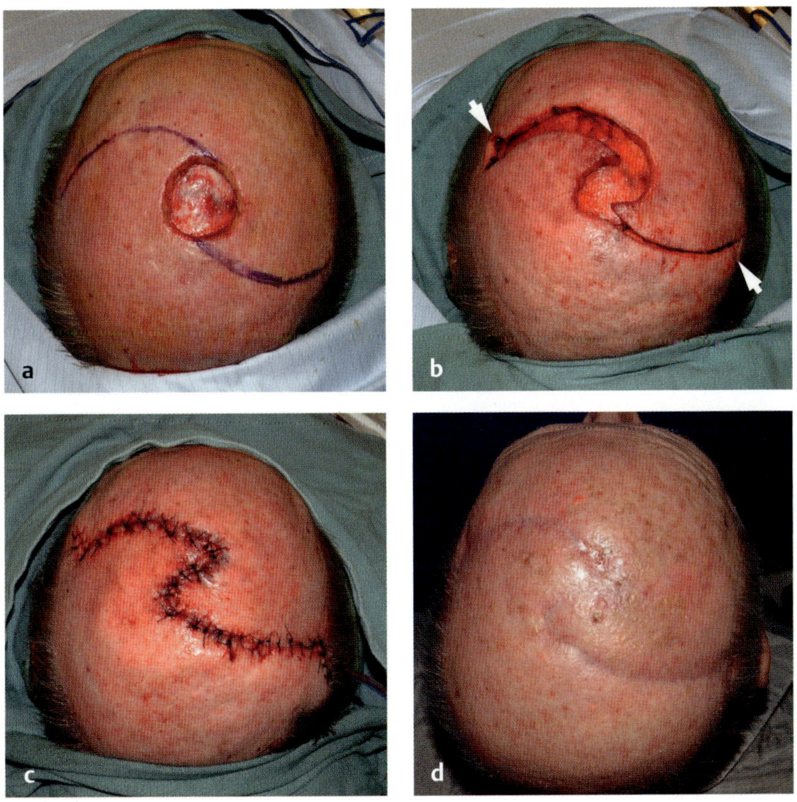


**Fig. 9.4** **(a)** Scalp defect following resection of a cutaneous malignancy. **(b)** Design of double opposing rotation flaps. The *arrows* indicate Burow's triangles excised away from the base of the flap, to avoid a standing cone or "dog-ear" deformity while preserving maximum blood supply to the flaps. **(c)** Immediate and **(d)** late postoperative results.

## Tissue Expansion

Tissue expansion is a technique that can augment the amount of tissue available for reconstruction of a defect using local scalp flaps. The use of tissue expansion is often limited in oncologic situations when there is an urgent need for resection, eliminating the possibility of pre-expanding scalp tissue prior to performing the reconstruction. Intraoperative expansion of scalp tissues, which acutely stretches existing tissues (i.e., mechanical creep), has been described, but this approach yields substantially less gain than staged tissue expansion, which generates actual new tissues (i.e., biological creep). More commonly, tissue expansion is employed in an elective, delayed setting, such as part of a staged plan to reconstruct an area of alopecia or a skin-grafted defect. The maximum theoretical size of a defect that can be closed with a tissue-expanded flap is 50% of the scalp surface area.[2] Radiated scalp tissues are generally considered a contraindication to use of tissue expanders due to the high rate of complications, such as infection, dehiscence, and tissue-expander exposure.

Tissue expanders may be rectangular, round, or crescentic. In scalp reconstruction, often more than one tissue expander is placed at a time, to enable completion of the reconstruction in a single operation following the expansion process. Preoperatively, tissue expanders that are larger than the anticipated defect size should be selected, and the scalp flap that will be used at the second stage should be predetermined. The tissue expander should be placed using an access incision that can be incorporated into the eventual scalp flap, or at least the incision should be planned so as not to interfere with the blood supply to the planned flap, such as placing it away from the base of the flap. A subgaleal pocket is created that is ~ 1 to 2 cm larger than the expander itself, and at least 1 to 2 cm away from the incision, to decrease the risk of wound dehiscence and extrusion.[3] A separate pocket at some distance from the first pocket is created for the filling port, thus minimizing the chance for migration of the valve or puncture of the prosthesis. Initial filling of the tissue expander intraoperatively is advisable to help stabilize the implant position, but not so much as to compromise scalp tissue vascularity. Closed suction drains should be used to minimize seroma formation, which can predispose to periprosthetic infection.

Tissue expansion is generally commenced 2 to 3 weeks after device placement, and it is performed serially thereafter on a weekly or every-other-week basis. The expanded scalp should ultimately measure ~ 20% greater than the defect size to account for tissue recoil during rotation or advancement. The second stage, involving tissue expander removal and scalp flap reconstruction, is then performed approximately 4 weeks after completion of expansion. At the time of flap reconstruction, the implant capsule may be scored, but it is not removed to minimize injury to the underlying subgaleal blood supply. After incisions have healed, any residual standing cone deformities can be removed at a subsequent revision procedure.

## Skin Grafts

Skin grafts may be used to reconstruct scalp defects of all sizes provided that the wound has a well-vascularized bed. While skin grafts are easily performed, they do not bear hair, and they may result in a contour deformity that may be especially more noticeable in the scalp, where the skin is thick. Primary closure or local scalp flaps should be considered first whenever possible. For reliable skin graft take, the pericranium must be intact prior to skin grafting **(Fig. 9.5)**. When bare calvarium without pericranium is exposed,

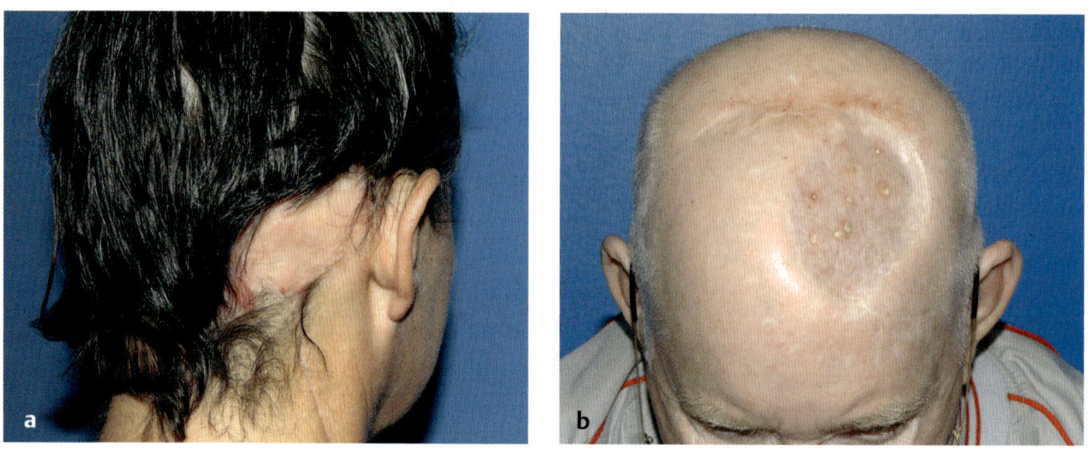


**Fig. 9.5** **(a)** Split- or full-thickness skin grafts will take readily on pericranium. **(b)** They will also adhere to bare calvarium, particularly if the bone has been burred down to expose vascular channels continuous with the diploic space, but they are prone to breakdown with time.

fascia from adjacent scalp tissue may be advanced or rotated into the wound as a galeal, temporoparietal, or pericranial flap to allow for application of a skin graft. An alternative approach is to remove the outer table of the calvarium with a bur to expose the vascular diploic space. Shortcomings of this latter approach include potential skin graft instability and a poor aesthetic outcome. Skin grafts should be avoided in the setting of prior radiation therapy due to diminished vascularity of the wound bed, which will likely decrease graft survival. If postoperative radiation therapy is anticipated, flap reconstructions may be more effective than skin grafts, which may slough or break down during and after treatment.

For full-thickness scalp defects that are too large for closure with a local scalp flap, skin grafts and scalp flaps may be used in combination. In these cases, the scalp flap is raised in a subgaleal plane and is used to reconstruct the defect, and then the donor site is skin grafted. Although this approach results in a potentially large skin-grafted donor site, the technique can achieve durable reconstruction for very large defects in patients who are not candidates for microsurgical reconstruction **(Fig. 9.3c)**.

### Regional Flaps

Regional flaps are, in general, infrequently used in scalp reconstruction due to the limited number of donor flaps in close enough proximity to the scalp. The temporoparietal fascia flap and temporalis muscle flap can be used for defects within or adjacent to the temporal region, and they are usually combined with a skin graft. The pedicled trapezius muscle or myocutaneous flap can be used to reconstruct defects of the occipital region. The trapezius flap can also be used for more distant scalp defects when it is performed as an extended flap using tissue from the middle third and lower third of the posterior trunk. However, the muscle is usually quite narrow in this region and cutaneous paddles are also usually limited in size if primary closure of the back donor site is planned.

## Scalp Reconstruction: Microsurgical Techniques

Free flap reconstruction of scalp defects is necessary when local options are inadequate. Local options may be rendered unsuitable for various reasons, most commonly the defect size and/or as a result of prior radiation therapy or surgery. Preoperatively, a defined reconstructive plan should be devised that includes selection of an appropriate flap donor site and recipient vessels. In addition, the patient should be optimized medically, considering the longer duration and greater complexity of a microsurgical reconstruction. We recommend preparation of the recipient blood vessels prior to flap harvest, especially when their presence and location will impact flap choice and dissection technique (e.g., recipient vessels that are distant from the defect may require dissection of a longer free flap pedicle than usual or may incur the need to harvest vein grafts). This can also minimize ischemia time when it is necessary to reposition the patient between flap harvest and microvascular anastomosis/flap inset.

### Recipient Vessel Selection

Recipient vessels should be selected that have adequate size and that are in close proximity to the defect. The superficial temporal vessels fulfill these requirements and are commonly used in microsurgical scalp reconstruction.[4] Located in the preauricular area, the superficial temporal vessels are relatively superficial and typically palpable just anterior to the root of the helix. When they are used, vein grafts are rarely necessary. Great care should be exercised during dissection, as the superficial temporal vessels can be thin-walled and fragile. Proximal dissection to the level of the auricular tragus, where the superficial temporal blood vessels are usually greater than 2.5 mm in diameter, may be necessary to minimize vessel size mismatch with the free flap blood vessels if they are of fairly large caliber.

The occipital artery is another axial vessel of the scalp that is sometimes used in microsurgical scalp reconstruction. It is most suited for posterior defects, and it is usually used in combination with the internal jugular vein or one its branches as the recipient vein. The occipital artery has a relatively small caliber that can sometimes preclude its use for microvascular anastomosis. Attention must be paid to postoperative positioning to avoid compression of the anastomosis at the base of the neck. The occipital vein usually runs in close proximity or even parallel to the occipital artery and drains either into the postauricular vein or directly into the internal jugular vein. It is also usually of small caliber, and consideration should be given to use of either the external or internal jugular veins.

When use of intrinsic vessels of the scalp is not possible, the facial vessels or other branches of the external carotid system may also be used as recipient arteries. The internal jugular vein and its branches are usually used concurrently as recipient veins. In these cases, the flap will usually need to traverse the preauricular or postauricular region. Intervening facial or scalp tissue is usually widely undermined or incised to accommodate the flap. It is often more straightforward to bridge this area with the flap itself, rather than tunnel the flap beneath native skin or scalp, to prevent compression of the pedicle as well as to minimize the flap pedicle length required to reach the defect. When tunneled, a generous subcutaneous tunnel should be made that takes into consideration postoperative edema.

## Free Flap Selection

Many flaps have been described for use in microsurgical scalp reconstruction.[5,6] In the scalp, a long pedicle is desirable due to the limited number of recipient vessels that are in close proximity. Muscle free flaps covered with skin grafts as well as flaps with a cutaneous paddle may be used. The most commonly used flaps include the latissimus dorsi, serratus anterior, rectus abdominis, radial forearm, anterolateral thigh, and omental free flaps. In our experience, muscle free flaps with skin grafts atrophy over time, but they have proven as durable in the long term as cutaneous free flaps even when a concurrent calvarial reconstruction is performed or in the context of postoperative radiation therapy. In either case, protruding hardware or sharp bony edges must be avoided to prevent wound breakdown and exposure. In obese patients, muscle flaps with skin grafts may be more appropriate, although most cutaneous free flaps can be thinned primarily or secondarily to achieve acceptable aesthetic results. Another option is an omental free flap, although we consider this a secondary option, mainly due to the need for a laparotomy to harvest the flap. Other factors that should guide flap selection include the defect size as it pertains to donor-site closure, donor-site morbidity, and the ability to employ a two-team approach for flap harvest and recipient-site preparation. Details of flap harvest can be found in the respective chapters dealing with each specific flap, while information pertinent to scalp reconstruction is presented here.

### *Latissimus Dorsi Flap*

The latissimus dorsi flap is usually our preferred option for large microsurgical scalp reconstructions **(Fig. 9.6)**. It is a thin flap that closely approximates

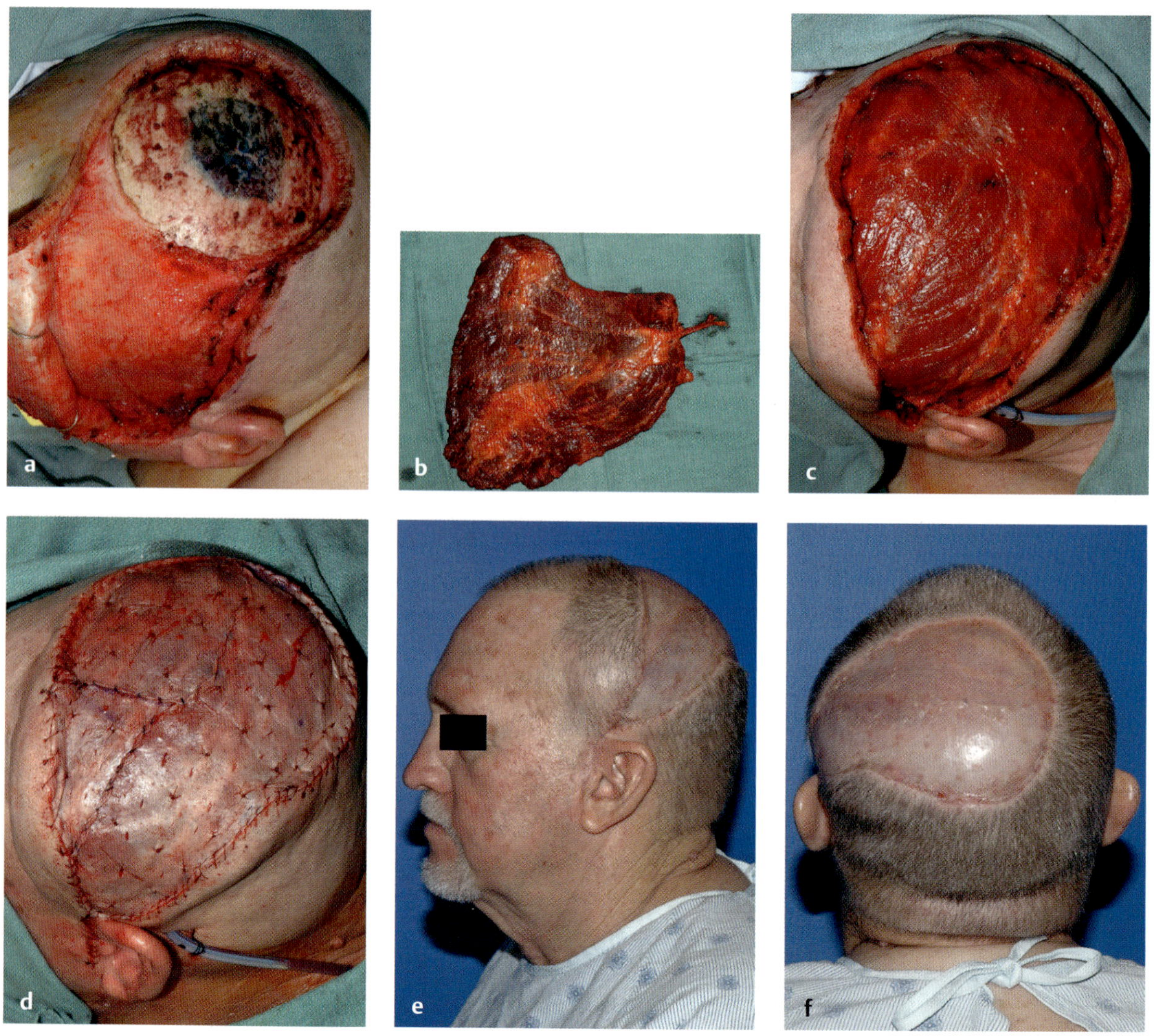

**Fig. 9.6** **(a)** Large scalp defect requiring free flap reconstruction. **(b)** A latissimus dorsi muscle free flap. **(c)** Flap inset with anastomosis to the left superficial temporal blood vessels. **(d)** Coverage with an unmeshed split-thickness skin graft. **(e,f)** Postoperative result.

the thickness of scalp tissue (once denervation atrophy has occurred), it has a large surface area, and it possesses a reasonably long vascular pedicle. The latissimus dorsi is usually harvested as a muscle-only flap and covered with a split-thickness skin graft when used for scalp reconstruction. A myocutaneous flap can be used, although in some patients this can result in excessive bulk and limits the flap width to ~ 8 cm if the donor site is to be closed primarily. In most patients, a single latissimus dorsi muscle flap is sufficient to cover all but the largest scalp defects (subtotal or total defects). If additional tissue is necessary, the serratus anterior muscle, whose blood supply is a branch of the thoracodorsal system, can be harvested with the flap.

The latissimus dorsi muscle originates from the iliac crest inferiorly and the lower thoracic and lumbar vertebrae medially, and it inserts onto the humerus. It measures ~ 25 × 35 cm. The latissimus dorsi flap has two dominant sources of blood supply from the thoracodorsal vessels in the axilla, and perforating vessels from the posterior intercostal vessels in the lumbar region. In free flap reconstruction, only the thoracodorsal vessels are used. The thoracodorsal blood vessel pedicle usually measures 8.5 cm in length. The thoracodorsal vessels arise from the subscapular vessels, and pedicle length may be as long as 10 cm if the subscapular vessels are included. The thoracodorsal nerve accompanies the pedicle and is divided in scalp reconstruction.

The latissimus dorsi muscle is typically harvested with the patient in lateral decubitus position. The ipsilateral upper extremity is included in the surgical field to allow for manipulation during surgery. When the latissimus dorsi flap is harvested, the arm is abducted and flexed anteriorly at the shoulder to provide wide exposure for pedicle dissection. If recipient vessels in the neck are utilized, the arm can then be extended at the shoulder and placed by the patient's side to provide access during microvascular anastomosis. In some cases, repositioning may be necessary to achieve the best access to the defect and to the recipient blood vessels for microvascular anastomosis. Position changes should be factored into the operative time when discussing the case with the patient and with the anesthesia team preoperatively.

When insetting the latissimus dorsi muscle flap, as well as other muscle flaps, we usually undermine the edges of the scalp defect 1 to 2 cm and tuck the flap beneath the free edges of the scalp.[7] This provides a more durable closure that is less prone to wound dehiscence. A temporary heaped up appearance results around the margins of the reconstruction, but the contour rapidly improves within a few weeks of surgery as the muscle undergoes atrophy from denervation and disuse.

The proximal portion of the latissimus dorsi muscle flap, near its humeral insertion, is usually thicker than the distal portion. Dividing the muscle several centimeters distal to the tendinous humeral insertion in an oblique manner, while taking care not to injure the vascular pedicle, can improve the contour of the proximal portion of the flap, often eliminating the need for secondary debulking to improve the cosmesis of the reconstruction. Intramuscular dissection of the flap pedicle in this region can also extend its functional length. If the flap remains bulky at its proximal end, we usually wait at least 3 months for the flap to undergo spontaneous atrophy prior to considering any surgical revisions.

We prefer to apply unmeshed, thick (0.012 to 0.016 inch), split-thickness skin grafts to muscle free flaps to maximize the durability as well as the cosmesis of the reconstruction, which can be quite good, particularly in bald patients. To minimize seroma formation, slits can be cut into large skin grafts at intervals ("pie-crusting") and multiple interrupted "quilting" sutures can be used to secure the graft to the underlying muscle free flap, which also prevents shearing of the graft from the muscle.

Loss of latissimus dorsi muscle function has minimal effect on an otherwise healthy patient. However, in patients dependent on upper extremity function for crutch use or bed to wheelchair transfer, alternative donor sites may need to be considered. To minimize donor-site morbidity, for smaller defects, the muscle may be split and based on either the transverse or descending branch of the thoracodorsal artery. It is usually easier to harvest the lateral muscle based on the descending branch, while maintaining the medial muscle in situ where it is supplied by the perforating branches of the posterior intercostal vessels. Nerve branches that travel with the descending branch are divided, while those accompanying the medial branch are left in continuity to preserve its function. Postoperative seromas occur more frequently with latissimus dorsi flap harvest than with most other flaps, and closed suction drains should be used judiciously.

### *Serratus Anterior Flap*

The serratus anterior flap is useful for microsurgical reconstruction of smaller scalp defects. It is typically harvested as a muscle-only flap that is skin grafted (the skin paddle of the musculocutaneous serratus anterior flap is usually considered unreliable). The serratus anterior muscle originates from ribs 1 through 8 (and occasionally from rib 9 in some patients) and inserts onto the medial border of the scapula, resulting in eight to nine muscle slips. It measures ~ 20 × 15 cm. The superior four slips are supplied by the lateral thoracic vessels and are innervated by the long thoracic nerve, while slips five through nine are supplied by the serratus branch of the thoracodorsal vessels and are innervated by the serratus branch of the thoracodorsal nerve. This arrangement of neurovascular supply confers the ability to harvest the flap segmentally, which can minimize donor-site morbidity. To prevent scapular winging or impairment of shoulder function, typically the lower three to four slips of the serratus anterior muscle are harvested based on the thoracodorsal vessels, while the superior slips are spared, resulting in a flap that is usually 10 × 15 cm. The vascular pedicle to the serratus anterior flap may be lengthened by dissecting up to, and including, the subscapular vessels.

The serratus anterior flap can be harvested with the patient in the lateral decubitus or "sloppy" lateral position. As with latissimus dorsi flap harvest, it is helpful to include the ipsilateral upper extremity in the surgical field. The muscle is most commonly accessed through an incision overlying the muscle along the anterolateral chest. Both neurovascular pedicles lie on the superficial surface of the muscle, so care should be exercised during initial exposure of the flap. The muscle is then usually elevated along its deep surface from inferior to superior. Branches to the latissimus dorsi muscle from the thoracodorsal system are ligated to maximize pedicle length, leaving the latissimus dorsi muscle supplied by the perforating branches of the posterior intercostal vessels.

For very large defects, a chimeric muscle flap that includes the serratus anterior muscle and the latissimus dorsi muscle can be harvested based on the subscapular vessels (**Fig. 9.7**). In addition, when a calvarial defect is present, vascularized rib can be transferred with the serratus anterior flap. The sixth or seventh rib is usually selected and up to 16 cm of rib can be harvested along with the muscle. The rib may be split or the deep perichondrium left in situ to minimize donor morbidity and the risk of pneumothorax during harvest.

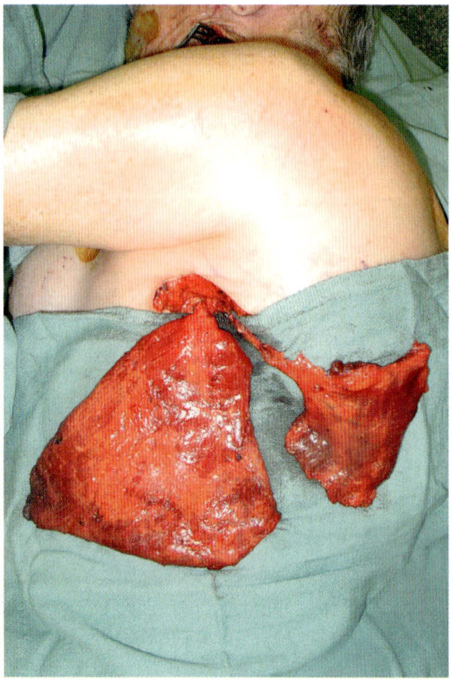

**Fig. 9.7** Latissimus dorsi muscle and serratus anterior muscle chimeric free flap based on the thoracodorsal artery and vein, which arise from the subscapular system, included in this dissection to increase pedicle length.

### *Rectus Abdominis Flap*

The rectus abdominis flap, like the latissimus dorsi and serratus anterior, is most commonly performed as a muscle free flap that is skin grafted. Although it can be performed as a myocutaneous flap with either a vertical or transverse skin paddle, the relatively thicker quality of abdominal soft tissues often compromises the aesthetic result. The rectus abdominis flap is long but has limited width; it is usually ~ 25 × 6 cm, which limits its use for very broad scalp defects. The rectus abdominis muscle attaches to the pubic symphysis inferiorly and the costal margin superiorly. It has a dual blood supply from the deep inferior epigastric artery, which serves as the basis for free flap reconstructions, and the superior epigastric artery. The deep inferior epigastric pedicle is 6 to 10 cm long and enters the muscle along its deep lateral aspect at approximately the level of the arcuate line. Intramuscular dissection of the proximal blood vessels, if the full length of muscle is not needed, can increase the functional length of the pedicle.

Harvest of the rectus abdominis flap is performed with the patient supine, through either a vertical midline or paramedian incision. When it is used as a myocutaneous flap, it can have either a vertically oriented or transversely oriented skin paddle, which is usually determined based on consideration of donor-site closure. In either case, the design of the skin paddle should include the periumbilical region, where most of the major musculocutaneous perforators are concentrated. After dissection through the subcutaneous tissues, the fascia is incised, and the muscle is released circumferentially along its entire length from the rectus sheath. The pedicle is identified along the deep surface of the muscle inferolaterally, and typically it is dissected down to its origin from the external iliac vessels.

The primary disadvantage of rectus abdominis flap harvest is donor-site morbidity, which can result in an abdominal bulge, hernia, or weakness. The risk of abdominal bulge can be minimized by meticulous layered closure of the anterior rectus sheath. When a myocutaneous flap is performed, it is advisable to harvest the flap in a fascia-sparing manner, with inclusion of only a minimal amount of fascia around musculocutaneous perforators. Careful dissection of the flap from its posterior aspect can help reduce the risk of a postoperative hernia. Placement of mesh should be considered in patients who are obese or who have had prior abdominal surgery that has compromised the quality of their fascia.

## Calvarial Reconstruction: Autologous Techniques

Autologous methods of reconstruction involve the use of either nonvascularized bone grafts or vascularized bone flaps. Nonvascularized bone grafts are readily harvested, most commonly from the calvarium or rib. Their use requires the presence of well-vascularized soft tissue coverage from which graft revascularization occurs. The use of nonvascularized bone grafts is limited to relatively small defects without contamination or infection.

Calvarial bone grafts are a convenient option since they may be obtained from within the same operative field.[12] The grafts are harvested as split grafts comprising the outer table of the calvarium, preferably from the parietal region posterior to the coronal suture, where the skull is the thickest. To harvest the graft, a trough is burred around the planned harvest site, and a saw or osteotome is used to remove the outer table of the calvarium. Grafts should not be harvested closer than 1.5 cm to the midline to avoid injury to the sagittal sinus. The amount of available graft can be limited, particularly when the defect and the donor site are in close proximity. Care should be taken not to violate the inner table or dura during harvest.

An extracranial technique may also be employed to harvest cranial bone grafts. With this approach, a craniotomy is performed and the outer and inner tables of the skull are split on a back table. The method of delamination is similar, with the use of saws and osteotomes to split the bone along the medullary space. The inner table is then returned to the donor site and the outer table is utilized as graft, and both of them are secured to native calvarium with wires or plates and screws. Although a craniotomy is required with this technique, there is less potential for injury to intracranial structures during harvest, which may be especially relevant in elderly or young patients.

The ribs are another source of nonvascularized bone grafts for calvarial reconstruction. Compared with calvarial bone grafts, rib grafts allow grafts of larger dimensions to be obtained. Rib grafts are usually harvested through an anterolateral or anterior chest wall incision centered over the seventh or eighth rib. In males, an incision directly over the rib is used, while in females an inframammary incision is preferable. Typically, no more than two to three adjacent ribs are harvested to prevent chest-wall instability or deformity. Grafts are sometimes obtained from alternating ribs to minimize donor-site morbidity. Once the ribs are exposed, the grafts are harvested in a subperiosteal plane to prevent injury to the underlying pleura. The grafts are then usually shaped with a rib bender to match the curved contour of the skull, and then they are fixated with plates and screws to the surrounding calvarium. Gaps between individual rib grafts can be filled with bone chips or hydroxyapatite bone cement. The use of rib grafts for calvarial reconstruction is limited primarily by donor-site morbidity.

Vascularized bone flaps have an intrinsic blood supply that broadens their applications in comparison to nonvascularized bone grafts. They can be reliably used in contaminated and radiated wounds, and they can be used to reconstruct larger defects than bone grafts, although their use is limited by donor-site availability. Both pedicled and free bone flaps have been used in calvarial reconstruction. Pedicled transfer of the outer calvarial table based on the superficial temporal vessels has been described, where the superficial temporal fascia and periosteum are preserved to maintain connections between the vascular pedicle and the transferred bone. However, more commonly, vascularized bone flaps are performed as free tissue transfers. Vascularized rib can be transferred with the serratus anterior muscle flap, as described above. This is particularly useful in cases of composite defects that have both soft tissue and bony components. The chest-wall morbidity associated with rib graft harvest is similar to that with use of the serratus myo-osseous free flap.

## Calvarial Reconstruction: Alloplastic Techniques

Calvarial reconstruction can also be performed using a variety of alloplastic materials, most commonly titanium mesh, polymethylmethacrylate, calcium phosphate ceramics, high-density porous polyethylene, and prefabricated polymer implants **(Fig. 9.9)**.[12,13] Compared with autologous methods of reconstruction, alloplastic materials are in abundant supply and have no associated donor-site morbidity, but they are subject to the risk of prosthetic infection, which may preclude their use in contaminated or infected wounds.

Titanium mesh is a metal alloy with many properties that make it well suited for calvarial reconstruction. It is easily contoured, is noncorrosive, allows for fluid egress, and is relatively resistant to infection. One of the disadvantages of titanium mesh is creation of scatter artifact on CT and MRI scans.

Polymethylmethacrylate (PMMA) is a high-molecular-weight polymer that is also commonly used for calvarial reconstruction. It is formed by means of an exothermic reaction when liquid meth-

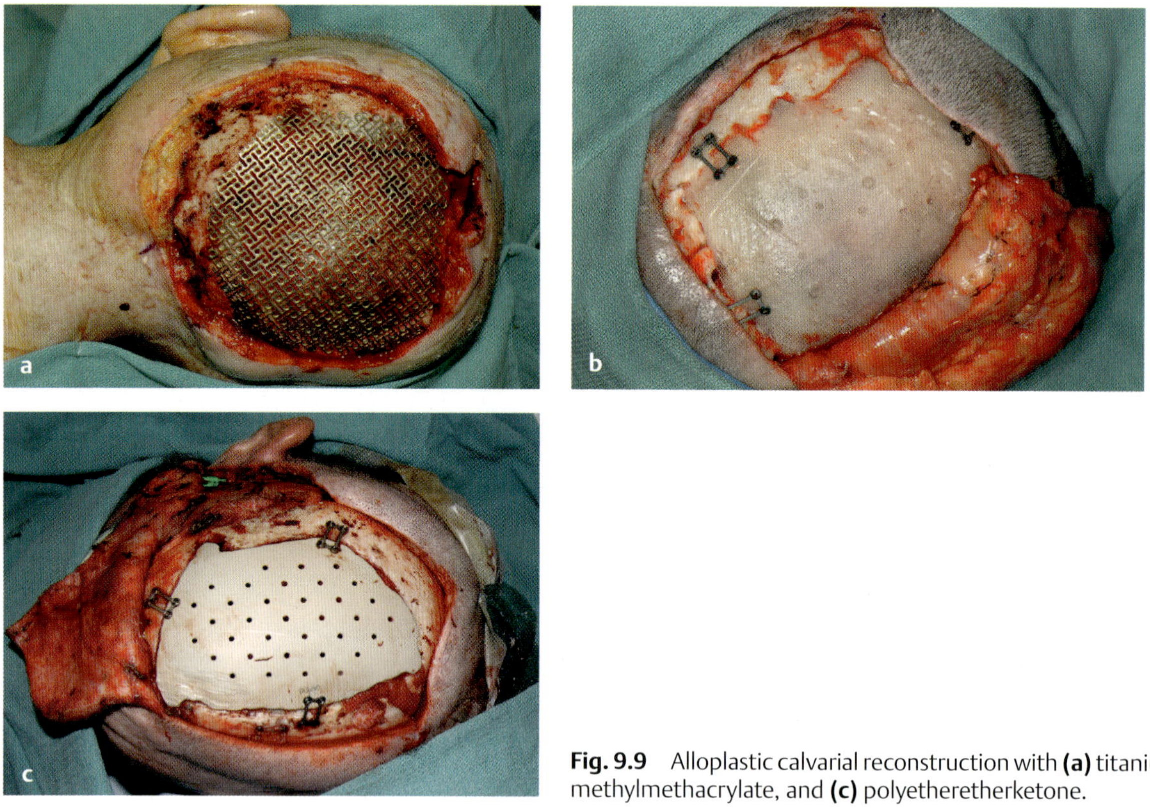

**Fig. 9.9** Alloplastic calvarial reconstruction with **(a)** titanium mesh, **(b)** polymethylmethacrylate, and **(c)** polyetheretherketone.

ylmethacrylate monomer is added to powdered methylmethacrylate polymer, during which care should be taken to cool the implant with continuous irrigation to prevent local tissue damage. PMMA can be strengthened by combining it with titanium mesh during implant formation.

Calcium phosphate ceramics, such as hydroxyapatite and calcium phosphate bone cements, are porous materials that are osteoconductive and provide a scaffold for bony ingrowth. Hydroxyapatite comes in either particulate or block form, whereas bone cements come as powders that are mixed with a solution intraoperatively to result in a moldable putty that hardens into a structurally stable implant. In our experience, calcium phosphate materials seem to be more prone to developing late infection.

High-density porous polyethylene implants are rigid, readily fixated, and come in a variety of shapes and sizes. Their porosity provides a framework into which tissue ingrowth can occur, which results in implant integration without capsule formation. However, although tissue ingrowth can stabilize implant position, it can make implant removal difficult in cases of exposure or infection. To decrease the risk of exposure or infection, coverage beneath a layer of periosteum or fascial envelope, in addition to skin, is advisable.

Prefabricated polymer implants based on CT data are a relatively recent advancement in calvarial reconstruction. Polyetheretherketone (PEEK; Synthes, West Chester, PA) is an example of such a biomaterial, and it possesses high tensile strength and resistance to degradation. Since prefabricated polymer implants are custom made for a patient's specific calvarial defect, they are most useful in delayed reconstructions, when the exact calvarial defect is known. If used for immediate calvarial reconstruction, the PEEK implant should be made slightly larger than the anticipated defect, as its edges can be readily burred down with standard surgical cutting burs to adjust its shape to fit.

## Algorithm

Several factors must be considered when planning scalp and calvarial reconstruction. The chief determinants of reconstructive method are the defect size and the quality of local tissue **(Fig. 9.10)**. For small defects, primary closure or local scalp flaps (when primary closure is not achievable) usually produce a better aesthetic outcome than skin grafting. Other secondary factors that should be considered to help guide the treatment strategy include the patient's medical condition and the status of the calvarium. Patients with poor overall prognosis or significant comorbidities but sizable defects may be better managed with large scalp flaps and back grafting of the donor site, rather than free flap reconstruction. Concurrent reconstruction of a calvarial defect may favor use of a free flap

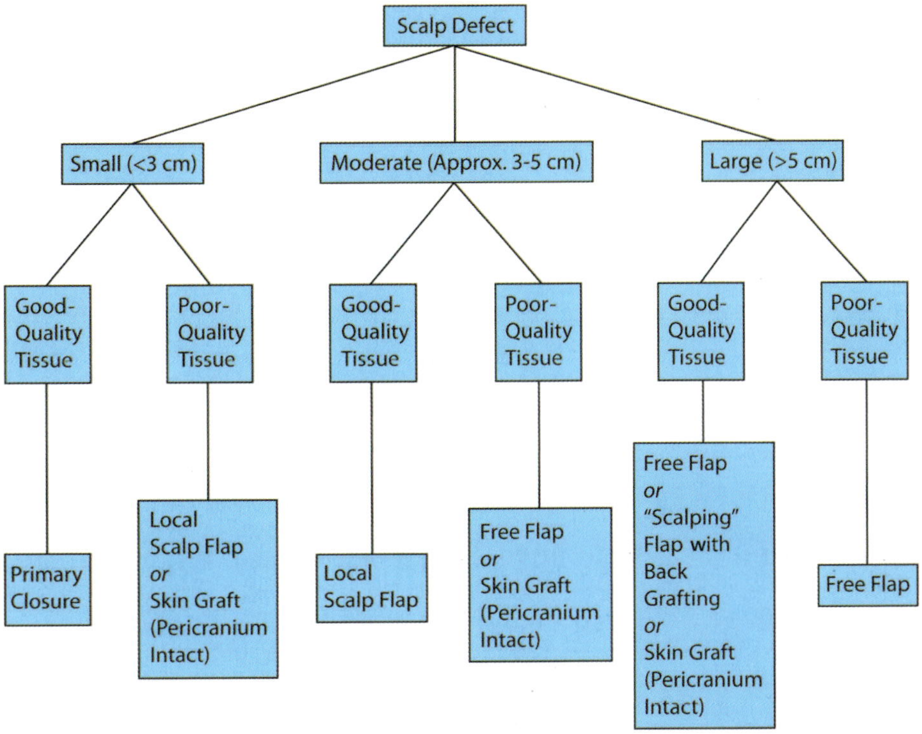


**Fig. 9.10** Algorithm for scalp reconstruction. Recommendations for reconstruction are based on approximate wound dimensions as well as the quality of remaining scalp tissue. Poor-quality tissue includes scalp tissue that has been previously radiated or operated upon and is of generally poor vascularity, increasing the risk for necrosis. Skin grafting is best reserved for wounds with intact pericranium at their base.

for scalp reconstruction to provide well-vascularized, tension-free scalp coverage, because wound dehiscence over nonvascularized bone or an alloplast usually requires removal of the cranioplasty.

## ■ Complications

Wound dehiscences can occur as a result of excessive tension; impaired healing in diabetes mellitus, with corticosteroid use, or with radiation therapy; diminished tissue vascularity from prior surgery; and improper flap design. Small wounds without exposed structures may be managed with local wound care and allowed to heal by secondary intent. Larger wounds may require skin grafting or readvancement of prior flaps. In some instances, an additional reconstruction may be required.

Infection is fortunately uncommon in the scalp due to its robust vascularity, but patients who undergo an alloplastic calvarial reconstruction may be at higher risk. In these cases, a trial of systemic antibiotics should be undertaken initially. If the clinical response is inadequate, the cranioplasty may have to be explanted and calvarial reconstruction performed in delayed fashion after resolution of the infection.

Partial and complete flap loss can occur with both local scalp flaps and free flaps. With local scalp flaps, flap loss usually occurs as a result of excessive tension and/or inadequate blood supply. Care should be taken to include at least one axial vessel and preferably more than one for large flaps, with excision of standing cones only secondarily after all wounds have healed. Free flap loss is usually secondary to a problem with the microvascular anastomosis and must be explored at the first sign of compromise to salvage the reconstruction. Caution should be exercised in the area of soft tissue closure over the anastomosis, as inelastic scalp tissues may compress the pedicle, especially when soft tissue edema increases postoperatively. It may be advisable to utilize free flap tissues to loosely cover the anastomosis, which can then be revised at a later stage.

## ■ Postoperative Care

The postoperative management of patients undergoing scalp reconstruction is an important component of the overall reconstructive outcome. Drains should be routinely used, even if a cranioplasty has been performed, since wide soft tissue undermining predisposes to fluid accumulation. The head should be elevated to minimize and facilitate resolution of soft tissue edema. Pressure should be relieved from the surgical sites postoperatively for at least 1 to 2 weeks. This may be particularly challenging when the surgical site extends onto the posterior scalp, and use of padding, alteration of patient positioning, or even application of a halo device may be necessary. Skin grafts should be immobilized with bolster dressings, except when combined with a free muscle flap, in which case a nonadherent dressing is placed and manipulated only by members of the surgical team. In cases of concomitant calvarial reconstruction, patients must be examined for signs of CSF leak or neurologic infection.

## ■ Case Examples

Case 1. A 74-year-old man presented with a recurrent squamous cell carcinoma of the scalp (**Fig. 9.11a**). He required wide local excision down to the calvarium, resulting in a 9 × 15 cm defect (**Fig. 9.11b**). Because the entire latissimus dorsi muscle was not needed for reconstruction, a split-latissimus dorsi muscle free flap was harvested, preserving the medial portion of the muscle, including its innervation via the thoracodorsal nerve (**Fig. 9.11c**). The superficial temporal vessels were explored but were deemed unacceptable for microvascular anastomosis. Therefore, the cheek was undermined in a subcutaneous plane and the anastomoses to the facial vessels were performed using saphenous vein grafts (**Fig. 9.11d**). The patient received postoperative radiation therapy and demonstrated a healed reconstruction with good contour 6 months later (**Fig. 9.11e**).

Case 2. An 81-year-old man presented with a recurrent malignant fibrous histiocytoma of the scalp following several prior resections (**Fig. 9.12a**). A composite resection of scalp and calvarium was performed. The calvarium was reconstructed with titanium mesh (**Fig. 9.12b**). A latissimus dorsi muscle free flap was then used for reconstruction of the scalp (**Fig. 9.12c**). The remaining scalp was undermined ~ 2 cm circumferentially, and the latissimus dorsi muscle was "tucked" beneath the scalp edge to provide a secure closure. Although a slight bulge from the muscle was visible initially, the contour deformity rapidly dissipated without need for later debulking. A "thick" (0.015 inch) split-thickness skin graft was applied and secured with multiple quilting sutures (**Fig. 12.11d**). The reconstruction remained intact after postoperative radiation therapy (**Fig. 12.11e**).

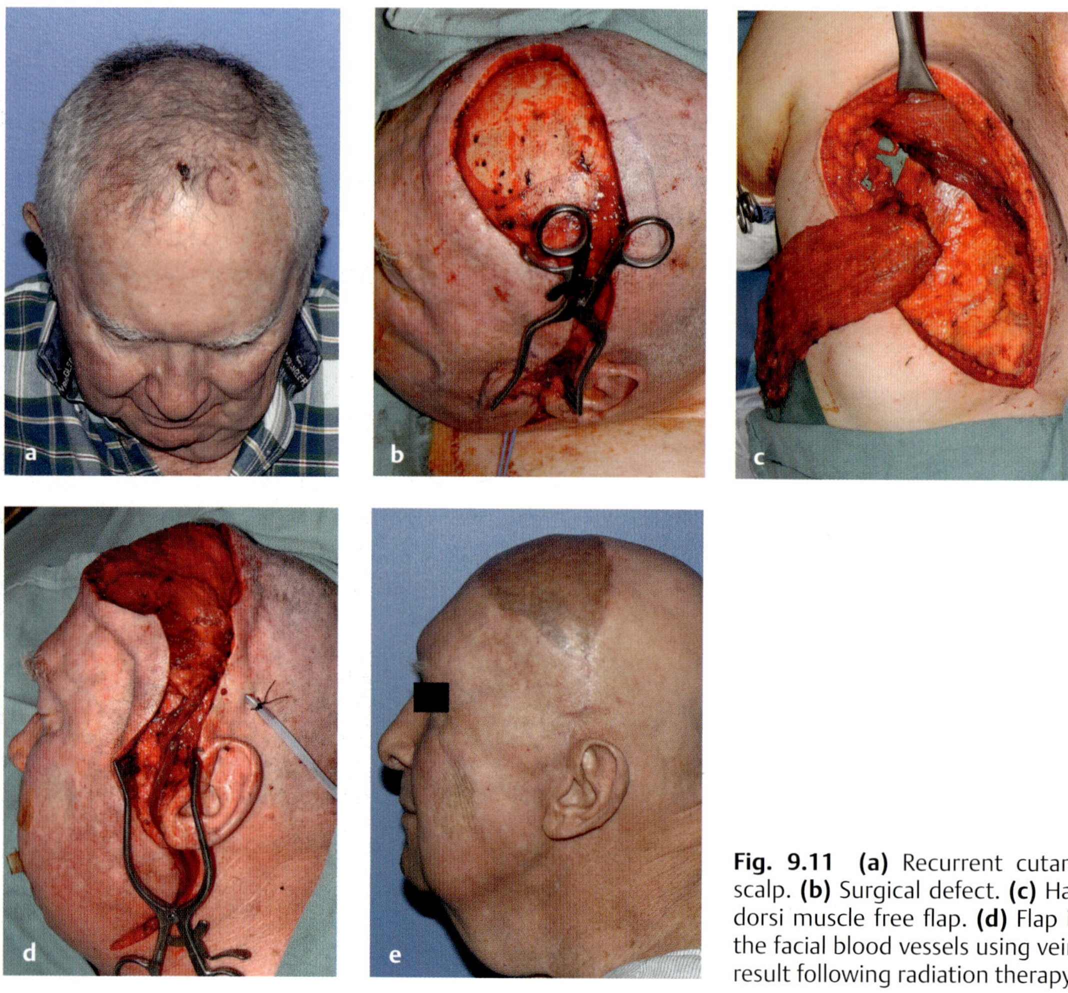

**Fig. 9.11** **(a)** Recurrent cutaneous malignancy of the scalp. **(b)** Surgical defect. **(c)** Harvest of a split–latissimus dorsi muscle free flap. **(d)** Flap inset with anastomosis to the facial blood vessels using vein grafts. **(e)** Postoperative result following radiation therapy.

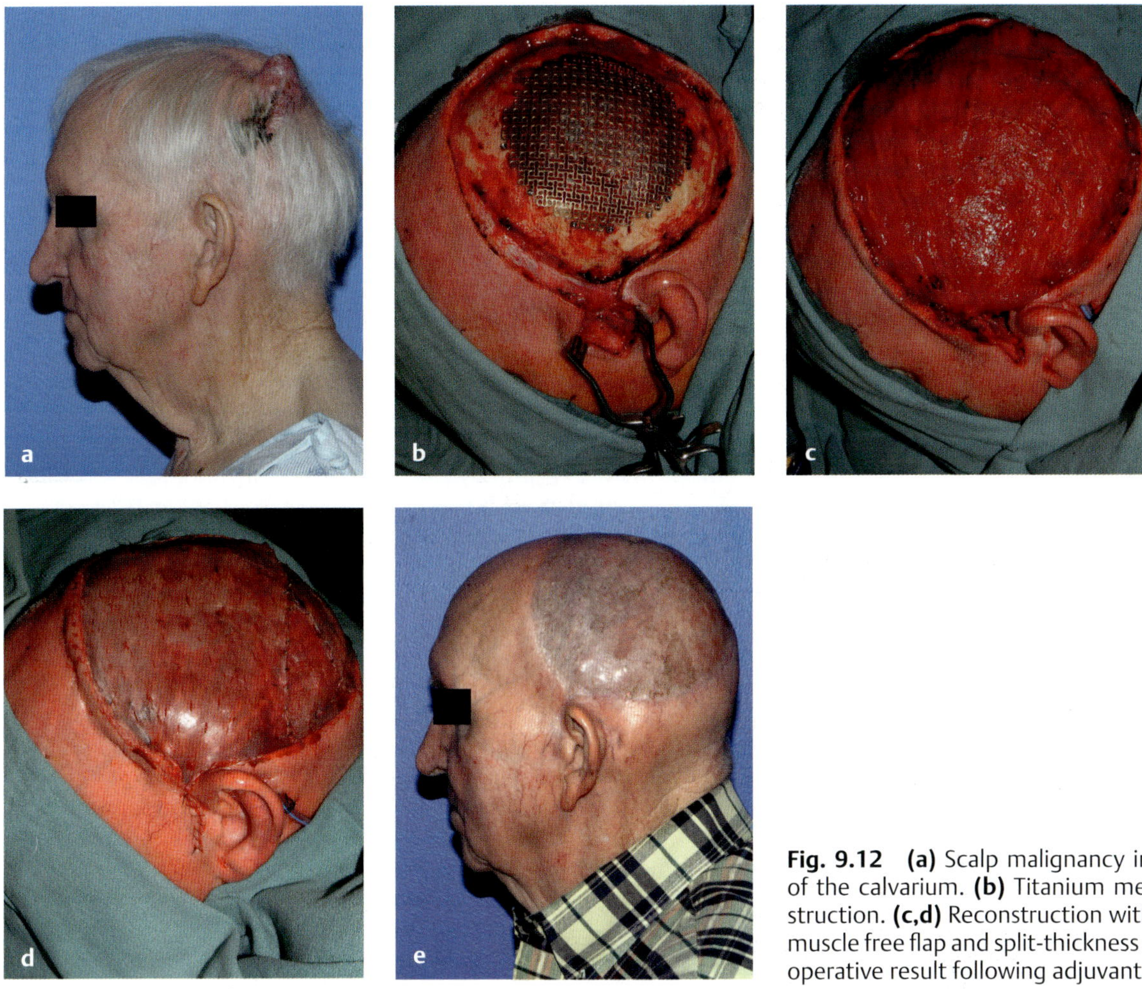


**Fig. 9.12** **(a)** Scalp malignancy invading the cortex of the calvarium. **(b)** Titanium mesh calvarial reconstruction. **(c,d)** Reconstruction with a latissimus dorsi muscle free flap and split-thickness skin graft. **(e)** Postoperative result following adjuvant radiation therapy.

## Pearls and Pitfalls

- Primary closure of scalp defects is generally limited to wounds measuring less than 3 cm in diameter owing to the limited elasticity of the scalp.
- Local scalp flaps should be designed as broadly based rotation-advancement flaps that incorporate at least one axial blood vessel.
- Reconstruction with local scalp flaps can be enhanced through the use of galeal scoring and skin grafting of the donor site.
- Tissue expansion has a limited role in oncologic reconstruction where immediate coverage of structures is needed.
- The latissimus dorsi free flap is often the preferred option for microsurgical scalp reconstruction due to its long vascular pedicle, large surface area, and low donor-site morbidity.
- The superficial temporal vessels should be utilized when possible for free flap reconstruction due to their reliability and the infrequent need for vein grafts due to their proximity to most scalp defects.
- Calvarial reconstruction for bony defects greater than ~ 3 cm in diameter should be considered to protect cranial contents and to restore scalp contour.
- Alloplastic materials, including titanium mesh and polymethylmethacylate, are straightforward and effective means of calvarial reconstruction.
- When scalp and calvarial defects coexist, reconstruction of both components in a single stage can usually be performed safely and effectively.
- When possible, scalp incisions should be planned so that they do not lie over graft materials.

## Expert Commentary *by Michael R. Zenn*

Scalp reconstruction is challenging due to the unique structures in the cranium and its anatomical location. Defects range from simple skin loss to full-thickness loss with exposed dura, and the reconstructive solution to each is different. The etiology of scalp wounds is also varied and can affect the options for reconstruction. The authors practice at a tertiary cancer center, and the emphasis of the chapter is oncologic microscopic reconstruction. My experience with scalp wounds includes trauma and infection as well as cancer, and accordingly my emphasis on the full reconstructive spectrum offers a different viewpoint.

Since the scalp is exposed to the world, cosmesis is an important consideration when contemplating scalp reconstructive options. The principle of "replacing like with like" is important, and often large defects of the scalp can be reconstructed with local tissue rearrangements utilizing scoring of the galea and transposition flaps, such as the yin–yang **(Fig. 9.3)**, double opposing semicircular flaps[14] **(Fig. 9.13)** and even the time-tested three- or four-flap techniques described by Orticochea.[15] Due to the incredible vascularity of the scalp, large scalp flaps can be rotated into position and back-grafted with split-thickness skin grafts, often solving difficult scalp wounds quickly, although with less than ideal cosmesis **(Fig. 9.14)**.

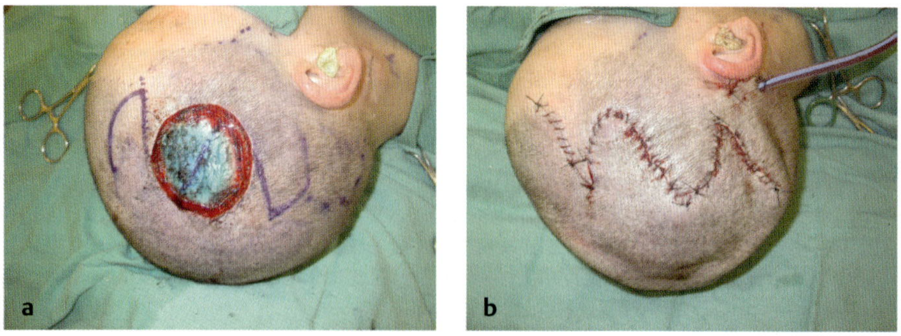

**Fig. 9.13** **(a)** A 43-year-old patient with a wide excision of a scalp melanoma. Local flaps in the form of doubleopposing semicircular flaps are utilized for closure. By incorporating z-plasties and scoring the galea, tissue transposition can be performed and no tissues are discarded. **(b)** After transposition and closure.

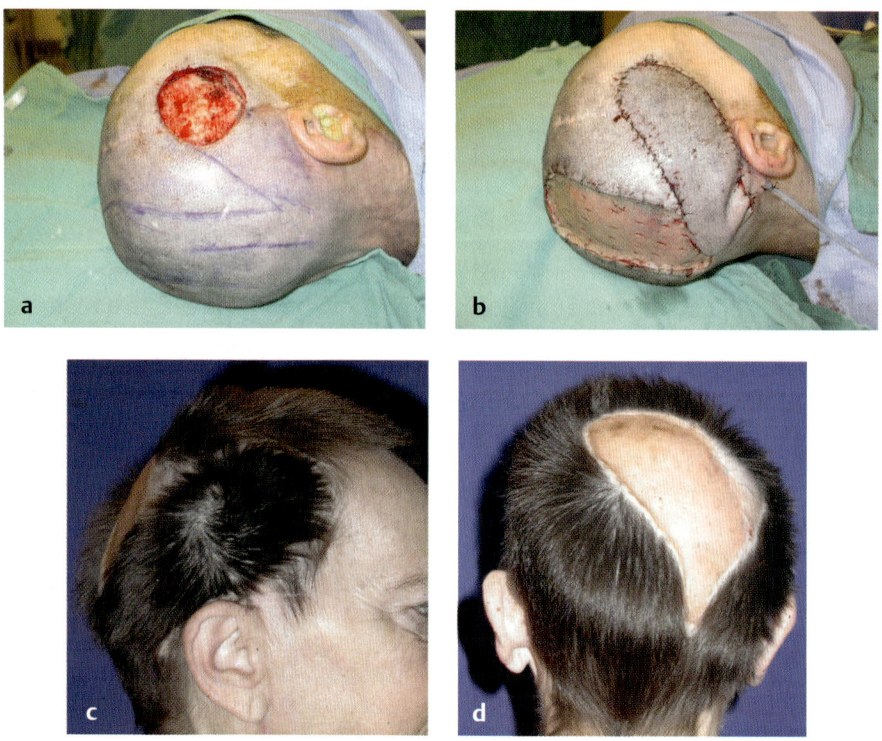

**Fig. 9.14** **(a)** A 66-year-old patient with a chronic wound after squamous cell carcinoma resection and irradiation. A transposition of scalp is planned on the occipital artery, which is located by Doppler exam and marked. **(b)** Tension-free rotation and inset of the flap are performed and the rotational dog-ear is left for future revision if needed. A skin graft will take well in the nonirradiated bed of the donor site. **(c)** Lateral view of flap at 6 months. **(d)** Posterior view of donor-site skin graft at 6 months.

The role of tissue expansion is underemphasized in this chapter. Often, with large oncologic resections, there is no time for the expansion process. This is not the case with scalp defects of other etiologies, where there is time for expansion prior to reconstruction or where wounds can be temporized with skin grafts while secondary expansion can be performed for eventual removal of the grafts. The cosmesis of scalp reconstruction with hair-bearing scalp is unsurpassed, and the scalp itself should always be considered as the ideal donor site. Unless previously irradiated, even small areas of residual hair-bearing scalp can be expanded over time and used for reconstruction (**Fig. 9.15**). The rule of thumb for scalp expansion is to place as many large expanders as possible and expand more than you think you need. Once flaps are expanded, galeal scoring becomes treacherous and is not recommended, because of the risk of devascularization and avulsion.

Radiation is a standard treatment for cutaneous malignancies of the scalp, especially in elderly patients with comorbidities preventing more complex reconstructive procedures. In such cases, with exposed bone, one can use the standard technique of burring the outer table of the skull and skin grafting. Since the area is irradiated, revascularization of the skin graft is often delayed and the grafts fail. In such cases, one can preliminarily place Integra Dermal Regeneration Template (Integra LifeSciences, Inc., Plainsboro, NY), which revascularizes over a period of weeks. This can be augmented with hyperbaric oxygen so that a nicely vascularized bed is created and skin grafting can be successful.[16]

The number of regional flaps for scalp reconstruction is limited. The trapezius flap was a workhorse flap prior to the era of microsurgical reconstruction, and it still has some use today. As mentioned in the chapter, it is mainly limited to the occipital region (**Fig. 9.16**). The flap is favorable because the rotation of the flap is toward its transverse cervical blood supply. Drawbacks include sacrifice of a functional muscle and scapular instability. The skin paddle of the myocutaneous flap is reliable over the

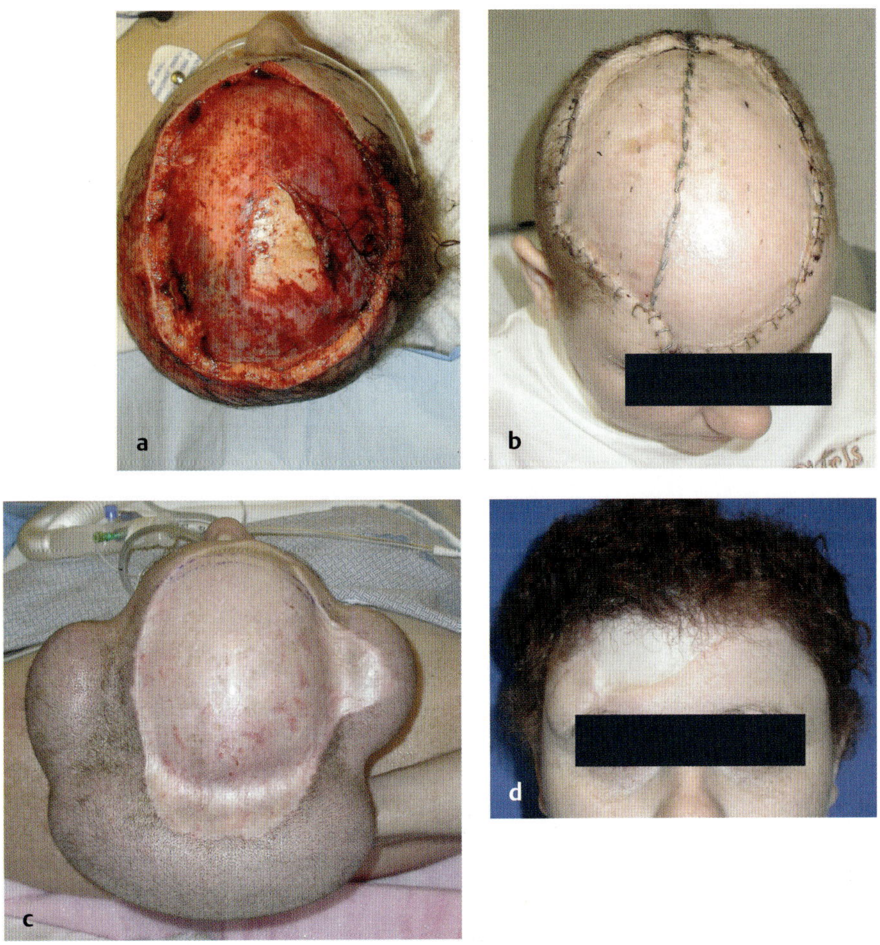

**Fig. 9.15** **(a)** A 25-year-old patient who sustained a scalp avulsion injury and a failed replantation. **(b)** After failed attempt at replantation of the scalp, skin grafting of the defect was performed. **(c)** Multiple large expanders were placed at all sites of hair-bearing skin and were over-expanded. **(d)** Six months after completion of scalp reconstruction. The patient later underwent forehead expansion and removal of her remaining forehead skin graft.

muscle and can be extended beyond the muscle by delay procedures or inclusion of the dorsal scapular branch of the transverse cervical artery.[17]

The chapter nicely covers microsurgical reconstruction of the scalp. I would only add that other flaps not mentioned exist for soft tissue and autogenous calvarial reconstruction and should also be considered:

- ALT flap with iliac crest (based on the ascending branch of the lateral femoral circumflex artery)
- Deep circumflex iliac artery flap with inner table of iliac bone
- Latissimus dorsi muscle with vascularized rib
- Parascapular flap with lateral scapular bone

My final pearls relate to the difficulty of finding recipient vessels for microvascular transfer. As mentioned in the chapter, the superficial temporal vessels should be the first choice when available. When these vessels appear diminutive, it is worth further proximal dissection into the substance of the parotid. This dissection often yields larger-caliber vessels. When they are not suitable as recipient vessels, an arteriovenous (AV) loop with saphenous vein graft should be considered. In these cases, I recommend harvesting the vein first and setting up the loop to neck vessels (facial or lingual artery, and internal jugular vein branch or external jugular vein) and letting blood circulate while the flap is harvested. The AV loop can safely be used as immediate recipient vessels for the flap. One should also consider the use of the descending lateral circumflex femoral system as an AV graft; this system offers a better range of vessel diameters for best caliber match and incurs a more limited access scar in the leg.[18]

Finally, the clinical problem of an infected bone flap or cranioplasty is a difficult management problem that almost always requires removal and delayed cranioplasty. Be aware of the "sunken flap syndrome" that this situation creates. I learned about this with a recent case of neurologic deterioration in a patient with a large free flap and no bony reconstruction due to infection.[19] The proposed mechanism of the syndrome is unprotected exposure of the brain to atmospheric pressure, and symptoms were resolved with urgent cranioplasty.

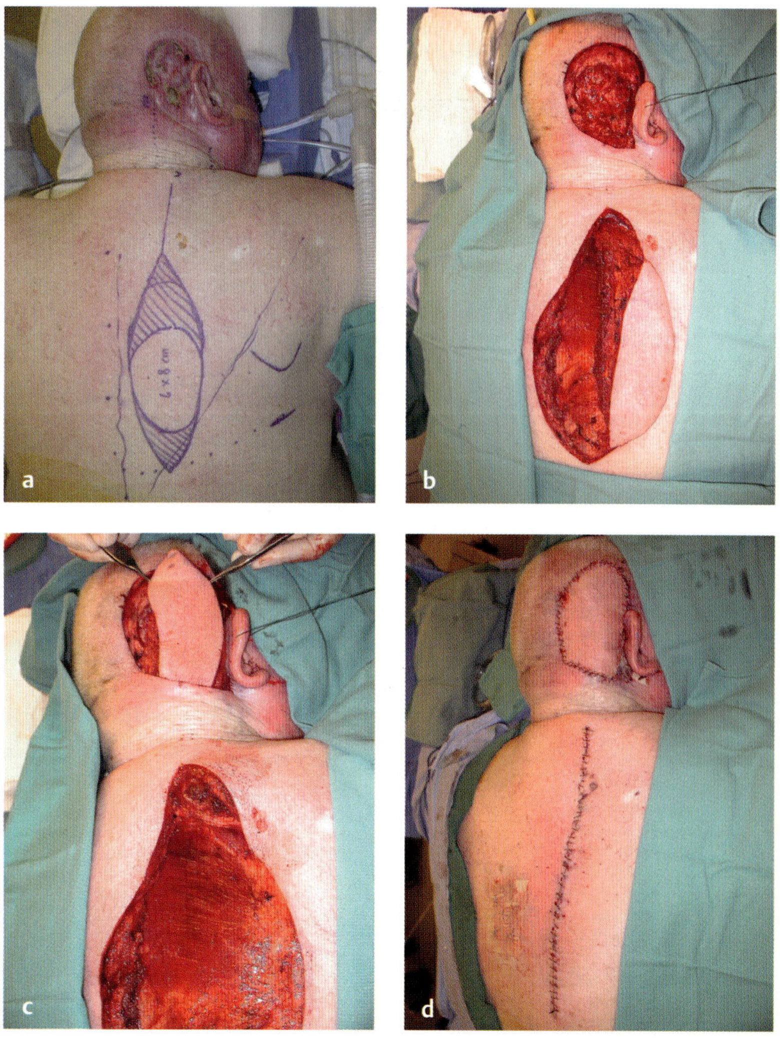

**Fig. 9.16** **(a)** A 71-year-old male with a history of sarcoma resection, irradiation of the right mastoid area, and failed skin graft reconstruction who underwent trapezius myocutaneous flap reconstruction. Exposed irradiated bone and the proposed trapezius flap with its skin paddle overlying the muscle are seen. **(b)** The flap is elevated on the transverse cervical vessels. **(c)** The flap is rotated and transposed through a subcutaneous tunnel. **(d)** Flap inset and primary donor-site closure.

## References


1. Bilkay U, Kerem H, Ozek C, Erdem O, Songur E. Alopecia treatment with scalp expansion: some surgical fine points and a simple modification to improve the results. J Craniofac Surg 2004;15(5):758–765
2. Chao AH, Yu P, Skoracki RJ, Demonte F, Hanasono MM. Microsurgical reconstruction of composite scalp and calvarial defects in patients with cancer: a 10-year experience. Head Neck 2012;34(12):1759–1764
3. Halvorson EG, Cordeiro PG, Disa JJ, Wallin EF, Mehrara BJ. Superficial temporal recipient vessels in microvascular orbit and scalp reconstruction of oncologic defects. J Reconstr Microsurg 2009;25(6):383–387
4. Hussussian CJ, Reece GP. Microsurgical scalp reconstruction in the patient with cancer. Plast Reconstr Surg 2002;109(6):1828–1834
5. Leedy JE, Janis JE, Rohrich RJ. Reconstruction of acquired scalp defects: an algorithmic approach. Plast Reconstr Surg 2005;116(4):54e–72e
6. Lesavoy MA, Dubrow TJ, Schwartz RJ, Wackym PA, Eisenhauer DM, McGuire M. Management of large scalp defects with local pedicle flaps. Plast Reconstr Surg 1993;91(5):783–790
7. Lipa JE, Butler CE. Enhancing the outcome of free latissimus dorsi muscle flap reconstruction of scalp defects. Head Neck 2004;26(1):46–53
8. Losken A, Carlson GW, Culbertson JH, et al. Omental free flap reconstruction in complex head and neck deformities. Head Neck 2002;24(4):326–331
9. Lutz BS, Wei FC, Chen HC, Lin CH, Wei CY. Reconstruction of scalp defects with free flaps in 30 cases. Br J Plast Surg 1998;51(3):186–190
10. Moreira-Gonzalez A, Jackson IT, Miyawaki T, Barakat K, DiNick V. Clinical outcome in cranioplasty: critical review in long-term follow-up. J Craniofac Surg 2003;14(2):144–153
11. Newman MI, Hanasono MM, Disa JJ, Cordeiro PG, Mehrara BJ. Scalp reconstruction: a 15-year experience. Ann Plast Surg 2004;52(5):501–506, discussion 506
12. Tadros M, Costantino PD. Advances in cranioplasty: a simplified algorithm to guide cranial reconstruction of acquired defects. Facial Plast Surg 2008;24(1):135–145
13. van Driel AA, Mureau MA, Goldstein DP, et al. Aesthetic and oncologic outcome after microsurgical reconstruction of complex scalp and forehead defects after malignant tumor resection: an algorithm for treatment. Plast Reconstr Surg 2010;126(2):460–470
14. Keser A, Sensöz O, Mengi AS. Double opposing semicircular flap: a modification of opposing Z-plasty for closing circular defects. Plast Reconstr Surg 1998;102(4):1001–1007
15. Arnold PG, Rangarathnam CS. Multiple-flap scalp reconstruction: Orticochea revisited. Plast Reconstr Surg 1982;69(4):605–613
16. Gonyon DL Jr, Zenn MR. Simple approach to the radiated scalp wound using INTEGRA skin substitute. Ann Plast Surg 2003;50(3):315–320
17. Zenn M, Jones G. Trapezius flap. In: Reconstructive Surgery: Anatomy, Technique, and Clinical Applications. St. Louis, MO: Quality Medical Publishing; 2012: 694–725
18. Zenn MR, Pribaz J, Walsh M. Use of the descending lateral femoral circumflex artery and vein for vascular grafting: a better alternative to an arteriovenous loop. Plast Reconstr Surg 2010;126(1):140–142
19. Chalouhi N, Teufack S, Fernando Gonzalez L, Rosenwasser RH, Jabbour PM. An extreme case of the syndrome of the trephined requiring the use of a novel titanium plate. Neurologist 2012;18(6):423–425

# 10 Facial Nerve Reconstruction

*Matthew M. Hanasono*

## Introduction

Division or resection of the facial nerve results in an inability to contract the superficial musculature of the face. Functionally, this condition is associated with an inability to close and protect the eye, to show expression, and to maintain oral competence, which can interfere with drinking, eating, and speech. The most common cause of facial paralysis is idiopathic (Bell's palsy), which resolves spontaneously in the majority of cases. In other cases, facial paralysis may be genetic (e.g., Möbius's syndrome), developmental (e.g., craniofacial microsomia), or traumatic. In head and neck surgery, removal of a vestibular schwannoma (acoustic neuroma) may involve excision of a portion of the facial nerve and is a common source of referral for facial nerve reconstruction. Other oncologic procedures that may involve facial nerve division or excision include parotidectomy and temporal bone resection.

## Anatomy

The facial nerve emerges from the stylomastoid foramen, which is located anterior to the styloid process. The posterior belly of the digastric muscle is a surgical landmark, with the facial nerve lying ~ 1 cm deep to the insertion of the digastric muscle into the mastoid bone. The tip of the tragal cartilage (tragal pointer) is another landmark, with the nerve lying ~ 1.0 to 1.5 cm anterior and inferior. Within the parotid gland, the facial nerve divides into two main trunks, supplying the upper and lower facial muscles, respectively. As the facial nerve exits the gland, there are between 8 and 15 branches making up the five divisions of the facial nerve: temporal, zygomatic, buccal, marginal mandibular, and cervical, which control various muscle of the face **(Fig. 10.1, Table 10.1)**. Beyond the parotid gland, there is significant arborization, with multiple internuncial branches.

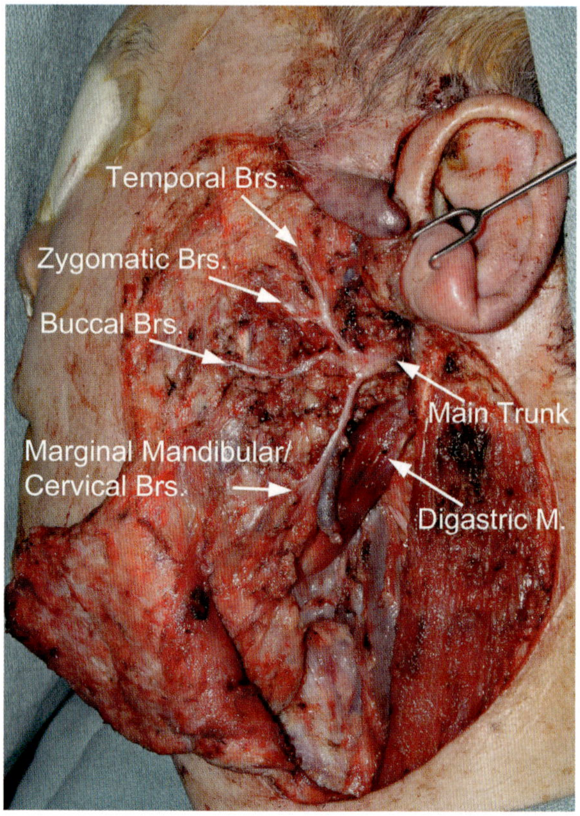


**Fig. 10.1** Left facial nerve following superficial parotidectomy. The facial nerve usually divides into upper and lower divisions within the parotid gland, then further divides into 8 to 15 branches that innervate the temporal, zygomatic, buccal, marginal mandibular, and cervical regions.

## Preoperative Assessment

The cause and time course of paralysis must be elucidated during the preoperative evaluation because they have a bearing on the outcome and help to determine what procedures are indicated. In cases where the facial nerve remains in continuity follow-

**Table 10.1** Muscles innervated by branches of the facial nerve and their functions

| Nerve branch | Muscle(s) | Action |
|---|---|---|
| Temporal | Frontalis<br>Corrugator supercilii<br>Procerus | Raises brows<br>Lowers and furrows brows<br>Lowers medial brow/wrinkles nasal skin |
| Temporal and zygomatic | Orbicularis oculi | Closes eyelids |
| Zygomatic and buccal | Zygomaticus major | Elevates corner of mouth |
| Buccal | Zygomaticus minor<br>Levator labii superioris<br>Levator labii superioris alaeque nasi<br>Nasalis<br>Risorius<br>Buccinator<br>Levator anguli oris<br>Orbicularis oris | Elevates upper lip<br>Elevates upper lip and nasolabial fold<br>Elevates nasolabial fold and nasal ala<br>Flares nostrils<br>Widens mouth<br>Widens mouth and compresses cheek<br>Elevates corner of mouth<br>Closes lips |
| Buccal and marginal mandibular | Depressor anguli oris | Lowers corner of mouth |
| Marginal mandibular | Depressor labii inferioris<br>Mentalis | Lowers lower lip<br>Tenses and elevates chin |
| Cervical | Platysma | Lowers corners of mouth |

ing surgery, neurapraxia may occur that can take up to a year to recover and is usually observed, although some temporary static procedures, mostly involving eye protection, can be helpful. Beyond 12 months, spontaneous recovery is usually unlikely and intervention is indicated. In other cases, the patient presents prior to tumor resection and must be counseled about the need for facial nerve repair or grafting as well as static and dynamic procedures for reanimation. Occasionally, facial nerve division or resection is unplanned prior to oncologic surgery, but reconstruction becomes indicated intraoperatively due to unexpected tumor involvement or inadvertent injury.

The patient is examined for facial muscular tone and volitional movement. If the level of injury is not known, the exam can also help in pinpointing the site of injury. If the facial nerve is divided within the temporal bone or intracranially, there may be a deficit in taste due to loss of chorda tympani function, or hyperacusis due to loss of stapedius muscle function. During the exam, the patient is asked to raise the eyebrows, close the eyes, smile, pucker the lips, and show the lower teeth to assess function of each of the major facial nerve branches. The eye on the paralyzed side is assessed for degree of closure, the presence of Bell's phenomenon, which aids in corneal protection, and signs of corneal exposure or abrasions. A "snap test" is performed to assess lower lid tone, and the presence of epiphora is noted. Loss of the nasolabial crease, deviation of the philtrum, commissure depression, and deviation of the lips and nose toward the normal side are signs of lack of facial muscular tone. The vector of mouth movement on the unaffected side is also recorded in preparation for either static suspension or dynamic smile reconstruction.

Because the House-Brackmann[1] grading system was designed to assess global facial nerve dysfunction rather than function of individual branches, its usefulness in extracranial nerve injury is limited. However, it remains a popular means of communicating facial nerve dysfunction, so it is often recorded in the medical record. The House-Brackmann grading system rates facial nerve function from I to VI. Briefly, Grade I is characterized by normal facial nerve function, Grade II is characterized by slight weakness on close inspection but normal symmetry at rest, Grade III is characterized by moderate dysfunction and obvious but not disfiguring asymmetry with movement but normal symmetry at rest, Grade IV is characterized by moderate to severe dysfunction and obvious or disfiguring asymmetry with movement but still normal symmetry at rest, Grade V is characterized by severe dysfunction with barely perceptible motion and asymmetry at rest, and Grade VI represents no facial movement. Recording the specific degree of function (either descriptively or using a percentage of normal) for each of the facial regions is more useful and accurate when there is differential injury to the temporal, zygomatic, buccal, and marginal mandibular nerve branches.

The more distal the facial nerve injury, the more arborization of the nerve branches makes it unnecessary to repair the nerve. A rough guide is that division of a nerve branch distal to the lateral orbit does not usually need to be repaired. Proximal transection of the nerve should be repaired, although the risk for synkinesis is higher. Repair within 72 hours of the injury takes advantage of the fact that the distal nerve stump can still be stimulated, resulting in muscular contraction, if the distal nerve is not easily identified.

The remaining cranial nerves should also be examined, and deficits should be addressed appropriately. Imaging studies, such as computed tomography (CT) and magnetic resonance imaging (MRI), can be useful in cases where the diagnosis is uncertain or to predict the extent of facial nerve resection so that the appropriate procedures can be planned. Electromyographic studies can be useful in predicting whether spontaneous recovery will occur as well as in assessing whether viable motor endplates exist if a delayed nerve repair or cranial transfer is being considered.

## Facial Nerve Repair

For nerve transections and resection of small segments, immediate direct nerve repair is indicated to provide the best results in terms of motor function. When resections are larger and the nerve cannot be repaired directly, interpositional or "cable" nerve grafting is indicated **(Fig. 10.2)**. Cable nerve grafts can be obtained by sacrifice of the great auricular nerve, branches of the cervical plexus at the C3 and C4 levels, or the sural nerve. When concomitant soft tissue reconstruction with an anterolateral thigh free flap is being performed, it is also convenient to harvest the lateral femoral cutaneous nerve as a graft.

Results of facial nerve repair following treatment for malignancy have been documented in only a few studies.[2,3,4,5] We observed at least some facial nerve recovery in 75% of patients (with < 12 months of facial nerve paralysis and in whom the proximal and distal ends of the facial nerve could be located) who underwent nerve graft repair occurring at a mean time of 7.7 months postoperatively. Recovery was observed even in patients with prior weakness or paralysis, postoperative radiation, and advanced age **(Fig. 10.3)**.[5] Iseli et al[3] reported at least some facial nerve recovery at a median time of 6.2 months postoperatively in 97% of their series of 33 patients who underwent facial nerve grafting, although their patient population contained a different mix of follow-up time, preoperative function, age, and radiation history. Taken together, these results argue for performing facial nerve repair whenever feasible in all patients who have not experienced motor endplate degeneration, regardless of the presence of risk factors for poor reinnervation, based on the assumption that even some recovery results in improved appearance and function.

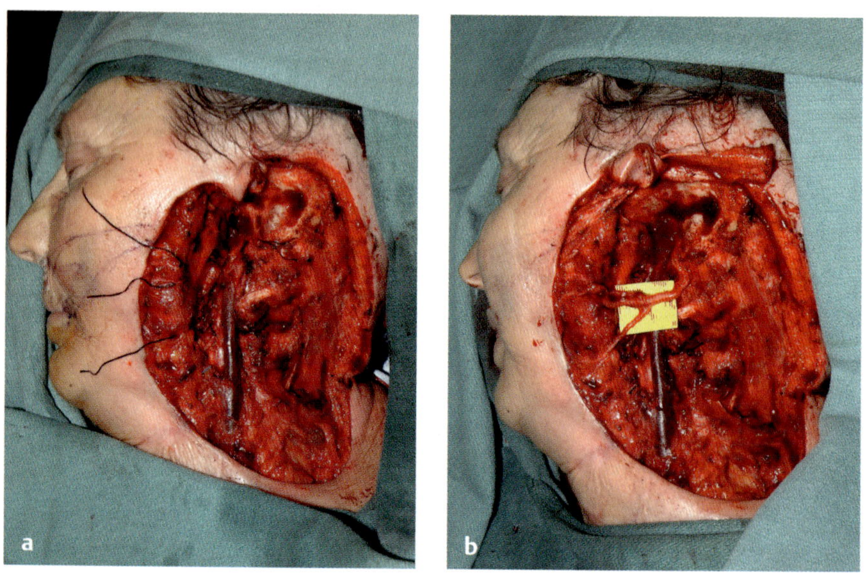


**Fig. 10.2** **(a)** Following radical parotidectomy and temporal bone resection, the proximal end and distal branches of the left facial nerve have been tagged with silk sutures. **(b)** Multiple nerve graft strands or single nerve graft strands that branch can be utilized as interpositional or "cable" nerve grafts to guide axonal regrowth for reinnervation of the facial muscles.

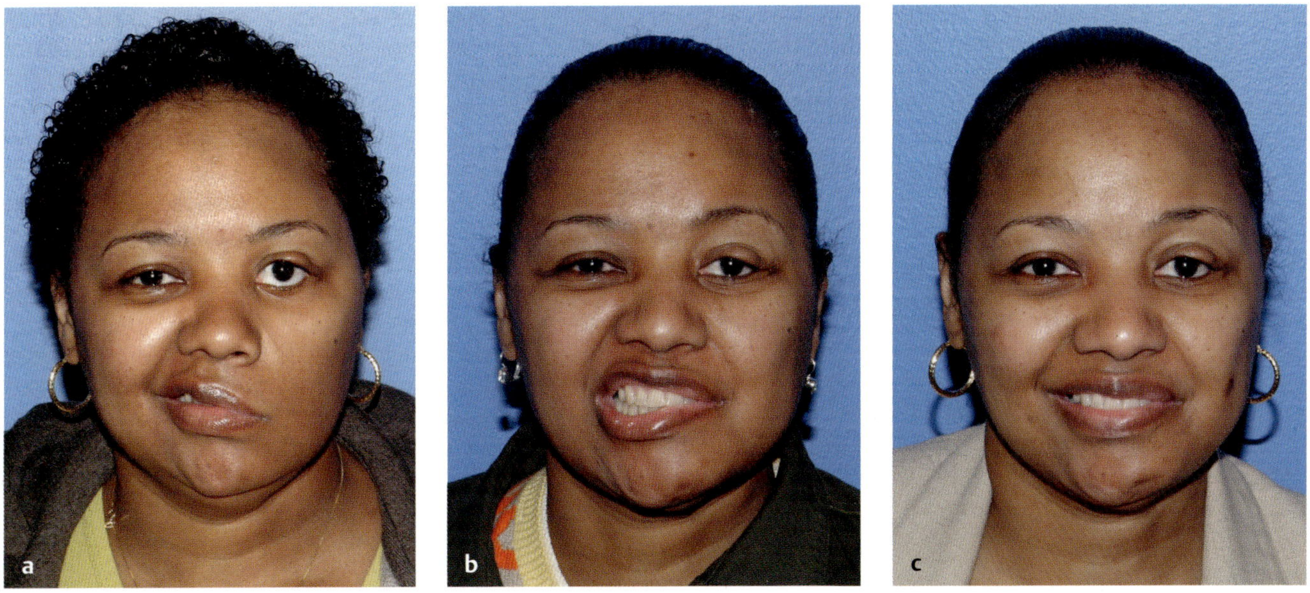


**Fig. 10.3** **(a)** Patient following parotidectomy with facial nerve resection at the main trunk. The facial nerve was reconstructed with a cable nerve graft. **(b)** At 6 months, the patient developed return of function (House-Brackmann Grade IV). **(c)** By 12 months, the patient had near-normal facial movement (House-Brackmann Grade II).

## ■ Nerve Transfer

When there is no proximal facial stump, immediate dynamic reanimation can be performed by coapting the distal facial nerve to the hypoglossal or masseteric nerves. This may serve as the definitive procedure for facial reanimation, or it may act as a "babysitter" procedure to keep the facial muscles from atrophying while awaiting axonal growth through cross-facial nerve graft(s). When the hypoglossal or masseteric nerve is used as a "babysitter," the nerve anastomosis is later taken down and replaced with a cross-facial nerve graft in ~ 6 to 12 months.

Hypoglossal–facial nerve transfer has been used to restore resting tone to the face.[6,7,8] The hypoglossal nerve is readily found running deep to the posterior belly of the digastric muscle and superficial to the external carotid artery **(Fig. 10.4)**. An end-to-end anastomosis has the disadvantage of causing unilateral tongue paralysis, with concomitant impairment of speech and swallowing function. An end-to-side anastomosis, usually via an interposition graft, is one way of decreasing the morbidity of this procedure. In end-to-side grafting, the epineurium is locally removed and some (25 to 30%) of the hypoglossal nerve axons are transected so that they may grow into the distal facial nerve. Speech and swallowing morbidity as well as synkinesis and mass motion with tongue movement have been shown to be greatly reduced using an end-to-side technique. In general, the innervation produced by this technique is not robust and it is used as a babysitter or as an adjunct to other techniques.

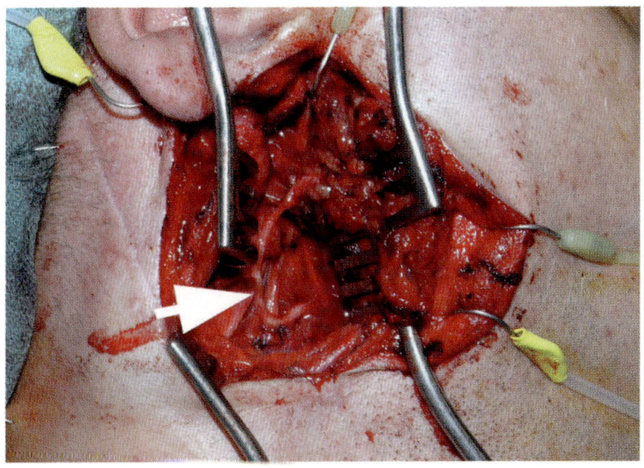

**Fig. 10.4** A nerve graft (*arrow*) has been used to connect the hypoglossal nerve, which lies deep to the posterior belly of the digastric muscle, to the distal cut end of the facial nerve.

A procedure that has more recently become popular is the use of the masseteric branch of the trigeminal nerve for dynamic facial reanimation.[9,10,11,12] The trigeminal nerve exits the intracranial cavity via the foramen ovale and passes over the lateral pterygoid muscle and through the coronoid notch of the mandible to enter the posterior surface of the masseter muscle near its origin beneath the zygomatic arch. It is found by careful lysis of the masseteric muscle fibers beginning at the posterior border of the mandible **(Fig. 10.5)**. The nerve usually takes an oblique course within the deep substance of the muscle, traveling from posterior superior to anterior inferior. Following the nerve distally allows adequate

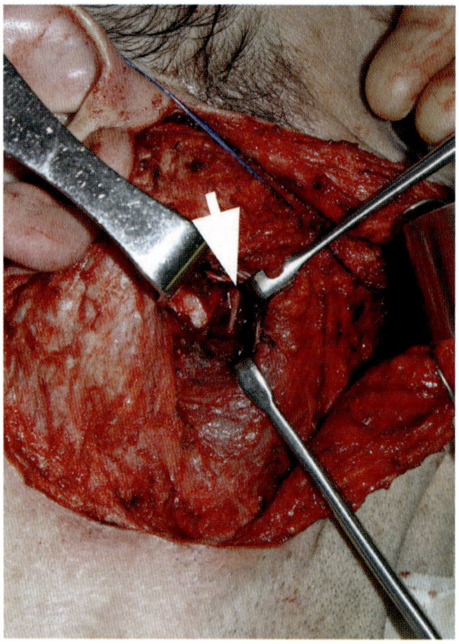

**Fig. 10.5** The masseteric branch of the trigeminal nerve (*arrow*) is identified by careful separation of the masseter muscle fibers, beginning at the posterior border of the mandibular ramus. The nerve exits the skull base, passes between the condyle and coronoid process of the mandible, and lies on the deep surface of the masseter muscle.

length to be gained for direct anastomosis either to the main facial nerve trunk, when it is intact, or to the zygomatic and buccal branches, which are usually preferentially selected for reinnervation due to their important expressive and sphincteric functions.

Sacrifice of the masseteric nerve does not result in functional problems with mastication, probably owing both to the sparing of proximal masseteric nerve fibers and to the redundant function of the masseter and temporalis muscles. The masseteric nerve has a strong motor impulse, which provides strong muscular activation and a fast reinnervation time, usually within 3 months. Unlike the hypoglossal nerve, the masseteric nerve is located close to the route of the facial nerve, which usually means that interpositional nerve grafting is unnecessary.

Patients can learn to activate the facial muscles by focusing on tongue or jaw contraction after hypoglossal or masseteric nerve transfer, respectively. With either procedure, synkinesis can occur, as can unwanted activation during mastication and speech. Cerebral cortical adaptation can occur after rehabilitation with masseteric nerve transfer, and emotional nerve activation has been reported.[10,11,12] The spinal accessory nerve has also been described as a donor nerve, but its use is uncommon due to the high degree of morbidity associated with the loss of motor function that accompanies its sacrifice, resulting in shoulder drop and pain. Additionally, control of facial movement independent of neck and shoulder function appears to be very difficult. The phrenic nerve has also been used for facial reanimation but can cause marked contraction with coughing, laughing, and deep inspiration, and use of the phrenic nerve is contraindicated in patients with pulmonary disease. In our practice, the spinal accessory and phrenic nerves are considered last resorts.

Cross-facial nerve grafting has the advantage of providing natural emotional activation without retraining.[13,14,15] In cross-facial nerve grafting, motor axons from the contralateral normal facial nerve grow through interpositional nerve grafts to reinnervate sectioned nerves on the paralyzed side. In this procedure, one or more nerves on the normal side are sacrificed and connected to a nerve graft, which is tunneled subcutaneously to the affected side of the face. Exposure of the contralateral normal nerve is usually performed through a facelift incision and elevation of a skin flap; nerve branches are identified and mapped as they exit the anterior edge of the parotid gland and travel toward the muscles of facial expression. The sural nerve is the most commonly used donor nerve for cross-facial nerve grafting owing to its length, availability, minimal donor-site morbidity, axonal density, and ease of harvest.

Intraoperative mapping of the contralateral normal side is performed using a nerve stimulator to identify redundant branches of the facial nerve that innervate the same groups of muscles. Grafting of zygomatic and buccal nerve branches have been described most frequently, again because of their relatively more valuable functions and contribution to symmetry in repose. If a dominant nerve is identified, it is spared, and secondary branches that produce weaker amplitude contractions when stimulated are preferred as donor nerves, to minimize the risk of denervating the donor side. The course of the interposition nerve grafts is usually within the upper lip or lower lip soft tissue.

Cross-facial nerve grafting has been described as either a one-stage or a two-stage procedure. Single-stage procedures reduce the number of surgeries required and patients may benefit from faster reinnervation. In a two-stage procedure, nerve graft(s) are sutured to the donor nerve branch on the normal side and tunneled to the affected side and left there. Axonal growth is typically estimated to be ~ 1 mm per day, which provides a rough guide for the amount of time needed before the second stage is performed. Nerve growth can sometimes be followed clinically by the presence of Tinel's sign along the nerve graft. For practical purposes, usually 6 to 12 months elapse before the second stage is performed. In the second stage, the distal end of the nerve graft is exposed, the nerve is trimmed sharply to remove any neuroma, and then the nerve is sutured to the distal portion of the severed facial nerve on the paralyzed side. An advantage of two-stage procedures is that the severed facial nerve can be grafted to the masseteric or hypoglossal nerves as babysitter nerves while waiting for cross-facial axonal growth.[16] This at least theoretically serves to keep the facial motor units viable due to earlier reinnervation from the babysitter nerves.

The main disadvantage of cross-facial nerve grafting is that results are inconsistent, not only between surgeons, but also for single surgeons using the same technique. Undesirable weakening of the normal contralateral side is a potential risk that can be avoided by locating and using nondominant branches as donor nerves. Grafting of distal nerve branches, rather than of the proximal facial nerve trunk, minimizes the risk for synkinesis and facilitates spontaneous emotional facial movement without the need for retraining. Muscle excursion is also usually less strong than with masseteric or hypoglossal nerve transfer. Because the regenerating axons must cross two suture lines and travel longer distances than ipsilateral donor nerves, reinnervation is slow and usually only partial. Best results for cross-facial nerve grafting are usually achieved when the nerve injury is recent (< 6 months), with limited motor endplate degeneration and muscle atrophy.

## Free Muscle Transfer

In many situations, facial nerve repair or nerve transfers are not feasible, because either the ends of the facial nerve cannot be located or too much time has elapsed since facial nerve injury or sacrifice, during which the motor endplates of the affected facial muscles have degenerated and the muscles have undergone atrophy and fibrosis, generally around 12 to 18 months. In such cases, the best option is functional muscle transplantation, which involves performing free tissue transfer of a given donor muscle and performing a motor neurorrhaphy either to a branch of the contralateral facial nerve or to the ipsilateral masseteric nerve. The most commonly transferred muscles include the pectoralis minor (as described by Terzis and Manktelow[17]), the latissimus dorsi (as described by Dellon and Mackinnon[18]), and the gracilis (as described by Harii et al[19]). Generally, 10 to 12 cm of muscle length is needed, and the muscle should provide adequate excursion without being too thick so as to not create an unappealing bulge in the side of the face it is used.

The gracilis muscle free flap is our preference due to its predictable anatomy, thinness, and minimal donor-site morbidity. It is probably the most commonly used donor muscle for facial reanimation and has the most data supporting its use. The gracilis muscle is located between the adductor longus (anterior) and adductor magnus (posterior) muscles. It originates at the anterior margin of the pubic symphysis and ramus of the ischium and inserts on the medial surface of the tibia. The vascular pedicle, which is a branch of the medial circumflex femoral artery, is located ~ 10 cm inferior to the pubic symphysis. The motor nerve (anterior branch of the obturator nerve), entering the muscle at a 45 degree angle to the long axis of the muscle, can be dissected proximally to the obturator foramen of the pelvis or even into the retroperitoneum to achieve up to 8 to 10 cm in length. It is also located at a 45 degree angle to the vascular pedicle, which enters the muscle perpendicularly at the same site as the nerve and arborizes into many branches.

The muscle is harvested with the patient's leg in the frog leg position **(Fig. 10.6)**. The adductor longus can be palpated with the thigh abducted. A longitudinal incision is made two to three fingerbreadths posterior to the adductor longus muscle, and the gracilis muscle should be readily identified. The pedicle and nerve lie deep to the adductor longus muscle, which is retracted anteriorly. The muscle is split longitudinally, because the entire circumference of the muscle will be too bulky and is unnecessary for establishing facial movement. The segment of muscle should be dissected with an intact motor nerve supply. Before the muscle is divided proximally and distally, temporary sutures are placed at 2 cm intervals to mark the length of muscle at rest so that it can be inset in the face under equal, or slightly more, tension.

The muscle is transferred to the face, which is exposed via a facelift (or parotidectomy) incision. Distally, it is secured to the oral commissure (modiolus) and orbicularis oris of the upper and lower lips, as well as the nasolabial crease. The facial artery and vein are used as recipient vessels when they are available. The obturator nerve is connected either to a previously placed cross-facial nerve graft or to the nerve to the masseter muscle, depending on the reconstructive approach. The muscle is then attached proximally to the zygomatic arch periosteum along a vector of pull that mimics the natural vector of smile in the contralateral face.

The advantages and disadvantages of cross-facial versus masseteric nerve innervation for free muscle transfer are the same as those discussed above for nerve transfer for facial nerve repair.[20] The choice of donor nerve is made on a case-by-case basis, with some surgeons preferring cross-facial nerve grafting in pediatric patients and the masseteric nerve in adults. The masseteric nerve has the advantages of not requiring a two-stage procedure and providing stronger contraction with essentially no donor-site morbidity. The disadvantage is that muscle contraction will not be spontaneous with facial movement of the contralateral side and that undesirable contraction can occur with chewing. However, many patients are able to train themselves to smile and to limit unintended muscle contraction over time, some even without conscious thought.

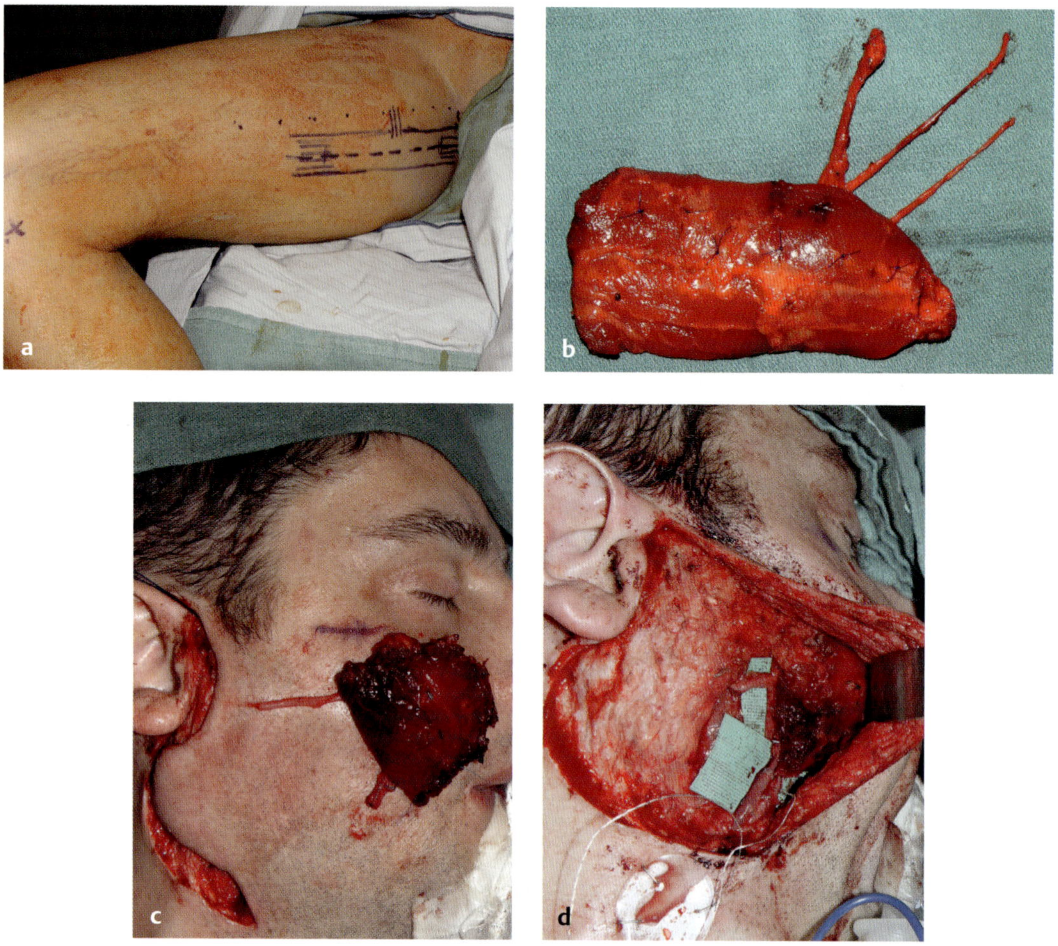

**Fig. 10.6 (a)** The gracilis muscle is harvested with the leg in abduction. It lies directly posterior and parallel to the adductor longus muscle, which is easily palpated. **(b)** A longitudinally split portion of the gracilis muscle with the vascular pedicle and two nerve branches attached. Both nerves were stimulated to ensure that they supplied the harvested portion of the muscle and could be used for dual innervation from the masseteric nerve and a cross-facial nerve graft. **(c)** Planned position of the gracilis muscle flap with its fibers oriented in the appropriate vector to create a symmetrical smile with the contralateral, normal side of the face. **(d)** The vascular pedicle is anastomosed to the facial artery and vein and a neurorrhaphy was performed to the masseteric nerve in this case.

Cross-facial nerve grafting has the advantage of allowing spontaneous function without the need for retraining. Its disadvantages are that it is a two-stage procedure with risk of contralateral face denervation, and it generally results in weaker muscle contraction than that associated with using the masseteric nerve as the donor nerve. When cross-facial nerve grafting is performed, the author usually makes a small incision lateral to the nasolabial crease and spreads the subcutaneous tissues until two branches of the facial nerve are located **(Fig. 10.7)**. The incision can also be hidden in the nasolabial crease for cosmesis, and the tissues lateral to the incision are explored for the buccal nerve branches. Nerves are stimulated with a handheld stimulator to confirm that they innervate the lip elevator muscles and that they are redundant so that division of one will not result in denervation of the normal side of the face. One of the branches is cut and a sural nerve graft is coapted to the proximal end with an epineural suture repair.

The nerve graft is then tunneled across the upper lip to the contralateral side. The free end of the graft is marked with a colored suture and is banked in the preauricular region of the contralateral face, accessed via a facelift incision, which will be reused for the muscle free flap transfer. At the time of second-stage surgery, the distal end of the graft can be biopsied to ensure that axonal growth has occurred. Single-stage muscle transfer with cross-facial innervation has been described, with encouraging results, although there is a theoretical risk of muscle atrophy and motor endplate degeneration occurring during the long time period that elapses while axonal regrowth into the muscle flap is occurring.[21]

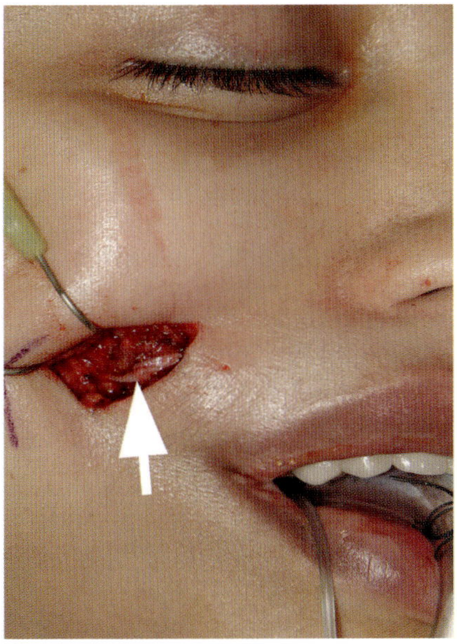

**Fig. 10.7** A buccal branch of the normally functioning facial nerve is divided and a neurorrhaphy is performed to a sural nerve graft (*arrow*). The nerve graft is tunneled subcutaneously to the affected side of the face. Prior to sacrifice of the buccal branch, a second branch is identified and stimulated to ensure that the lip elevator muscles are still adequately innervated.

## Static Facial Reanimation

Facial nerve rehabilitative procedures can also be of great help to patients and incur a low rate of complications requiring revision surgery. Immediate rehabilitation has the advantage of sparing the patient some of the morbidity of facial paralysis, especially during and immediately after adjuvant therapy, when further surgery may be risky. Rose[22] and Deleyiannis et al[23] have shown that facial nerve recovery is not prevented by facial paralysis rehabilitative procedures performed at the time of the initial surgery and believe static procedures complement nerve repair. Golio et al[24] also did not find a higher rate of complications nor an effect on symptomatic improvement in eye exposure in patients who had early periocular surgeries for facial nerve rehabilitation, before radiation therapy was administered, compared with patients who had the same procedures in a delayed setting.

### Brow/Forehead

Eyebrow symmetry can be attained by disabling the intact contralateral normal frontal branch with a neurectomy. The problem with this approach is that the brows may become too ptotic and create a tired or stern appearance and, in some individuals, interfere with the visual field in upward gaze. Chemodenervation with botulinum toxin of the contralateral nonparalyzed side of the frontalis and other facial muscles to improve symmetry is a temporary procedure that is also widely utilized. If favorable functional and aesthetic results are achieved, then permanent denervation with neurectomy can be performed.

A browlift procedure is more commonly performed in the cancer population, where the mean age and, consequently, the incidence of natural brow ptosis are relatively high. An endoscopic or pretrichial browlift may be sufficient in mild cases of asymmetry, but a direct (just above the brow) or indirect (within a mid-forehead rhytid) approach generally results in a much greater degree of correction **(Fig. 10.8)**. A skin excision is performed to

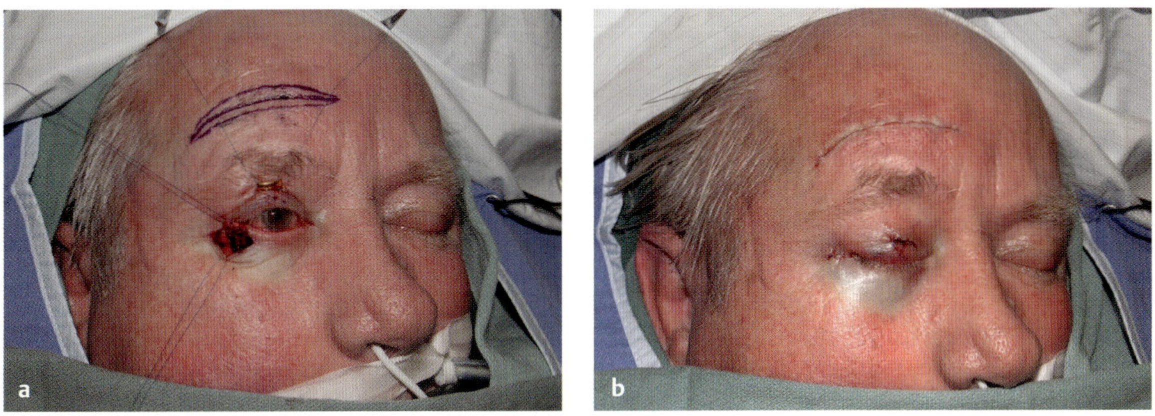

**Fig. 10.8** **(a)** A gold upper eyelid weight is about to be inserted superficial to the tarsal plate through a small incision made in the upper eyelid crease. A lateral canthoplasty (tarsal strip procedure) and indirect browlift are also being performed. The weight is secured with fine (7–0) permanent sutures to the perichondrium of the tarsus. **(b)** Immediate postoperative appearance.

elevate the skin appropriately for symmetry with the contralateral side as measured when the patient is awake with the eyes open. Overcorrection is sometimes needed if the patient tends to have a hyperactive contralateral frontalis muscle (due to natural senile brow ptosis), or a bilateral procedure can be performed. The frontalis muscle is also suspended to the frontal periosteum before the skin is closed with polydioxanone or permanent sutures. The resulting scars are usually acceptable, particularly in elderly patients and in men with prominent brows.

## Upper Eyelid

Patients with facial nerve paralysis have difficulty closing the affected upper eyelid, but they can open it normally because the levator palpebrae superioris, which is innervated by the oculomotor nerve (III), is still intact. Gold eyelid weights can be very reliable, with low rates of exposure (under 10% in a series of 104 gold implants reported by Rofagha and Seiff).[25] The gold eyelid implants are generally available in weights from 0.6 to 1.8 g, graduated in 0.2 g increments. Ideally, the appropriate weight is chosen preoperatively in the office by taping sample implants to the upper lid and observing for complete eye closure.

In general, a 1.0 g weight is usually the appropriate starting point, and it is chosen when facial paralysis does not exist at the time of preoperative evaluation. If the weight turns out to be inappropriate, it can be easily exchanged for another weight at a later date, under local anesthesia in the office if need be, to avoid delaying adjuvant treatment. Alternatively, gold eyelid weight placement can be performed in a delayed manner and eye closure can be managed with nonsurgical methods, such as lubrication and lid taping. Also, as facial nerve function improves following nerve repair or nerve transfer, eyelid weights can be removed or downsized. Platinum weights are also available and have the advantage of being smaller because of the greater density of platinum compared with gold.

Placement is via a small incision made in the supratarsal crease. A precise pocket is dissected superficial to the tarsal plate as close as possible to the lid margin. The gold weight is secured to the perichondrium using 7–0 polypropylene sutures (**Fig. 10.8**). The incision is closed with a 6–0 absorbable running suture.

## Lower Eyelid

Lower lid laxity resulting in ectropion is most frequently treated with lid-tightening procedures, such as lateral canthoplasty using a tarsal strip technique (**Fig. 10.9**). In this procedure, a lateral canthotomy is made with scissors; then a lower lid cantholysis is performed by cutting the lower lid canthal tendon. This should free the lower eyelid. A subciliary incision is made and a short skin flap is elevated. The

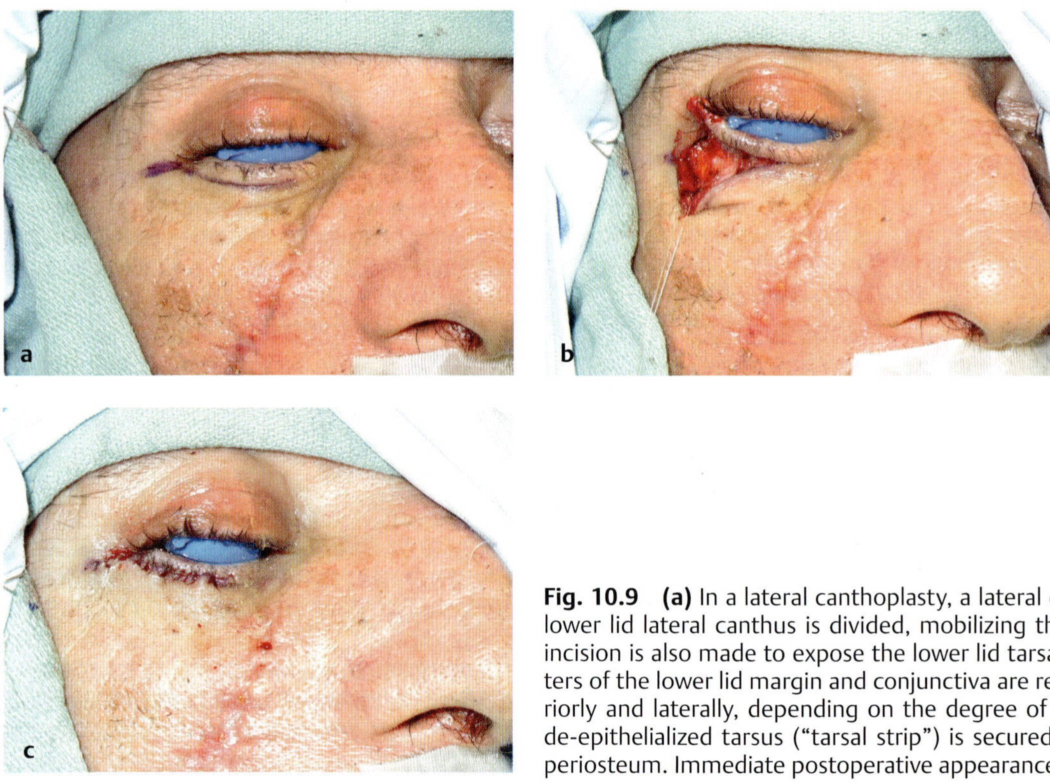

**Fig. 10.9** **(a)** In a lateral canthoplasty, a lateral canthotomy is planned. The lower lid lateral canthus is divided, mobilizing the lower eyelid. A subciliary incision is also made to expose the lower lid tarsal plate. **(b)** Several millimeters of the lower lid margin and conjunctiva are removed and advanced superiorly and laterally, depending on the degree of correction needed. **(c)** The de-epithelialized tarsus ("tarsal strip") is secured to the upper, inner orbital periosteum. Immediate postoperative appearance.

amount of canthal suspension is estimated by pulling on the canthal tendon in a lateral-superior vector. The lid margin is excised and the conjunctiva is removed based on the amount of advancement anticipated. A horizontal mattress suture with long-lasting absorbable suture (e.g., polydiaxanone) or permanent suture (e.g., polypropylene) is used to suspend the denuded “tarsal strip” to the inner, upper lateral orbital periosteum, by Whitnall’s tubercle. The suture is tied so that the knot faces superficially, away from the globe surface. Excess skin is conservatively trimmed, then the subciliary incision and lateral canthotomy are closed with fine absorbable suture, such as fast-absorbing gut.

The lateral canthoplasty occasionally needs to be repeated for recurrent ectropion, particularly in elderly patients. Combining the lateral canthoplasty with a lateral tarsorrhaphy in which a few millimeters of both upper and lower lid margins are denuded and a suture is used to create a lid adhesion (tying the knot laterally, away from the cornea), can be used to treat severe ectropion and lagophthalmos, but it horizontally narrows the lid aperture, which can be cosmetically unappealing. In some cases, even after fairly aggressive lid tightening with a lateral canthoplasty, there is residual medial lagophthalmos. A medial canthoplasty can augment the lateral canthoplasty by using sutures to plicate or suspend the lax medial canthal tendon to the medial orbital periosteum. Care needs to be taken not to constrict or suture through the upper and lower tear duct canaliculi when performing a medial canthoplasty.

For recalcitrant lower lid ectropion, a fascial sling or palmaris longus tendon sling can be used to suspend the entire lower lid. This procedure corrects both lateral and medial ectropion. Alternately, the lower lid can be elevated by placing a cartilage graft beneath the lower lid tarsus, as a mechanical bolster to increase lower lid stiffness. This cartilage is placed via a subciliary incision, after which a skin–muscle flap is elevated off the tarsal plate and conjunctiva. The naturally curved conchal cartilage works well as graft material for this purpose. A hard palate mucosal graft, placed into a transverse conjunctival incision at the lower border of the tarsal plate, can also be used to functionally lengthen and simultaneously stiffen the lower eyelid. Some authors have favored transposition of a portion of the temporalis muscle or its fascia to pull the upper and lower lids laterally to produce eye closure. However, the motion is abnormal and may not correct the lid position and lagophthalmos completely.

## Cheek and Lips

A flaccid cheek and downturned lower face with an adynamic commissure not only may be the most disconcerting sign associated with facial paralysis but also can interfere with speech and oral competence, as well as nasal breathing due to nasal alar collapse. Both static and dynamic (described previously) procedures have been designed to address the lower face. Static procedures consist of subcutaneous fascia or tendon graft suspension. The author prefers to use fascia lata of the thigh because of its abundance and the fact that it can be harvested simultaneously with preparation of the anterolateral thigh free flap, which is often used for concurrent soft tissue reconstruction, through the same donor-site incision **(Fig. 10.10)**.[26] Others have described using the plantaris tendon, which is present

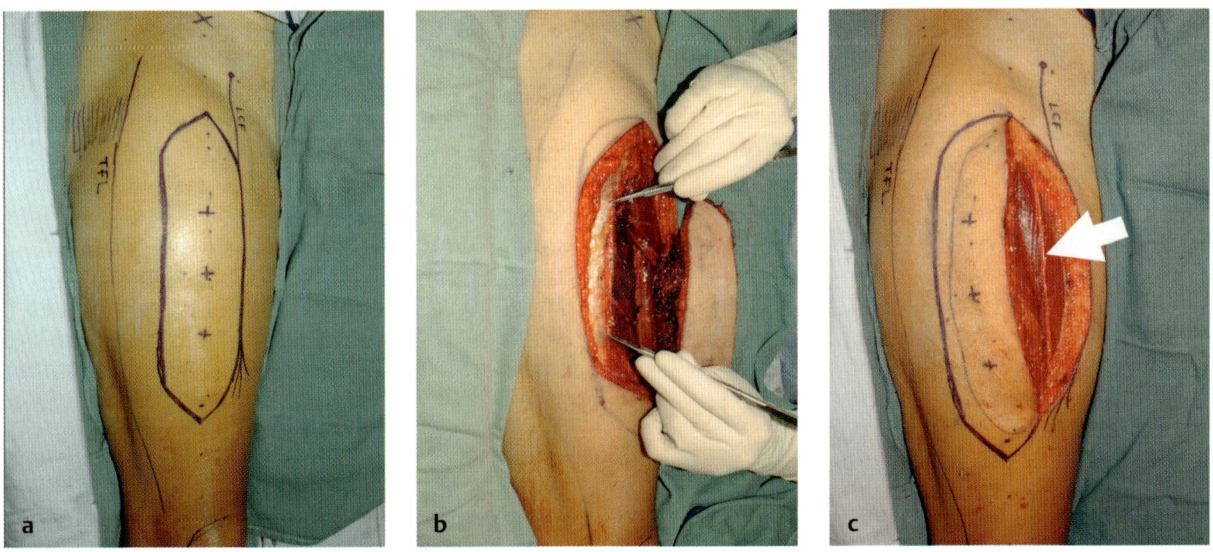


**Fig. 10.10** **(a)** The anterolateral thigh free flap is a favored donor site for soft tissue reconstruction of parotidectomy and temporal bone defects. **(b)** A strip of fascia lata is harvested from the same donor-site incision. **(c)** The lateral femoral cutaneous nerve (*arrow*) also can be harvested from the anterolateral thigh free flap donor site and used as a nerve graft.

in ~ 85% of patients and can be obtained through a short transverse incision just behind the medial malleolus.

The author usually uses several grafts or splits a single graft into several slips distally to suspend the oral commissure, upper lip at the nasolabial crease, and the nasal ala (**Fig. 10.11**). The graft is tunneled from a preauricular incision to each of these target areas. A small counter incision at each site is made and the distal slips of the graft, which are of differing lengths as needed to produce the required amount of pull to create the desired symmetry with the contralateral side, are secured to the deep investing fascia and dermis with permanent suture. The slip that goes to the oral commissure is further split so that it attaches to the orbicularis muscles of the upper and lower lips and the modiolus at the commissure. The counter incisions are closed first; then the proximal fascia graft(s) are secured to the zygomatic arch periosteum under tension in the appropriate vector needed to match the contralateral direction of muscular movement. Overcorrection is desirable, because the amount of suspension rapidly decreases over the first 2 weeks following surgery, after which it usually stabilizes.

If necessary, retightening of the graft can be performed by re-opening the preauricular incision and freeing up the graft with limited dissection, then resuspending it to the zygomatic arch periosteum. In the author's experience, the distal fixation to the commissure, nasolabial crease, and nasal ala remains secure and revision is usually very successful. It is also the author's preference to perform a fascial/tendon sling procedure concurrently with nerve repair/grafting when the degree of reinnervation is not expected to be great or there is substantial facial tissue laxity (e.g., due to old age), rather than to watch and wait, since a secondary sling procedure runs the risk of disrupting healing nerve repairs and grafts. Unilateral or differential bilateral rhytidectomy can also be performed in patients with substantial skin laxity to help with symmetry and overall appearance.

In unilateral facial paralysis, the paralyzed lower lip is higher than the contralateral side due to absence of lower lip depressor function normally generated by the marginal mandibular branch of the facial nerve. The contralateral normally functioning lower lip depressors can be temporarily paralyzed with botulinum toxin to restore symmetry to the smile. If permanent correction is desired, a myomectomy or marginal mandibular neurectomy can be performed, either through a facelift type incision or a direct incision approximately one fingerbreadth below the lower mandibular border. The marginal mandibular nerve can be reliably located beneath the platysma muscle running transversely across the superficial surface of the facial vein.

## Reconstructive Algorithm

Our reconstructive algorithm is summarized in **Fig. 10.12**. In the author's practice, all patients undergoing a division of the facial nerve are considered for

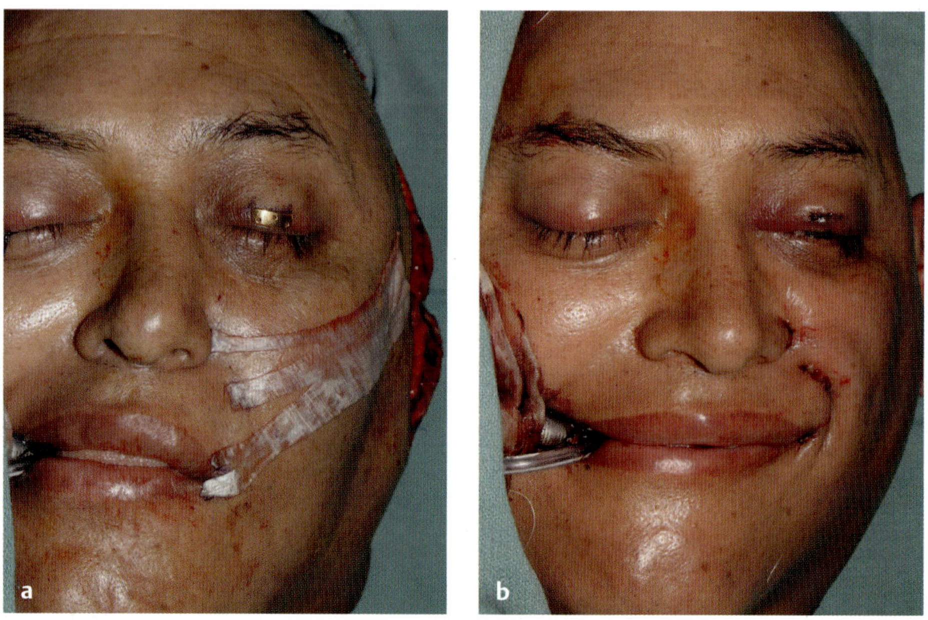

**Fig. 10.11** **(a)** A fascia lata graft from the thigh is used for static reanimation of the lower face. The graft is split into separate slips to suspend the nasal ala, nasolabial fold, and the corner of the mouth to the periosteum of the zygoma. **(b)** Immediate postoperative appearance. A gold upper eyelid weight was also placed.

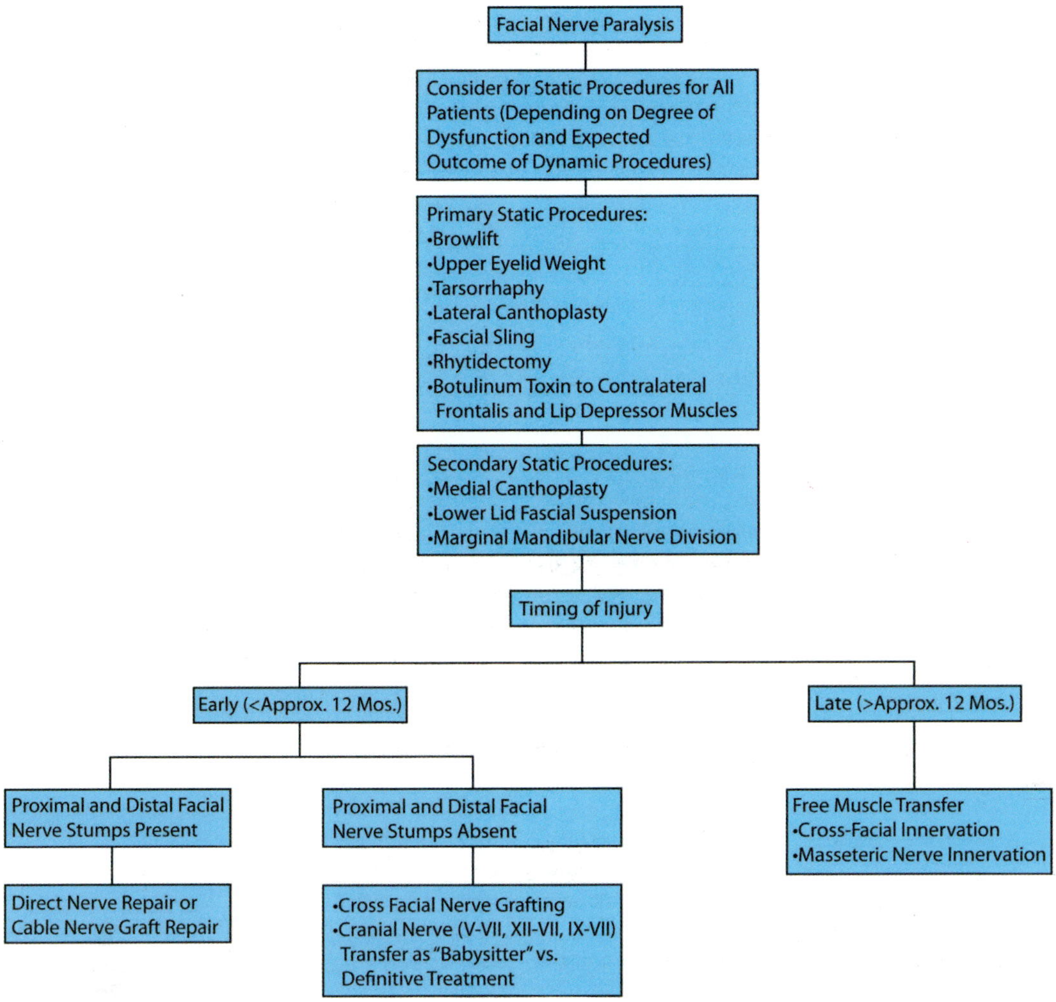


**Fig. 10.12** Algorithm for addressing facial nerve defects in head and neck cancer patients.

static procedures, regardless of whether dynamic procedures are planned. If the outcome of dynamic procedures is expected to be favorable, static procedures are not performed. However, in many patients, only partial return of function is expected after the dynamic procedure and usually after a relatively long delay, or the outcome is unpredictable. In those cases, static procedures are discussed with the patient. Static procedures can be performed secondarily if the degree of dysfunction and disfigurement is unknown or hard to predict preoperatively. However, in the cancer population, the author frequently performs static procedures immediately after tumor resection because the opportunity for secondary procedures is limited by the need to proceed with adjuvant therapy.[5] Performing simultaneous static procedures even if dynamic procedures are also performed can spare the patient much of the morbidity of facial nerve paralysis, including superior visual field obstruction, corneal exposure, epiphora, nasal obstruction secondary to alar collapse, speech impairment, and oral incompetence, during recovery from surgery and while undergoing adjuvant therapy. Static procedures are especially indicated in the elderly population because of skin and ligamentous laxity associated with senescence, and many patients may even benefit from bilateral procedures to correct problems with the contralateral, nonparalyzed side. Eyelid weight placement is often reversed or the weight is downsized if facial nerve function returns following successful nerve repair, grafting, or transfer.

With regard to dynamic procedures, nerve repair and cable nerve grafting are performed whenever the proximal and distal facial nerve stumps can be identified. If not, nerve transfer is considered. Free muscle transfer has usually been performed as a secondary procedure, mainly due to the considerable length of surgery for skull base resection and soft and bony tissue flap reconstruction. However, in selected cases, immediate dynamic reconstruction with a muscle free flap innervated by nerve coaptation to the masseteric nerve can be considered.

The list of procedures discussed above is by no means exhaustive. However, the procedures described have proven to be the most useful in treating patients with oncologic facial nerve paralysis.

## Postoperative Care

Patients should be counseled about wearing eye protection when blinking is impaired. The eyes should be lubricated frequently with hydroxypropyl methylcellulose eye drops during the day and a more viscous ointment during the night. When passive eye closure is incomplete, the eye can be taped laterally (rather than over the cornea) or a moisture chamber can be obtained. Patients especially at risk for exposure keratitis and corneal ulceration are those with combined cranial nerve V and VII deficits with an absent corneal reflex and decreased corneal sensation.

The benefit of physical therapy for facial nerve recovery following repair has not been well studied. There are significant variations in technique and there are limited outcome data using validated quantitative measurements. Retraining following nerve transfer or motorized free muscle flap reconstruction is likely of benefit. When the masseteric nerve is used to supply either the facial muscles or a muscle free flap, the patient must learn to create facial movement by biting down on the ipsilateral side of the jaw. Eventually, many patients can learn to move their face even without clenching the teeth and some can develop a spontaneous smile.

## Future Directions

Vascularized nerve transfer in which a nerve and its nourishing blood vessels are used as an interpositional conduit between a donor nerve and the distal facial nerve recipient have been described. It is hypothesized that the enhanced viability of interpositional nerve tissue results in improved reinnervation. Limited case series are promising, but the technique has been evaluated by only a limited number of centers.

The ideal repair involves regrowth of the appropriate facial nerve axon, of which there are ~ 11,000, back to the original end organs. Improving regeneration of neurites, growth of axons along their original pathways (which may be obstructed by scar tissue), and preservation of functional facial muscular end organs are all strategies for achieving better outcomes.

## Case Example 1

A woman presented with a right parotid cancer and paralysis of the temporal branch of her right facial nerve. She was treated with a right parotidectomy, including resection of the overlying facial skin and her facial nerve **(Fig. 10.13)**. Her skin and right facial soft tissues were reconstructed with an anterolateral thigh free flap. The lateral femoral cutaneous nerve was used as a source of nerve grafts, and two zygomatic branches and two lower-division branches of her facial nerve were repaired. Temporal branches were not available for repair due to the extent of her resection. She also underwent a right upper eyelid gold weight placement, direct browlift, and fascia lata sling. She received postoperative chemotherapy and radiation. Six months after completing radiation, she underwent revision of her browlift, lateral canthoplasty, and free flap reconstruction. Two years after surgery, she had nearly symmetrical function of muscles innervated by the zygomatic and buccal branches of her facial nerve.

## Case Example 2

A woman with a history of recurrent adenoid cystic carcinoma of the right external ear was treated with subtotal auriculectomy, lateral temporal bone resection, and parotidectomy, sacrificing the facial nerve. The defects initially were reconstructed with a temporalis muscle flap and a skin graft; then, after the patient completed radiation therapy, she received a fascial sling for static suspension. After repeated wound-healing problems involving the auricular remnant, she was referred for completion auriculectomy and soft tissue reconstruction **(Fig. 10.14)**. Additionally, the

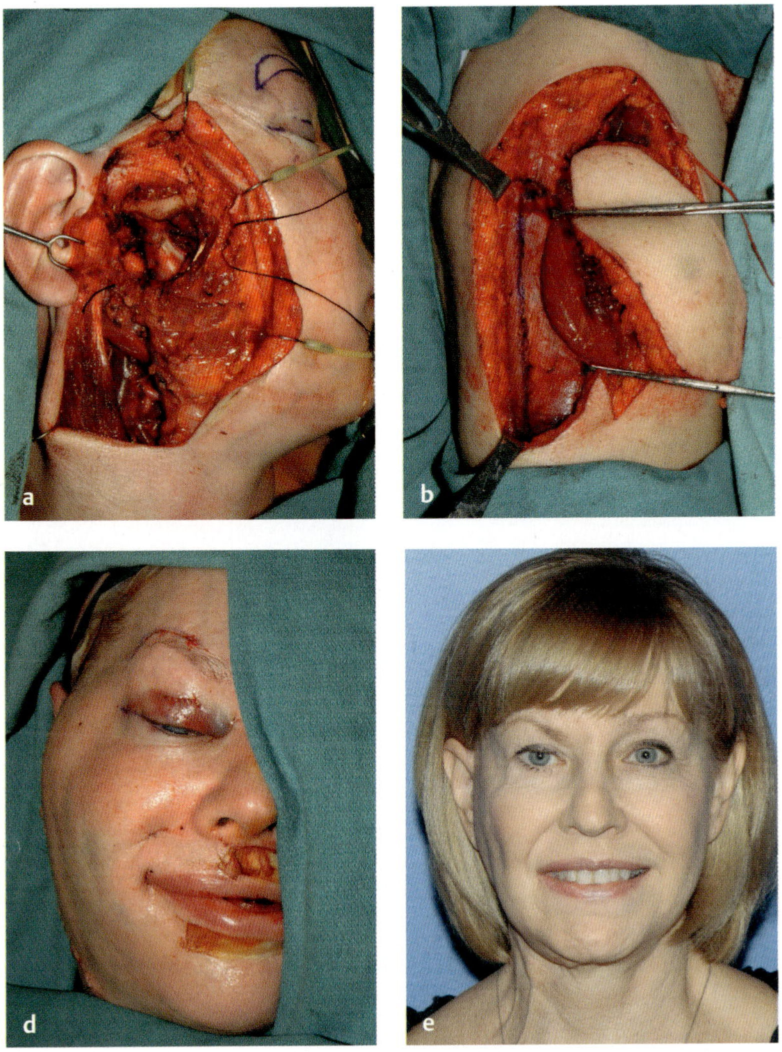

**Fig. 10.13** **(a)** A radical parotidectomy and selective neck dissection have been performed. The proximal facial nerve and distal zygomatic and buccal branches have been tagged with silk suture. **(b)** An anterolateral thigh free flap is dissected for soft tissue reconstruction and a fascial graft is harvested from the same donor-site incision. **(c)** The free flap and fascia graft are inset. **(d)** Immediate postoperative appearance. An upper eyelid gold weight and a direct browlift were also performed. **(e)** Postoperative appearance at ~ 1 year, with return of lower facial motor function. The fascia graft does not interfere with facial animation.

patient desired dynamic facial reanimation. She underwent a cross-facial nerve graft procedure in which a neurorrhaphy was performed between one of the buccal branches of her left facial nerve and a sural nerve graft, via an external cheek incision. Six months later, she underwent a free gracilis muscle transfer with neurorrhaphy to the cross-facial nerve graft and vascular anastomosis to the facial artery and vein. She also underwent removal of the auricular remnant and soft tissue reconstruction with a deep inferior epigastric perforator flap. One year later, the patient had spontaneous contraction of her gracilis muscle during smiling.

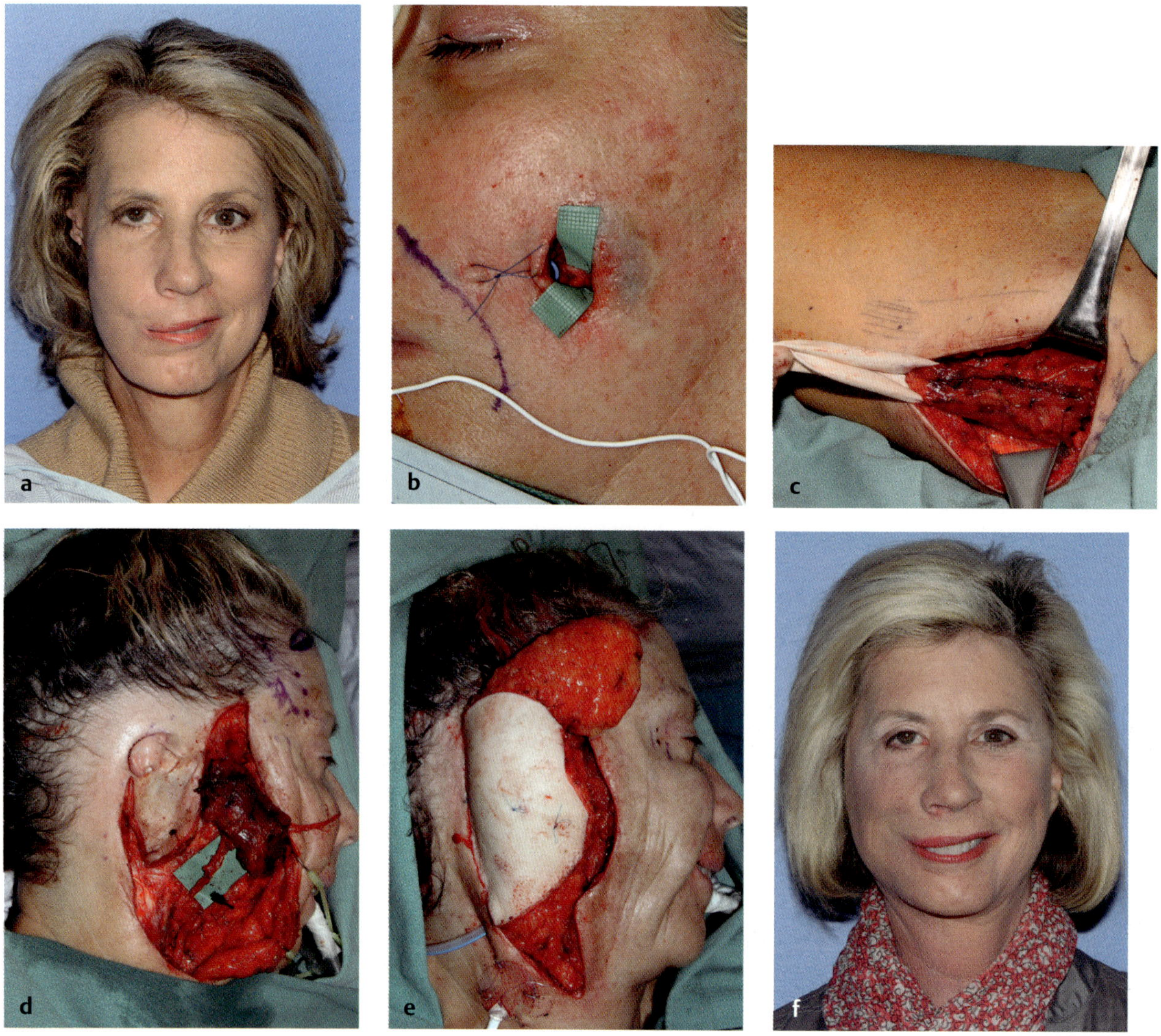

**Fig. 10.14** **(a)** Patient who has previously undergone a temporal bone resection, near-total auriculectomy, and facial nerve resection. **(b)** In the first stage of reconstruction, two buccal branches of the normal contralateral facial nerve were identified and their function was verified with a nerve stimulator. One of the branches is sacrificed and a neurorrhaphy is performed to a sural nerve graft, which is tunneled to the other side of the face. **(c)** In the second stage of reconstruction, a gracilis muscle free flap is harvested for dynamic facial reanimation. **(d)** The gracilis muscle is revascularized following anastomosis with the facial artery and vein and is reinnervated by coaptation of the anterior branch of the obturator nerve to the cross-facial nerve graft. **(e)** A deep inferior epigastric perforator flap is performed for soft tissue reconstruction. **(f)** Postoperative appearance at ~ 18 months showing contraction of the gracilis muscle to create a spontaneous smile.

## Pearls and Pitfalls

- All patients undergoing oncologic surgery that may include resection or division of the facial nerve should be examined preoperatively for facial nerve function and should be counseled accordingly about the potential need for reconstructive procedures.
- In most cases, if facial nerve continuity is not disrupted, the patient should be observed for at least a year before surgical procedures are performed, with the exception of selected static procedures involving eye protection.
- Direct facial nerve repair or cable nerve grafting should be attempted in virtually all patients when the proximal and distal stumps of the facial nerve are available, including in the setting of prior weakness, advanced age, or planned radiation therapy.
- When the proximal facial nerve is not available for repair/grafting, the distal nerve(s) can be grafted to redundant contralateral facial nerve branches or ipsilateral "donor" nerves, including the masseteric (V), hypoglossal (XII), or spinal accessory (IX) nerve.

- The masseteric nerve has become the preferred donor nerve for facial nerve transfer due to its effectiveness in producing strong contractions and minimal donor-site morbidity.
- Cranial nerve transfer can be used as a definitive procedure for facial nerve reconstruction or as a "babysitter" to help prevent motor endplate degeneration and muscle atrophy while awaiting axonal growth through cross-facial nerve graft(s).
- Free muscle transfer can be used to reanimate the lower face, mimicking the action of smiling while also providing tension on the corner of the mouth to prevent loss of oral competence and facial symmetry.
- Commonly used muscle free flaps for dynamic facial reanimation include the gracilis, latissimus dorsi, serratus anterior, and pectoralis minor muscles.
- Motor reinnervation of muscle free flaps can be achieved by utilizing a cross-facial nerve graft from a buccal branch of the contralateral facial nerve, usually in a two-stage procedure, or in a single stage using the masseteric nerve.
- Static procedures, such as browlift, upper eyelid gold weight placement, lateral canthoplasty, and fascial slings, should be considered for all patients with facial paralysis resulting from oncologic resection, even in patients undergoing dynamic procedures, depending on the degree of facial nerve functional impairment and expectations for recovery. Elderly patients with age-related brow ptosis, lower eyelid laxity, and skin redundancy, in particular, may benefit from immediate static corrective procedures while awaiting partial or even total return of facial nerve function.

## Expert Commentary *by Michael Klebuc*

It is a pleasure to provide commentary as an adjunct to this well-structured, thoughtful, and practical chapter outlining a comprehensive approach to the surgical rehabilitation of the paralyzed face. The author's treatment of the paralyzed face in many ways mirrors the current practice in our center; however, there are several distinct differences that may be of interest to the reader. Additionally, the author provides an array of surgical pearls in the chapter that warrant restating in an effort to reinforce their significance.

The author has stated the importance of early intervention with regard to traumatic transection of the facial nerve. The severed distal branches of the facial nerve can often be stimulated for 48 to 72 hours after injury. The retained excitability can prove very beneficial for identifying these fine structures and we make a concerted effort to explore these injuries within 48 hours to capitalize on this phenomenon. Furthermore, there is significant arborization of the facial nerve anterior to a vertical line extending down from the lateral canthus, and lacerations to the zygomatic and buccal branches of the facial nerve typically recover well in this zone even if a formal repair is not performed. It is likely that good tissue re-approximation brings the nerve ends into close enough proximity for the regenerative process to move forward. Regardless, facial lacerations as well as intentional and unintentional surgical transections, even in this region, should be explored under the surgical microscope and, if proximal and distal nerve stumps are identified, should be repaired without tension, using nerve grafts if necessary. Frontal and marginal mandibular branches do not demonstrate the same level of arborization and should be repaired or grafted if possible. Sometimes, soft tissue trauma and contamination will prohibit immediate nerve repair. In this situation, the transected nerve ends are tagged with nonabsorbable suture and repair is delayed until the wound management is completed. There is a biologic, regenerative advantage to performing the nerve repairs within 1 month of the date of injury, and this should be considered when formulating a treatment plan.[27]

The authors have described the use of the great auricular nerve for interposition nerve grafting. This is a workhorse nerve graft donor; however, care must be taken in head and neck cancer cases to verify the nerve has not been infiltrated by tumor. Alternatively, one can harvest the proximal, central portion of the sural nerve where it courses between the gastrocnemius muscles. In an adult, this will yield a nerve graft 10 to 12 cm long that is devoid of branches. In the majority of patients this harvest technique preserves the lateral branch of the sural nerve emanating from the common peroneal nerve, thereby preserving sensation of the lateral malleolus. If a large amount of nerve graft is required, the saphenous nerve and the medial antebrachial cutaneous nerve can provide additional sources of graft material.

The author also discussed the evolving role of the motor nerve branch to the masseter with regard to reanimating the paralyzed face. The masseteric nerve has been: (1) utilized to power free muscle flaps, (2) transferred directly to the facial nerve (V–VII), and (3) combined with cross-facial nerve grafts as a babysitter.[12]

A series of topographic landmarks have been described that facilitate nerve dissection.[28] The main trunk of the motor nerve to masseter can be reliably identified at a point 3 cm in front of the tragus and 1 cm below the zygomatic arch. It is important to note that the masseter muscle has three distinct lobes, and the nerve courses along the superficial surface of the deep lobe within the substance of the muscle and does not run along the muscle's deep surface as depicted in many anatomy textbooks. The masseteric nerve has a dense population of myelinated motor fibers, with ~ 2700 and 1500 axons in the main trunk and descending branch, respectively.[29] The descending branch is most frequently transferred as it can be adequately mobilized to reach zygomatic and buccal branches of the facial nerve without interposition grafting. Additionally, preservation of the proximal masseteric nerve branches is important to prevent extensive muscle atrophy that can produce a cosmetic deformity at the mandibular angle.

The masseteric to facial nerve (V–VII) transfer can be an effective technique for restoring motion in the midface when the proximal stump of the facial nerve is unavailable for interposition grafting in the presence of intact distal branches and viable muscles of facial expression. The isolated V–VII transfer can produce powerful commissure excursion; however, it often results in poor facial resting tone and an effaced nasolabial fold. The addition of static procedures should be considered when performing the V–VII transfer, especially in the elderly patient.

In our facial paralysis center, cross-facial nerve grafts (CFNGs) are frequently utilized in conjunction with the V–VII transfer in an effort to improve resting tone and spontaneity. This is undertaken in a single stage utilizing nerve conduction mapping of the unaffected side to guide the sites of distal nerve repair on the silent hemiface. The V–VII transfer is left permanently intact, even after cross-facial reinnervation occurs, as it provides a major contribution to the overall result. This also holds true when the hypoglossal nerve is utilized as a babysitter (XII–VII transfer). In this scenario, a two-stage approach is beneficial. Much of the previous surgery has been performed in the neck, thereby limiting scar in the anterior parotid region. The facial nerves can be identified and stimulated in this region, clarifying their precise function. Branches of interest are then selectively transected and united with the CFNG. Insufficient nerve graft fascicles will be available to hit all potential targets and the XII–VII transfer should be left intact, as it often provides some resting tone and function via the untransected branches.[16] Unfortunately, the V–VII with CFNG is difficult to perform in two stages due to scarring from the previous parotid dissection and the potential for injury to the V–VII portion of the reconstruction.

The masseteric nerve has also found favor for its synergy with smiling. In long-term follow-up of patients with free muscle flap facial reanimation innervated by the masseteric nerve, Manktelow et al[30] found that 85% could create a smile without clenching their teeth and 59% felt their smile was spontaneous. The ability of the masseteric nerve to yield reflexive, effortless facial motion is supported by a series of anatomical findings. Embryologic evidence suggests that a subset of individuals have facial nerve fibers coursing within the motor pathway of the trigeminal nerve.[31] This neural connectivity has also been confirmed via EMG. Schaverien et al[32] have demonstrated electrical activity in the masseter muscle in 40% of test subjects when both volitional and involuntary smiles are elicited. Neural plasticity and the proximity of chewing and smiling centers on the cortical motor strip also have a well-described beneficial influence.

Another advantage of using the masseteric nerve for free muscle transfer innervation is that the reconstruction can be achieved in a single procedure, and the dense population of motor axons allows for the use of small muscle flaps, limiting midfacial bulk. Typically, one-third to one-quarter of the diameter of the gracilis muscle is utilized. Care must be taken to avoid large muscle flaps, because they can create an overpowered, unnatural grimace. This stands in contrast to muscle flaps innervated by CFNGs, where larger segments of muscle are frequently harvested to compensate for the more limited axonal input.

If CFNGs are employed for free muscle transfer innervation, it has been our practice to fully explore the donor facial nerve by identifying branches through a preauricular incision. This more extensive exploration is advocated on the grounds that it avoids the nasolabial fold incision that is generally unacceptable in the pediatric patient while providing access to larger, more proximal, facial nerve branches whose function has been compared with their neighbors' and has been carefully mapped. Regardless, it is interesting how consistently the most desirable facial nerve branch for smile reconstruction is identified at Zuker's point,[33] a point halfway along a line drawn from the helical root to the oral commissure. Typically, in this vicinity two or three large zygomatic branches producing a forceful smile are encountered. The largest branch is usually isolated for selective transection and anastomosis to the CFNG. Selection of the smaller, weaker branches will usually result in an underpowered free muscle flap following the second stage of the reconstruction. Regardless of which source of innervation is chosen to power the flap, great care must be taken to anchor the flap several millimeters medial to the modiolus and nasolabial fold to accommodate for the inevitable lateral drift that occurs during the healing process.

Eyelid weights can be a very effective in the treatment of paralytic lagophthalmos. Weights of various sizes can be applied to the upper eyelid with two-sided tape. The weight that produces complete eye closure without ptosis is selected. Skin-colored, external eyelid weights can also be purchased by patients and worn at home, giving them a chance to determine the benefit of the device and to select the most effective size. The most frequent error is selecting a weight that is too light and does not achieve full blink or complete eye closure. In our center, 1.4 g and 1.6 g weights are the most frequently utilized devices. During placement the weight should be slightly medialized in relation to the cornea and limbus. As mentioned by the author, the weight must be anchored with nonabsorbable sutures to prevent motion and to counter the potential of the implant to barrel roll.

Lastly, the lower lip is a frequently ignored and undertreated portion of the facial paralysis deformity. Neurotoxins have been successfully used to weaken the lower lip depressor muscles on the unaffected side, transiently enhancing symmetry. This effect can be made permanent if the patient desires by performing a partial excision of the depressor labii inferioris via an intraoral approach, avoiding visible external scars.[34] Care must be taken to prevent injury to the mental nerve, which can produce bothersome lower lip anesthesia.

In closing, I again commend Dr. Hanasono on an outstanding chapter and hope the reader will find this short commentary of value when approaching the surgical rehabilitation of the paralyzed face.

## Case Example

A 15-year-old male presented with congenital facial paralysis (Möbius's syndrome; **Fig. 10.15**). Bilateral facial reanimation was undertaken in two stages utilizing endoscopy-assisted free gracilis muscle flaps **(Fig. 10.16)** innervated by the descending branch of the masseteric nerve **(Fig. 10.17)**. Flap perfusion was provided by the superficial temporal artery and vein. The dense population of myelinated motor fibers in the masseteric nerve allowed for the use of small muscle flaps **(Fig. 10.18** and **Fig. 10.19)** that achieved full commissure excursion while avoiding excess bulk in the cheeks **(Fig. 10.20** and **Fig. 10.21)**.

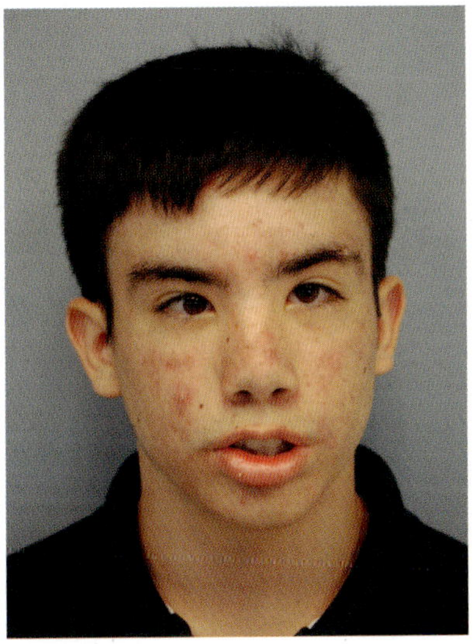

**Fig. 10.15** Bilateral congenital facial paralysis (Möbius's syndrome).

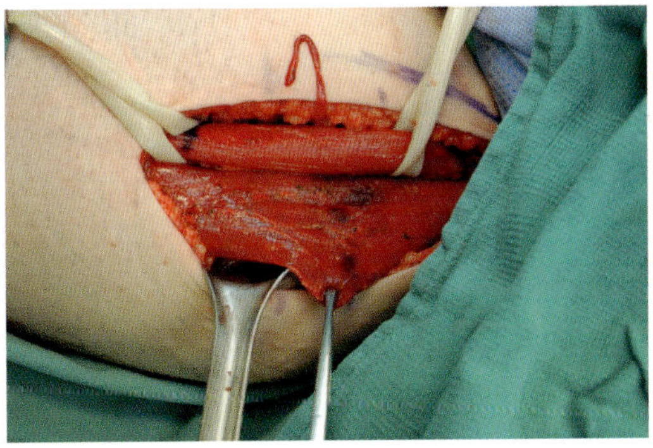

**Fig. 10.16** Small free muscle flap—one-quarter of the gracilis muscle diameter.

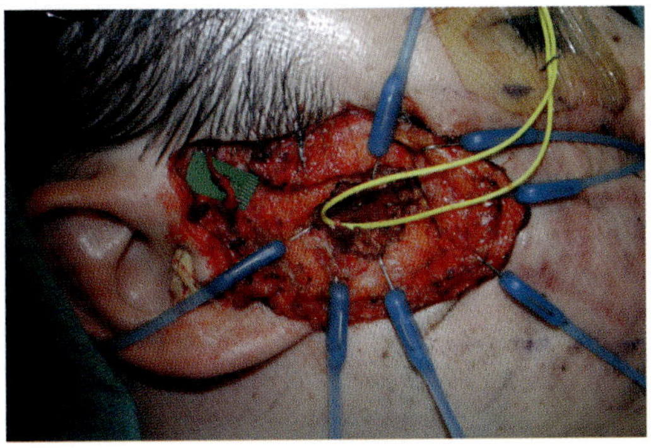

**Fig. 10.17** Descending branch of the masseteric nerve and the superficial temporal vessels isolated via a limited preauricular incision.

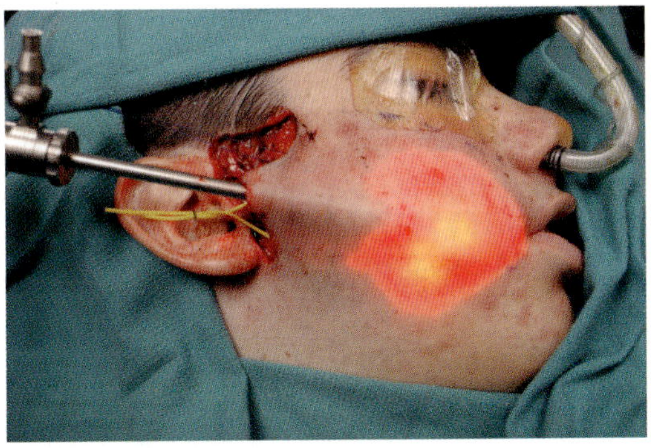

**Fig. 10.18** Endoscopy-assisted placement of anchoring sutures near the commissure.

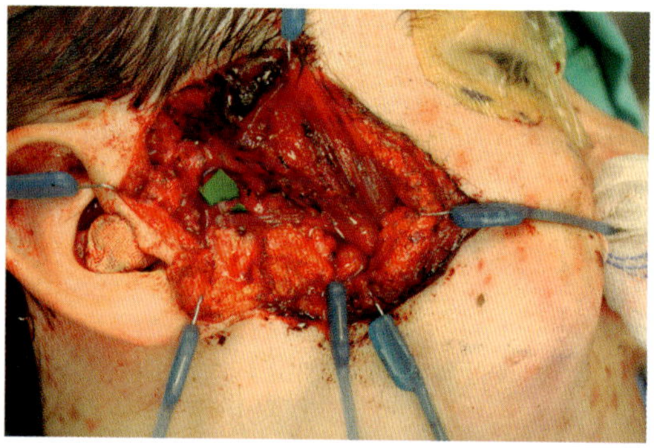

**Fig. 10.19** Insetting free gracilis muscle flap.

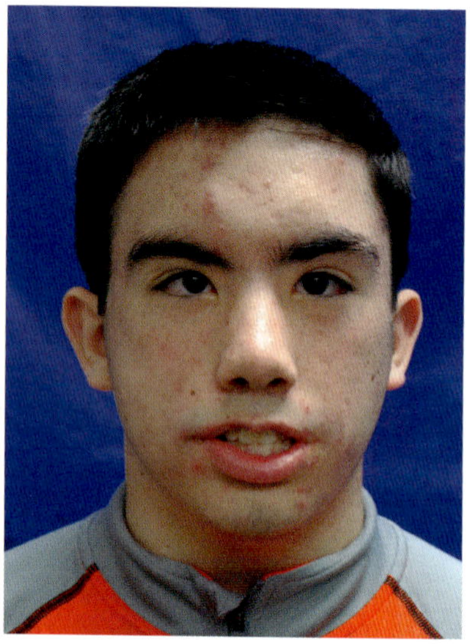

**Fig. 10.20** Postoperative photo in repose.

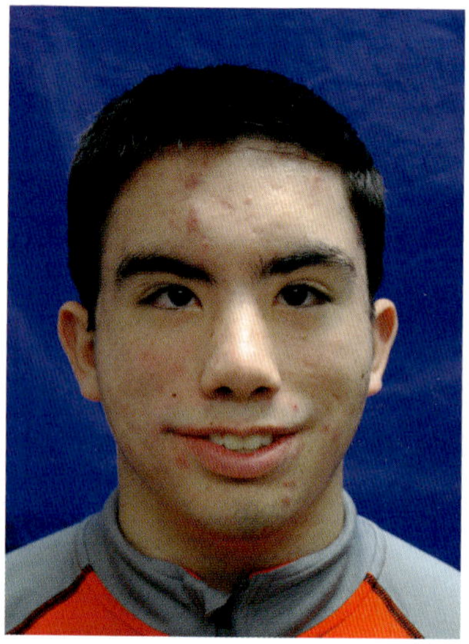

**Fig. 10.21** Postoperative photo with animation.

## References


1. House JW, Brackmann DE. Facial nerve grading system. Otolaryngol Head Neck Surg 1985;93(2):146–147
2. Brown PD, Eshleman JS, Foote RL, Strome SE. An analysis of facial nerve function in irradiated and unirradiated facial nerve grafts. Int J Radiat Oncol Biol Phys 2000;48(3):737–743
3. Iseli TA, Harris G, Dean NR, Iseli CE, Rosenthal EL. Outcomes of static and dynamic facial nerve repair in head and neck cancer. Laryngoscope 2010;120(3):478–483
4. Gidley PW, Herrera SJ, Hanasono MM, et al. The impact of radiotherapy on facial nerve repair. Laryngoscope 2010;120(10):1985–1989
5. Hanasono MM, Silva AK, Yu P, Skoracki RJ, Sturgis EM, Gidley PW. Comprehensive management of temporal bone defects after oncologic resection. Laryngoscope 2012;122(12):2663–2669
6. Korte W. Nerve grafting: facial nerve on hypoglossal. Dtsch Med Wochenschr 1903;29:293–295
7. Conley J. Hypoglossal crossover—122 cases. Trans Sect Otolaryngol Am Acad Ophthalmol Otolaryngol 1977;84(4 Pt 1):ORL-763–ORL-768
8. Koh KS, Kim J, Kim CJ, Kwun BD, Kim SY. Hypoglossal-facial crossover in facial-nerve palsy: pure end-to-side anastomosis technique. Br J Plast Surg 2002;55(1): 25–31
9. Spira M. Anastomosis of masseteric nerve to lower division of facial nerve for correction of lower facial paralysis. Preliminary report. Plast Reconstr Surg 1978;61(3):330–334
10. Manktelow RT, Tomat LR, Zuker RM, Chang M. Smile reconstruction in adults with free muscle transfer innervated by the masseter motor nerve: effectiveness and cerebral adaptation. Plast Reconstr Surg 2006;118(4):885–899
11. Coombs CJ, Ek EW, Wu T, Cleland H, Leung MK. Masseteric-facial nerve coaptation—an alternative technique for facial nerve reinnervation. J Plast Reconstr Aesthet Surg 2009;62(12):1580–1588
12. Klebuc MJ. Facial reanimation using the masseter-to-facial nerve transfer. Plast Reconstr Surg 2011;127(5):1909–1915
13. Anderl H. Reconstruction of the face through cross-face nerve transplantation in facial paralysis. Chirurgia Plastica 1973;2:17–45

14. Scaramella LF. Anastomosis between the two facial nerves. Laryngoscope 1975;85(8):1359–1366
15. Baker DC, Conley J. Facial nerve grafting: a thirty year retrospective review. Clin Plast Surg 1979;6(3):343–360
16. Terzis JK, Tzafetta K. The "babysitter" procedure: minihypoglossal to facial nerve transfer and cross-facial nerve grafting. Plast Reconstr Surg 2009;123(3):865–876
17. Terzis JK, Manktelow RT. Pectoralis minor: a new concept in facial reanimation. Plast Surg Forum 1982;5: 106–110
18. Dellon AL, Mackinnon SE. Segmentally innervated latissimus dorsi muscle. Microsurgical transfer for facial reanimation. J Reconstr Microsurg 1985;2(1):7–12
19. Harii K, Ohmori K, Torii S. Free gracilis muscle transplantation, with microneurovascular anastomoses for the treatment of facial paralysis. A preliminary report. Plast Reconstr Surg 1976;57(2):133–143
20. Birgfeld C, Neligan P. Surgical approaches to facial nerve deficits. Skull Base 2011;21(3):177–184
21. Kumar PA, Hassan KM. Cross-face nerve graft with free-muscle transfer for reanimation of the paralyzed face: a comparative study of the single-stage and two-stage procedures. Plast Reconstr Surg 2002;109(2):451–462, discussion 463–464
22. Rose EH. Autogenous fascia lata grafts: clinical applications in reanimation of the totally or partially paralyzed face. Plast Reconstr Surg 2005;116(1):20–32, discussion 33–35
23. Deleyiannis FWB, Askari M, Schmidt KL, Henkelmann TC, VanSwearingen JM, Manders EK. Muscle activity in the partially paralyzed face after placement of a fascial sling: a preliminary report. Ann Plast Surg 2005;55(5):449–455
24. Golio D, De Martelaere S, Anderson J, Esmaeli B. Outcomes of periocular reconstruction for facial nerve paralysis in cancer patients. Plast Reconstr Surg 2007;119(4): 1233–1237
25. Rofagha S, Seiff SR. Long-term results for the use of gold eyelid load weights in the management of facial paralysis. Plast Reconstr Surg 2010;125(1):142–149
26. Hanasono MM, Sacks JM, Goel N, Ayad M, Skoracki RJ. The anterolateral thigh free flap for skull base reconstruction. Otolaryngol Head Neck Surg 2009;140(6): 855–860
27. May M. Trauma to the facial nerve. Otolaryngol Clin North Am 1983;16(3):661–670
28. Borschel GH, Kawamura DH, Kasukurthi R, Hunter DA, Zuker RM, Woo AS. The motor nerve to the masseter muscle: an anatomic and histomorphometric study to facilitate its use in facial reanimation. J Plast Reconstr Aesthet Surg 2012;65(3):363–366
29. Coombs CJ, Ek EW, Wu T, Cleland H, Leung MK. Masseteric-facial nerve coaptation—an alternative technique for facial nerve reinnervation. J Plast Reconstr Aesthet Surg 2009;62(12):1580–1588
30. Manktelow RT, Tomat LR, Zuker RM, Chang M. Smile reconstruction in adults with free muscle transfer innervated by the masseter motor nerve: effectiveness and cerebral adaptation. Plast Reconstr Surg 2006;118(4):885–899
31. Baumel JJ. Trigeminal-facial nerve communications. Their function in facial muscle innervation and reinnervation. Arch Otolaryngol 1974;99(1):34–44
32. Schaverien M, Moran G, Stewart K, Addison P. Activation of the masseter muscle during normal smile production and the implications for dynamic reanimation surgery for facial paralysis. J Plast Reconstr Aesthet Surg 2011;64(12):1585–1588
33. Dorafshar AH, Borsuk DE, Bojovic B, et al. Surface anatomy of the middle division of the facial nerve: Zuker's point. Plast Reconstr Surg 2013;131(2):253–257
34. Hussain G, Manktelow RT, Tomat LR. Depressor labii inferioris resection: an effective treatment for marginal mandibular nerve paralysis. Br J Plast Surg 2004;57(6):502–510

# 11 Principles of Multidisciplinary Care in Head and Neck Cancer Treatment

*Steven S. Chang and Randal S. Weber*

## Introduction

The field of head and neck oncology is evolving rapidly. This evolution is a result of both the explosion of knowledge regarding the molecular biology of head and neck cancers and the coinciding development of novel treatments. These changes, coupled with continued advancements in biotechnology, have led to increasingly complex management of the head and neck cancer patient. It is not the goal of this chapter to provide the reader with a complete understanding of head and neck oncology. The purpose of this chapter is to introduce the principles of contemporary management of the head and neck cancer patient. The framework of modern cancer care is the multidisciplinary care team. In this chapter, we provide the rationale for the team and describe its members and how each member ideally contributes to the care of the patient. Last, we summarize the general treatment principles of head and neck oncology.

## Rationale for the Multidisciplinary Team Approach

Head and neck cancer treatment is extremely nuanced. Each subsite and histology **(Table 11.1)** has a unique treatment paradigm that involves various combinations of chemotherapy agents, radiation regimens, and surgical approaches.[1,2,3] Each discipline brings to the patient an in-depth knowledge of its respective modality. Multidisciplinary care extends beyond treatment of the cancer; it involves many ancillary services that are essential to successful cancer treatment, with the overarching goals being to cure the disease, to preserve critical structures, and, whenever possible, to preserve or restore form and function. For example, a larynx-sparing treatment is ineffective if, at the completion of treatment, the larynx is anatomically preserved but functionally the patient is unable to swallow without a feeding tube or to breathe without a tracheostomy. Coordination of the treating disciplines and participation by rehabilitation experts improve the functional outcomes. Treatment for cancer involves restoration or rehabilitation of speech, swallowing, breathing, hearing, vision, and appearance. One of the challenges in caring for head and neck cancer patients is the relative rarity of the disease. The multidisciplinary model of head and neck cancer care by its nature is complex, but it can improve the quality and efficiency of care and decrease treatment costs.

## The Members of the Multidisciplinary Team

The multidisciplinary team has many members. The primary players for treatment are usually head and neck surgeons, radiation oncologists, and medical oncologists, but optimizing treatment for head and neck cancer requires a very large group of additional clinicians and ancillary staff. These services include, but are not limited to, dentistry, ophthalmology, speech-language pathology, medical oncology (sarcoma, melanoma, squamous specialties), radiation oncology (sarcoma, melanoma, squamous specialties), endocrinology, thoracic surgery, nutrition/dietary therapy, physical and occupational therapy, radiology (interventional and neuroradiology), nuclear medicine, pathology, anesthesiology, medicine, reconstructive surgery, intraoperative nursing, intraoperative surgical technicians, postoperative nursing, social workers, and discharge planners. Each member is important at different stages of the patient's care.

**Table 11.1** Major subsites and histologies in head and neck cancer

| Major Subsites in Head and Neck Cancer |
|---|
| 1. Aerodigestive<br>a. Nasopharynx<br>b. Paranasal sinus/nasal cavity<br>c. Oral cavity<br>I. Lip<br>Ii. Buccal<br>Iii. Hard palate<br>Iv. Alveolar<br>V. Retromolar trigone<br>d. Oropharynx<br>I. Soft palate<br>Ii. Tonsil<br>Iii. Base of tongue<br>e. Hypopharynx<br>f. Larynx<br>I. Supraglottic<br>Ii. Glottic<br>Iii. Subglottic<br>G. Trachea<br>2. Skin<br>3. Endocrine organs<br>4. Bone and cartilage<br>5. Orbital/lacrimal<br>6. Salivary gland<br>a. Parotid<br>b. Submandibular<br>c. Lingual<br>d. Minor |
| **Major Histologies in Head and Neck Cancer** |
| • Squamous cell carcinoma<br>• Salivary malignancy<br>• Thyroid cancer<br>• Parathyroid cancer<br>• Melanoma<br>• Basal cell carcinoma<br>• Sarcoma<br>• Bone/cartilage-derived malignancy<br>• Odontogenic malignancy<br>• Lymphoma<br>• Neuroendocrine cancer<br>• Metastases (e.g., renal cell carcinoma, lung cancer) |

## The Multidisciplinary Team Leader and Patient Evaluation/Treatment Planning

Participation by members of the multidisciplinary team differs for each cancer patient depending upon the patient's needs. The head and neck surgeon usually is the first member of the team to see the patient for evaluation, and he or she serves as the team leader or "captain of the ship." The head and neck surgeon coordinates care, organizing diagnostic evaluations and consultations. In all cases, however, care of the patient should be collaborative, and treatment recommendations should be in accordance with evidence-based guidelines.

The head and neck surgeon performs a complete history and physical examination, focusing on smoking habits, alcohol consumption, weight loss, and medical condition. Consultations with dentistry, radiation, medical oncology, speech-language pathology, and reconstructive surgery are obtained as indicated. All members of the treatment team should meet the patient prior to final treatment recommendations, allowing each clinician to assess the patient's pretreatment status and tumor. The initial visit serves to facilitate any postoperative care that is required. Additionally, diagnostic studies are obtained, which usually include a CT or MRI scan of the head and neck, chest imaging, modified barium swallow, and blood studies. Once the appropriate work-up is completed and the members of the team have all had an opportunity to evaluate the patient, it is the responsibility of the surgeon to present the patient at a multidisciplinary tumor conference, where a plan of care is formulated. At a follow-up visit, the head and neck surgeon presents the recommendations to the patient. Central to the multidisciplinary care model is communication. Group meetings facilitate efficient, frequent, and open communication among the team members. Frequent discussions between the head and neck surgeon and the patient are important.

Central to all the planning and coordination of care is to avoid delays in the patient's treatment initiation. The goal is to begin treatment within 2 to 4 weeks of the initial evaluation, to avoid progression of disease. Postoperative complications, such as fistula, leaks, hematoma, and flap failures, can cause delays in further treatment and compromise care. In most instances, adjuvant radiotherapy is ideally initiated 4 weeks after surgery.[4,5]

The preoperative assessment by the head and neck surgeon, which is the second visit, accomplishes several goals. The head and neck surgeon reviews all test results, confirms pathology results, and reviews radiology images and laboratory reports. Careful review of each consultant's recommendations (surgical, medical, and ancillary) is mandatory. A pathologist and radiologist who specialize in the head and neck are essential for accurate treatment planning. With all the information available, the head and neck surgeon then provides a treatment recommendation and discusses with the patient the goals of treatment and anticipated outcome. The goal of surgical treatment is removal of locoregional disease. The head and neck surgeon's responsibility is to discuss with the patient the goal of therapy, the likelihood of complete tumor removal and disease control, and the anticipated functional outcome.

In addition, the head and neck surgeon must coordinate postoperative adjuvant therapy, such as radiation or chemotherapy. This responsibility should extend beyond the surgical procedure; the head and neck surgeon must coordinate speech and swallowing therapy, visiting nursing, social work, physical therapy, and nutrition therapy. Every patient presents challenges, and anticipating those challenges facilitates the treatment course and avoids delays in care.

Tumors of the upper aerodigestive tract present difficult challenges. Preoperatively, the surgeon must discuss with the anesthesiologist how the airway should be managed. Options include standard laryngoscopy and oral intubation. If visualization of the larynx is felt to be difficult, awake fiberoptic intubation should be considered. If fiberoptic intubation is not feasible, an awake tracheostomy is the best option to secure the airway. Communication among the entire team is imperative. The benefits of performing a tracheostomy are that the airway is secured, it is a low-risk procedure, it facilitates weaning from mechanical ventilation, and often it makes intraoral surgeries easier. Additionally, if a patient has upper airway reconstruction and requires additional operations, instrumentation of the reconstructed airway for re-intubation is not necessary. The downsides of the tracheostomy include patient discomfort, temporary inability to speak, requirement for a competent caregiver after hospital discharge, and possible delays in speech/swallow rehabilitation. In most surgeries of the upper aerodigestive tract that require reconstruction, securing the airway with a tracheostomy for the perioperative course is the best approach.

A second important consideration is nutritional support. Assessment by a speech-language pathologist (SLP) is vital in decision making. The SLP can provide insight into the patient's preoperative ability to swallow and in some cases predict the postoperative risk of aspiration. The reconstructive surgeon is also important in decision making. Generally, the reconstructive surgeon decides when the postoperative swallow evaluation is permissible and when it is safe to test the suture line with a swallow test. Options for perioperative alimentation include oral swallow, nasal feeding tube, or percutaneous gastrostomy tube (PEG). The decision should be jointly made by the head and neck surgeon and the reconstructive surgeon.

Another important aspect of the dialogue between the head and neck surgeon and reconstructive surgeon is to provide a reasonable estimate of the defect size and a time estimate for the resection. Anticipated resection of soft tissue and/or bone is essential to communicate. A good reconstructive surgeon allows the ablative surgeon to confidently remove any tumor to widely negative margins. Ultimately, the extent of surgery is determined by what is required for complete tumor extirpation; however, it is incumbent upon the head and neck surgeon to alert the reconstructive surgeon of the predicted size of the defect and of any deviation from the plan. It is also the responsibility of the reconstructive surgeon to inform the ablative surgeon when no reasonable reconstructive options exist. Whenever possible, concurrent two-team surgery is preferred to reduce the overall operative time for the patient. Shorter operative time has been shown to reduce postoperative complications and to increase the likelihood that the patient will not require extended mechanical ventilation. In some cases, the teams must work sequentially when there is inadequate operative field separation. In general, combined cases should be considered for a first start whenever possible, to avoid having to operate late into the evening. Extending late in the day usually requires exchange of the surgical support team, which is not ideal. In some cases, it is advisable to discuss the skin incisions with the reconstructive surgeon to avoid losing the ability to perform local rotation flaps.

## The Surgical Team

Intraoperatively, the head and neck surgeon has the responsibility for the coordination and communication of patient care. The benefits of an experienced team who work together on a frequent basis cannot be overemphasized. Assembling an operating room team who routinely participate in these highly specialized surgeries and who are familiar with the procedures and instruments greatly reduces operative times. For example, in patients with an oral cavity lesion, it is preferable to use nasal intubation, which allows much better visualization for resection, and the anesthesia team must be comfortable with all intubation techniques needed to care for patients with altered airway anatomy. It is also the responsibility of the head and neck surgeon to alert the anesthesia team to possible difficulties with each patient. When the ablation and flap harvest proceed concurrently, separate scrub teams must be available for each team. For craniofacial resections with reconstruction, separate scrub teams for head and neck surgery, reconstructive surgery, and neurosurgery are necessary. Patient positioning and room setup are vital for efficient two-team surgery **(Fig. 11.1)**. Communication and team hand-offs are critical to ensure safe transitions of care. The complexity of multiteam cases increases the risk for instrument, needle, and sponge miscounts. The anesthesia team

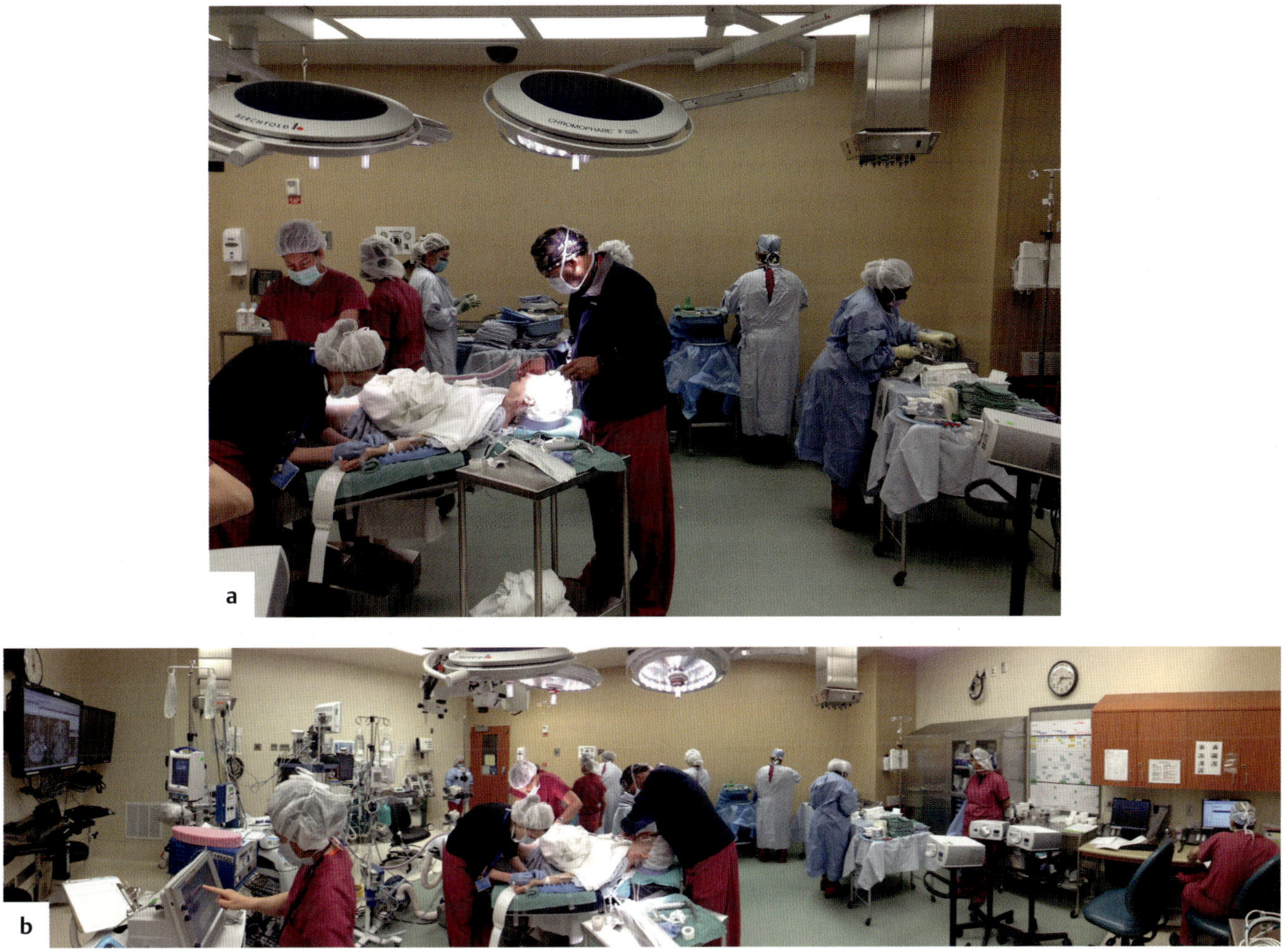

**Fig. 11.1** **(a)** The patient is turned 180 degrees away from the anesthesia team for maximal access to the head and neck region and free flap harvesting. Note the four scrub teams, each with a complete surgical set. In this case, four teams were involved in the surgical plan (head and neck surgery, neurotology, neurosurgery, plastic surgery). **(b)** Panoramic view of the operating room setup for the same patient. Note arrangement of the scrub team and anesthesia teams. Also the microscope is mounted to the ceiling for swift access and transitions of care. Not shown in this image are the stereotactic image guidance system and neurosurgical microscope, which are outside the room.

should be continually updated on unusual or unexpected blood loss or any airway issues. Conversely, the anesthesia team should continually update the surgical team regarding use of paralytics, fluid management, deep vein thrombosis prophylaxis, and antibiotic prophylaxis.

The head and neck surgeon should strive to complete the extirpation in a reasonable interval to allow for timely completion of the reconstruction. The overarching goal is to complete the entire procedure as safely and efficiently as possible. The ablative surgeon must facilitate the reconstructive procedure by ensuring proper vessel handling and preservation. Whenever possible, the common facial vein or other internal jugular tributaries are preserved for use as recipient blood vessels for microvascular free flaps. Similarly, branches of the external carotid, including the facial artery and the superior thyroid artery, are preserved. The recipient vessels should be handled gently. Cross-clamping with hemostats should be avoided. Adequate vessel length must also be preserved to facilitate manipulation during microvascular anastomosis.

## ■ Head and Neck Surgeon—Postoperative Responsibilities

In the postoperative period, the head and neck surgeon is responsible for coordinating care among the various services. In cases that involve free tissue transfer reconstruction, the care and observation of flap viability are the responsibility of the reconstructive team. The head and neck surgeon is responsible for fluid and electrolyte management, nutritional support, and coordination of subspecialty medical services. In the postoperative period, the head and neck surgeon coordinates discharge and support services, again in collaboration with the reconstructive team. When fluid overload occurs, administration of diuretics is always discussed with the reconstructive surgeon prior to administration. Rapid fluid shifts must be avoided. Too vigorous diuresis can potentially result in venous collapse and flap loss.

Perioperative care is facilitated by critical pathway order sets, which are standard order sets that ensure that no aspect of care is overlooked and that prevent omissions and deviations from the normal course of care. Critical care pathway order sets are created with multidisciplinary input, and critical care pathways increase the efficiency of patient care and facilitate communication between teams. Critical care pathways have been demonstrated to decrease resource utilization while improving quality and safety. Creating critical pathways must allow flexibility to accommodate individual patient needs as necessary.

Postdischarge visits are also multidisciplinary and should include the head and neck surgeon, reconstructive surgeon, SLP, nutritionist, and physical therapist. In the preparation for adjuvant therapy, the patient should be referred to dental oncology, radiation oncology, and medical oncology. In general, postoperative adjuvant therapy should commence within 4 to 6 weeks of surgery. Follow-up with the reconstructive surgeon is necessary for any late-occurring wound problems or when flap revision is necessary to improve function or cosmesis. Dental oncology follow-up is necessary for completion of dental rehabilitation (such as implants) or if early osteoradionecrosis develops, requiring local débridement.

Finally, long-term outpatient tumor surveillance of the patient is primarily the responsibility of the head and neck surgeon. In general, our cancer surveillance protocol for the first 2 years after treatment is a visit every 2 to 3 months. After the second year, visits are extended to every 6 months, until 5 years after treatment. At each visit, several studies are obtained: a CT or MRI scan of the primary site, chest X-ray, and thyroid function tests. Additionally, a PET scan or ultrasound may be obtained as indicated.

## General Head and Neck Surgical Oncology Principles

The surgical plans for patients are determined by both the histology of the tumor and the goal of therapy based upon the clinical evaluation. En bloc resection with widely negative margins (confirmed by intraoperative frozen section when possible) is the goal for malignant or high-grade lesions.[6] The guiding principle of surgical resection is that the first resection attempt is has the best chance of cure. In cases where the surgical plan is for salvage after either induction or previous therapy, it is necessary to resect to the pretreatment margin to ensure clearance of the disease.[7]

In general, indications for postoperative radiation therapy are pathological identification of perineural invasion, lymph node metastasis, advanced tumor stage, vascular invasion, close (< 5 mm) surgical margins, or extracapsular tumor spread. These factors are essentially indications that there may be microscopic disease left behind after surgery. To prevent postoperative progression of disease, radiation is normally started within 4 weeks of surgery. Indications for postoperative chemotherapy are generally for the following pathological findings: a grossly positive margin, extracapsular spread of tumor, or multiple lymph node involvement. Chemotherapy is normally given in addition to radiation as a radiosensitizer.

For further study, the National Comprehensive Cancer Network provides continuously updated guidelines for cancer care in an algorithmic format. The guidelines are a great resource for expert advice and evidence-based care of head and neck cancers.

## References


1. Forastiere AA, Goepfert H, Maor M, et al. Concurrent chemotherapy and radiotherapy for organ preservation in advanced laryngeal cancer. N Engl J Med 2003;349(22):2091–2098
2. Forastiere AA, Zhang Q, Weber RS, et al. Long-term results of RTOG 91-11: a comparison of three nonsurgical treatment strategies to preserve the larynx in patients with locally advanced larynx cancer. J Clin Oncol 2013;31(7):845–852
3. Wolf GT; The Department of Veterans Affairs Laryngeal Cancer Study Group. Induction chemotherapy plus radiation compared with surgery plus radiation in patients with advanced laryngeal cancer. N Engl J Med 1991;324(24):1685–1690
4. Bonner JA, Harari PM, Giralt J, et al. Radiotherapy plus cetuximab for locoregionally advanced head and neck cancer: 5-year survival data from a phase 3 randomised trial, and relation between cetuximab-induced rash and survival. Lancet Oncol 2010;11(1):21–28
5. Ang KK, Harris J, Wheeler R, et al. Human papillomavirus and survival of patients with oropharyngeal cancer. N Engl J Med 2010;363(1):24–35
6. Scholl P, Byers RM, Batsakis JG, Wolf P, Santini H. Microscopic cut-through of cancer in the surgical treatment of squamous carcinoma of the tongue. Prognostic and therapeutic implications. Am J Surg 1986;152(4): 354–360
7. Zafereo ME, Hanasono MM, Rosenthal DI, et al. The role of salvage surgery in patients with recurrent squamous cell carcinoma of the oropharynx. Cancer 2009;115(24): 5723–5733

# 12 Recipient Vessel Dissection

*Matthew M. Hanasono*

## ■ Introduction

The availability of recipient arteries and veins with sufficient caliber and blood flow within the vicinity of the defect site is paramount to success in microvascular free flap surgery. The vascular anatomy of the head and neck is complex, with numerous potential recipient arteries and veins. Dissection of adequate recipient vessels may be difficult given the high density of vital structures within the head and neck region, and especially with prior surgery and/or radiation. In circumstances in which local vessels are not available, or are of inadequate quality, distant vessels, in the contralateral neck or outside the head and neck region, must be considered.

## ■ Anatomy

Knowledge of neck anatomy is important not only to efficiently locate suitable recipient vessels for free flap reconstruction, but also to avoid potential complications, such as injury to critical neurovascular structures. Care must be taken to spare cranial nerves, particularly those that control facial and head and neck movement, mastication, deglutition, and speech. In the setting of altered anatomy after neck dissection and/or radiation therapy, preservation of these structures may be challenging.

The branches of the external carotid artery, from proximal to distal, are the superior thyroid, ascending pharyngeal, lingual, facial, occipital, posterior auricular, superficial temporal, and maxillary artery, which is also known as the internal maxillary artery **(Fig. 12.1)**. Most commonly, either the facial artery or the superior thyroid artery is selected as the recipient artery.[1,2] The occipital artery is occasionally useful as a recipient vessel, particularly for occipital scalp and posterior neck reconstructions. The ascending pharyngeal artery is not commonly used because it comes off the external carotid medially and is usually of very small caliber, as is the posterior auricular artery. The external carotid artery itself may serve

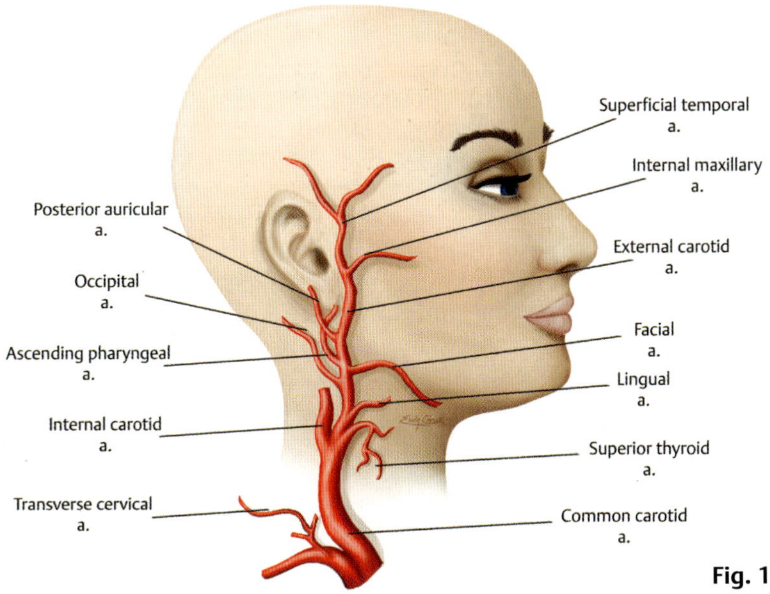


**Fig. 12.1** Head and neck arterial anatomy.

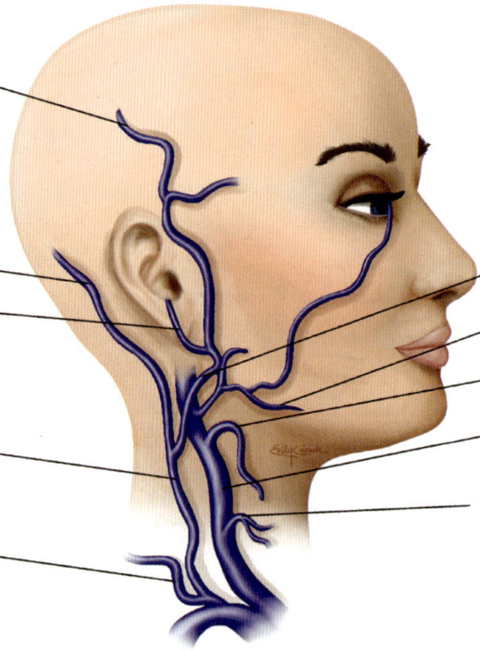


**Fig. 12.2** Head and neck venous anatomy.

as a recipient artery, often with very good vessel length and large diameter. When possible, this vessel is used as a recipient artery distal to its lower branches to preserve vascularity to the head and neck. The superficial temporal artery is located most cephalad and is often employed in reconstruction of the upper third of the face and in scalp reconstruction.

Venous anatomy in the neck is more variable **(Fig. 12.2)**. The internal jugular vein originates from the jugular foramen as a continuation of the sigmoid sinus at the skull base and travels medial to the sternocleidomastoid muscle, eventually draining into the subclavian vein. The internal jugular vein usually receives multiple branches, including the retromandibular vein, the common facial vein, the lingual vein, the pharyngeal vein, the superior thyroid vein, the middle thyroid vein, and the occipital vein. Many of these branches may share a common origin.[3] The external jugular vein lies deep to the platysma muscle, but superficial to the sternocleidomastoid muscle. It is formed by the joining of a branch of the retromandibular vein and the posterior auricular vein. Use of the anterior jugular vein, which empties into either the external jugular or subclavian vein, as a recipient vessel has not been well documented in the literature, most likely due to its frequent ligation in neck dissection, low flow, and susceptibility to flow interruption by compression.

## ■ Preoperative Considerations

Microvascular reconstruction of head and neck defects is often significantly more challenging in patients who have previously undergone neck dissection and/or radiation therapy to the neck.[3,4] A history of neck dissection or preoperative radiation therapy may result in the absence of recipient blood vessels adequate for successful free tissue transfer. Fibrosis and scarring may also make dissection tedious, obliterating tissue planes and increasing the friability of blood vessels. Consideration must be given to the possibility of extended operating times, the need to perform interposition vein grafting, and the need to dissect recipient vessels either in the contralateral neck or outside the head and neck area.

During the preoperative evaluation, in addition to being questioned about a history of prior neck dissection and irradiation, the patient should be queried regarding trauma or other neck surgery. A history of cerebrovascular disease or known carotid stenosis also raises the risk of inadequate arterial inflow as well as the need for extremely gentle handling of the common and internal carotid arteries during surgery. Preoperative carotid ultrasound or angiography may be indicated. A history of cervical spine disease or cervical fusion may limit the ability to position the neck to gain access to recipient blood vessels.

# ■ Operative Approach

## Cervical Recipient Blood Vessel Dissection

Recipient vessels are generally well exposed after concurrent primary tumor resection and neck dissection. The type and extent of neck dissection will determine what vessels are available for microvascular anastomosis. The facial artery is usually ligated just above the digastric tendon after the submandibular gland has been removed as part of the neck dissection and may be usable as a recipient artery (**Fig. 12.3**). Often, it will need to be dissected and transposed from under the digastric muscle and hypoglossal nerve to gain adequate length. The lingual artery, which is located just anterior to the facial artery or arises from a common trunk, may be another good option for use as a recipient artery.

The external jugular vein is frequently ligated high in the neck during neck dissections, but the remnant may be long enough and in good enough condition for use as a recipient vein. The common facial vein is usually ligated and may be available for use as a recipient vein using an end-to-end anastomotic technique. When the internal jugular vein has been ligated, it may still be possible to perform an end-to-end anastomosis to the remaining vein, if the size mismatch is not too great, or an end-to-side microvascular anastomosis to the stump, if the mismatch is significant.[5]

When a concurrent neck dissection has not been performed, a limited-access incision may be made just below the inferior border of the mandible over the palpable pulsations of the facial artery and result in exposure of the facial artery and vein above the submandibular gland (**Fig. 12.4**). Typically used for midfacial reconstructions, exposure of these vessels allows the anastomosis to be performed without need for further dissection of the neck. One caveat to this approach is that the caliber of the vessels may be small at this level. Otherwise, a transverse incision is made approximately two fingerbreadths below the inferior border of the mandibular body and is placed in a cervical rhytid if possible. The platysma muscle is exposed and divided. Subplatysmal flaps then are elevated. The marginal mandibular nerve lies within the superficial layer of the deep cervical fascia, superficial to the submandibular gland and common facial vein, below the inferior border of the mandible (**Fig. 12.5**). Care should be taken to identify and protect this nerve or to avoid dissection above the inferior border of the submandibular gland.

The facial vessels are usually readily identified below the submandibular gland, which is a lobular structure located partially below the lower border of the mandibular body. The facial vein travels superficial to the submandibular gland, while the facial artery usually travels within, or deep to, the gland.

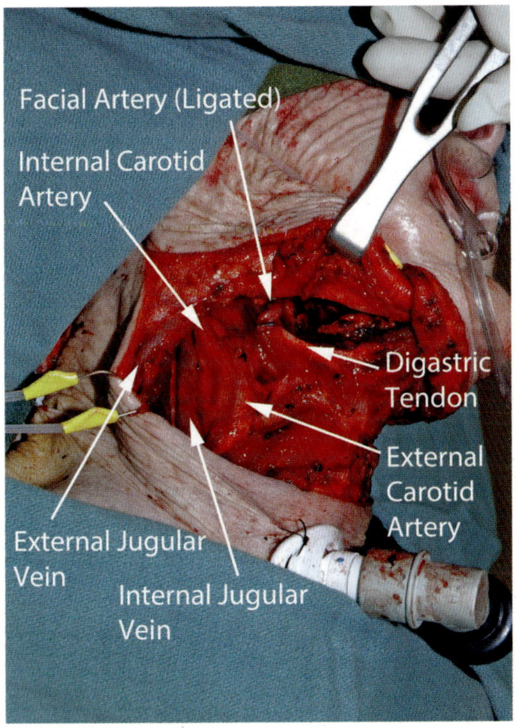


**Fig. 12.3** Exposure of the cervical arteries and veins in the right neck after a selective neck dissection. The facial artery has been ligated superior to the digastric tendon and the submandibular gland has been excised. The internal and external jugular veins are visible.

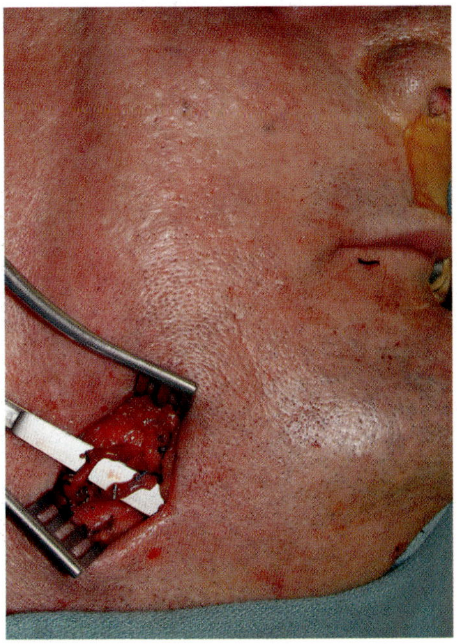

**Fig. 12.4** Exposure of the facial artery and vein through a limited-access incision along the inferior border of the mandibular body.

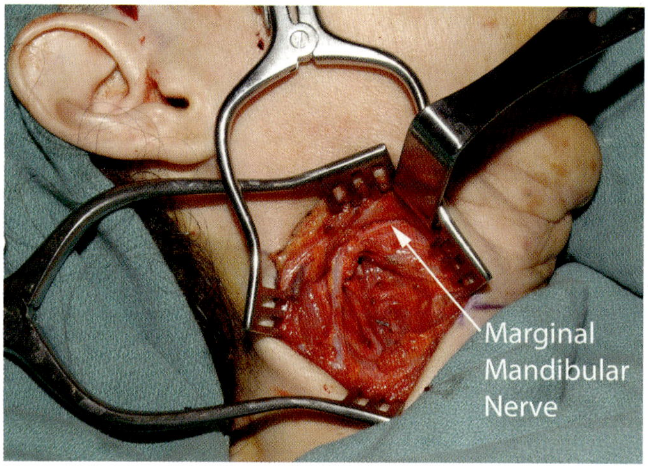


**Fig. 12.5** Exposure of the upper cervical vessels is performed by making a transverse incision one to two fingerbreadths below the inferior border of the mandible. Subplatysmal flaps have been elevated and the marginal mandibular nerve is visible within the superficial layer of the deep cervical fascia.

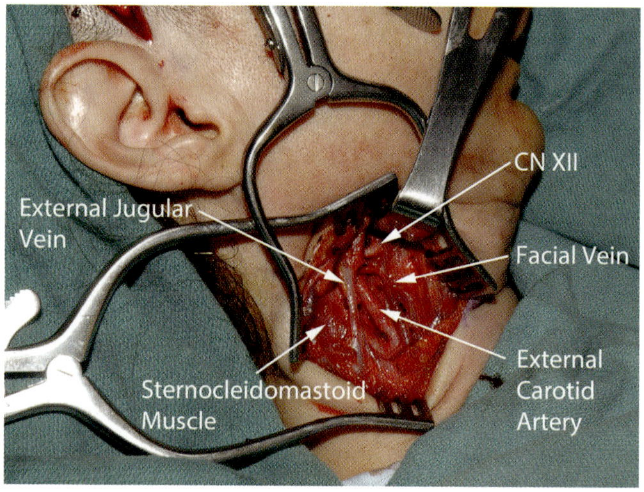


**Fig. 12.6** The deep cervical fascia and submandibular gland have been retracted and the facial artery is seen traveling beneath the hypoglossal nerve.

If the distal facial vessels are inadequate in caliber, flow, or location, then exposure of the internal jugular vein and the external carotid artery should be performed. Care is taken not to inadvertently interrupt the external jugular vein, which lies superficial to the sternocleidomastoid muscle.

The carotid sheath is exposed by retraction of the sternocleidomastoid muscle posteriorly. The spinal accessory nerve will be encountered entering the sternocleidomastoid muscle on its medial surface, superiorly, and should be spared. The internal jugular vein is located posterior and lateral within the carotid sheath, which is opened sharply. The common carotid artery, carotid bulb, internal carotid artery, and external carotid artery can be identified by dissecting fibrofatty tissue just medial and anterior to the internal jugular vein. The vagus nerve, which lies between the internal jugular vein and the carotid artery, is carefully preserved. Additionally, the ansa cervicalis, which is a loop of nerves that arise from the hypoglossal nerve anteriorly and the cervical spinal nerves (C2 and C3) posteriorly that supply the strap muscles, should be spared if possible. Transection of the ansa cervicalis may adversely affect deglutition, since these nerves are responsible for laryngeal elevation during swallowing. The ansa cervicalis lies on the superficial surface of the internal jugular vein and carotid artery. The distal branches of the external carotid artery lie beneath the posterior belly of the digastric muscle, which can be retracted superiorly for exposure **(Fig. 12.6)**. The hypoglossal nerve lies deep (medial) to the posterior belly of the digastric muscle, but superficial (lateral) to the external carotid artery and must be preserved.

## Superficial Temporal Blood Vessel Dissection

The superficial temporal vessels are accessed through a separate incision in the preauricular area. This incision is usually "zigzagged" so that it lies within the preauricular skin crease, to minimize visibility of the postoperative scar **(Fig. 12.7)**. The vessels are usually palpable just anterior to the upper margin of the auricular helix. Careful, atraumatic dissection is important since the superficial temporal vein is very thin-walled and can easily be damaged. The superficial temporal vessels are usually of small caliber unless they are dissected proximally, into the parenchyma of the parotid gland, to the level of the earlobe. Dissection is usually terminated at this point to avoid injury to the facial nerve. The proximal vessels are usually of good caliber for microvascular anastomosis, averaging 1.8 to 2.7 mm for the artery and 2.1 to 3.3 mm for the vein.[6]

## Locating Recipient Blood Vessels in the Previously Operated and/or Irradiated Neck

When the pedicle length is inadequate to reach the recipient vessels, vein grafting or construction of a temporary arteriovenous loop is required **(Fig. 12.8)**. This is particularly pertinent to cases in which the ipsilateral neck has undergone prior surgery and/or radiation and the contralateral neck must be used as a source of recipient blood vessels. Although some

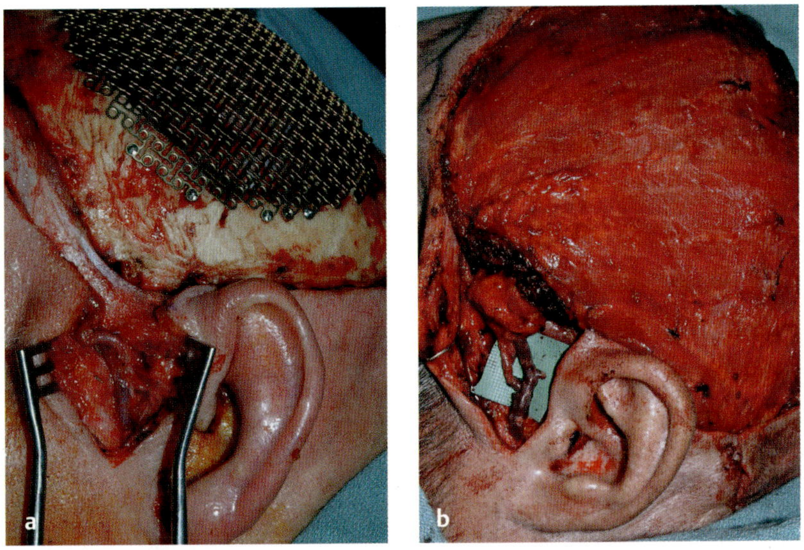


**Fig. 12.7** **(a)** Exposure of the superficial temporal artery and vein through a preauricular incision. **(b)** Microvascular anastomosis to the superficial temporal vessels for a latissimus dorsi muscle free flap used for scalp reconstruction.

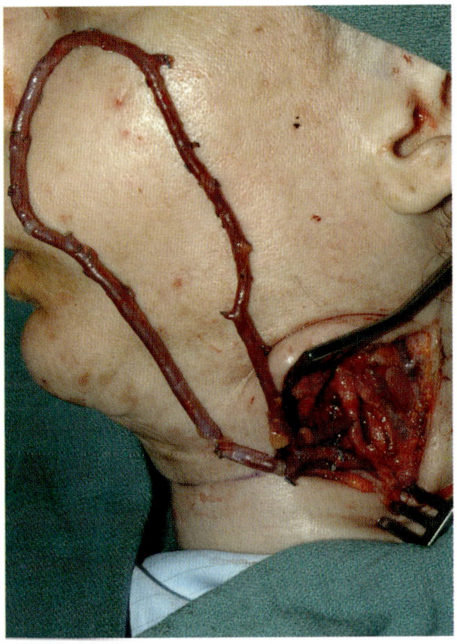

**Fig. 12.8** A temporary arteriovenous loop is created between the external carotid artery and internal jugular vein using a saphenous vein graft. When the microvascular free flap is ready for transfer, the loop is divided and the anastomoses are made to the cut ends of the vein graft.

studies suggest a higher incidence of flap failure when vein grafts or temporary arteriovenous loops are used in head and neck reconstruction, others have shown outcomes equivalent to outcomes with free flaps performed without vein grafts.[4] When possible, it is most prudent to use flaps with long pedicles or to orient the flap in such a way as to avoid vein grafts. Nevertheless, a short interpositional vein graft is preferable to performing the microvascular anastomosis under tension or with an unfavorable pedicle geometry that causes the vessels to become kinked.

Arteriovenous loops can be employed for microvascular anastomosis as a one-stage procedure in which a loop is created and divided at the time of free tissue transfer, essentially the same as performing separate vein grafts to the recipient artery and vein. Alternatively, a two-stage procedure may be employed in which the arteriovenous loop is created and then is followed by free tissue transfer at a second operation. Several small series have reported variable success rates, ranging from 60 to 100%, with the two-stage procedure.[2,7] However, based on the high success rates with using a one-stage procedure or direct use of interposition vein grafts without formation of a loop, there seems to be little need to delay reconstruction to allow loop maturation.[4,8]

The use of the transverse cervical artery and vein has also proven to be a valuable strategy when the upper cervical vessels cannot be used. These vessels are usually preserved during a selective neck dissection but may be ligated or injured during a modified radical or radical neck dissection. The transverse cervical artery arises medially in the neck from the thyrocervical trunk, or occasionally from the subclavian artery directly. The transverse cervical vein drains into the external jugular vein or the subclavian vein. The cervical incision is usually extended with a

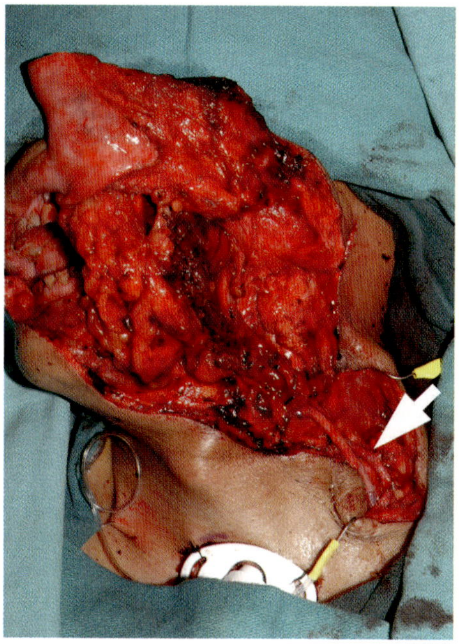

**Fig. 12.9** Use of the transverse cervical artery and vein in the posterior triangle of the left neck for microvascular anastomosis (*arrow*).

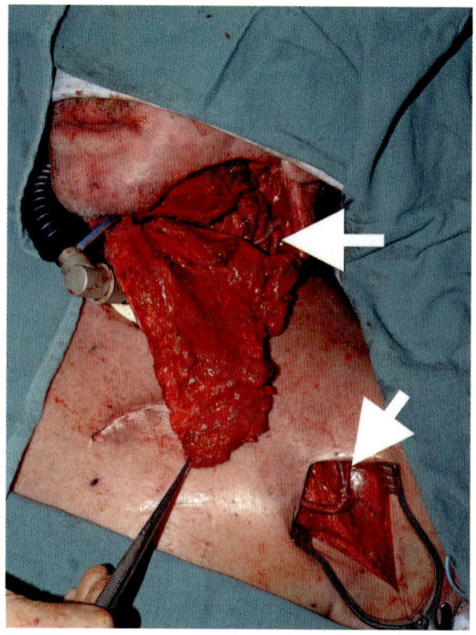

**Fig. 12.10** Use of the left cephalic vein for recipient vessel anastomosis (*arrows*). The vein is transposed to the neck, taking care not to kink or twist the vessel.

downward incision in the direction of the ipsilateral acromial process, or a separate supraclavicular incision can be made **(Fig. 12.9)**. The omohyoid muscle, which is identified lateral to the posterior border of the sternocleidomastoid muscle and just superior to the clavicle, is a surgical landmark for the transverse cervical artery and vein, which are deep to the muscle within the loose supraclavicular fatty tissue.[9] An alternative to using the transverse cervical vein is use of the proximal external or internal jugular veins.

The cephalic vein can be an excellent source of venous drainage in head and neck microvascular surgery. Advantages of the cephalic vein are that it requires only a single venous anastomosis, provides a long pedicle, lies outside the zone of radiation or prior surgery, and is associated with a generous diameter for microvascular anastomosis.[10,11] The cephalic vein is located in the deltopectoral groove and is traced distally adjacent to the lateral bicipital groove **(Fig. 12.10)**.

The use of the internal mammary vessels for head and neck surgery has not commonly been reported but is well known in breast reconstruction with autologous free tissue transfer.[12] The internal mammary vessels are usually located by removal of the second or third costal cartilage after division of the overlying pectoralis muscle **(Fig. 12.11)**. Inferior to the third rib, the caliber of the vein diminishes significantly and is usually less than 1.5 mm.

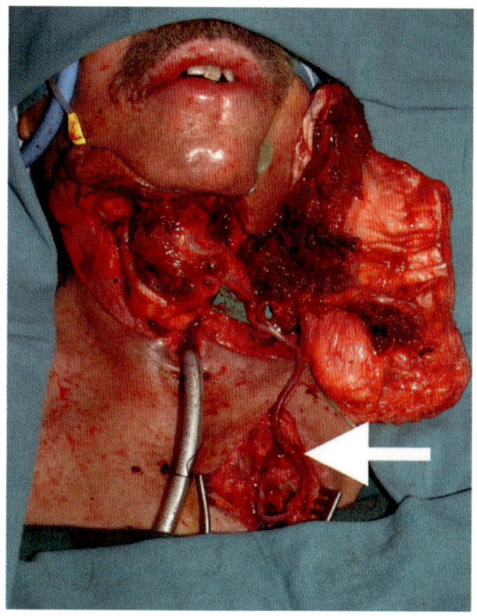

**Fig. 12.11** Use of the left internal mammary artery for microvascular anastomosis (*arrow*).

The thoracoacromial artery and vein have also been described as potential recipient vessels in head and neck reconstruction.[11,13] The thoracoacromial artery arises from the axillary artery and divides into acromial, deltoid, clavicular, and pectoral branches. Use of the pectoral branch of the thoracoacromial trunk for end-to-end anastomoses obviously prevents use of the pedicle pectoralis major muscle or myocutaneous flap as a secondary flap for reconstruction. However, in cases where the pectoralis major muscle flap has already been transferred and adequate healing has taken place, division and use of the pectoral branches, which remain well preserved within the perivascular fat pad, as recipient vessels has been reported.[13]

### Multiple Free Flaps

Cases requiring multiple free flap reconstruction may pose an even greater challenge for finding adequate recipient blood vessels in close proximity to the defects. Use of the distal pedicle of one flap for anastomosis to a second flap has been described.[14] However, for unclear reasons, this technique is generally felt to be associated with an increased flap loss rate. Some authors have speculated that thromboembolism from the first anastomosis affects the second anastomosis, others have suggested that a steal phenomenon might play a role in reducing perfusion to the second flap, and still others feel that flap loss is due to the difficulty of positioning the second flap without kinking of the pedicle. Transfer of a second flap onto a branch of another free flap pedicle has also been reported without complications.[8] The use of the pedicle of a failed or excised flap as the recipient vessel for a second flap with comparable success rates to the initial procedure has also previously been described.[15]

## Complications

Potential recipient vessels should always be assessed for location, direction, caliber, blood flow, and the quality of the vessel wall. The microvascular surgeon must be cognizant of surgical trauma, proximal ligation, and the possibility of vessel occlusion related to radiation fibrosis or vascular disease. Vessels may need to be trimmed back proximally to an area of adequate caliber and patency. Mild to moderate perivascular fibrosis due to prior radiation or surgery is not usually a contraindication to usage, as long as blood flow is adequate.

The external jugular vein has been associated with higher rates of venous thrombosis in some studies, but not in others.[16] Theoretical reasons for higher rates of thrombosis may include surgical trauma and even ligation during neck dissection, low flow, and susceptibility to external compression due to its superficial location. If the external jugular vein is to be used, it should be checked for patency with heparinized saline irrigation, and it should be dissected completely from the surface of the sternocleidomastoid muscle to avoid potential pivot points where the vessel may kink during head movement. In addition, all sources of potential compression, such as snug tracheostomy ties, should be avoided during the postoperative healing period.

Injury to the marginal mandibular branch of the facial nerve, great auricular and other cervicospinal sensory nerves, hypoglossal nerve, ansa cervicalis, spinal accessory nerve, and vagus nerve are all potential complications of neck recipient vessel preparation. The spinal accessory nerve originates posterior to the jugular vein, enters the medial surface of the sternocleidomastoid muscle, and exits its posterior border just superior to the great auricular nerve after giving off motor branches to the muscle. Sacrifice of the spinal accessory nerve is debilitating, resulting in shoulder drop, pain in the glenohumeral joint, and weakness, with limited movement in the shoulder due to loss of trapezius muscle function.

The possibility of a chyle leak from either the thoracic duct in the left neck or the accessory thoracic duct in the right neck also exists, particularly with dissection of the transverse cervical artery and vein within the supraclavicular region of the neck. If a chyle leak is identified, an attempt may be made to repair it with microvascular suture. Otherwise, the duct is ligated. When a chyle leak is recognized after surgery as an accumulation of milky fluid beneath the skin flap, an attempt may be made to treat it conservatively with closed suction drainage and dietary modifications (i.e., a medium-chain triglyceride diet should decrease the volume of chyle).[17] If conservative management is unsuccessful, operative re-exploration is indicated.

Care must also be exercised in dissecting the internal jugular vein. A large inadvertent venotomy may result in not only severe hemorrhage, but also a life-threatening air embolism. Ligation of the internal jugular vein can result in severe facial edema, although this is usually transient when the ligation is only unilateral. Similarly, a gentle technique is required when manipulating the carotid artery. In patients with atherosclerosis, there is risk for dislodging atheromatous plaques, resulting in cerebrovascular insult. Pressure on the carotid bulb may also result in bradycardia or even asystole. Bradycardia usually ceases when manipulation of the carotid bulb stops, but it can also be remedied by periadventitial injection of 2% lidocaine.[18]

## Pearls and Pitfalls

- Knowledge of head and neck anatomy is important, not only for finding adequate recipient vessels for head and neck free flap reconstruction, but also to avoid potential complications during neck exploration, such as injury to critical neurovascular structures.
- Location of adequate recipient vessels may be challenging, especially after prior surgery and/or radiation.
- In some cases, interposition vein grafting may be necessary to reach recipient vessels in the contralateral neck. In other cases, it may be best to locate vessels outside the head and neck area.
- Alternative regional vessels include the transverse cervical vessels, cephalic vein, internal mammary vessels, and thoracoacromial vessels.
- In reoperative microsurgery, previously used recipient vessels can often be reused, when the pedicle to the prior free flap can be safely transected.

## References


1. Nahabedian MY, Singh N, Deune EG, Silverman R, Tufaro AP. Recipient vessel analysis for microvascular reconstruction of the head and neck. Ann Plast Surg 2004;52(2):148–155, discussion 156–157
2. Shima H, von Luedinghausen M, Ohno K, Michi K. Anatomy of microvascular anastomosis in the neck. Plast Reconstr Surg 1998;101(1):33–41
3. Hanasono MM, Barnea Y, Skoracki RJ. Microvascular surgery in the previously operated and irradiated neck. Microsurgery 2009;29(1):1–7
4. Jacobson AS, Eloy JA, Park E, Roman B, Genden EM. Vessel-depleted neck: techniques for achieving microvascular reconstruction. Head Neck 2008;30(2):201–207
5. Graham BB, Varvares MA. End-to-side venous anastomosis with the internal jugular vein stump: a preliminary report. Head Neck 2004;26(6):537–540
6. Shimizu F, Lin MP, Ellabban M, Evans GRD, Cheng MH. Superficial temporal vessels as a reserve recipient site for microvascular head and neck reconstruction in vessel-depleted neck. Ann Plast Surg 2009;62(2):134–138
7. Angel MF, Chang B, Clark N, Wong L, Ringelman P, Manson PN. Further clinical use of the interposition arteriovenous loop graft in free tissue transfers. Microsurgery 1993;14(8):479–481
8. Hanasono MM, Weinstock YE, Yu P. Reconstruction of extensive head and neck defects with multiple simultaneous free flaps. Plast Reconstr Surg 2008;122(6):1739–1746
9. Yu P. The transverse cervical vessels as recipient vessels for previously treated head and neck cancer patients. Plast Reconstr Surg 2005;115(5):1253–1258
10. Horng SY, Chen MT. Reversed cephalic vein: a lifeboat in head and neck free-flap reconstruction. Plast Reconstr Surg 1993;92(4):752–753
11. Harris JR, Lueg E, Genden E, Urken ML. The thoracoacromial/cephalic vascular system for microvascular anastomoses in the vessel-depleted neck. Arch Otolaryngol Head Neck Surg 2002;128(3):319–323
12. Urken ML, Higgins KM, Lee B, Vickery C. Internal mammary artery and vein: recipient vessels for free tissue transfer to the head and neck in the vessel-depleted neck. Head Neck 2006;28(9):797–801
13. Aycock JK, Stenson KM, Gottlieb LJ. The thoracoacromial trunk: alternative recipient vessels in reoperative head and neck reconstructive microsurgery. Plast Reconstr Surg 2008;121(1):88–94
14. Wei FC, Celik N, Chen HC, Cheng MH, Huang WC. Combined anterolateral thigh flap and vascularized fibula osteoseptocutaneous flap in reconstruction of extensive composite mandibular defects. Plast Reconstr Surg 2002;109(1):45–52
15. Nakayama B, Kamei Y, Toriyama K, Hyodo I, Hasegawa Y, Torii S. Usefulness of a first transferred free flap vascular pedicle for secondary microvascular reconstruction in the head and neck. Plast Reconstr Surg 2002;109(4):1246–1253
16. Chalian AA, Anderson TD, Weinstein GS, Weber RS. Internal jugular vein versus external jugular vein anastamosis: implications for successful free tissue transfer. Head Neck 2001;23(6):475–478
17. de Gier HH, Balm AJ, Bruning PF, Gregor RT, Hilgers FJ. Systematic approach to the treatment of chylous leakage after neck dissection. Head Neck 1996;18(4):347–351
18. Babin RW, Panje WR. The incidence of vasovagal reflex activity during radical neck dissection. Laryngoscope 1980;90(8 Pt 1):1321–1323

# 13 Postoperative Care and Management of Surgical Complications

*Peirong Yu*

## Postoperative Care

### General Postoperative Care

After major head and neck tumor ablation and microsurgical reconstruction, patients are usually kept in the surgical intensive care unit overnight, sedated, and placed on a ventilator, which they are weaned off the next morning, as tolerated, and then are transferred to a flap floor when they are deemed stable. The advantage of having patients sedated overnight is to avoid unnecessary agitation and vomiting, which may result in increased risk of hematoma or flap compromise. The disadvantage of keeping patients sedated and on a ventilator overnight is the need for high volumes of intravenous fluids because of the sedation and paralysis. Sedation and paralysis often cause hypotension and require intravenous fluid resuscitation because vasopressors are generally considered contraindicated after free flap surgery. Therefore, patients may become fluid overloaded, which can cause significant cardiopulmonary complications in those with minimal cardiopulmonary reserve. In recent years, we have had increasing numbers of patients spontaneously breathing without ventilator support after surgery. These patients recover faster and develop fewer cardiopulmonary complications with significantly shorter length of stay. Deep vein thrombosis (DVT) and delirium tremens prophylaxis are given as indicated.

### Airway Care

Most patients have a tracheostomy, and routine tracheostomy care is provided. In particular, frequent airway suctioning is need. Once the patient is off the ventilator, humidified air/oxygen is provided through a T-piece connected to the tracheostomy tube or a tracheostomy mask. Care should be taken not to blow cold air directly onto the flap. Downsizing the tracheostomy tube is usually performed on postoperative day 4 or 5, and decannulation is usually possible within 1 or 2 weeks. If aspiration is present, such as following base of tongue and oropharyngeal reconstruction, decannulation is usually delayed.

### Feeding

An oral diet can be resumed on postoperative day 1 or 2 if the oral cavity or pharyngeosophagus was not involved in surgery. In patients with oral cavity or pharyngoesophageal reconstruction, oral intake is delayed for 1 to 6 weeks depending on the location and type of reconstruction. During that time, enteral feeding, usually through a Dobhoff feeding tube placed through the nose to the stomach, can be started on postoperative day 1. For most oromandibular, tongue, and oropharyngeal reconstructions, a modified barium swallow (MBS) study is performed by the speech pathologists, usually on postoperative day 7, to evaluate swallowing function, possible suture line leaks, and aspiration. In patients with no leaks or aspiration, a liquid diet is started and then quickly advanced to a soft or regular diet as tolerated. Patients should rinse their mouths frequently with saline or chlorhexidine gluconate solution for several weeks. In patients with leaks or aspiration upon swallowing, oral intake is withheld and an MBS study is repeated in 2 weeks or longer, as clinically indicated. In previously irradiated patients who have undergone pharyngoesophageal reconstruction with a fasciocutaneous flap, such as the anterolateral thigh flap or radial forearm flap, an MBS is usually performed 4 to 6 weeks after reconstruction to allow adequate time for the skin flap to heal if prior radiotherapy was given. In patients without prior radiation, an MBS is performed 2 weeks after surgery. With a jejunal flap reconstruction, MBS is performed around 7 days after surgery if no prior radiotherapy was given. In patients with prior radiotherapy, MBS is delayed for another week. After a normal MBS, a liquid diet is given for 3 days and then is advanced to soft diet if tolerated. When an asymptomatic leak is detected by MBS, an oral diet is withheld for 2 more weeks and MBS is repeated.

When long-term tube feeding is indicated, the nasogastric feeding tube is converted to the gastrostomy tube under fluoroscopy (percutaneous fluoroscopic gastrostomy, PFG) or a percutaneous endoscopic gastrostomy (PEG) can be performed in the beginning of the case. The nutritional service is usually consulted for the management of enteral feeding, such as the selection of formulas and types of feeding (continuous or bolus feeding).

## Activities and Donor-Site Care

Early ambulation is important to prevent DVT and pulmonary complications. Patients are encouraged to get out of bed and to sit in a chair on postoperative day 1 or when they are off the ventilator and fully awake. Ambulation usually starts on postoperative day 2. No special activity limitations are required with flaps that are not from the lower extremity. After harvest of the anterolateral thigh flap with primary closure, no activity limitations are necessary. If the donor-site closure requires skin grafting, patients can ambulate with a knee immobilizer to prevent knee flexion during walking. Once the skin grafts have taken, which is usually determined on postoperative day 5 or 6, patients can ambulate as tolerated without a knee immobilizer. After harvest of the fibula flap, a posterior splint or fracture boot is placed in the lower extremity whether skin grafting is required or not. Patients are encouraged to ambulate on postoperative day 2 with assistance, with the splint on and partial weight bearing with a walker. The leg should be elevated above the heart when the patient is not ambulating. The splint is taken down on postoperative day 3 if no skin grafting was required at the donor site, or on postoperative day 6 if skin grafting was required.

## Antibiotics

Broad-spectrum antibiotics, such as ampicillin-sulbactam, are usually used prophylactically. Postoperatively, antibiotics are usually continued for 3 days or longer, as indicated. However, there is no consensus about how long antibiotics should be used postoperatively after a prolonged surgery and reconstruction. In patients who are allergic to penicillin, use of a combination of clindamycin and ciprofloxacin is our preference.

## Wound Care

Neck and facial incisions are usually covered with antibiotic ointment and left open to air without any dressings. No particular wound care is needed if the incisions are clean; otherwise, the incisions can be cleaned with normal saline or hydrogen peroxide twice a day and antibiotic ointment can be applied after each cleaning. Patients can take showers when drains are removed and skin grafts are healed.

## Flap Monitoring

The first 24 hours after free flap surgery is the critical time for flap monitoring since the majority of failures occur during that time.[1,2] Our recommendation for flap monitoring is shown in **Table 13.1**.

Numerous methods have been described for flap monitoring.[3,4,5,6,7,8,9,10] Clinical observation of a visible free flap is the gold standard method against which other monitoring systems are generally measured. However, even the most experienced observer may have difficulty in assessing certain flaps, and monitoring systems are of significant value in these situations and in the assessment of buried flaps. The ideal monitor should be easy to perform, reliable, noninvasive, objectively repeatable, promptly reactive to blood flow changes, appropriate for continuous monitoring, inexpensive, and "fool proof" for unskilled observers. It is important that the surgeon show the nurse what the healthy flap looks like when the patient arrives in the recovery room or intensive care unit after surgery, because this appearance serves as the baseline for subsequent flap monitoring. The nurse should then show the next shift of nurses how the healthy flap should look, and so on. The nurses are instructed to call the doctors when there is a change from the baseline. We primarily use clinical assessment in conjunction with either handheld or implantable Doppler (Cook-Swartz implantable Doppler or coupler flow-Doppler). None of the adjunctive methods is ideal. Careful clinical assessment is imperative.

**Table 13.1** Frequency of flap monitoring: The MD Anderson recommendation

| Timing | Frequency |
|---|---|
| First 72 hours | Every hour |
| Days 4–5 | Every 2 hours |
| After Day 5 | Every 4 hours |

## Monitoring Buried Flaps

Although the handheld or implantable Doppler devices can be used to monitor buried flaps, their reliability remains a major concern.[11] One way to monitor a buried flap is to leave part of the flap outside the incision for clinical assessment. This part can be removed at beside before the patient is discharged from the hospital. This is commonly the practice when the jejunal flap is used for pharyngoesophageal reconstruction.[12] A small segment of the jejunum based on a separate branch of the mesentery vessel is externalized **(Fig. 13.1)**. Similarly, a part of the anterolateral thigh flap, either skin or muscle, based on a separate perforator or muscular branch, can be externalized for monitoring **(Fig. 13.2)**. A small segment of the radial forearm flap or ulnar artery perforator flap can also be externalized **(Fig. 13.3)**. Flap tissue of 2 × 3 cm or slightly larger is recommended for effective monitoring.[13]

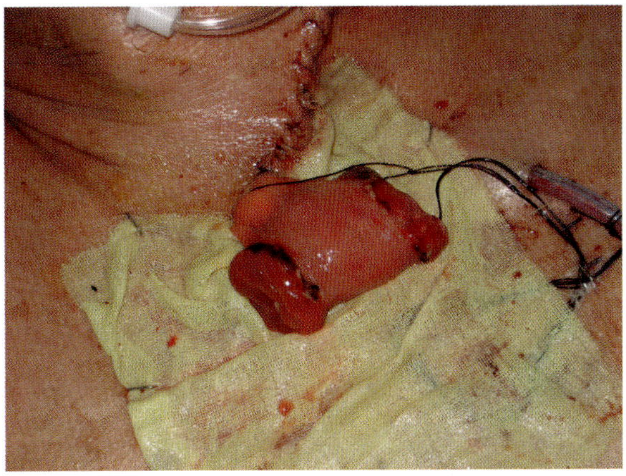

**Fig. 13.1** Monitoring a buried jejunal flap. A segment of jejunum based on two or three terminal mesentery branches is externalized through the neck incision for monitoring purposes. This segment is easily excised at the bedside before the patient is discharged from the hospital.

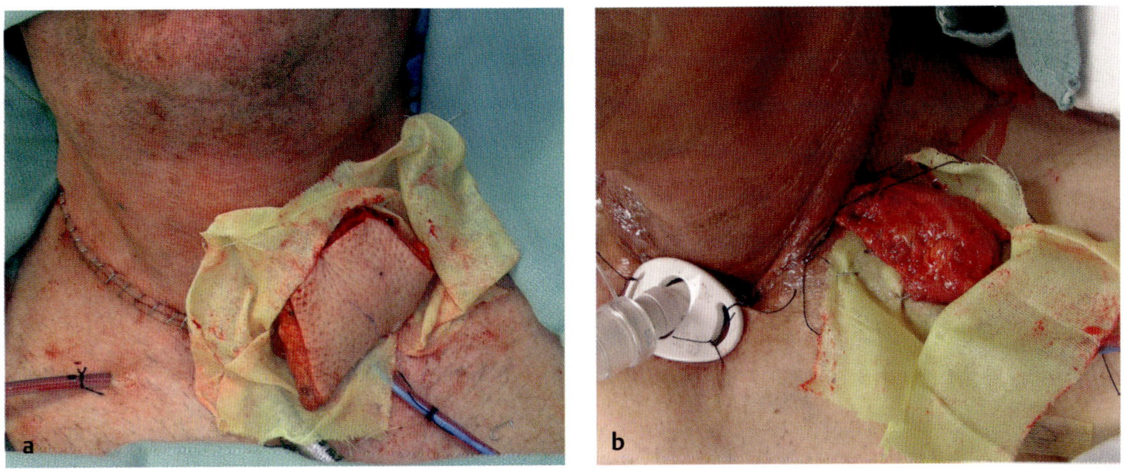

**Fig. 13.2** **(a)** Monitoring a buried anterolateral thigh (ALT) flap. A separate skin paddle based on a second cutaneous perforator is externalized through the neck incision for monitoring purposes, similar to the jejunal flap concept. **(b)** The monitoring skin is excised at bedside before discharge. In the absence of additional cutaneous perforators, a segment of the vastus lateralis muscle based on a muscular branch can be externalized for monitoring. The pink color of the muscle is easy to assess.

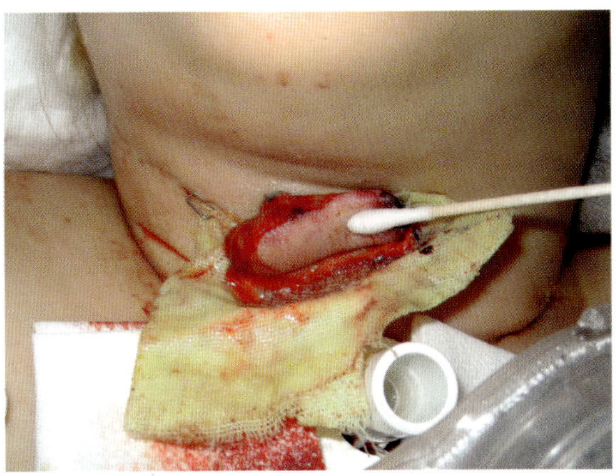

**Fig. 13.3** Monitoring a buried radial forearm flap. A small distal skin paddle of the radial forearm flap after de-epithelializing a strip of skin, or a separate proximal skin paddle based on a perforator, can be externalized. Similarly, a separate skin paddle based on a second perforator of the ulnar artery perforator flap can be externalized for monitoring.

## ■ Managing Surgical Complications

Surgical complications can occur at the donor site and recipient site (head and neck sites). In the recipient site, the most common surgical complications in the immediate postoperative period include flap pedicle thrombosis, hematoma, wound infection, wound dehiscence, and orocutaneous or pharyngocutaneous fistula. In the donor site, common complications include hematoma, seroma, wound infection, wound dehiscence, and loss of skin grafts.

### Pedicle Thrombosis

In our experience at MD Anderson Cancer Center, the prevalence of vascular compromise after head and neck free flap construction is 3.7% and the incidence of flap failure is 2.1%.[2] Venous thrombosis is more common than arterial thrombosis **(Table 13.2)**. Most failures occur in the first 24 hours **(Fig. 13.4)**. The most common cause for arterial failure is technical difficulties due to diseased vessels, small artery, and size mismatch. The most common cause for venous failure is mechanical compromise, such as kinking, tension, twisting, and compression. Overall, the flap salvage rate was 61% when flap compromise occurred within 72 hours and only 13% when it occurred more than 72 hours after surgery.[2]

When a flap compromise is suspected, immediate surgical exploration is mandatory. The incision is reopened and the vascular anastomoses are inspected for possible thrombosis or mechanical obstruction. If the venous congestion is the result of mechanical causes without thrombosis inside the vein, correction of the causes should immediately resolve flap congestion. The flap insetting and the position of the vascular pedicle should be carefully redone to correct these factors. If thrombosis is present, the anastomosis should be excised and thrombectomy should be performed. The vessels should be thoroughly irrigated with heparinized saline. An intravenous dose of 2500 to 3000 units of heparin is usually given before the thrombectomy. For simple mechanical obstructions or thrombosis, it is not necessary to continue heparin postoperatively. For difficult thrombosis or rethrombosis, we usually prefer a low-dose heparin intravenous infusion for 3 to 5 days at 500 units per hour. The diseased or injured segment of the vessel should be excised and replaced with a vein graft if necessary.

If no venous outflow is observed after establishing the arterial inflow, thrombosis may be present in the microcirculation within the flap. To dissolve the microthrombi, thrombolytic agents, such as tissue plasminogen activator (TPA), can be injected into the pedicle artery, either via opening a side branch or using a 30-gauge needle. There is no established dosage of TPA for free flap salvage. We typically start with 2 to 4 mg diluted to 1 mg/mL, based on our own experience. A repeat injection can be given after 20 minutes or so if needed. In the meantime, the surgical field should be gently irrigated with warm saline and covered with a warm towel to avoid vessel spasm. It may take 20 to 30 minutes for the flap to regain perfusion after such management. Once good venous outflow is obtained, the vein can be left open to drain out the thrombolytic agents in the flap before re-anastomosing the veins to avoid systemic effect of thrombolytic agents.

**Table 13.2** Timing of arterial and venous failures

| | **Artery** | | **Vein** | |
|---|---|---|---|---|
| **Timing** | Occlusion | Failure | Occlusion | Failure |
| < 24 hours | 8 | 7 | 14 | 4 |
| 24–48 hours | 2 | 0 | 3 | 1 |
| 48–72 hours | 1 | 0 | 5 | 1 |
| 72 hours–7 days | 1 | 1 | 7 | 5 |
| > 7 days | 0 | 0 | 2 | 2 |
| Total | 12 | 8 (67%) | 31 | 13 (42%) |

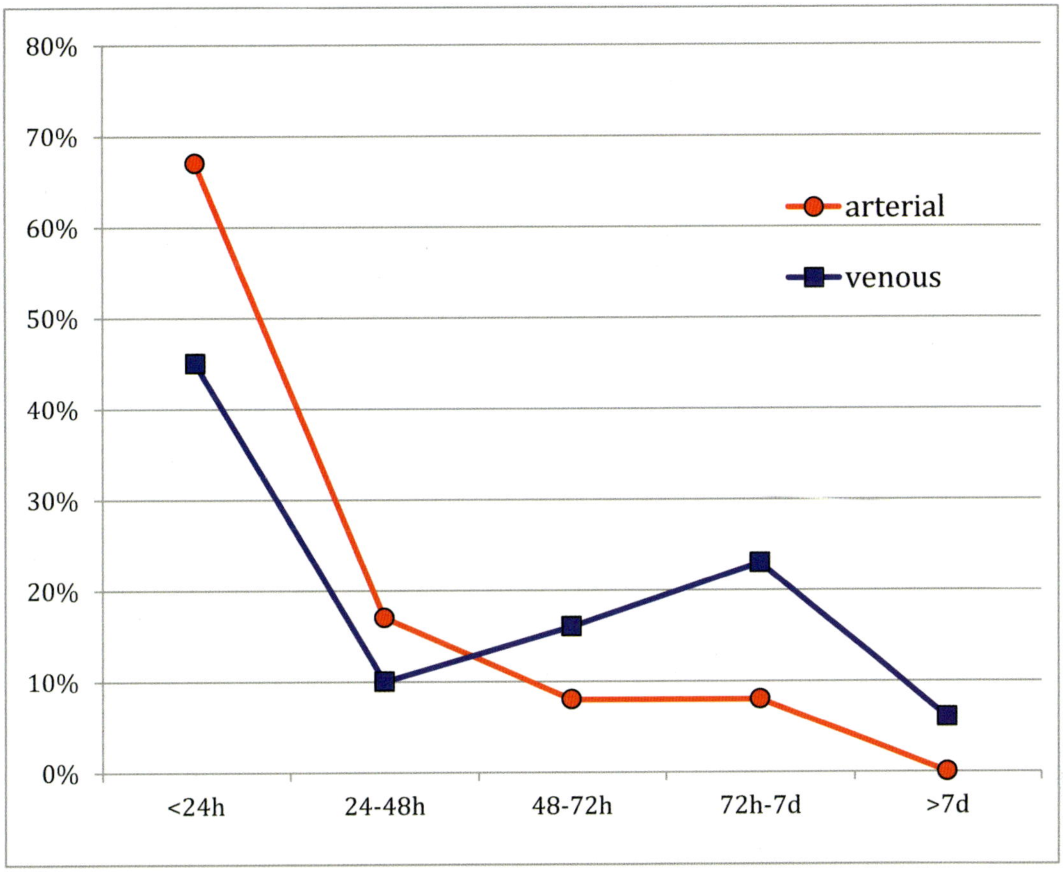


**Fig. 13.4** Timing of arterial and venous compromise following free flap reconstruction for head and neck defects at the MD Anderson Cancer Center between 1996 and 2005.

## Hematoma

Reasons for hematoma include general oozing from the surgical bed, inadequate cautery or ligation of the vessels, and reopening of the vessels after hypertension or agitation. Hematoma in the head and neck region should be evacuated immediately in the operating room because most, if not all, hematomas will get infected due to long exposure and contamination. In addition, hematoma can compress the flap pedicle, causing pedicle thrombosis, or it may be a sign of thrombosis of the vein at the anastomosis, causing blood to ooze from the flap. Thorough exploration of the surgical field should be performed, and the flap vascular pedicle should also be explored for bleeding. After hematoma evacuation and proper hemostasis, the entire surgical field should be thoroughly irrigated with normal saline and possibly antibiotic-containing saline to minimize the risk of infection. Care should be taken not to irrigate the saline directly on the vascular pedicle, which may cause spasm and thrombosis.

Large hematomas in the donor site should be explored, while small hematomas without active bleeding can be observed. Such hematomas will usually liquefy after 7 to 10 days, and increased drainage of dark blood can be observed in donor-site drains.

## Wound Infection

Neck wound infection usually occurs between 5 and 10 days after surgery, most commonly around 6 or 7 days. The infection rate is reported to be between 10% and 20% after a major surgery and reconstruction. The main reason for such a high wound infection rate is the prolonged contamination at the time of surgery. Any dead space, nonviable tissue, or hematoma can cause infection; therefore, they should be taken care of promptly. Including a small amount of flap muscle can be a very effective way to eliminate dead space and minimize infection. Thorough irrigation of the wound at the end of surgery is also important. Several liters of normal saline or antibiotic solution may be needed to irrigate a large wound.

Although many patients manifest with a fever, increased white blood cell count, and erythema and swelling around the incision, clinical manifestations may be very subtle in some patients, such as the elderly, diabetic, and immunocompromised. Once an early infection is suspected, incision and drainage in the operating room with adequate exposure should be performed, followed by thorough débridement and irrigation. Cultures should be taken during surgical exploration. Intravenous antibiotic therapy is also initiated. For early wound infections without dead space, the neck incision can potentially be closed primarily over a drain or only a small portion of the incision left open for dressing changes after a thorough débridement. Incision and drainage of the wound infection should not be delayed, because infection may cause flap pedicle thrombosis and flap loss. Thrombosis due to infection is extremely difficult to salvage.

## Wound Dehiscence or Skin Graft Loss

Small wound dehiscence either at the donor site or recipient site can be managed with dressing changes to allow secondary healing. Surgical closure of the wound dehiscence in the head and neck region is unlikely to succeed. Partial skin graft loss at the donor site can also be managed with dressing changes. Large areas of skin graft loss or wound dehiscence can be managed with a vacuum-assisted closure (wound VAC).

## Leaks and Fistulas

Leaks are defined as radiographic leaks without a clinical fistula, while a fistula is defined as a clinically evident fistulation between the oropharyngeal cavity and the outside skin. Leaks are discovered during an MBS study. Small leaks without clinical infection or fistula can be observed conservatively and oral intake must be delayed. A repeat MBS is performed 2 weeks later to re-evaluate the leak. Most leaks heal spontaneously within 2 weeks.

Small fistulas can also be observed conservatively, and they should heal spontaneously within 2 to 4 weeks. Large leaks with fluid collection, dead space, or infection should be taken care of surgically. Serial irrigation and débridement may be necessary. After débridement, a muscle flap, such as a sternocleidomastoid muscle or pectoralis major muscle flap, can be used to obliterate the dead space, which should also be placed over the flap dehiscence from the oral or pharyngeal mucosa. Attempt to close the dehiscence at this stage is usually unsuccessful and may cause more tearing of the surrounding tissue. A muscle flap can effectively heal dehiscence and fistulas.

## Pearls and Pitfalls

- Meticulous postoperative care is critical not only to patient recovery but also to prevent flap loss due to unsatisfactory fluid volume status and problems with positioning, which can cause pedicle or flap compression.
- Clinical monitoring for flap color, temperature, turgor, and capillary refill continues to be the gold standard.
- Emergent return to the operating room is essential for flap salvage.
- Flap salvage requires accurate diagnosis of the etiology of flap compromise so that measures can be taken to correct the inciting event and to prevent it from recurring.
- Hematomas should generally all be evacuated and explored, since they can be associated with ongoing blood loss, infection, pedicle compression, or venous obstruction.
- Early purulent infections should be incised and drained, then irrigated and débrided in the operating room, since infections can lead to pedicle thrombosis as well as systemic illness. Culture-directed antibiotics should also be administered.

### References

1. Chen KT, Mardini S, Chuang DC, et al. Timing of presentation of the first signs of vascular compromise dictates the salvage outcome of free flap transfers. Plast Reconstr Surg 2007;120(1):187–195
2. Yu P, Chang DW, Miller MJ, Reece G, Robb GL. Analysis of 49 cases of flap compromise in 1310 free flaps for head and neck reconstruction. Head Neck 2009;31(1):45–51
3. Cho BC, Shin DP, Byun JS, Park JW, Baik BS. Monitoring flap for buried free tissue transfer: its importance and reliability. Plast Reconstr Surg 2002;110(5):1249–1258
4. Fernando B, Young VL, Logan SE. Miniature implantable laser Doppler probe monitoring of free tissue transfer. Ann Plast Surg 1988;20(5):434–442
5. Kind GM, Buntic RF, Buncke GM, Cooper TM, Siko PP, Buncke HJ Jr. The effect of an implantable Doppler probe on the salvage of microvascular tissue transplants. Plast Reconstr Surg 1998;101(5):1268–1273, discussion 1274–1275
6. Rand RP, Cramer MM, Strandness DE Jr. Color-flow duplex scanning in the preoperative assessment of TRAM flap perforators: a report of 32 consecutive patients. Plast Reconstr Surg 1994;93(3):453–459
7. Raskin DJ, Erk Y, Spira M, Melissinos EG. Tissue pH monitoring in microsurgery: a preliminary evaluation of continuous tissue pH monitoring as an indicator of perfusion disturbances in microvascular free flaps. Ann Plast Surg 1983;11(4):331–339

8. Solomon GA, Yaremchuk MJ, Manson PN. Doppler ultrasound surface monitoring of both arterial and venous flow in clinical free tissue transfers. J Reconstr Microsurg 1986;3(1):39–41
9. Swartz WM, Izquierdo R, Miller MJ. Implantable venous Doppler microvascular monitoring: laboratory investigation and clinical results. Plast Reconstr Surg 1994;93(1):152–163
10. Swartz WM, Jones NF, Cherup L, Klein A. Direct monitoring of microvascular anastomoses with the 20-MHz ultrasonic Doppler probe: an experimental and clinical study. Plast Reconstr Surg 1988;81(2):149–161
11. Rosenberg JJ, Fornage BD, Chevray PM. Monitoring buried free flaps: limitations of the implantable Doppler and use of color duplex sonography as a confirmatory test. Plast Reconstr Surg 2006;118(1):109–113, discussion 114–115
12. Reece GP, Bengtson BP, Schusterman MA. Reconstruction of the pharynx and cervical esophagus using free jejunal transfer. Clin Plast Surg 1994;21(1):125–136
13. Ferguson RE Jr, Yu P. Techniques of monitoring buried fasciocutaneous free flaps. Plast Reconstr Surg 2009; 123(2):525–532

# 14 Management of Osteoradionecrosis of the Mandible

*Peirong Yu*

## Introduction

Osteoradionecrosis (ORN) of the mandible is a serious complication of radiotherapy that causes significant morbidity and loss of quality of life. The definition of ORN is still somewhat controversial. The general consensus is that ORN is defined as an area of nonhealing bone persisting for several months (2 to 6 months) in the absence of recurrent tumor.[1,2] Furthermore, early stages of ORN can present without evidence of intraoral mucosal disruption.

Not all patients who undergo radiation therapy in the head and neck region will develop ORN. It is difficult to determine which subset of patients is at risk for developing ORN. The prevalence ranges from 5 to 15%.[3,4] When chemotherapy is added to radiotherapy, the incidence of ORN may be increased, whereas the use of intensity-modulated radiotherapy may reduce it.[5] Factors that are thought to affect the development of ORN include size and intraoral location of the tumor, dose of radiation, mandibular surgery, dental extractions, infection, immune status, and malnutrition.[6] Many patients with oral cancer have other serious systemic diseases and have often had a long history of alcohol and tobacco misuse. These, combined with poor nutrition and unsatisfactory oral hygiene, place such patients at high risk of developing ORN.

The goals of treating ORN are to prevent progression of early ORN and to eliminate the irradiated, irreversibly damaged tissue and to replace it with well-vascularized tissue.

## Mechanisms of Osteoradionecrosis

### Radiation-Induced Cell Injury

At the cellular level, radiation causes direct DNA damage via the formation of hydroxyl free radicals. Because the effect of radiation on DNA occurs during mitotic division, the guiding principle in radiation therapy is targeting cancer cells with high mitotic activity and cell turnover; therefore, early radiation injury is the result of depletion of cells that have a high mitotic rate. Late radiation injury develops in cells that have a longer cell cycle and protracted cell turnover, so late effects do not manifest until much later in time. Several studies have shown that a radiation dose of greater than 54 Gy or 66 Gy is significantly associated with ORN.[7,8]

Radiation-induced bone injury begins as reactive hyperemia and subsequent inflammation, a potentially reversible stage.[6,9,10] As injury progresses, microvascular thrombosis and loss of osteocytes occur, causing osteoclastic resorption and reduced bone regeneration. The combination of death of osteoblasts, failure of osteoblasts to repopulate, and excessive proliferation of myofibroblasts results in a reduction in bony matrix and its replacement with fibrous tissues. Finally, progressive fibrosis results in mechanical destabilization and subsequent pathologic fracture.

ORN affects the mandible more often than the maxilla or any other bones of the head and neck. The location of ORN within the mandible varies based on dentition, blood supply, and surgical trauma.[11] The body of the mandible is most commonly affected, followed by the angle, symphysis, and ramus. The dominant blood supply to the body of the mandible is the inferior alveolar artery, and radiation causes obliteration of this artery. The most vulnerable site of the mandibular body is the premolar, molar, and retromolar cortex, owing to the lack of muscular attachments and primary dependence on the inferior alveolar artery for its blood supply.[7,12]

## Clinical Presentation

ORN can develop spontaneously or as the result of a traumatic insult. Spontaneous ORN usually occurs late. ORN, however, can develop quickly following even minor injury.[13] This can occur after dental extraction, surgical biopsy, chronic irritation due to ill-fitting dental appliances, or by exposure of irradiated bone secondary to overlying soft tissue necrosis. The majority of patients develop ORN within the first 3 years of completing radiation therapy.[7]

The radiation injury in ORN extends far beyond bone and affects all tissue types. There is mucosal disruption and dysfunction, salivary gland failure resulting in decreased production of salivary enzymes, xerostomia, parotid inflammation, and fibrosis. Soft tissue contracture and temporomandibular joint (TMJ) dysfunction cause trismus, which further affects oral hygiene and causes worsening of ORN.

Several ORN classifications have been described.[4,14] It is generally accepted that early (stage I) ORN involves only the superficial cortical bone, with minimal soft tissue ulceration. The majority of patients with stage I ORN may be treated with conservative management. Stage II involves both the cortical bone and underlying medullary bone. In stage III, there is diffuse involvement of the mandible that causes fracture and fistula formation.

Diagnosis of ORN can be established by clinical manifestations and imaging studies. Clinical presentations of ORN include: (1) pain, which is present in 90% of patients; (2) exposed bone, which is present in 50 to 60% of patients; (3) trismus, present in 40 to 50% of patients; (4) pathologic fractures; and (6) orocutaneous fistula.

Radiologic evaluation includes a Panorex plain film to evaluate the entire mandible for cortical erosion and fracture. CT scan of the head and neck can be useful in evaluating soft tissue involvement, potential tumor recurrence, and status of the neck for recipient vessel selection. A biopsy of the area is performed to exclude the possibility of tumor recurrence, as up to 10% of ORN patients may harbor recurrent disease.[7]

# ■ Treatment of Osteoradionecrosis of the Mandible

The best treatment for ORN is prevention. The first step is to identify potential risk factors in all patients undergoing radiation therapy. Maintaining adequate oral hygiene, fluoride supplement treatments, properly fitting oral appliances, and frequent intraoral exams and follow-up visits with dental oncologists are the mainstays of preventative care for radiated patients. Dental health is particularly important in the prevention of ORN. Thorough dental screening must be performed prior to radiation therapy to identify teeth with caries or gingival disease that might serve as portals for chronic irritation and wounds that can lead to ORN. Addressing these problems prior to radiation therapy, with extractions in a nonradiated field, is far preferable to postradiation dental extractions. Postradiation dental extractions have a higher rate of complications from nonhealing sockets that allow exposed alveolar bone to become desiccated and necrotic. In the event that postradiation dental surgery becomes necessary, perioperative hyperbaric oxygen (HBO) therapy has been shown to reduce the incidence of ORN.[15]

Stage I ORN usually responds well to conservative care, while a Stage III ORN will require radical débridement and free flap reconstruction. Patients with Stage II ORN are usually managed with conservative therapy first, including antibiotics, débridement, sequestrectomy, HBO, and pharmacotherapy.[16,17] Cases of refractory Stage II ORN may need surgical resection and reconstruction.

## Hyperbaric Oxygen Therapy

HBO, first described in the early 1980s, had a much more prominent role in treating ORN due to the limited surgical options at the time. The rationale for using HBO is that saturating the oxygen level to superphysiologic levels may augment oxygen tension in tissues and improve wound healing. Marx was an early pioneer of the use of HBO therapy for ORN and the Marx protocol is still widely used today.[1] His protocol was designed to identify patients who would respond to HBO without surgery and to recognize patients with progressive disease who would require surgical intervention. The outcomes of HBO therapy, however, remain controversial. Several studies, including a randomized controlled study, have shown no benefit of HBO.[11,18,19]

## Pharmacotherapy

The use of antioxidant and antifibrotic drugs has been popularized recently for prophylaxis and treatment of ORN. Pentoxifylline is a notable candidate. It is a methylxanthine derivative that exerts an anti-TNFa effect, increases erythrocyte flexibility, dilates blood vessels, and inhibits inflammatory reactions in vivo. Pentoxifylline is combined with tocopherol for antifibrotic effect. Tocopherol counteracts the reactive oxygen species that were generated during oxidative stress by protecting cell membranes against peroxidation of lipids, against partial inhibition of TGF-b1, and against expression of procollagen genes, thus reducing fibrosis.[20] The two drugs act synergistically as potent antifibrotic agents and have been shown to be effective in the treatment of ORN.[21]

## Surgical Management

### Indications for Surgery

1. Intractable pain unresponsive to conservative treatment. Surgical resection of necrotic bone provides immediate relief of pain.
2. Pathologic fractures
3. Orocutaneous fistula
4. Osteomyelitis

### Goals of Surgical Management

1. Control of pain
2. Control of infection
3. Thorough débridement: removal of all dead bone and soft tissue.
4. Repair of orocutaneous fistula
5. Reconstruction of bony defects
6. Restoration of function and form

### Preoperative Assessment and Surgical Planning

Thorough understanding of the bony and soft tissue defect is essential for surgical planning. A head and neck CT scan is required to assess the extent of bone necrosis and to rule out cancer recurrence. A CT scan will also provide information about neck recipient blood vessels for free flap reconstruction. ORN with orocutaneous fistulas is often associated with the worst frozen neck. Reconstruction can be extremely difficult, and a careful operative plan is of paramount importance. Medical evaluation is also important, since surgery can be difficult and lengthy. Donor-site assessment usually includes fibula, anterolateral thigh flap, and radial forearm donor sites. For through-and-through defects, more than one free flap may be needed for reconstruction. Functional and aesthetic outcomes for through-and-through defects are usually suboptimal. The patient and family need to be well informed. Long-term antibiotic therapy is also required before and after surgery; usually, a 6-week course is given.

### Clinical Classification of Mandibular Osteoradionecrosis Defects

Mandibular ORN is a complex surgical problem. Reconstruction of ORN defects depends on the extent of bony involvement and on the soft tissue involvement. To guide reconstruction, a simple and practical classification system was created by the author (**Table 14.1**). Type I is a segmental bony defect. It is further divided into Ia and Ib according to the extent of soft tissue defect. Type II is a posterior defect or hemimandibular defect. Similarly, it is further classified as IIa and IIb based on the extent of soft tissue defect. A careful surgical plan should be formed for each individual patient depending on the type of defect.

**Table 14.1** Classification of mandibular osteoradionecrosis defects and treatment options by type

| Defect | Type Ia | Type Ib | Type IIa | Type IIb |
|---|---|---|---|---|
| Bony defect | Segmental | Segmental | Posterior or hemimandibular | Posterior or hemimandibular |
| Condyle | Intact | Intact | Removed | Removed |
| Mucosal defect | Yes | Yes | Yes | Yes |
| External skin defect | No | Yes | No | Yes |
| Option 1 | Fibular bone-only flap | Two-skin-island fibular or fibular OC + soleus | Fibular OC or iliac crest osteocutaneous flap | Two-skin-island fibular or fibular OC + soleus |
| Option 2 | Iliac crest or scapula | Double free flaps (fibular OC + ALT, fibular OC + RFF) | ALT with or without VL | ALT with two skin islands or one-skin-island ALT with VL |
| Option 3 | | Fibular OC + Pec flap | | |
| Option 4 | | Remove condyle, two-skin-island ALT | | |

ALT, anterolateral thigh; OC, osteocutaneous; Pec, pectoralis major; RFF, radial forearm flap; VL, vastus lateralis muscle.

## Management of Mandibular Osteoradionecrosis Defects by Type

### Type Ia Defects

A type Ia defect is typically a lateral segmental defect with an intact condyle **(Fig. 14.1)**. Because of the intact condyle and ramus, this type of defect is best reconstructed with a bone flap to maximize function. Our preferred flap is the fibular osteocutaneous flap with a skin paddle to reconstruct the intraoral soft tissue defect **(Fig. 14.2)**. Because of the fibrosis, one should always expect the intraoral mucosal defect to be larger than it appears. Therefore, a larger skin paddle should be planned. In this type of defect, neck fibrosis is mild or moderate and ipsilateral recipient vessels are usually available in the external carotid system, such as the facial or lingual artery and the facial vein or internal jugular vein. Near-normal oral function and reasonable aesthetic results can be expected after reconstruction.

### Type Ib Defects

Because of soft tissue defects both intraorally and externally, type Ib defects are more difficult to reconstruct. In addition, these patients usually have long-standing orocutaneous fistulas and repeated episodes of osteomyelitis **(Fig. 14.3)** resulting in

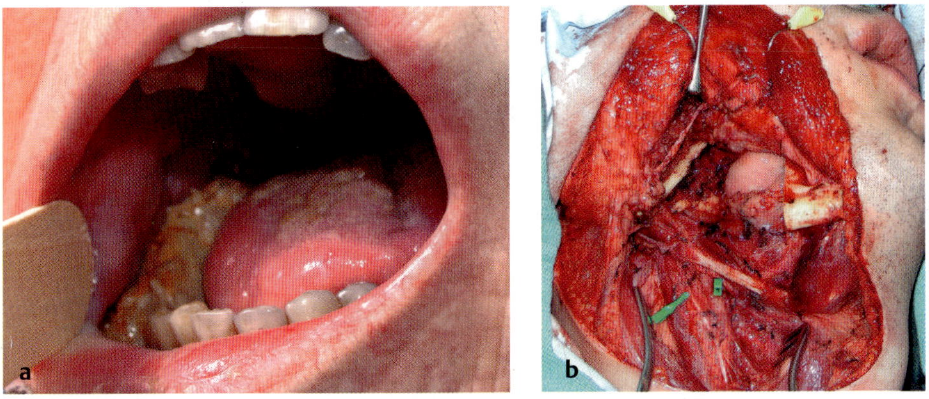

**Fig. 14.1** **(a)** Osteoradionecrosis (ORN) involving the body and retromolar trigone of the right mandible. **(b)** Surgical resection of ORN in this patient resulted in a lateral segmental defect, a type Ia defect.

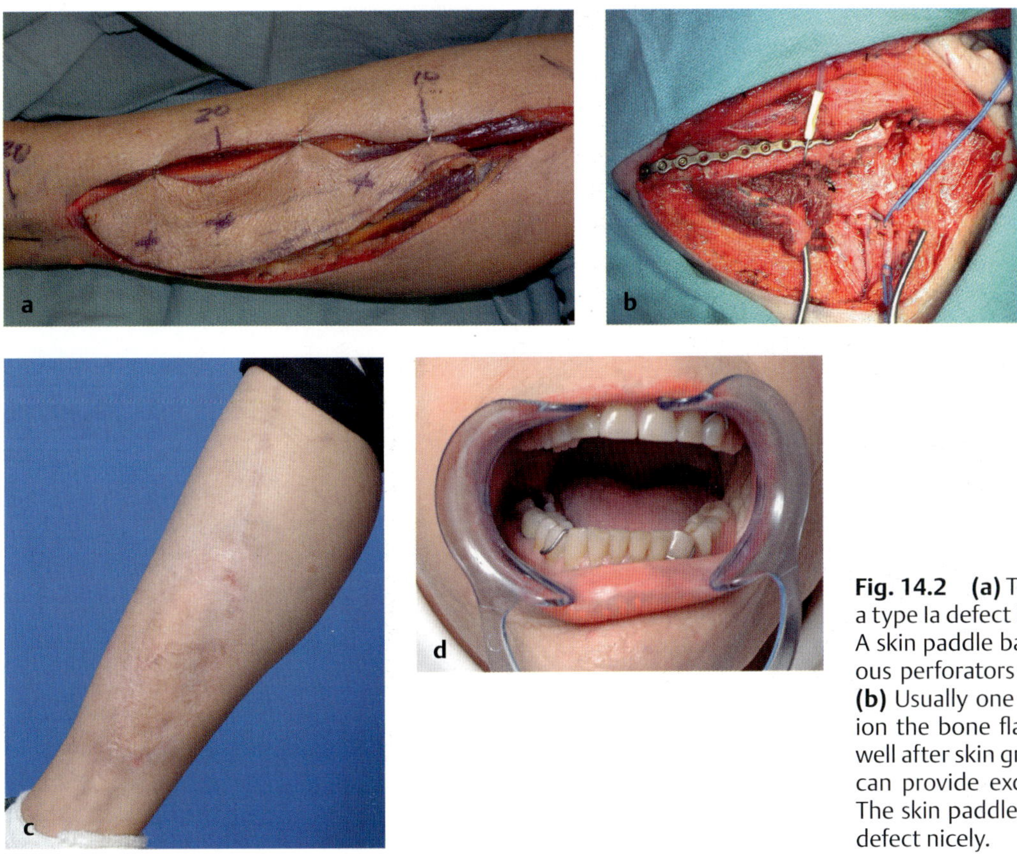

**Fig. 14.2** **(a)** The preferred flap to reconstruct a type Ia defect is a fibular osteocutaneous flap. A skin paddle based on the distal septocutaneous perforators is included for intraoral lining. **(b)** Usually one osteotomy is required to fashion the bone flap. **(c)** Donor site usually heals well after skin grafting. **(d)** Bone reconstruction can provide excellent occlusion and function. The skin paddle covers the intraoral soft tissue defect nicely.

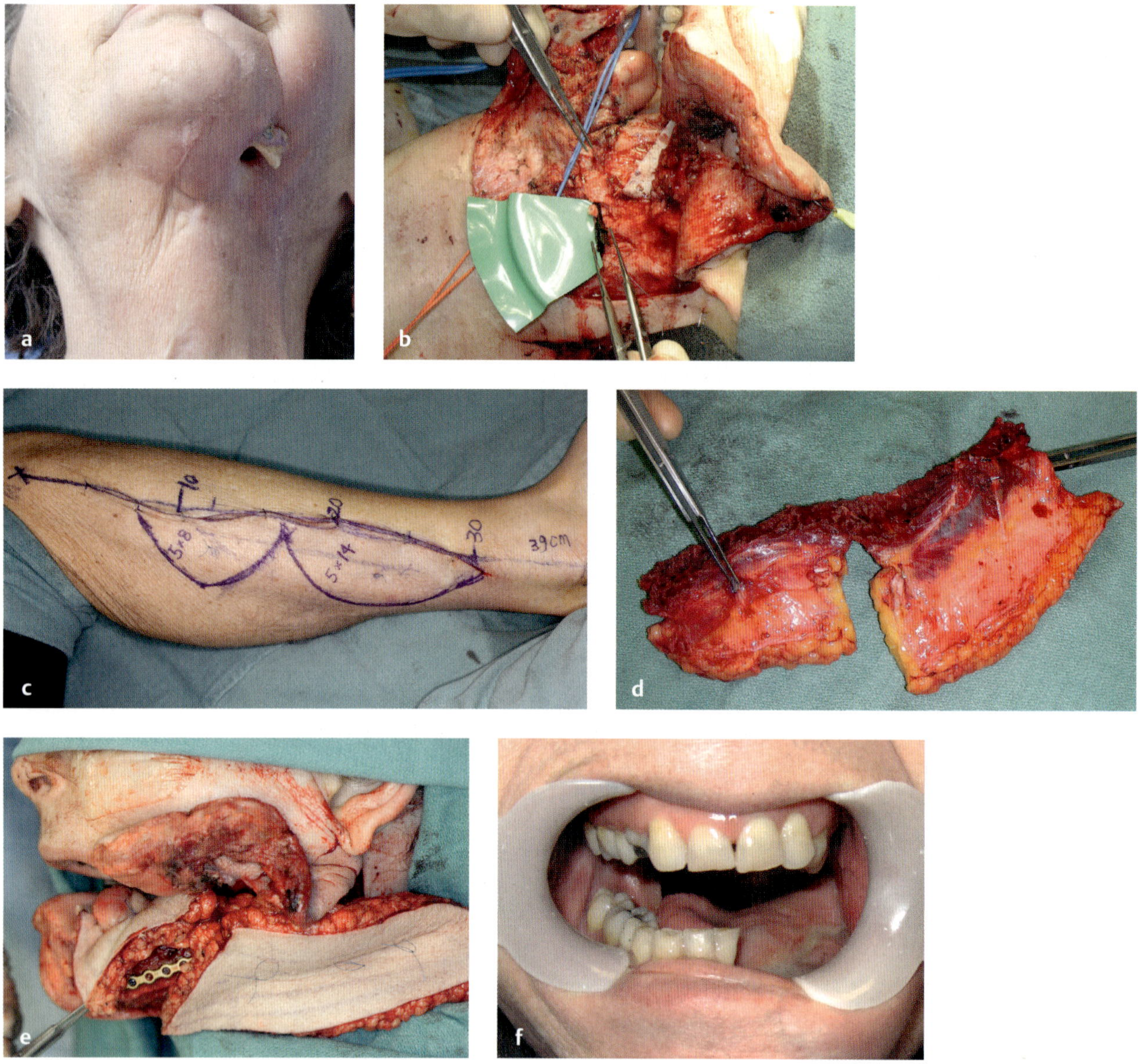


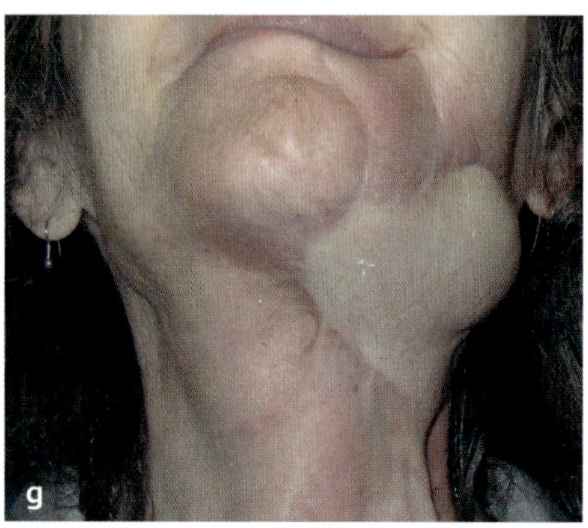


**Fig. 14.3** **(a)** A patient with a type Ib defect. Fracture, osteomyelitis, and orocutaneous fistula are present. **(b)** Surgical resection resulted in a through-and-through defect. **(c,d)** A two-skin-island fibular osteocutaneous flap was designed. **(e)** The distal skin paddle was used for intraoral lining and the second proximal skin paddle was used for external skin coverage. **(f,g)** Both the external and intraoral skin paddles healed well.

severe neck fibrosis, which makes recipient vessel dissection extremely difficult. The goals of reconstruction are to provide bone continuity as well as intraoral coverage and external neck resurfacing. The reconstructive options are as follows.

### Option 1. Two-Skin-Island Fibular Osteocutaneous Flap

The reconstruction would be simplest if a single flap could provide all three components: bone, intraoral coverage, and external resurfacing. We have shown in our recent study that the fibular flap can potentially meet these requirements.[22] Two distinct groups of peroneal artery perforators are present in the lateral aspect of the lower leg along the fibular flap territory **(Fig. 14.4)**. The distal perforators, ranging from one to three in number, are located in the third quarter of the fibular length **(Fig. 14.5)**. These perforators are the primary perforators for the traditional fibular flap skin paddle. This skin paddle is usually used for the intraoral mucosal defect due to its thinness and close association with the bone segment that is used for mandibular reconstruction. A distinct proximal perforator can also be found at one-third of the length from the fibular head. A skin paddle based on this perforator is usually independent from the bone (the proximal bone is usually discarded) and can be easily turned outward for external neck resurfacing. Since the perforator to the second skin paddle is usually quite a distance away from the first one, it can reach a defect that is also distant from the intraoral defect **(Fig. 14.6)**.

Because of the chronic frozen neck, recipient vessels may be hard to find. The external carotid system is still the first option to explore. The lingual artery is usually available, while the facial artery usually has been removed at the previous surgery. The external carotid artery itself can be used as a recipient artery. The internal jugular vein is usually available as a

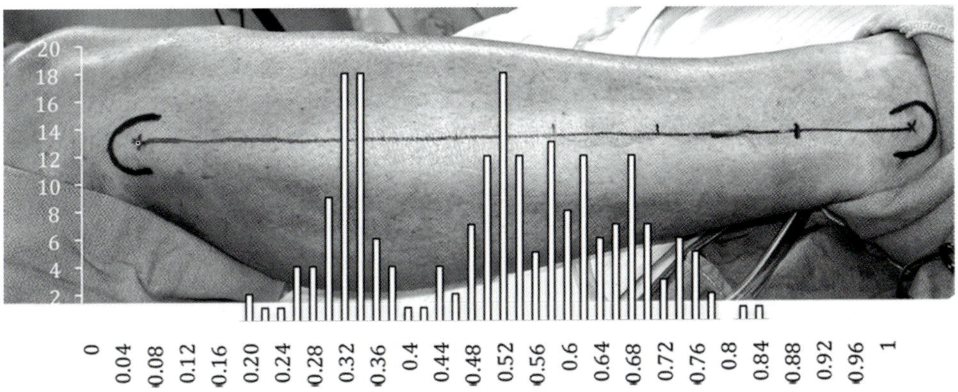


**Fig. 14.4** Peroneal artery perforator distribution. Two distinct groups of perforators are present. The distal perforators are located within the third quarter of the fibula and the proximal one at one-third the distance from the fibular head.

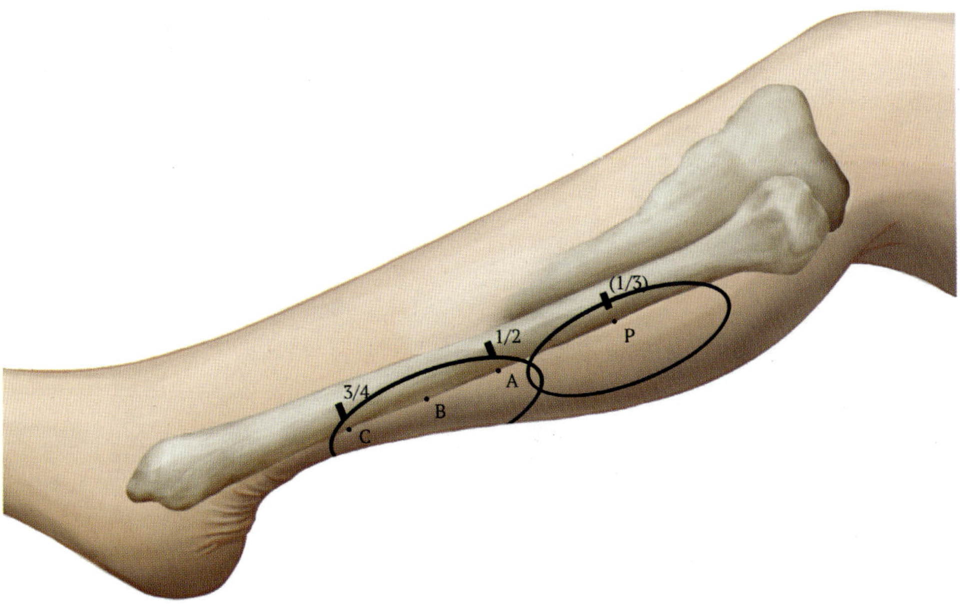


**Fig. 14.5** Two separate skin paddles can be designed based on the two distinct groups of perforators.

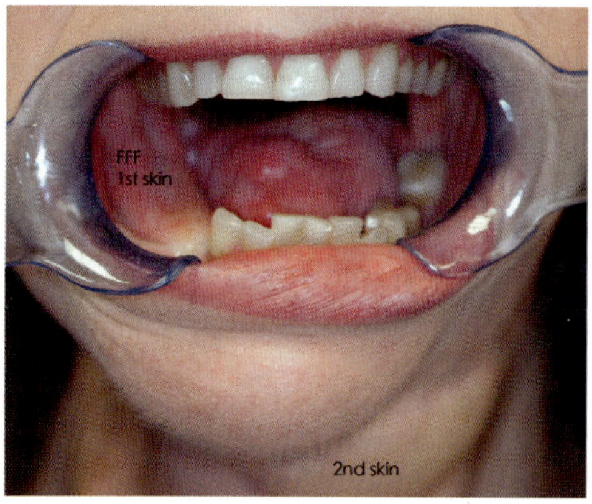


**Fig. 14.6** The second proximal skin paddle is usually outside the fibular bone segment. It can be used to cover an external defect at a distance from the bone defect.

recipient vein. If it has been removed during a previous neck dissection, the external jugular vein in the lower neck would be the second choice. If the external carotid system is not available, the transverse cervical vessels are explored over the clavicle, as is discussed in another chapter. The contralateral neck vessels can also be used.

### *Option 2. One-Skin-Island Fibular Osteocutaneous Flap with Soleus Muscle and Skin Grafting*

The proximal peroneal artery perforator is usable in 85 to 90% of patients. In some patients, this perforator is absent, is too small, or originates form a different source vessel (posterior tibial artery or popliteal artery). In these situations, inclusion of some of the soleus muscle proximally can provide additional coverage. The skin paddle is usually placed intraorally and the muscle is placed extraorally with split-thickness skin grafting **(Fig. 14.7)**. Since the soleus muscle pedicle is more proximally located, away from the skin paddle, there is more freedom to position the muscle away from the bone defect if necessary. Skin grafts on the soleus muscle heal well.

### *Option 3. Double Free Flap Reconstruction*

Larger defects may exceed the skin paddle size the fibular flap can provide, requiring a second flap. In some cases, a second free flap may give better functional outcomes (for example, for a simultaneous tongue reconstruction). Depending on the size of the defects, the second soft tissue free flap can be placed either intraorally or externally. The anterolateral thigh flap is the most commonly used second flap for this purpose **(Fig. 14.8)**. This flap can be harvested from the same leg as the fibular flap. The fibular osteocutaneous flap is usually harvested first. Insetting and revascularization of the fibular flap are performed first, before the anterolateral thigh flap. If a thinner and/or smaller flap is needed, the radial forearm flap or a lateral arm flap can be used **(Fig. 14.9)**. Both the radial forearm and lateral arm flap provide better color match with the facial skin, while the anterolateral thigh flap is usually much lighter than facial skin color.

The disadvantage of double free flap reconstruction is certainly the complexity. In addition, availability of recipient vessels may be limited and additional recipient vessel sites may need to be explored **(Fig. 14.8a)**. If planned well, a second free flap may add only 2 hours of operating time, not much longer than performing a pedicled pectoralis major flap.

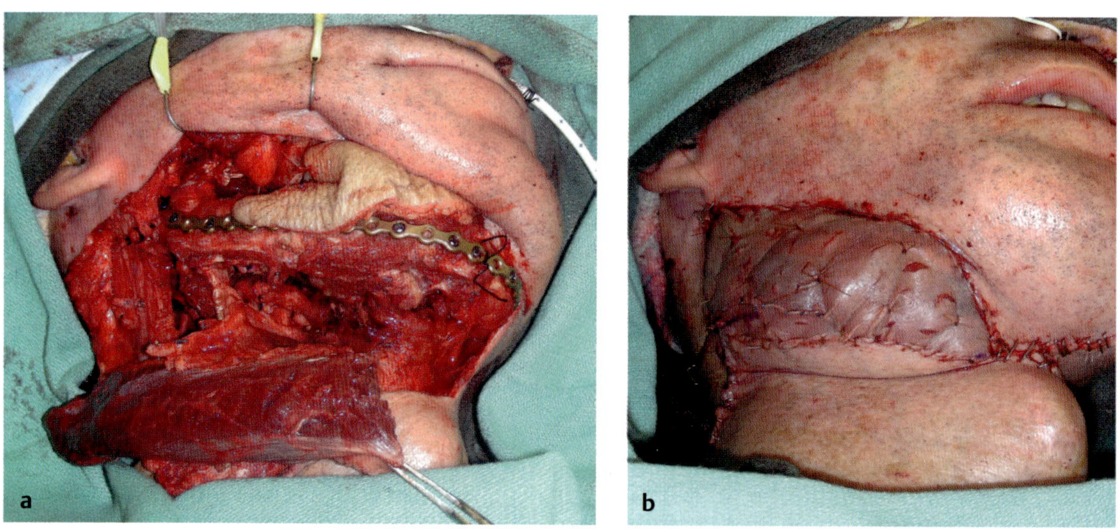


**Fig. 14.7** (**a**) The soleus muscle can be included in the fibular flap for external skin coverage with split-thickness skin grafting, (**b**) while the skin paddle is used for intraoral coverage.

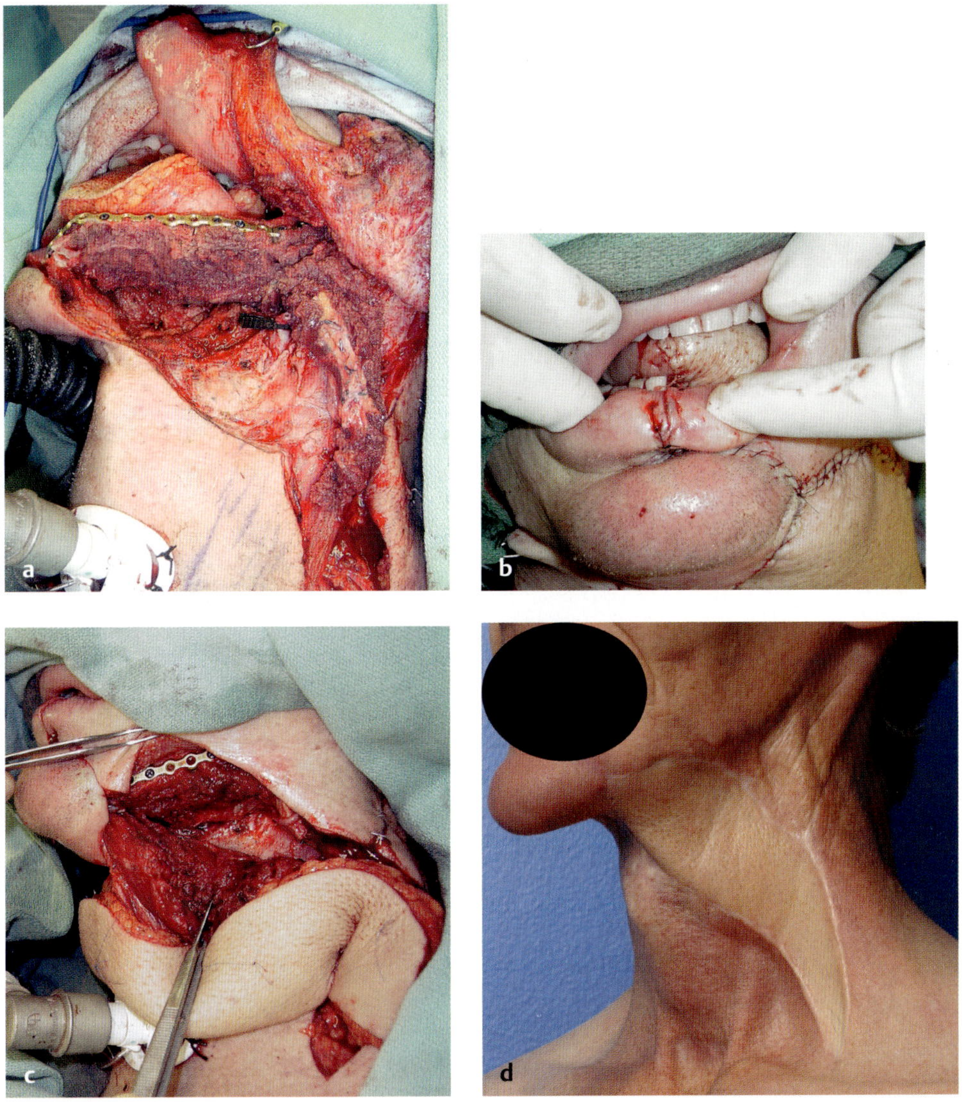


**Fig. 14.8** **(a,b)** Double free flap reconstruction of a type Ib defect. In this patient, a fibular osteocutaneous flap was used for bone reconstruction with the skin paddle for intraoral coverage. **(c,d)** An anterolateral thigh free flap was used for external skin coverage. **(a)** Recipient vessels included the external carotid artery and the transverse cervical vessels.

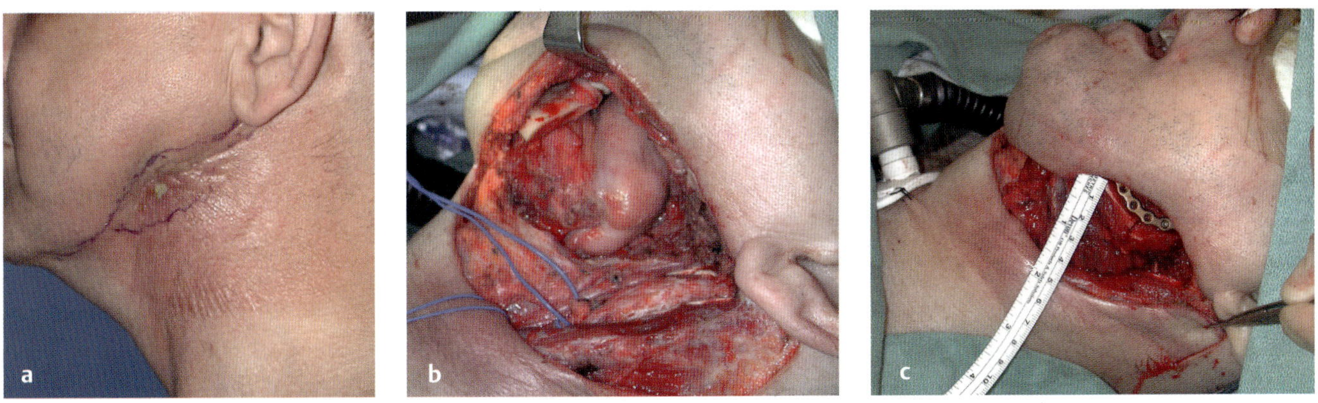


**Fig. 14.9** (**a,b**) Another patient with osteoradionecrosis of the lateral mandible with a type Ib defect. **(c)** A fibular osteocutaneous flap was used for bone and intraoral reconstruction. (*Continued on page 196*)

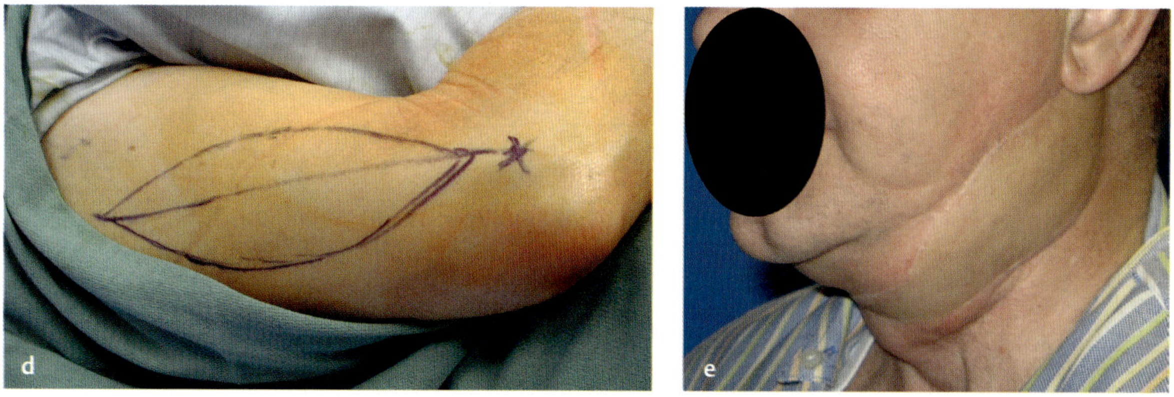

Fig. 14.9 (*Continued*) **(d)** A second flap, a lateral arm free flap, was used for external skin coverage. **(e)** The lateral arm flap has a better color match with cheek skin.

### *Option 4. Fibular Osteocutaneous Flap with a Pectoralis Major Muscle or Myocutaneous Flap*

The pectoralis major flap can be used for external skin coverage while the fibula flap skin paddle is used for intraoral coverage. The pectoralis major muscle can reach the upper neck and along the mandibular border (**Fig. 14.10**). In male patients, a skin paddle can be included. In female patients, the design and reliability of the skin paddle can be a problem. We prefer using the muscle alone with skin grafting. To increase the arc of rotation and also minimize the bulk in the lower neck, the vascular pedicle should be islanded and the proximal muscle not included.

The main disadvantage of using the pectoralis muscle is the downward force exerted as the muscle atrophies and fibroses, potentially causing neck contracture and displacement of the lower lip resulting in drooling and oral incompetence. The muscle bulk in the neck can also be aesthetically unpleasing, especially if the flap is not islanded.

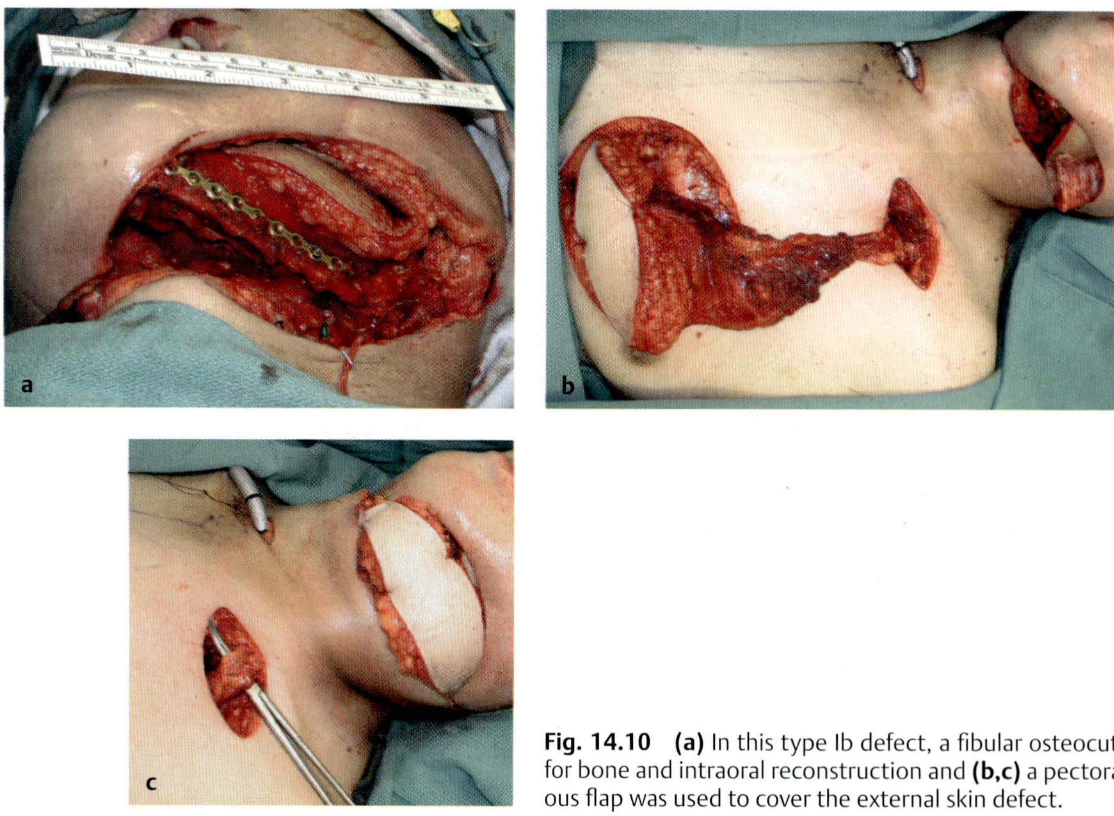

**Fig. 14.10** **(a)** In this type Ib defect, a fibular osteocutaneous flap was used for bone and intraoral reconstruction and **(b,c)** a pectoralis major myocutaneous flap was used to cover the external skin defect.

### *Option 5. Convert to a Posterior or Hemimandibulectomy Defect by Removing the Ramus and Condyle and Reconstructing It with a Soft Tissue Flap*

In patients who are not good candidates for a vascularized bone flap or double free flap, soft tissue flap reconstruction is acceptable for posterolateral defects. The condyle and remaining ramus should be removed to convert a segmental mandibular defect into a posterior or hemimandibulectomy defect. Common soft tissue flap options include a two-skin-island anterolateral thigh flap **(Fig. 14.11)** and a rectus abdominis myocutaneous flap. In high-risk patients, a pedicled pectoralis major myocutaneous flap can be considered.

## Type II Defects

In type II defects, the condyle and ramus are removed. The defect may extend all the way to the parasymphysis, although most defects end in the anterior or mid body of the mandible **(Fig. 14.12)**. Without the condyle, the importance of bony reconstruction is much lower. Bone reconstruction may minimize the jaw deviation and provide better occlusion and slightly better definition of the jaw line compared with soft tissue flap reconstruction. Functional outcomes are, however, similar. In the setting of ORN, especially in the presence of infection and for through-and-through defects, reconstruction with soft tissue flaps may have fewer postoperative complications and quicker recovery.[23]

Common bone flaps for posterior defects are the fibular flap and the iliac crest flap. The iliac crest flap may be a good option for posterior defects because of its natural shape and thus no need for osteotomies. Our preferred soft tissue flap is the anterolateral thigh flap, while the rectus abdominis flap is a good alternative.

## Mandibulectomy Without Reconstruction

In selected patients in whom complex reconstruction is impractical, the necrotic bone may be surgically débrided and the wound left to heal secondarily **(Fig. 14.13)**. Obviously, only lateral or posterior defects can be managed without reconstruction. The defects are usually of limited length, with minimal soft tissue defect. Severe fibrosis around the mandible is present. Such fibrosis may actually help stabilize the remaining bone to avoid severe deformity. This option is reserved for patients with very severe neck fibrosis who are not good candidates for free

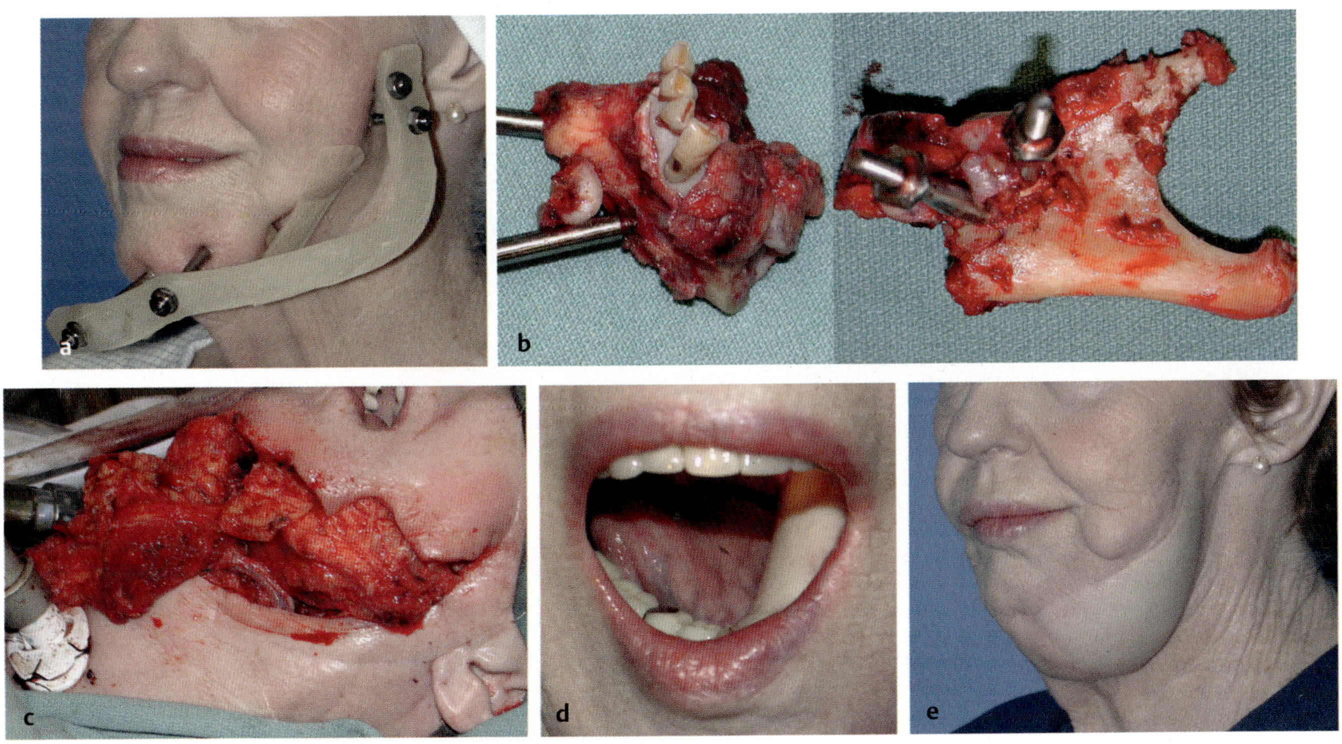

**Fig. 14.11** **(a)** A patient with osteoradionecrosis of the body of the mandible and was placed on an external fixator for more than 1 year. The necrotic bone was resected. **(b)** The condyle was also removed, converting a type Ib defect into a type IIb defect. **(c)** A two-skin-island anterolateral thigh flap was used to reconstruct the hemimandibulectomy defect. **(d,e)** Both skin paddles healed well, with reasonable occlusion and appearance, and with good mouth opening and function.

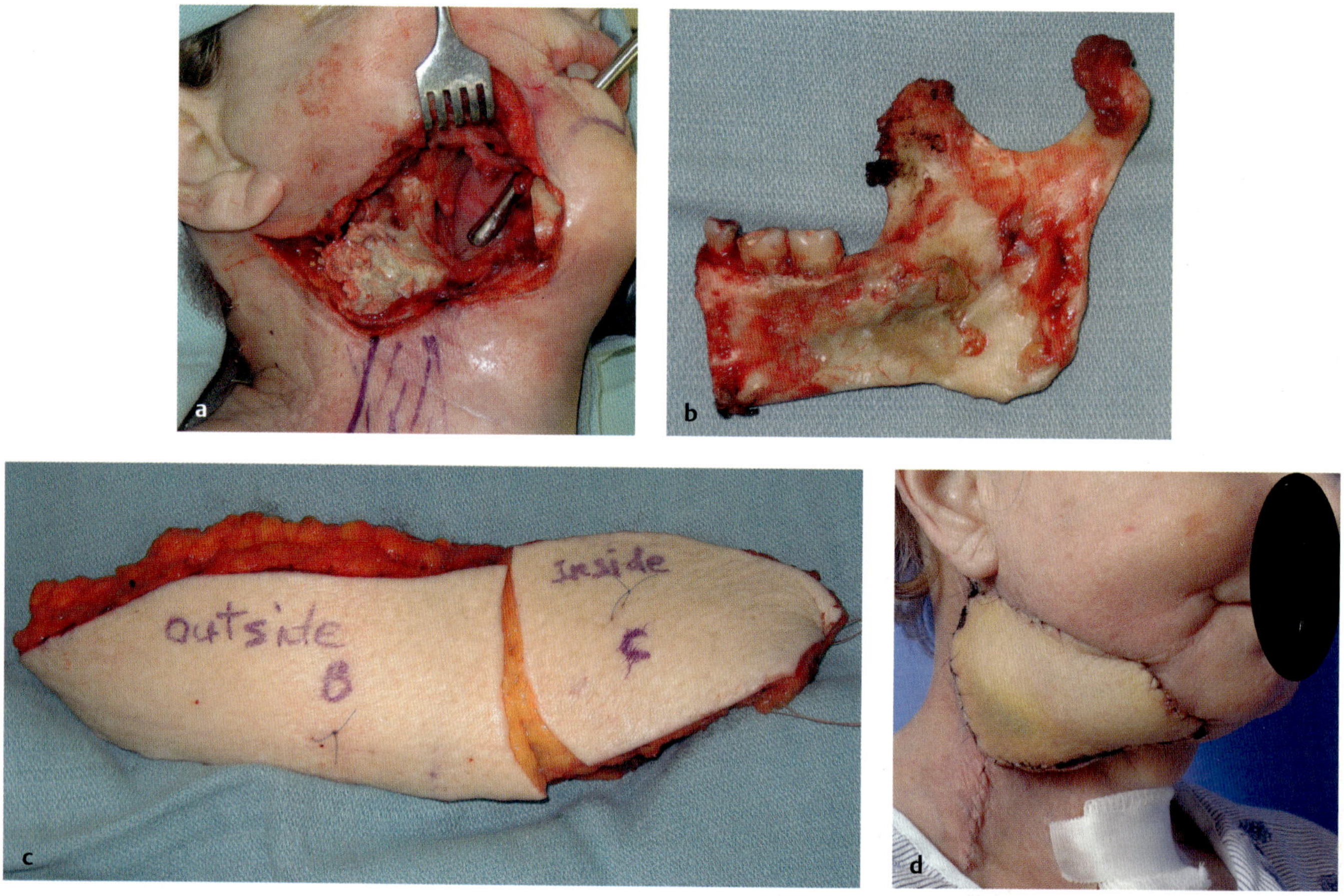


**Fig. 14.12** (**a,b**) A type IIb posterior defect after surgical resection of an osteoradionecrosis with infection. (**c,d**) A two-skin-island anterolateral thigh flap was used to reconstruct this through-and-through defect.

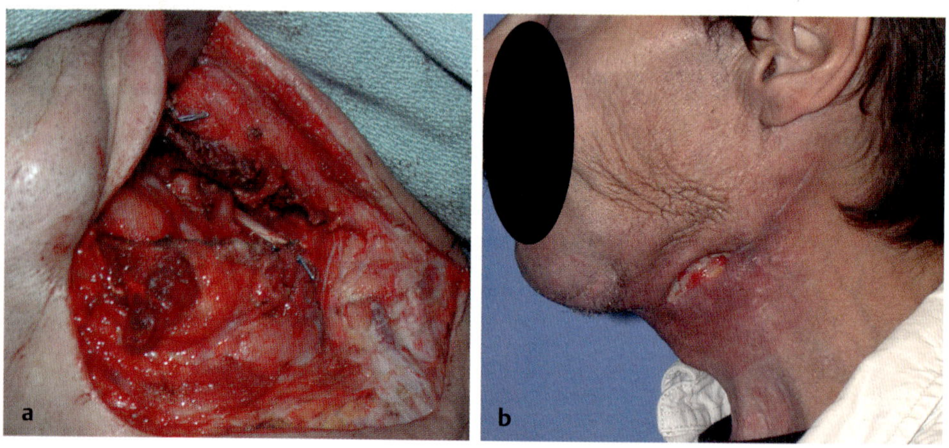


**Fig. 14.13** **(a)** A high-risk patient with posterior mandibular osteoradionecrosis and severe neck fibrosis but minimal soft tissue defect. **(b)** After a posterolateral mandibulectomy, the defect was left to heal secondarily without any form of reconstruction. Postoperative photographs showed reasonable appearance and function.

## Pearls and Pitfalls

- In addition to radiation, causes of ORN are multifactorial and may include concurrent chemotherapy, dental infections, dental extractions, mandibular surgery, tobacco and alcohol use, and malnutrition.
- Early-stage ORN is usually treated conservatively with oral hygiene and topical or systemic antibiotics.
- More advanced (stage II) ORN is managed with débridement, dental sequestrectomy, antibiotics, and, possibly, pharmacotherapy and/or hyperbaric oxygen therapy.
- Stage III and refractory stage II ORN usually require radical débridement and free flap reconstruction.
- Intractable pain, pathologic fractures, fistulas, and osteomyelitis are the usual indications for mandibulectomy and flap reconstruction.
- Patients with ORN and a fistula often need double skin paddle, skin paddle and muscle, or double free flap reconstruction.
- Due to compromised healing capacity, difficult recipient-vessel dissection, and medical comorbidities, reconstruction for ORN is often more difficult than reconstruction for cancer.
- A good understanding of recipient-vessel anatomy is required for free flap reconstruction, which may include a search for alternate recipient blood vessels if the ipsilateral external carotid artery and internal jugular vein and their branches are encased in scar tissue or are otherwise unavailable.
- While re-establishing oral function is not a given following surgery, a theoretical advantage of replacing irradiated, necrotic bone is the ability to provide dental restoration with osseointegrated implants into nonirradiated free flap bone.

## References


1. Marx RE. Osteoradionecrosis: a new concept of its pathophysiology. J Oral Maxillofac Surg 1983;41(5):283–288
2. Beumer J, Harrison R, Sanders B, Kurrasch M. Osteoradionecrosis: predisposing factors and outcomes of therapy. Head Neck Surg 1984;6(4):819–827
3. Lyons A, Ghazali N. Osteoradionecrosis of the jaws: current understanding of its pathophysiology and treatment. Br J Oral Maxillofac Surg 2008;46(8):653–660
4. Notani K, Yamazaki Y, Kitada H, et al. Management of mandibular osteoradionecrosis corresponding to the severity of osteoradionecrosis and the method of radiotherapy. Head Neck 2003;25(3):181–186
5. Kuhnt T, Becker A, Bloching M, et al. Phase II trial of a simultaneous radiochemotherapy with cisplatinum and paclitaxel in combination with hyperfractionated-accelerated radiotherapy in locally advanced head and neck tumors. Med Oncol 2006;23(3):325–333
6. Bras J, de Jonge HK, van Merkesteyn JP. Osteoradionecrosis of the mandible: pathogenesis. Am J Otolaryngol 1990;11(4):244–250
7. Goldwaser BR, Chuang SK, Kaban LB, August M. Risk factor assessment for the development of osteoradionecrosis. J Oral Maxillofac Surg 2007;65(11):2311–2316
8. Lee IJ, Koom WS, Lee CG, et al. Risk factors and dose-effect relationship for mandibular osteoradionecrosis in oral and oropharyngeal cancer patients. Int J Radiat Oncol Biol Phys 2009;75(4):1084–1091
9. Sanger JR, Matloub HS, Yousif NJ, Larson DL. Management of osteoradionecrosis of the mandible. Clin Plast Surg 1993;20(3):517–530
10. Jereczek-Fossa BA, Orecchia R. Radiotherapy-induced mandibular bone complications. Cancer Treat Rev 2002;28(1):65–74
11. Annane D, Depondt J, Aubert P, et al. Hyperbaric oxygen therapy for radionecrosis of the jaw: a randomized, placebo-controlled, double-blind trial from the ORN96 study group. J Clin Oncol 2004;22(24):4893–4900
12. Murray CG, Daly TE, Zimmerman SO. The relationship between dental disease and radiation necrosis of the mandible. Oral Surg Oral Med Oral Pathol 1980;49(2):99–104
13. Tobey RE, Kelly JF. Osteoradionecrosis of the jaws. Otolaryngol Clin North Am 1979;12(1):183–186
14. Schwartz HC, Kagan AR. Osteoradionecrosis of the mandible: scientific basis for clinical staging. Am J Clin Oncol 2002;25(2):168–171
15. Marx RE, Johnson RP, Kline SN. Prevention of osteoradionecrosis: a randomized prospective clinical trial of hyperbaric oxygen versus penicillin. J Am Dent Assoc 1985;111(1):49–54
16. Wong JK, Wood RE, McLean M. Conservative management of osteoradionecrosis. Oral Surg Oral Med Oral Pathol Oral Radiol Endod 1997;84(1):16–21
17. Ang E, Black C, Irish J, et al. Reconstructive options in the treatment of osteoradionecrosis of the craniomaxillofacial skeleton. Br J Plast Surg 2003;56(2):92–99
18. Gal TJ, Yueh B, Futran ND. Influence of prior hyperbaric oxygen therapy in complications following microvascular reconstruction for advanced osteoradionecrosis. Arch Otolaryngol Head Neck Surg 2003;129(1):72–76
19. D'Souza J, Goru J, Goru S, Brown J, Vaughan ED, Rogers SN. The influence of hyperbaric oxygen on the outcome of patients treated for osteoradionecrosis: 8 year study. Int J Oral Maxillofac Surg 2007;36(9):783–787
20. Delanian S, Balla-Mekias S, Lefaix JL. Striking regression of chronic radiotherapy damage in a clinical trial of combined pentoxifylline and tocopherol. J Clin Oncol 1999;17(10):3283–3290
21. Delanian S, Depondt J, Lefaix JL. Major healing of refractory mandible osteoradionecrosis after treatment combining pentoxifylline and tocopherol: a phase II trial. Head Neck 2005;27(2):114–123

22. Yu P, Chang EI, Hanasono MM. Design of a reliable skin paddle for the fibula osteocutaneous flap: perforator anatomy revisited. Plast Reconstr Surg 2011;128(2): 440–446
23. Hanasono MM, Zevallos JP, Skoracki RJ, Yu P. A prospective analysis of bony versus soft-tissue reconstruction for posterior mandibular defects. Plast Reconstr Surg 2010;125(5):1413–1421
24. Baumann DP, Yu P, Hanasono MM, Skoracki RJ. Free flap reconstruction of osteoradionecrosis of the mandible: a 10-year review and defect classification. Head Neck 2011;33(6):800–807

# 15 Dental and Facial Prosthetic Rehabilitation

*Theresa M. Hofstede, Patricia C. Montgomery, and Richard C. Cardoso*

## Introduction

Patients undergoing ablative surgical resection and reconstruction for head and neck cancers have functional and aesthetic challenges. Fortunately, their self-confidence and quality of life can often be enhanced with prosthetic rehabilitation. Intraoral and extraoral prostheses frequently restore a level of form and function that may not be possible with reconstruction flaps alone. Reconstruction flaps, particularly bone-containing flaps, can often provide an excellent foundation for prosthetic rehabilitation. To achieve optimal results, the maxillofacial prosthodontist and anaplastologist should be part of the multidisciplinary team caring for the patient and have an active role in the rehabilitative treatment planning. This chapter discusses extraoral and intraoral prosthetic rehabilitation of the head and neck cancer patient, in coordination with surgical reconstruction.

## Extraoral Prosthetic Rehabilitation

### Preoperative Evaluation

Conventional facial prostheses include nasal, orbital, and auricular prostheses. Successful prosthetic rehabilitation of these craniofacial defects requires communication among the patient, the surgical team, and maxillofacial prosthetic team. Good communication better prepares the patient for the physical and psychological changes ahead. During the preoperative evaluation, the maxillofacial team should discuss the design and fabrication process, time frame for completion, types of prosthetic materials available, prosthesis longevity, the associated costs, and necessary commitment to facial hygiene and prosthetic care. The patient's aesthetic expectations should be met with an honest discussion of realistic outcomes. Preoperative photographs of the patient should be taken to provide a record of facial features that will aid in visualizing the size and contours of the future prosthetic. In some cases, a facial moulage (impression) can be made of the affected area before surgical ablation if there is minimal anatomical distortion and the process is not traumatic to the patient. This impression will yield a dental stone replica, which can be utilized for measurements and as a potential template in the future.

Cases involving osseointegrated craniofacial implant–retained facial prosthetics require substantial preoperative planning prior to implant placement. Assessment of the bone available for implantation is essential to preoperative planning. The quality and volume of the bone, hygiene, thickness of the soft tissue cover, and use of radiation therapy may affect the outcomes of craniofacial implant rehabilitation.[1,2,3,4,5,6,7,8,9] Surgical templates can be fabricated by the prosthetic rehabilitation team to ensure proper placement of the implant(s) in the available bone. Computer-aided design software utilizing computed tomographic (CT) data for implant placement planning may be particularly useful in areas where bone stock is limited and/or where exact implant placement and angulation are necessary.

### General Surgical Guidelines and Prosthetic Rehabilitation

The success of a facial prosthesis depends upon the tissue or "platform" that the prosthesis will contact. The ideal postsurgical site varies based on the type of facial prosthesis needed, such as an orbital, auricular, or nasal prosthesis. In the case of a head and neck cancer patient, control of the cancer precedes concerns for aesthetics; hence, treatment of disease takes priority. However, an ablative procedure performed without an understanding of maxillofacial prosthodontic enhancement may provide a cure for the disease yet leave the patient orally and aesthetically handicapped.[10] Facial defects resulting from ablative and reconstructive surgery can be enhanced with surgical rehabilitative principles utilized to optimize prosthetic success. These general principles are:

1. Smooth bony margins to allow for soft tissue coverage without flap abrasion.
2. Place a split-thickness skin graft (STSG) on exposed bone or periosteum not covered with free tissue or a pedicle flap. An STSG resists the abrasive forces of prostheses much better than respiratory mucosa, granulation tissue, or secondary intention epithelialization. STSG replacement of respiratory mucosa also decreases mucous secretion and crust formation in the defect, thus improving hygiene and retention.
3. Remove unsupported tissue tags, as they are difficult to capture in their correct anatomical position during the impression procedure. Prostheses fabricated over tissue tags frequently are overcontoured and less aesthetically pleasing.
4. Reconstruct facial defects with tissues that best match the tissue surrounding the recipient bed in color and texture. Tissue with excessive hair growth can interfere with prosthesis retention, and laser hair removal may be necessary.
5. Sufficient space must be maintained for an adequately contoured prosthesis, especially in the orbit. Excessively bulky flaps can obliterate the space required. Flap revision may be necessary to provide adequate space for a better outcome.

A successful facial prosthesis depends on several factors—support, stability, and retention—of which retention is a primary component.[11] Prostheses can be retained by anatomical-mechanical undercuts, intraoral–extraoral communication, adhesives/tapes, extraoral osseointegrated implants, or a combination of these methods. Each form of retention has specific anatomical requirements, thus reinforcing the need for preoperative treatment planning from the entire multidisciplinary team.

## Extraoral Osseointegrated Implants

In 1977, Brånemark and Albrekttsson introduced percutaneous craniofacial implants for use with bone conduction hearing aids.[12] Today, facial prosthetic reconstruction based on osseointegrated implants is an important consideration for the retentive security of a facial prosthesis and can greatly facilitate accurate placement of the prosthesis on the remaining facial platform. Craniofacial implants are threaded, cylindrical titanium screws, which form a bond between the bone and the surface layer of titanium oxide (osseointegration). The implants engage an abutment, which provides the transmucosal or transdermal attachment for the facial prosthesis. There are two common prosthetic attachment components to consider for extraoral attachment to the abutment: bar construction with clips or magnetic attachment. Each requires specific placement guidelines and maintenance to ensure the success of the prosthesis.

Successful craniofacial implants require adequate volume and density of bone and proper orientation of the implants. For example, in total auriculectomy cases, the ideal position of implants for an auricular prosthesis is based on using the external ear canal as a focal point. The implants and the bar construction or magnets should be located underneath the proposed antihelix to achieve adequate depth and contour of the prosthesis (**Fig. 15.1** and **Fig. 15.2**).[13] Implant placement in this area may not be possible due to extensive surgery with temporal bone resection and flap placement, which can obliterate the ear canal. Placing implant(s) superiorly in the temporal bone will make the implant components visible, thereby producing poor prosthetic aesthetics. These implants may also interfere with the placement of a bone-anchored hearing device.

Orbital prostheses must rest within a concave defect for optimal aesthetic results. Implant placement for orbital prostheses is centered on the malar body, supra- or infraorbital rim, lateral rim, or a combination thereof. The implant placement should be concealed by the prosthesis and should not interfere with the complex contours needed for an orbital prosthesis. The angle of implant placement will affect the orientation of the implant abutment, which may hinder proper placement of the prosthetic components, resulting in poor aesthetics or the inability to utilize the implant (**Fig. 15.3**).

Implant placement for a nasal prosthesis is determined on an individual basis, as much of the bone surrounding the nasal defect has complex architecture and typically is too thin to support craniofacial implants.[14] Implants can be placed diagonally into the anterior nasal spine so that they engage the basal maxillary bone; however, placement is limited by the presence of teeth and a tooth root injury must be avoided. Implants that exit through the mobile skin tissue of the upper lip often have chronic irritation and thus should be avoided. Implants placed in the anterior part of the nasal floor should be spaced 8 to 10 mm apart and should exit through immobile

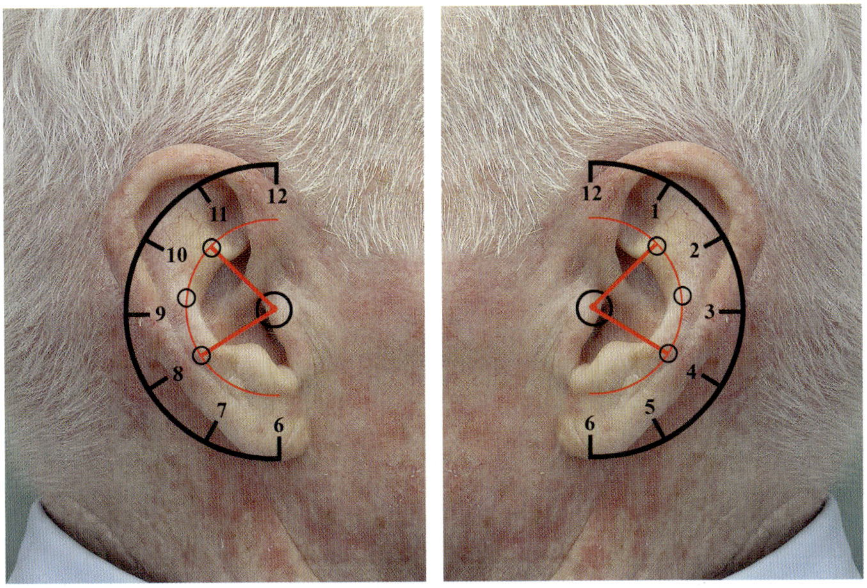


**Fig. 15.1** The size and depth of the defect, size and shape of the future prosthetic ear, position and number of implants, loading situation, mobility of the surrounding tissue, and age, ability, and hygiene of the patient should be considered in the planning stages. The size and shape of the ear prosthesis will ultimately determine the number of implants and implant placement. Prior to surgery, a surgical template can be fabricated by the facial prosthetic team to aid in implant placement. For optimal aesthetics, the implants should be placed directly under the antihelix to obtain adequate depth to camouflage the retentive components within the prosthesis. Generally, the ideal position is ~ 20 mm from the center of the external ear canal opening, or in the case of the atretic ear, the anticipated opening. On the right ear, the optimal positions are between 8 o'clock and 10:30. On the left ear, the optimal positions are between 4 o'clock and 1:30. The distance between the implants should be at least 15 mm, depending on the anatomical situation.[15]

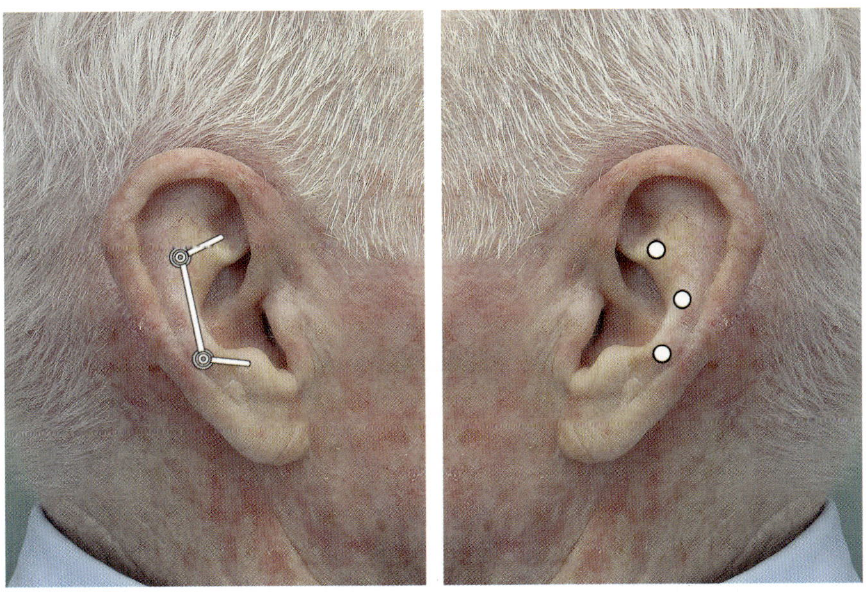

**Fig. 15.2** The size and shape of the ear prosthesis will ultimately determine the number of implants and implant placement. The placement of two implants is normally sufficient for satisfactory retention using the bar and clip retentive components. In some cases, it may be necessary for three implants to ensure satisfactory bar and clip retention of a large ear prosthesis. For magnetic retention, three implants are preferred, but two implants can be sufficient.

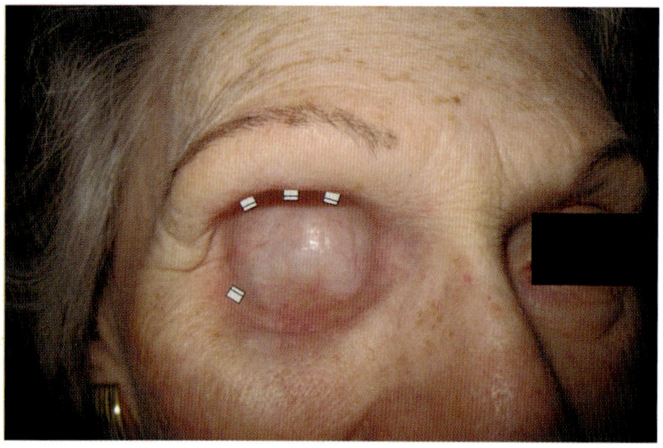

**Fig. 15.3** In patient cases that allow, individual magnets attached to the appropriate length of abutment in the upper and lower orbital rim are recommended for retention of an orbital prosthesis. It is more favorable to have more than two fixtures placed in both the upper and lower rims.[15] Bar construction with retentive clips is recommended for large orbital defects where proper cleaning around the abutments is possible.

tissue **(Fig. 15.4)**.[16] The literature suggests there is a higher incidence of implant failure in the nasal region due to chronic dermatitis of the peri-implant tissue, particularly in the glabellar region.[17,18]

Many variables must be considered in the placement of extraoral osseointegrated implants for the retention of an auricular, nasal, or orbital prosthesis.

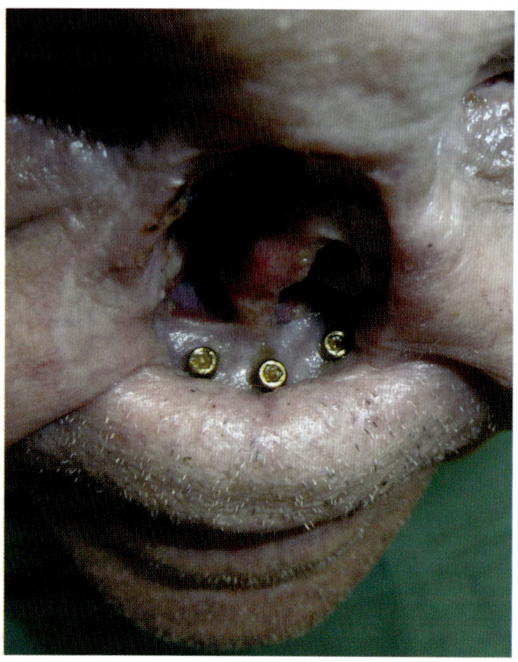

**Fig. 15.4** Endosteal implants can be used, based on individual cases, to retain nasal prostheses. To ensure adequate space for a substructure, remove the bony structures inside the nasal cavity and place a split-thickness skin graft. Implants should be placed vertically into the maxillary alveolar bone in edentulous patients to support a substructure for retention of a nasal prosthesis.

1. Implants should be placed prior to radiation therapy if at all possible due to risk of osteoradionecrosis, and greater implant failure rates in irradiated bone.[19] A healing time of 6 to 8 months is needed for osseointegration in irradiated bone, and hyperbaric oxygen therapy may be indicated to enhance wound healing.[20]
2. Poorly positioned implants may not be usable because they result in an overcontoured and ineffective prosthesis.
3. Hygiene of the defect and transmucosal tissue is an important consideration prior to implant placement. Patients who are unwilling or unable to maintain good hygiene should be considered for other forms of rehabilitation.
4. Stereolithographic models made from computed tomography (CT) scans are useful to evaluate the bone contours and thickness of the oral cavity and facial topography. The surgical guides made from these models are placed directly on the bone as a drill guide.

Determining and visualizing the retention of the future prosthetic ear, nose, or eye are essential to a successful prosthetic rehabilitation outcome.

## Postsurgical Evaluation

The patient should return to the maxillofacial prosthetic team postoperatively to evaluate healing, the extent of anatomical loss, and the determination of a time commitment. The prosthesis-bearing surface, and the presence of exposed bone, infection, granulation tissues, or a bulky soft tissue flap should be discussed with the reconstructive surgeon regarding revisions. Implant position can be evaluated to determine the future retentive mechanism. Gentle palpation of the surgical site can identify areas of tenderness, edema, and friable or bleeding tissue as well as evaluate tissue tone and mobility.[16] Hypermobile tissue surrounding the defect can significantly decrease prosthesis retention.

Prosthetic rehabilitation may be delayed if postoperative chemotherapy or radiotherapy is needed. If osseointegrated implants are placed at the time of surgery, an additional 6 to 8 months are needed for osseointegration before prosthetic rehabilitation can begin. This may be shortened to 4 to 6 months if the patient does not require radiation therapy. Treatment-related morbidities can include edema, tenderness, dermatitis, fibrosis, and flap atrophy. Prior to prosthetic rehabilitation, the defect and flap reconstruction should be dimensionally stable to ensure an accurate fit of the underlying tissue.

## Biomaterials

Elastomers have been used for almost 50 years to fabricate facial prostheses. These customized prostheses are intrinsically and extrinsically colored to mimic human skin shades with various pigments and afford good color stability. The surface texture of the silicone can be made to match the surface texture of the surrounding tissue, helping to create a lifelike prosthesis.[21,22] The success of any facial prosthesis depends on the physical and mechanical properties of the materials used. Since the 1960s, elastomeric polymers, such as silicone rubber, have been the biomaterial of choice.[23] The ideal mechanical properties of this biomaterial are durability, ease of manipulation, and flexibility similar to skin. The edges of the cured silicone can be thinned to accommodate movement when adhered to soft tissue. Limitations of silicone rubber include: poor edge strength, limited material longevity, discoloration over time, and the ability to support fungal growth. The average lifespan of the prosthesis is 1 year, due to degradation from daily use, adhesive application and removal, and fading from ultraviolet exposure.[24]

Acrylic resin is often utilized in facial prosthetics for substructures, with samarium cobalt magnets to help guide the prosthesis into place. It is also used to house the retentive components needed for implant-retained prostheses. Additionally, acrylic resin is used to fabricate an ocular prosthesis (prosthetic eye globe), used in an orbital prosthesis.

## Prosthetic Retention

Retention of the prosthesis can be accomplished by several methods, including medical-grade adhesives, double-sided tapes, acrylic resin substructures (with or without embedded magnets), anatomical undercuts, mechanical retention, and craniofacial osseointegrated implants. The type of retention is dictated by the patient's defect site, the quality of the underlying hard or soft tissue, tissue movement with facial expressions, and the contours. Retention cannot be achieved on friable, wet, or thin tissue. Problems with adhesive interaction with the skin can affect the longevity of the bond, can cause dermatologic sensitivity problems, and can affect the ability to completely remove the adhesive residue.[11,25] Maintenance of the skin and prosthesis requires considerable daily effort and dexterity by the patient. Patient acceptance of, and confidence in, the prosthesis rely upon predictable prosthesis retention.

## Common Types of Facial Prostheses

### Nasal Prosthesis

Partial or total nasal prostheses are commonly used to replace ablated nasal tissues for patients who undergo a partial or total rhinectomy when surgical reconstruction cannot be achieved **(Fig. 15.5)**. A successful nasal prosthesis depends upon these surgical enhancements to the nasal region:

1. All unsupported tissue tags, including alar tags, should be removed if future surgical reconstruction is not anticipated. Tissue tags are frequently out of anatomical location, making them difficult to incorporate into an aesthetic prosthesis.
2. The stability of a nasal prosthesis is enhanced if the nasal bones remain intact. This vertical support is also helpful for retaining eyeglasses.
3. The nasal septum should be reduced anteriorly to provide a concave defect that will accommodate an acrylic resin substructure, which will aid in prosthesis retention and orientation. This will also diminish the mucous discharge, which can contaminate the prosthesis and reduce the adhesive bond.
4. An STSG placed around the periphery of the defect reduces tissue movement and enhances adhesion by providing a surface without hair growth or glandular secretions.
5. Maintaining the anterior nasal spine and lip attachments can prevent migration of the lip superiorly.[26]

### Auricular Prosthesis

Partial or total auricular prostheses are desirable when a subtotal or total auriculectomy is necessary **(Fig. 15.6)**. In most cases, surgical reconstruction, particularly in the radiated field, rarely achieves an acceptable aesthetic result. Retention of the auricular prosthesis can be achieved with liquid medical-grade adhesives, medical-grade double-sided tapes, anatomical acrylic resin substructures, or osseointegrated implants. The location, contours, orientation, and retention of the prosthesis are often enhanced with total resection.

A successful auricular prosthesis depends on surgical enhancements to the recipient site.

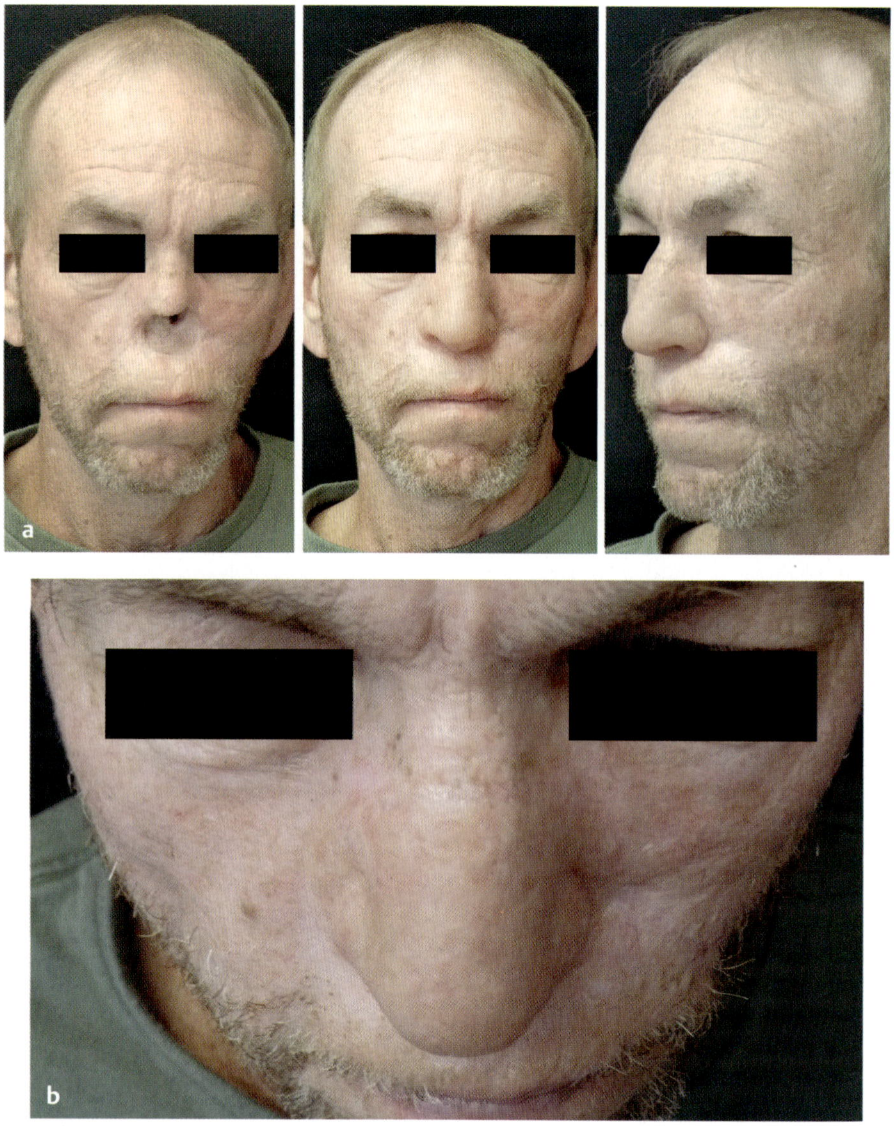

**Fig. 15.5** **(a)** The patient is a 55-year-old male with a history of basal cell carcinoma of the left nasal ala, columella, and anterior septum, with perineural invasion, who underwent a partial rhinectomy and anterior septectomy with a split-thickness skin graft (STSG) followed by postoperative radiation therapy. The nasal spine is intact, providing vertical support of the nasal prosthesis. The skin graft enhances adhesion of the liquid water-based adhesive used to retain the nasal prosthesis. **(b)** Close-up showing the detail of the extrinsic coloration of the silicone prosthesis

1. The recipient site should be flat or slightly concave for optimal aesthetics. Bulky reconstruction flaps should be thinned to allow for bilateral facial symmetry.
2. An STSG provides a smooth surface without hair growth. This enhances the adhesive bond to the skin.
3. The location, contours, orientation, and retention of the prosthesis are often enhanced with total resection. Distortion of tissue remnants following a partial resection can hinder aesthetics and bilateral symmetry, thus reducing the quality of the final prosthetic.
4. The tragus is beneficial tissue to maintain during a total auriculectomy, particularly if the position is not distorted. Orienting the prosthesis is easier with a stable anatomical landmark. Also, prosthetic margins are minimized and better concealed with the tragus in place.
5. The superior portion of the auricle has cartilaginous support but often becomes distorted following surgical closure. Eyeglass retention is still possible if the root of the helix adjacent to the tragus is preserved.
6. Surgical loss of the middle third of the pinna is sometimes necessary. The defect can be prosthetically restored but presents a placement and retention problem to some patients.

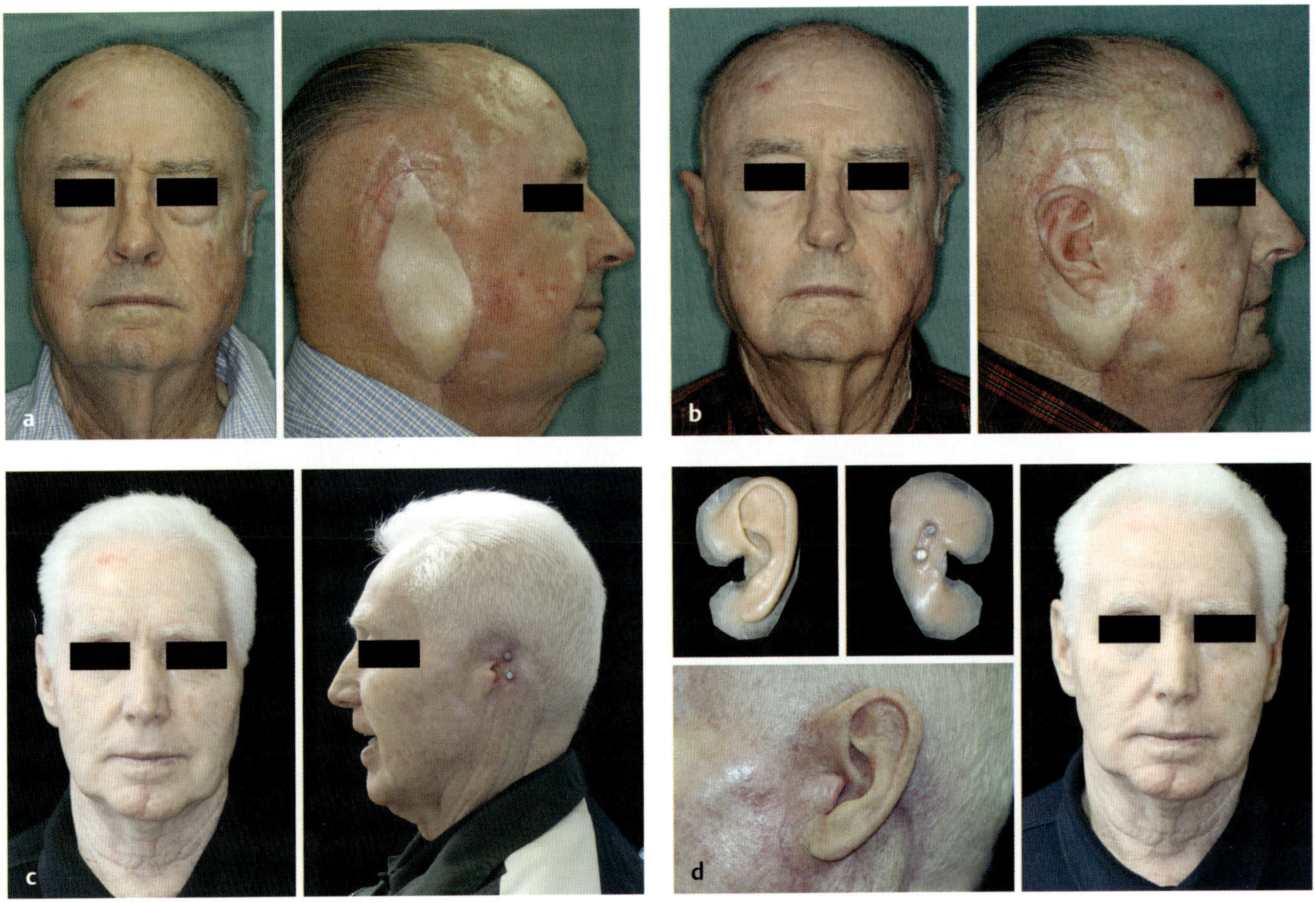

**Fig. 15.6** **(a)** The patient is a 73-year-old male with a history of recurrent squamous cell and basal cell carcinoma of the right external auditory canal who has undergone a total right auriculectomy, a temporal bone resection, parotidectomy, neck dissection, and free flap reconstruction, followed by postoperative external beam radiation therapy. Before beginning prosthetic rehabilitation, a procedure was done to revise the free anterolateral thigh flap to the head and neck region on the right and suction-assisted lipoplasty of the bulky contours of the lower aspect of the flap to balance bilateral symmetry. The patient was then ready to begin prosthetic rehabilitation. **(b)** The flat contours of the skin graft without a stable anatomical landmark presented a challenge for repeatable correct positioning of the auricular prosthesis. Retention of the prosthesis was achieved with the use of a medical-grade double-sided tape. **(c)** The patient is a 79-year-old male with a history of poorly differentiated carcinoma of the left outer ear who has undergone a left-sided auriculectomy, cervicofacial advancement flap, and placement of two osseointegrated implants for prosthetic rehabilitation. He did not require postoperative radiation therapy. **(d)** Silicone prosthesis before final extrinsic coloration with magnetic retention components in an acrylic substructure embedded into the silicone. Final silicone prosthesis was retained with magnets plus medical-grade double-sided tape for additional security of the borders to the skin.

7. The inferior half of the pinna and lobe are not beneficial for the retention or orientation of the prosthesis in most cases. The instability of these tissues is a challenge to capture in an impression.

## Orbital Prosthesis

The design and fabrication of an orbital prosthesis following an exenteration is one of the most aesthetically challenging and artistically demanding restorations (**Fig. 15.7**). The prosthesis must mirror the contralateral eye, beginning with the ocular prosthesis, followed by matching the unique contours of the eyelids and the surrounding tissue. The perfect recipient site is needed or an aesthetically correct orbital prosthesis is not possible. Retention of the orbital prosthesis can be achieved with liquid medical-grade adhesives, medical-grade double-sided tapes, acrylic resin substructures, or osseointegrated implants.

A successful orbital prosthesis also depends upon the surgical enhancements to the recipient site:

1. The eyelids should be resected; however, the eyebrow is maintained in the same position as

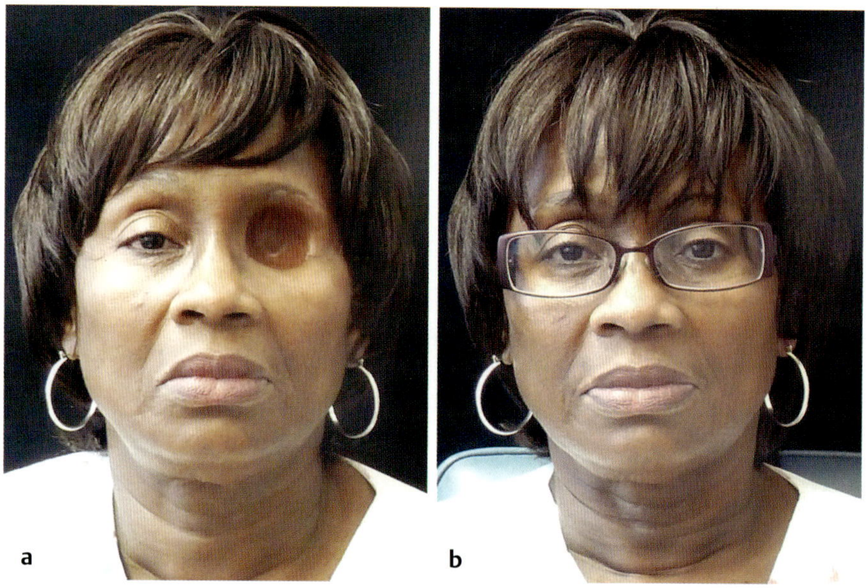

Fig. 15.7 The patient is a 63-year-old female with a history of recurrent squamous cell carcinoma of the left bulbar conjunctiva, caruncle, and lower palpebral conjunctiva who underwent a left orbital exenteration. **(a)** The concavity of her defect provides enough space for the globe-shaped ocular prosthesis to be correctly positioned within the orbital prosthesis, **(b)** resulting in excellent aesthetic results. Eyeglasses aid in disguising the borders of the prosthesis.

the contralateral eyebrow. The periorbital bony rim can aid in supporting the weight of the prosthesis and ideally should be preserved.

2. The margins of resected orbital bones should be smoothed and rounded to minimize tissue irritation and future bone exposure. Without support of the infraorbital rim, the prosthesis will drop, due to lack of support. In that case, reconstruction of the inferior bone is preferred.
3. Occluding the orbit with bulky flaps should be avoided if an orbital prosthesis is planned **(Fig. 15.8)**. A concave bony orbit lined with an STSG or thin flap is the ideal recipient site for an orbital prosthesis. This will provide an immobile tissue foundation, the depth required for mirror-imaging lifelike contours, and a good adhesive platform.

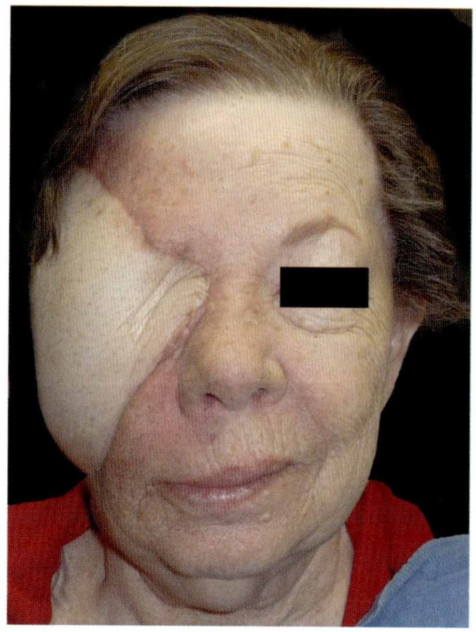

Fig. 15.8 Prosthetic restoration of an orbital defect is one of the most difficult restorative procedures. Bulky skin flaps that completely occlude the orbit do not allow for aesthetic restoration; therefore, a concavity defect lined with an STSG is preferable whenever possible.

# ■ Intraoral Prosthetic Rehabilitation

## Maxillary Defects

Resected lesions of the maxilla (maxillectomy) that are not reconstructed with surgical microvascular techniques require placement of an obturator. The oroantral/oral-nasal defects resulting from resection of the maxillary sinus, hard/soft palate, and alveolar ridge lead to unintelligible speech, impaired swallowing, and nasal regurgitation (unless the oral-nasal partition can be re-established). An obturator is a removable prosthesis that replaces all or part of the palate that is resected during the tumor ablative surgery.[27] The primary functions of an obturator are to re-establish the partition between the oral cavity and the sinus/nasal cavity, and to recreate the palatal contours for appropriate speech sounds.[28,29]

The size and location of the proposed surgical defect, the presence and condition of remaining teeth, and the remaining prosthesis-bearing surface are considerations for maxillary prosthetic rehabilitation with an obturator.[27] As the defect size increases, there is a decrease in the amount of residual palate and remaining teeth that can be utilized for retention.[28,29,30,31] This, in turn, decreases retention and stability of the prosthesis, which decreases functionality and overall patient satisfaction.[31,32,33] Osseointegrated endosseous implants placed in edentulous areas provide excellent support, retention, and stability to prostheses that otherwise would be compromised following tumor ablative procedures.[29,34,35] The use of radiation therapy postoperatively can, however, preclude implant placement due to the risk of later developing osteoradionecrosis. Important factors in the successful implant prosthetic rehabilitation following radiation therapy are radiation dose to proposed implant sites, time from radiation therapy to implant surgery, implant fixture and abutment length, available bone stock, and appropriate selection of implant sites.[29,30,36] The benefits of hyperbaric oxygen therapy to enhance wound healing in patients who require implant restoration remain controversial and are actively being studied.[37]

Prosthetic rehabilitation using an obturator prosthesis is divided into three phases: surgical, interim, and definitive.

## Surgical Obturator

A surgical obturator is a removable prosthesis, often without prosthetic teeth, placed at the time of surgery. The primary objective of this prosthesis is to restore the palatal continuity, which ultimately restores speech and swallowing function without nasal regurgitation. It also supports the surgical packing, which holds the STSG in place, and reduces postoperative bleeding. Surgical obturators often circumvent the need for a nasogastric feeding tube and decrease the duration of postoperative recovery or hospital stay. A patient's psychological status is improved with the ability to speak and eat immediately after surgery.[28,29,38,39]

## Interim Obturator

An interim obturator prosthesis is placed 5 to 10 days postoperatively, following removal of the surgical obturator/packing. During normal healing, the maxillectomy defect will continue to remodel, which leads to ongoing challenges of nasal regurgitation and hypernasality. To accommodate these changes, the interim obturator is modified with resilient polymethyl methacrylate material **(Fig. 15.9)**. Most often the interim obturator is fabricated with prosthetic teeth to establish appropriate lip and cheek contour during healing, and to reduce contracture of scar tissue.[28,29,38,39] A well-contoured, intimately fitting interim obturator can be modified and converted to a definitive obturator once the defect has become dimensionally stable.

## Definitive Obturator

A definitive obturator is fabricated once the maxillary defect is dimensionally stable.[27] Generally, a definite obturator can be fabricated 3 to 4 months after surgery; however, multiple factors may affect timing of fabrication, i.e., size of defect, the use and timing of postoperative radiation, prognosis for tumor, bone exposure, or progress of healing.[28] Missing teeth are replaced not only to maximize oral function, but also to restore facial symmetry. The definitive obturator prosthesis can be fabricated with a metal framework depending upon contours and condition of remaining teeth and patient expectations **(Fig. 15.10)**.

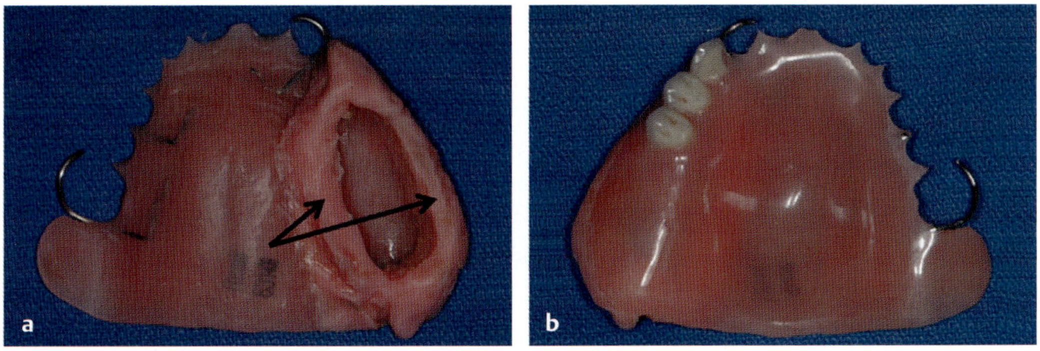


**Fig. 15.9 (a,b)** Interim obturator fabricated with wrought wire clasps embedded in an acrylic resin base. The resilient material (*arrows*) has been molded by the palatal defect and the adjacent muscles and is frequently modified during this healing phase.

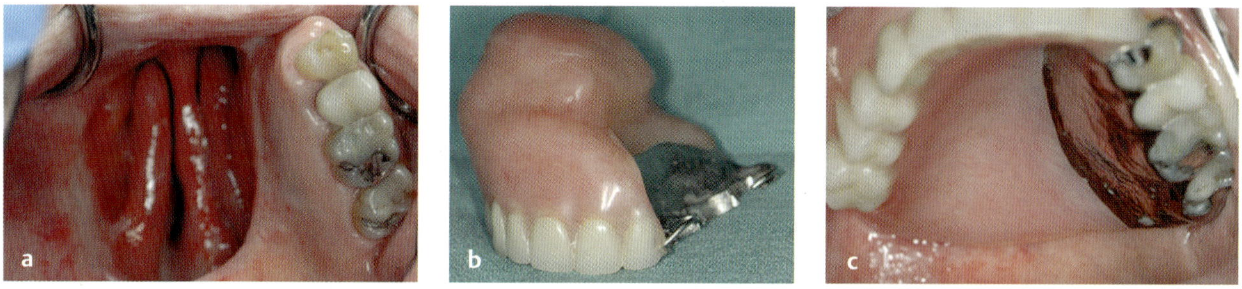

Fig. 15.10 (a) An extensive defect of the right maxilla and premaxilla creates functional and aesthetic challenges. (b,c) A definitive obturator fabricated from a cast framework and acrylic resin closes the defect and restores speech and swallowing function, as well as lip support.

As with any maxillofacial prosthesis, the remaining dentition is critical to the functionality of the prosthesis. Every effort should be taken to maintain and enhance the dentition. For patients who received postoperative radiation therapy, meticulous oral hygiene and daily fluoride therapy are required.[29,40]

### Pharyngeal Obturators

Patients who have extensive resections of the soft palate require obturation. Similar to hard palate obturators, pharyngeal obturators reestablish the partition between the oropharynx and nasopharynx (**Fig. 15.11**). The major distinction is that the remaining pharyngeal musculature must function against the obturator during normal speech and swallowing.[28] At the time of the surgical procedure, the surgeon and the maxillofacial prosthodontist must decide whether the remaining structure will be functional. It is often easier to rehabilitate a patient's speech and swallowing if the soft palate is removed completely, as compared with a partially functional or a totally nonfunctional soft palate.[29,31] This difficulty is related to restricted access to the oropharynx for adequate obturation.[31]

## Surgical Considerations to Enhance Obturator Rehabilitation

Difficulties in prosthetic rehabilitation can be minimized, or even eliminated, with careful surgical planning. Dental casts are usually fabricated preoperatively and are used for discussion between the head and neck surgeon and the maxillofacial prosthodontist. The proposed surgical margins should be determined so that an appropriately sized surgical prosthesis can be fabricated. The overall oral condition should be addressed, i.e., oral surgical needs and dental restorations that may be required. Teeth that are nonrestorable or have questionable prognoses require extraction, ideally at the time of the tumor ablative surgery.[29]

Several surgical recommendations should be considered to improve prosthetic outcome.

1. Osteotomies should be made through an edentulous area of the socket of an extracted tooth to prevent bone/tooth loss.[29]
2. An STSG should be placed in the maxillary defect; this will allow for formation of a scar band and provide retention of the obturator, as well as create a resilient prosthesis-bearing

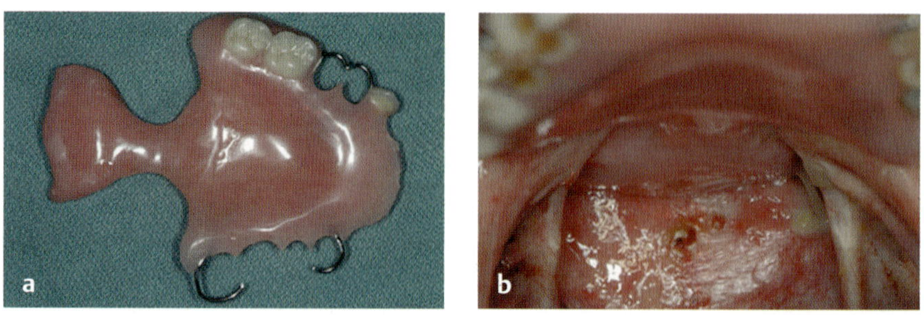

Fig. 15.11 (a) The pharyngeal obturator extends posteriorly at the level of the hard palate to separate the oropharynx from the nasopharynx. (b) The middle and superior constrictor muscles function against this extension to provide a seal during speech and swallowing.

surface. This will improve overall hygiene of the defect by decreasing the amount of mucous or crust formation and nasal polyp formation.[29,39]

3. Removal of the inferior and middle turbinates, even if they are unaffected, is recommended to allow for adequate superior extension of the prosthesis. The respiratory epithelium surrounding the turbinates is friable and will become a constant source of bleeding and irritation.[29,30,34,36]
4. The amount and architecture of the remaining maxilla will directly influence the support and stability of the prosthesis. In anterior lesions, an effort should be made to spare the maxillary tuberosity bilaterally, a primary prosthesis-bearing area. When the tuberosity cannot be spared, due to tumor extent, an effort should be made to spare the premaxilla for the same reason.[29,30,34,36]
5. An intraoral approach, as opposed to a Weber-Fergusson incision, allows for ease of manipulation of the lip and cheek postoperatively during the interim phase of obturation.[34,39]
6. If not affected by disease, the remaining palatal mucosa can be wrapped around the palatal osteotomy to provide a denture-bearing surface.

## Surgical Reconstruction of Maxillary Defects

Current microvascular techniques have facilitated surgical reconstruction of a maxillectomy defect, providing separation between the oral and nasal cavities. Function and cosmetics can be restored effectively with a surgical reconstruction; however, depending upon bulk and location of the reconstruction, it may preclude future prosthetic rehabilitation. If the flap occupies the space where the prosthetic teeth should be positioned, the prosthetic rehabilitation may not be possible without flap revision.

Successful prosthetic rehabilitation following surgical reconstruction of the maxilla requires an osseous element. The bone can support endosseous implants and also relay the occlusal force to the cranium to resist long-term resorption. The fibular flap is well suited for this type of reconstruction. The vertical height of a fibula has been found to range from 13.1 to 16.7 mm, with an average of 15 mm.[41,42,43] This, along with its bicortical configuration, is ideal for placement of endosseous implants. Many head and neck bony defects are considered suitable for fibular reconstruction, and functional rehabilitation can be optimal in these patients. Patients who receive implant-retained maxillary prostheses supported by implants placed into fibular reconstructions have near optimal mastication and speech.[44] Placement and orientation of the fibula are critical to the prosthetic success, as adequate space is necessary for prosthetic components and the prosthesis (**Fig. 15.12**). Presurgical collaboration between the surgeon and the prosthodontist, with possible use of stereolithographic models, is essential for prosthetic success (**Fig. 15.13**).

Soft tissue flaps, without an osseous component, often preclude the fabrication of a dental prosthesis. These reconstructions often lack the ability to support a prosthesis, resulting in a nonretentive and potentially nonfunctional prosthesis. Alveolar or bony support and immobile soft tissue are key elements in a functional prosthesis. The patient's desire for prosthetic rehabilitation should be taken into consideration at the treatment-planning phase; however, realistic expectations must be discussed. Soft tissue flaps are thought to best serve patients who are not interested in postsurgical prosthetic rehabilitation, those with a small posterior defect, and those, possibly, unable or unwilling to care for an obturator.[28]

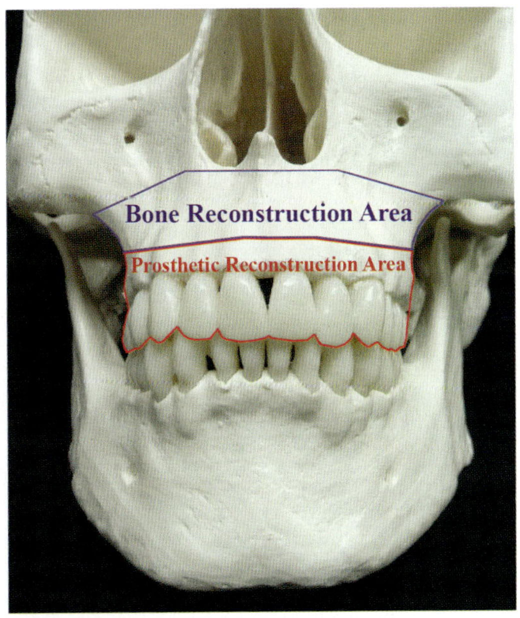


**Fig. 15.12** Maxillary reconstruction with an osteocutaneous flap requires careful presurgical planning. The bone should be positioned superiorly and should not invade the intended space for the prosthesis.

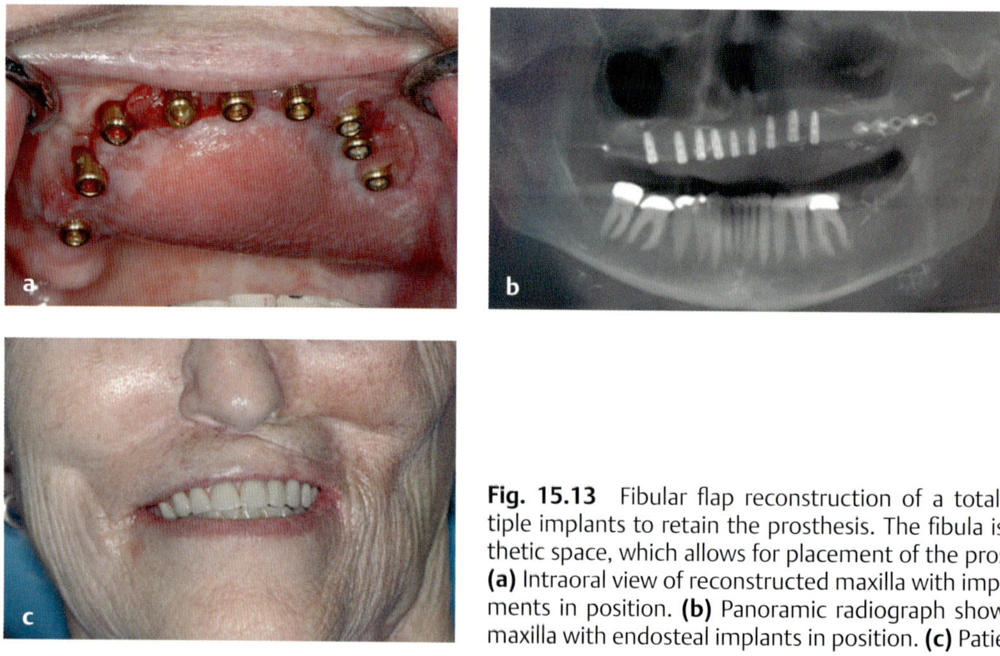

Fig. 15.13 Fibular flap reconstruction of a total maxillectomy defect, with multiple implants to retain the prosthesis. The fibula is positioned superior to the prosthetic space, which allows for placement of the prosthetic teeth in a natural position. **(a)** Intraoral view of reconstructed maxilla with implants uncovered and locater abutments in position. **(b)** Panoramic radiograph showing fibular reconstruction of the maxilla with endosteal implants in position. **(c)** Patient with completed restoration.

## Palatal Augmentation Prosthesis

The contours of the palate are important not only for speech sounds but also in deglutition. Articulation is accomplished by precise positioning of the tongue, lips, and cheeks against the palate, teeth, and other oral structures.[28] Deglutition, generally speaking, requires maximal contact of the tongue to the palate. Palatal augmentation prostheses recontour the hard palate to allow for improved lingual contact during speech and swallowing following either a partial or total glossectomy **(Fig. 15.14)**.[27]

The tongue is considered to be very adaptable to change; however, a direct correlation has been established between the amount of lingual tissue removed and impairment of articulation.[28] Patients who have speech and/or swallowing challenges postoperatively, even those with flap reconstructions, may benefit from this type of prosthesis. A review of the literature has shown that patients with severe restrictions in tongue-palate contact following resection had an improvement in speech (86%; 36 of 42 subjects) and swallowing (86%; 32 of 37 subjects) with the use of a palatal augmentation prosthesis.[45]

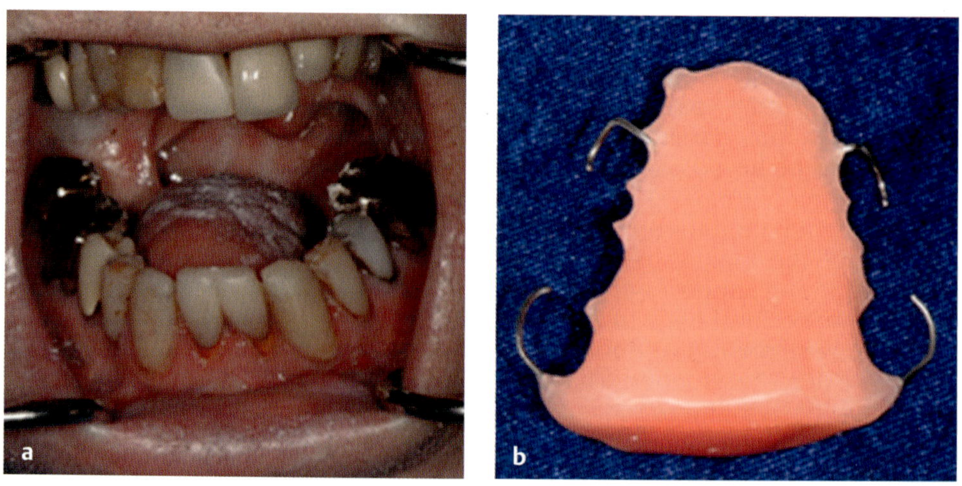

**Fig. 15.14** **(a)** The range of motion of the tongue is restricted following partial glossectomy and reconstruction. **(b)** The palatal augmentation seats on the palate and fills the void in the palatal vault where the tongue cannot touch. It provides a contact surface for speech and swallowing.

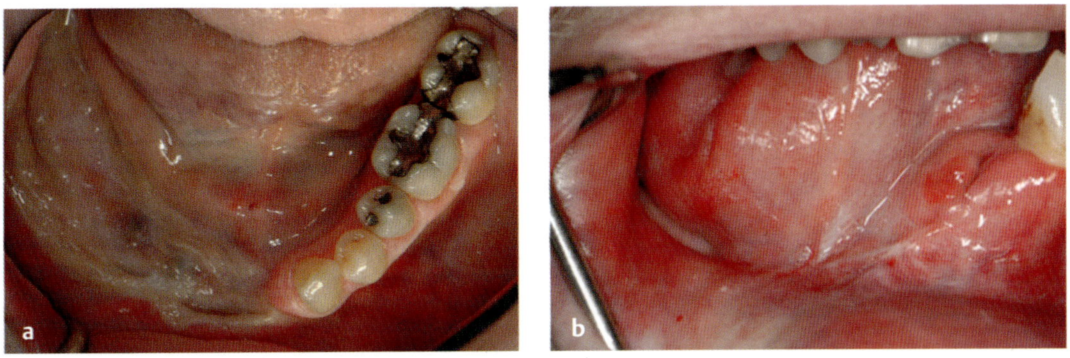

Fig. 15.15 **(a)** Well-healed STSG over a marginal mandibulectomy defect. This STSG provides a resilient, nonmobile foundation ideal for prosthesis placement. **(b)** Primary closure of the floor of mouth and the buccal mucosa creates a mobile mucosa that would dehisce if a mandibular resection prosthesis were placed onto it.

## Mandibular Defects

Mandibular defects secondary to tumor ablation create functional and aesthetic challenges. The magnitude varies with the extent of the resection and reconstruction. Frequently, speech, mastication, lip posture, bolus control, and occlusion are compromised. Prosthetic rehabilitation of the resected mandible can often improve these deficits. Retention, support, and stability of the mandibular resection prosthesis can be enhanced with the remaining mandibular teeth, endosteal implants, and a nonmobile soft tissue base. Surgical reconstruction of the mandibular defect can have a profound effect on the quality of the prosthetic rehabilitation.[46] Surgical enhancements to improve prosthetic outcomes include:

1. Placement of an STSG over a marginal mandibulectomy defect will provide optimal prosthetic-bearing surface **(Fig. 15.15a)**.[47] Primary closure of the floor of mouth and buccal mucosa will usually preclude prosthetic rehabilitation **(Fig. 15.15b)**.
2. Osteotomies made through tooth sockets, rather than interseptal bone, maintain osseous support of teeth adjacent to the resection site.
3. Maintain unaffected healthy teeth to aid in prosthesis retention and orientation of the prosthesis.
4. If possible, restore continuity defects of the mandible with osteocutaneous flaps to reduce facial defects and deviation of the mandible.
5. During the mandibular reconstruction, maintain the preoperative orientation of the remaining mandibular segments. This will optimize mandibular movement and occlusal orientation and minimize temporomandibular joint problems.
6. Position the osseous portion of the flap along the inferior border of the mandible to restore proper facial form. This also allows for adequate space for implant and prosthesis placement.

Patients with a defect of the alveolar ridge following a marginal mandibulectomy typically have limited morbidity, as the mandibular continuity and musculature are often intact. However, with the loss of the teeth and alveolar bone, masticatory function is reduced. Also, the lower lip can invert into the oral cavity if the resection involves the anterior mandibular segment **(Fig. 15.16)**. Mandibular resection prostheses will restore the occlusal table and masticatory function and provide adequate lip support. The prosthesis can be retained by the remaining teeth or osseointegrated implants **(Fig. 15.17)**. If, however, the patient is edentulous, meaningful retention of the mandibular resection prosthesis will be difficult, and placement of endosteal implants at the time of the surgery should be considered.

Mandibles reconstructed with an osteocutaneous flap can create additional challenges during prosthetic rehabilitation. The skin paddle of the flap can be bulky and mobile and have a fluctuant consistency. If multiple teeth remain in the mandible, a tooth and soft tissue retained mandibular resection prosthesis may be fabricated with reasonable results. Over time, the bulk of the skin paddle

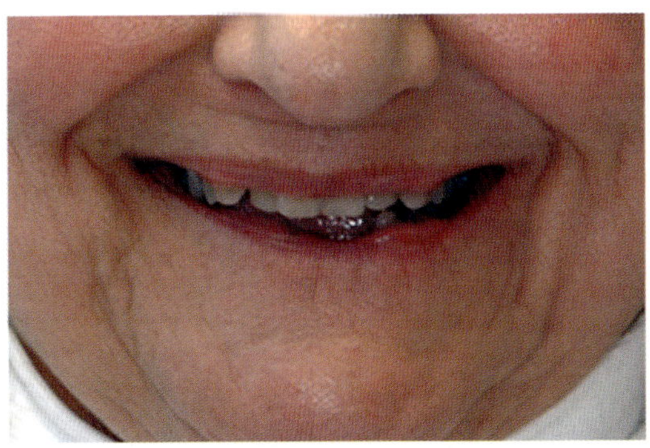

Fig. 15.16 Patient treated with a right marginal mandibulectomy due to a squamous cell carcinoma of the gingiva. The mandibular lip falls into the oral cavity without a prosthesis.

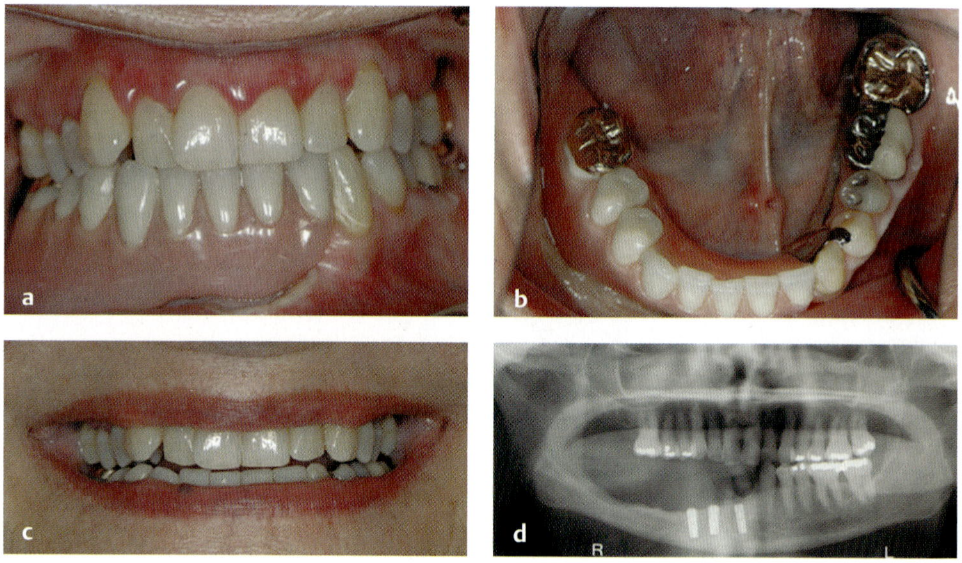

**Fig. 15.17** Mandibular resection prosthesis restoring a marginal mandibulectomy defect. This removable prosthesis is supported by the teeth and the bone under the skin graft and is retained by implants and clasps around the teeth. This optimal prosthetic foundation allows for restoration of function and aesthetics to a presurgical level. **(a)** Intraoral view of mandibular resection prostheses in position. **(b)** Occlusal view of mandibular resection prostheses in position area. **(c)** Aesthetic view of patient's smile. **(d)** Panoramic radiograph showing marginal mandibulectomy defect and implants in position.

under the prosthesis base may atrophy and provide a more stable base for the prosthesis **(Fig. 15.18)**. With multiple missing mandibular teeth, however, the retention of the prosthesis becomes more challenging. The placement of endosteal implants into the remaining mandibular bone or the osseous flap can greatly enhance prosthetic success.[35] Resected mandibles are frequently reconstructed with fibular flaps.[48] The osseous component of the flap is ideal for implant placement. Implants are typically placed as a two-stage procedure, following complete healing of the flap. The implants are placed into the fibula and allowed to heal for 3 to 6 months. They are then uncovered and the restorative abutments are placed. A surgical splint must also be placed at the time of uncovering to prevent healing of the skin paddle over the abutments **(Fig. 15.19)**. Following healing and maturation of the skin paddle around the abutments, the mandibular resection prosthesis can be fabricated **(Fig. 15.20)**.

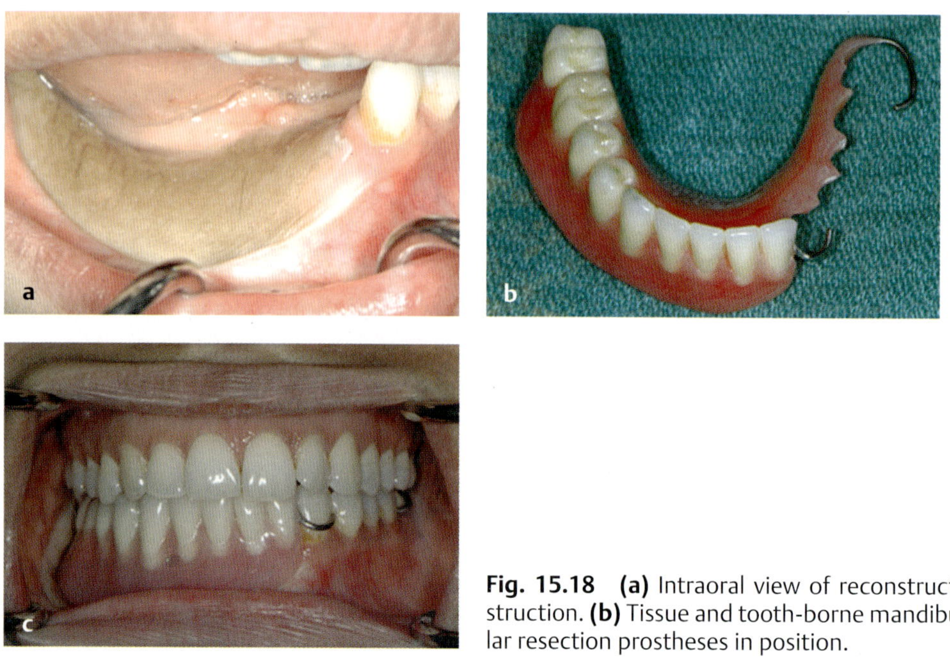

**Fig. 15.18** **(a)** Intraoral view of reconstructed mandible without implant reconstruction. **(b)** Tissue and tooth-borne mandibular resection prosthesis. **(c)** Mandibular resection prostheses in position.

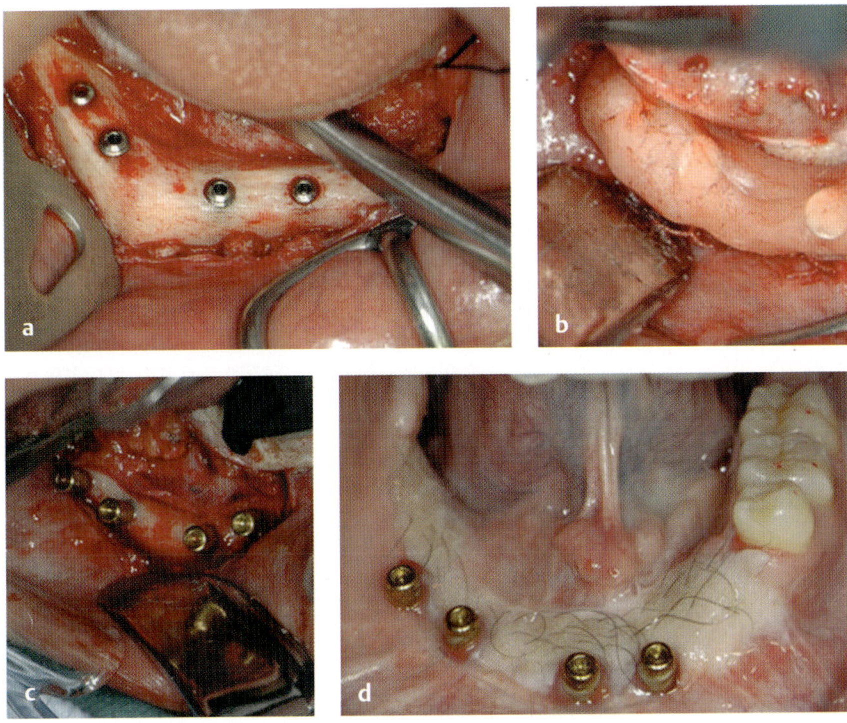

**Fig. 15.19** **(a)** Endosteal implants placed into the fibular flap of a reconstructed mandible. **(b)** Following adequate healing, the implants are uncovered and restorative abutments are screwed into the implants. **(c)** A surgical splint that clips onto the abutments is fabricated intraoperatively. This will prevent skin growth over the abutments. **(d)** The skin paddle has healed sufficiently for prosthetic fabrication.

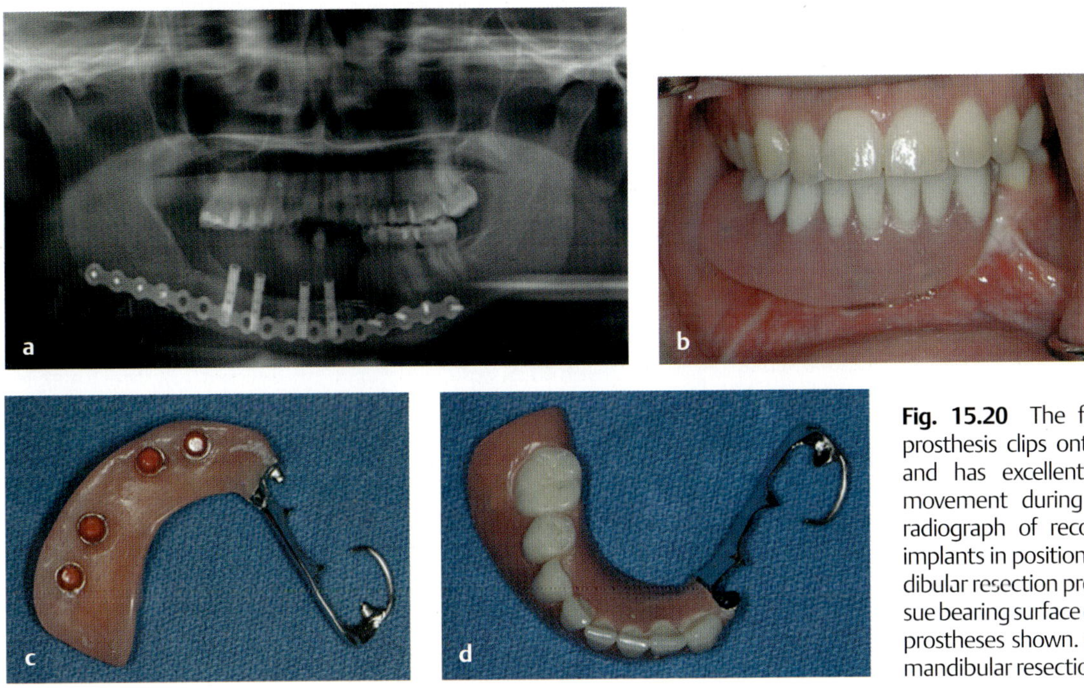

**Fig. 15.20** The final mandibular resection prosthesis clips onto the implant abutments and has excellent retention with minimal movement during function. **(a)** Panoramic radiograph of reconstructed mandible with implants in position. **(b)** Intraoral view of mandibular resection prostheses in position. **(c)** Tissue bearing surface of the mandibular resection prostheses shown. **(d)** Occlusal surface of the mandibular resection prostheses shown.

## Summary

The surgical reconstruction of tumor-ablated defects of the head and neck can sometimes fall short of providing functional and aesthetic outcomes. Extraoral and intraoral prosthetic rehabilitation can enhance functional and aesthetic outcomes, and provide a critical improvement of a patient's quality of life and sense of well-being. A sound and healthy tissue foundation for prosthetic placement and retention is crucial for success. Flap tissue should not obstruct the space that the prosthesis must occupy. Multidisciplinary planning and collaboration between the head and neck surgeon, reconstructive surgeon, and maxillofacial prosthodontist or anaplastologist are essential to optimize results. It is with such teamwork throughout the planning and treatment phases that optimal results can be achieved.

## References


1. Karayazgan B, Gunay Y, Atay A, Noyun F. Facial defects restored with extraoral implant-supported prostheses. J Craniofac Surg 2007;18(5):1086–1090
2. Karayazgan-Saracoglu B, Zulfikar H, Atay A, Gunay Y. Treatment outcome of extraoral implants in the craniofacial region. J Craniofac Surg 2010;21(3):751–758
3. Cervelli V, Bottini DJ, Arpino A, et al. Orbital reconstruction: bone-anchored implants. J Craniofac Surg 2006;17(5):848–853
4. Karakoca S, Aydin C, Yilmaz H, Bal BT. Survival rates and periimplant soft tissue evaluation of extraoral implants over a mean follow-up period of three years. J Prosthet Dent 2008;100(6):458–464
5. Leonardi A, Buonaccorsi S, Pellacchia V, Moricca LM, Indrizzi E, Fini G. Maxillofacial prosthetic rehabilitation using extraoral implants. J Craniofac Surg 2008;19(2):398–405
6. Jensen OT, Brownd C, Blacker J. Nasofacial prostheses supported by osseointegrated implants. Int J Oral Maxillofac Implants 1992;7(2):203–211
7. Schoen PJ, Raghoebar GM, van Oort RP, et al. Treatment outcome of bone-anchored craniofacial prostheses after tumor surgery. Cancer 2001;92(12):3045–3050
8. Wright RF, Zemnick C, Wazen JJ, Asher E. Osseointegrated implants and auricular defects: a case series study. J Prosthodont 2008;17(6):468–475
9. Beumer J III, Curtis TA, Marunick MT, et al. Restoration of facial defects: etiology, disability, and rehabilitation. In: Beumer J III, Curtis TA, Marunick MT, eds. Maxillofacial Rehabilitation: Prosthodontic and Surgical Considerations. St. Louis, MO: Ishiyaku Euroamerica; 1996:377–436
10. Martin JW, Lemon JC, King GE. Oral and facial restoration with prosthetics. In Knoll SS, ed. Reconstructive Plastic Surgery for Cancer. Mosby; 1996:130–138
11. Lemon JC, Chambers MS. Conventional methods of retention of facial prostheses. Paper presented at: First International Congress on Maxillofacial Prosthesis,1994.
12. Brånemark PI, Albrektsson T. Titanium implants permanently penetrating human skin. Scand J Plast Reconstr Surg 1982;16(1):17–21
13. Higuchi KW. Surgical principles of osseointegration. In: Branemark PI, Tolman DE, eds. Osseointegration in Craniofacial Reconstruction. Carol Stream, IL: Quintessence Publishing Co.; 1998:111–126
14. Miles BA, Sinn DP, Gion GG. Experience with cranial implant-based prosthetic reconstruction. J Craniofac Surg 2006;17(5):889–897
15. Bergstrom K. Anaplastological technique for facial defects. In: Branemark PI, De Oliveira MF, eds. Craniofacial Prostheses: Anaplastology and Osseointegration. Carol Stream, IL: Quintessence Publishing Co.; 1997:101–110
16. Hofstede TM, Montgomery PC, Jacob RF, Wesley PJ, Martin JW, Chambers MS. Prosthetic Rehabilitation. Cutaneous Malignancy of the Head and Neck: A Multidisciplinary Approach. San Diego, CA: Plural Publishing; 2011:587–599
17. Nishimura RD, Roumanas E, Moy PK, Sugai T. Nasal defects and osseointegrated implants: UCLA experience. J Prosthet Dent 1996;76(6):597–602
18. Scolozzi P, Jaques B. Treatment of midfacial defects using prostheses supported by ITI dental implants. Plast Reconstr Surg 2004;114(6):1395–1404
19. Ihde S, Kopp S, Gundlach K, Konstantinović VS. Effects of radiation therapy on craniofacial and dental implants: a review of the literature. Oral Surg Oral Med Oral Pathol Oral Radiol Endod 2009;107(1):56–65
20. Granstrom G. Osseointegration in the irradiated patient. In: Branemark PI, Tolman DE, eds. Osseointegration in Craniofacial Reconstruction. Carol Stream, IL: Quinessence Publishing Co.; 1998:95–108
21. Haug SP, Andres CJ, Munoz CA, Bernal G. Effects of environmental factors on maxillofacial elastomers: Part IV—Optical properties. J Prosthet Dent 1992;68(5):820–823
22. Kiat-Amnuay S, Mekayarajjananonth T, Powers JM, Chambers MS, Lemon JC. Interactions of pigments and opacifiers on color stability of MDX4-4210/type A maxillofacial elastomers subjected to artificial aging. J Prosthet Dent 2006;95(3):249–257
23. Heller HL, Mckinstry RE. Facial Materials. Fundamentals of Facial Prosthetics. Arlington, VA: ABI Professional Publications; 1995:79–97
24. Chen MS, Udagama A, Drane JB. Evaluation of facial prostheses for head and neck cancer patients. J Prosthet Dent 1981;46(5):538–544
25. Kiat-amnuay S, Gettleman L, Khan Z, Goldsmith LJ. Effect of adhesive retention on maxillofacial prostheses. Part I: skin dressings and solvent removers. J Prosthet Dent 2000;84(3):335–340
26. Marunick MT, Harrison R, Beumer J III. Prosthodontic rehabilitation of midfacial defects. J Prosthet Dent 1985;54(4):553–560
27. The glossary of prosthodontic terms. J Prosthet Dent 2005;94(1):10–92
28. Beumer J III, Marunick M, Garrett N, et al. Rehabilitation of maxillary defects. In: Beumer J III, Marunick M, Esposito SJ, eds. Maxillofacial Rehabilitation: Prosthodontic and Surgical Management of Cancer-Related, Acquired, and Congenital Defects of the Head and Neck. 3rd ed. Hanover Park, IL: Quintessence Publishing Co.; 2011:155–213
29. Chambers MS, Lemon JC, Martin JW. Surgical techniques to enhance prosthetic rehabilitation. In: Bailey BJ, Johnson JT, Newlands SD, eds. Head and Neck Surgery—Otolaryngology. 4th ed. Philadelphia, PA: Lippincott Williams and Wilkins; 2006:1853–1865
30. Lemon JC, Martin JW, Jacob RF. Prosthetic rehabilitation. In: Weber RS, Miller MJ, Goepfert H, eds. Basal and Squamous Cell Skin Cancers of the Head and Neck. Baltimore, MD: Williams and Wilkins; 1996:305–312
31. Jacob RF, King G. Indirect retainers in soft palate obturator design. J Prosthet Dent 1990;63(3):311–315
32. Okay DJ, Genden E, Buchbinder D, Urken M. Prosthodontic guidelines for surgical reconstruction of the maxilla: a classification system of defects. J Prosthet Dent 2001;86(4):352–363

33. Aramany MA. Basic principles of obturator design for partially edentulous patients. Part I: classification. J Prosthet Dent 1978;40(5):554–557
34. McCord JF, Michelinakis G. Systematic review of the evidence supporting intra-oral maxillofacial prosthodontic care. Eur J Prosthodont Restor Dent 2004; 12(3):129–135
35. Eckert SE, Desjardins RP. The impact of endosseous implants on maxillofacial prosthetics. In: Taylor TD, ed. Clinical Maxillofacial Prosthetics. Chicago, IL: Quintessence Publishing Co.; 2000:145–153
36. King GE, Jacob RF, Martin JW. Oral and dental rehabilitation. In: E. JM, ed. Complications in Otolaryngology and Head and Neck Surgery. Philadelphia, PA: BC Decker; 1986:131
37. Tumerdem-Ulug B, Kuran I, Ozden BC, et al. Does hyperbaric oxygen administration before or after irradiation decrease side effects of irradiation on implant sites? Ann Plast Surg 2011;67(1):62–67
38. Martin JW, Jacob RF, Larson DL, King GE. Surgical stents for the head and neck cancer patient. Head Neck Surg 1984;7(1):44–46
39. Teichgraeber J, Larson DL, Castaneda O, Martin JW. Skin grafts in intraoral reconstruction. A new stenting method. Arch Otolaryngol 1984;110(7):463–467
40. Martin JW, Austin JR, Chambers MS, Lemon JC, Toth BB. Postoperative care of the maxillectomy patient. ORL Head Neck Nurs 1994;12(3):15–20
41. Fukuda M, Takahashi T, Nagai H, Iino M. Implant-supported edentulous maxillary obturators with milled bar attachments after maxillectomy. J Oral Maxillofac Surg 2004;62(7):799–805
42. Funk GF, Arcuri MR, Frodel JL Jr. Functional dental rehabilitation of massive palatomaxillary defects: cases requiring free tissue transfer and osseointegrated implants. Head Neck 1998;20(1):38–51
43. Peng X, Mao C, Yu GY, Guo CB, Huang MX, Zhang Y. Maxillary reconstruction with the free fibula flap. Plast Reconstr Surg 2005;115(6):1562–1569
44. Schusterman MA, Reece GP, Miller MJ, Harris S. The osteocutaneous free fibula flap: is the skin paddle reliable? Plast Reconstr Surg 1992;90(5):787–793, discussion 794–798
45. Marunick M, Tselios N. The efficacy of palatal augmentation prostheses for speech and swallowing in patients undergoing glossectomy: a review of the literature. J Prosthet Dent 2004;91(1):67–74
46. Beumer J III, Marunick M, Silverman S, et al. Rehabilitation of tongue and mandibular defects. In: Beumer J III, Marunick M, Esposito SJ, eds. Maxillofacial Rehabilitation: Prosthodontic and Surgical Management of Cancer-Related, Acquired, and Congenital Defects of the Head and Neck. 3rd ed. Hanover Park, IL: Quintessence Publishing Co.; 2011:61–154
47. Schramm VL Jr, Johnson JT, Myers EN. Skin grafts and flaps in oral cavity reconstruction. Arch Otolaryngol 1983;109(3):175–177
48. Hidalgo DA. Fibula free flap: a new method of mandible reconstruction. Plast Reconstr Surg 1989;84(1):71–79

# 16 Robotic Reconstructive Surgery

*Amir Ibrahim, Karim A. Sarhane, F. Christopher Holsinger, and Jesse C. Selber*

## Introduction

Malignant lesions of the oropharynx and base of tongue are challenging to treat due to the complex functional anatomy. The frequent need for morbid procedures (e.g., lip and mandible splitting approaches) to resect such tumors has led to a shift in practice patterns toward primary combined chemotherapy and radiation[1,2] **(Fig. 16.1)**. However, toxicity rates following this approach can be very high, and functional status following treatment may be low.[3] Transoral Robotic Surgery (TORS) for minimally invasive resection of oropharyngeal malignancies has the benefits of locoregional control without the morbidity of a mandibulotomy or high-dose chemoradiation.[4,5] TORS has been shown to be an acceptable alternative to chemoradiation for the treatment of malignant lesions of the oropharynx, with equivalent oncologic control and improved functional outcomes in some series.[6]

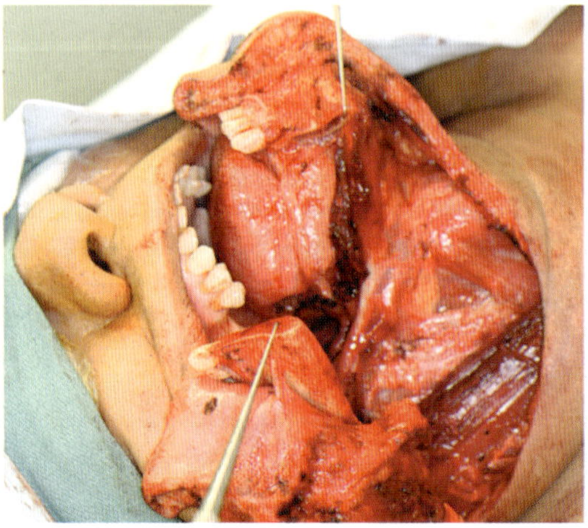

**Fig. 16.1** Traditional lip-splitting and mandibulotomy approach to oropharyngeal tumors. Not only is this approach associated with disfigurement, but also there is a late risk for osteoradionecrosis and fracture at the mandibulotomy site when radiation is combined with surgery.

Many TORS defects are left to heal by secondary intention, but when vital structures are exposed or functional anatomy is missing, reconstruction can serve an important role in minimal access resections. The challenge posed by these and other minimally invasive extirpations is that the anatomy of the oropharynx remains restricted and access is limited by the oral opening. For these cases, Transoral Robotic *Reconstructive* Surgery (TOR*R*S) has provided a useful adjunct. In this chapter, we discuss the clinical application of TOR*R*S to address defects created by minimal access resections, such as TORS or pull-through resections using only a small lateral pharyngotomy.

We start by revisiting the different paradigm shifts in the management of patients with head and neck cancer, then we discuss the rationale for, and rise of, TORS (resection). Next, the role of TOR*R*S (reconstruction) is described, along with preliminary guidelines for its clinical application. The surgical technique is briefly described, with some examples. We finish by contrasting the overall advantages of such medical innovation with its shortcomings, and we highlight the areas needing further improvements.

## Paradigm Shifts in the Management of Oropharyngeal Neoplasms

Management trends for head and neck cancer patients have evolved considerably over the past several decades—from wide surgical extirpation, to radiotherapy, to chemoradiotherapy, and in certain centers, minimally invasive surgical resection. This evolution was mostly guided by efforts to decrease treatment side effects and to optimize functional outcomes while ensuring tumor control.

Surgical extirpation of oropharyngeal tumors has historically been performed by dividing the mandible or splitting the lip, often leading to a significant rate of acute complications in comparison to primary radiotherapy[7,8]; furthermore, this approach necessitated extensive coverage (usually in the form of free flap reconstruction), and often still required adjuvant radiotherapy.[9] Consequently, standard of care shifted to primary radiotherapy,[8] often in association with chemotherapy.[10,11] Although good locoregional control is achieved, acute morbidity rates with the higher radiation doses and combination therapy were elevated[12,13]; severe mucositis, which notoriously accompanied intensity-modulated radiation therapy, is compounded by the toxicity of induction chemotherapy, resulting in acute grade ≥ 3 toxicity rates approaching 90%.[14,15] Delayed toxicity events (dysphagia, feeding tube dependence) have also been noted in several studies.[1,16]

TORS was intended to provide a surgical solution that mitigated the morbidity of the wide-open surgical approaches without incurring the drawbacks of chemoradiation. The technique allows surgeons to achieve complete resection of selected oropharyngeal, laryngeal, and hypopharyngeal tumors with much lower functional impairment than with traditional strategies. Furthermore, this technology is associated with less blood loss, fewer postsurgical complications, and shorter duration of hospitalization than traditional open procedures.[5] Early and mid-term reports have shown encouraging oncologic and functional outcomes.[17,18,19] TORS has been adopted at multiple centers and received FDA approval in 2009.[20]

## ■ The Role of TORRS

Despite improvements in morbidity over traditional techniques, TORS can still result in functionally compromising or unsafe postsurgical defects (depending on their size and anatomical location) if not followed by adequate reconstruction. The reconstructive challenge created by minimally invasive resections is that the cylinder of the oropharynx remains almost entirely closed, severely restricting access to oropharyngeal anatomy as reconstructive surgeons attempt to inset and contour vascularized tissue. In particular, the anatomical region between the uvula and the epiglottis is very difficult to approach without a mandibulotomy or wide pharyngotomy. Preserving a competent velopharyngeal sphincter, a watertight seal between the pharynx and neck, and adequate sensation and volume in the tongue base is necessary to optimize the physiological function of the oropharynx and to minimize functional deficits.[21,22] Defects that expose vital structures or resect functional anatomy require judicious reconstructive efforts to preserve function; these techniques range from local tissue rearrangement and closure to free tissue transfer.

The majority of small defects require no reconstruction at all and can be left to heal by secondary intention, with minimal functional limitations. Others, such as those in the deep tonsillar area and those extending to the soft palate, can require some form of tissue coverage, as they may result in carotid sheath or mandibular ramus exposure, oro- or pharyngocutaneous fistulas, and a potential for velopharyngeal incompetence. Some of these defects can be reliably reconstructed with facial artery myomucosal (FAMM) flaps, buccal rotation flaps, and a variety of other pharyngeal flaps (see Case 1). The authors reported the use of the robot to reconstruct a defect of the soft palate, tonsillar pillar, and pharyngeal wall with a FAMM flap in one patient in a case series describing robotic reconstruction.[23] Bonawiz et al[6] reported successful closure of defects of the soft palate in a series of five patients who underwent combined robotic-assisted resection of malignant lesions with immediate FAMM flap reconstruction.

Defects resulting from larger tumor resections are often topographically complex and may extend from the tip of the tongue all the way to the epiglottis, involving a significant pharyngeal component. When the resection cannot be completed with a transoral approach, a pharyngotomy is often added for the deepest component. Combining transoral robotic flap inset with manual inset through the pharyngotomy defect is also possible. In these cases, however, it is important to note that, although a pharyngotomy needs to be created, it is often smaller than the wide pharyngotomies traditionally required for accessing such tumors, since access to the upper pharynx is achieved robotically rather than through the neck. These larger defects benefit from a robotic transoral reconstructive approach (see Case 2).[24] The use of TORRS for challenging defects of the head and neck has been shown to be both feasible[25] and effective.[23] In addition, by taking this approach, plastic surgeons are able to provide reliable reconstructive support for the head and neck oncologic surgeon to robotically resect larger, deeper, and more complex tumors that would be very challenging to reconstruct through traditional methods.

## ■ Indications and Preoperative Evaluation

Reports on the use of TORRS so far have focused on feasibility, safety, and extent of applicability; no clear instructions incorporating patient and tumor factors have yet been put forth. The authors recently proposed an algorithm for the use of TORRS based on tumor site, tumor extent, and patient-specific factors.[17] The algorithm functions as a structural scheme into which future recommendations can be incorporated.

## Tumor Site

Tumor site is probably the most influential factor affecting the feasibility of a transoral robotic approach for resection and reconstruction. Lesions of the oral cavity are easily accessible manually and do not substantially benefit from TORS. An exception is lesions in the retromolar trigone; large tumors in this area are adjacent to the base of tongue (BOT), tonsil, and mandibular ramus. Due to the difficult location, a robotic approach can be advantageous in this setting for both resection and reconstruction. Local flaps, such as the FAMM flap, buccal fat pad flap, and buccal and pharyngeal mucosal transposition flaps, are good choices for many such cases. Free flaps are rarely used; not only is the area very restricted, but a free flap would entail dissecting and exposing the neck to the oropharynx. Unless there is a clear indication for free tissue transfer (such as prior radiation or resections), avoiding such methods is advocated.

Conversely, tumors located within the oropharynx (tonsil, BOT, soft palate) benefit substantially from TORS resection and reconstruction. Limited room to maneuver and poor visualization are obstacles to traditional surgical resection that are over come by the TORS system.[26,27] With the ascent of robotic technology, improved visualization and more precise instrumentation have allowed the resection of more complex and invasive tumors. Defects created by such large resections (where critical structures, such as the carotid sheath or bone, are exposed) are best addressed using robotic free flap reconstruction.[5,23] As for tumors involving the soft palate, free flaps or palatoplasties are usually performed; in select circumstances, similar functional outcomes may be attained with a prosthetic obturator.[28,29]

For tumors extending to the supraglottic larynx, reconstruction is guided by the extent of hypopharyngeal involvement and whether the lesion is located above or below the hyoid bone. In patients with a large oral opening, the supra- and infrahyoid areas can be directly attained, and TORS might not be required; free tissue transfer is also difficult in this area. However, in case the defect is large enough to require free flap reconstruction,[30] a tracheostomy is indicated.

## Tumor Extent

As mentioned previously, resection of small tumors (i.e., T1 and T2) can be allowed to heal by secondary intention; this approach is safe and results in satisfactory functional outcomes. As for larger lesions (i.e., T3, T4) or for posterior T2 tumors, or when the carotid sheath is exposed, a surgical fistula is created, or velopharyngeal compromise is anticipated to occur, vascularized tissue reconstruction is required to restore normal anatomy and to ensure good functional outcomes. Several these lesions may also undergo "hybrid" resections, i.e., combining a transoral approach with a small pharyngotomy; these cases are typically followed by a "hybrid" type of reconstruction, where TOR*R*S is performed and the deepest inset is completed through the neck.

## Prior Therapy

Irradiation damages local micro- and macrovasculature, making local flaps undesirable for reconstruction. Additionally, some recurrent cancers are treated with a second course of radiation therapy. In such cases, free tissue transfer is sometimes indicated even when defects might otherwise be small enough not to require coverage. This type of reconstruction brings in healthy vascularized tissue and allows for re-irradiation by ensuring a durable form of wound coverage.[21,25]

## Patient Factors

Patient performance status constitutes the primary determinant of the decision for any type of surgery. As obesity is reaching very high levels,[31] medical comorbidities, such as diabetes and vascular diseases, are increasing among all patient age groups. Such conditions compromise perfusion and wound healing, and, hence, increase the risk of dehiscence, infections, and other wound complications. Tight glycemic control in the pre- and postoperative period is fundamental. More frequently than obesity, however, head and neck cancer patients suffer from malnutrition, chronic cachexia, and muscle wasting. In addition to these factors, significant smoking history and poor cardiopulmonary status may also compromise the operative course of such patients, making them vulnerable to complications associated with long operative times. It is also important to consider the other preoperative patient variables that are associated with poor postoperative performance, such as anemia, coronary or peripheral vascular disease, dysphagia, or a history of recurrent aspiration.[32,33]

# ■ Surgical Technique

## Patient Positioning

TOR*R*S is usually combined with TORS, where patient positioning and set up is already optimized for robotic surgery. Patients are usually placed in the supine position and are supported with a shoulder roll, to provide adequate neck extension, and with a "doughnut" gel pad to ensure occipital scalp protection. Both upper and lower extremities are well padded to prevent nerve injury, especially in overweight and obese patients.[34] TED stockings and sequential compression devices are also applied to the lower extremities in an effort to minimize deep vein thrombosis.

## Robotic Setup

The setup for the robotic portion is similar for all TORRS cases.[23] The approach involves use of a mouth retractor. When the tongue base is not involved, a Dingman retractor is placed in the mouth to create a stable interdental opening and to provide lingual retraction.[35] When reconstruction of the BOT is required, the tongue must remain mobile; a cheek retractor is placed to maintain a stable frame, a mouth prop is used to create a wide interdental opening, and a suture is placed at the tip of tongue to allow manipulation **(Fig. 16.2)**. Two robotic arms and the endoscope are placed in the mouth, converging on the target pharyngeal anatomy, and the tumor is resected with the surgeon sitting at the robotic console. Occasionally, tumors are too large for a complete transoral resection, and, in these cases, a small lateral pharyngotomy can be added for additional exposure.[17]

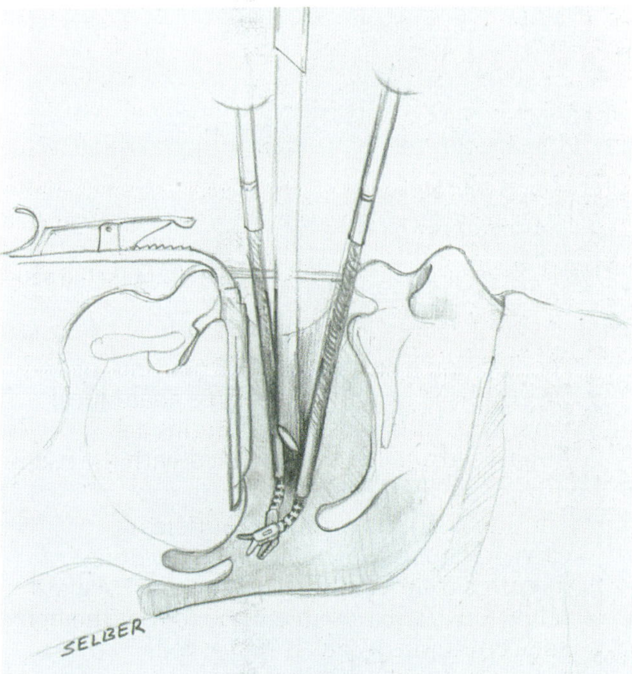


**Fig. 16.2** Diagram showing robotic setup for operating on oropharyngeal tumors. A Dingman oral retractor is utilized to keep the mouth open. Surgery is performed via two robotic arms and is visualized with an endoscope.

## Robotic Docking

The exact location and position of the patient side cart depends on the location of the defect. Since the robotic arms function best when the working area is lined up with the base, and when the arms are working back toward it, for defects located in the right tonsillar area it is recommended to position the robot at 45 degrees from the foot of the right side of the operating table. When the defect is in the left tonsillar area, 45 degrees from the foot of the left side is preferred. For central or posterior pharyngeal defects, either of these two positions is acceptable. In any case, the patient side cart should be against the base of the bed, to bring it as close as possible to the mouth. When operating on the palate, it is more convenient to bring the robot in from the head of the bed.

In all of these settings, the two robotic arms are aligned around a point converging at the target anatomy in the oropharynx. The shoulders of the three arms should be angled at 90 degrees, and the arms should form ~ 45 degree angles with the endoscope.

## Robotic Flap Inset

Following flap elevation, inset within the mouth is performed using two 8 mm needle drivers and 4–0 or 3–0 polyglactin sutures. Two needle drivers are preferable to a needle driver and grasper because it is sometimes necessary to throw sutures with both arms of the robot (depending on the angle and location within the oral cavity). The suture is trimmed to approximately 3 inches in length, to avoid extra suture material in the mouth. Interrupted sutures are placed and tied using human hands. Economy of motion is important because small movements at the tips of the instruments correspond to large movements more proximally; excursion of the robotic arms is limited by the area within the mouth retractor. On occasion, when the space is too restricted, such as in the glossopharyngeal sulcus, sutures can be placed robotically, taking advantage of the improved visualization and dexterity, and then tied down blindly by hand.

## Robotic Microvascular Anastomosis

Once the robotic portion of the inset is performed, the arms can be removed from the mouth, and instruments can be changed and then placed back in proximity to the neck vessels. Arms number 1 and number 2 are equipped with Black Diamond Micro forceps, rather than the larger jawed needle drivers used during the inset. A third arm is equipped with a "fine tissue forceps" attachment serving as a stationary assistant, and the surgeon is able to toggle back and forth between arms number 1 and number 3, depending on which one is being used to position the vessel and which is being used to sew. For anastomosis, 9–0 nylon sutures are commonly used.

Robotic microvascular anastomosis is a promising technique. The facial artery is the most utilized recipient artery. It courses beneath the hypoglossal nerve and underneath the digastric muscle, often under the body of the mandible. If the patient has a tracheostomy or ventilator tubing, the space available to perform the anastomosis may be confined. The robot's precision and visualization in restricted spaces addresses such issues and permits microanastomoses to be performed with much more physical convenience.

Due to lack of haptic or tactile feedback, careful attention to visual cues is vital, particularly when it comes to setting down the knot. It is important to maintain equal tension in both ends of the suture and to minimize movement of the anastomosis while tying (as this represents a differential in applied tension), and to only pull until the air in the knot disappears. These measures are essential to minimize vessel trauma. Due to poorly designed robotic microsurgical instruments with broad and flat tips and with diamond dust coating, attention is needed to avoid inadvertently cutting the suture.

## ■ TORRS Advantages

TORRS offers all the advantages of a robotic platform, which have made possible many surgical approaches that were previously technically difficult or unfeasible. They are briefly summarized below.

### Enhanced Precision

Computer-enhanced surgical technology is able to provide superhuman precision. The robotic platform completely eliminates fine tremors of the human hand through sophisticated hardware and software filters, and provides up to five times reduction in amplitude motion (motion scaling). These characteristics, in addition to better ergonomics and improved visual acuity, have led to a considerable enhancement of the surgeon's control of the instruments and tissues, allowing challenging procedures to be performed with more confidence.[36]

### Increased Dexterity

Robotic instruments provide increased degrees of freedom, which enhance the ability to handle arteries, veins, nerves, and other tissues with minimal trauma. In addition, unlike laparoscopy, the robotic platform is free of the fulcrum effect; thus, handling of the robotic arms is much more natural than laparoscopic surgery.[37]

### Enhanced Hand-Eye Coordination

The robotic visual system is equipped with three-dimensional optics at 10 times the magnification, which affords high-definition images. The three-dimensional view with depth perception is much more advanced than a conventional operating room camera (e.g., laparoscopic camera). The high-resolution images, coupled with increased degrees of freedom and improved dexterity, allow meticulous identification and dissection of fine anatomical structures; in addition, microanastomoses can be performed with enhanced precision and visualization.

### Ergonomic Positioning

Another highlight of the robot is ergonomic positioning. With the surgeon sitting remotely at a comfortably designed station, the robotic technology obviates the need to twist and turn in awkward positions, especially when operating in narrow visual fields (**Fig. 16.3**). In microsurgery, surgeons spend a lot of time working around structures to fit their hands in space; robotic microsurgery eliminates the need to work around tracheostomy tubes, under the mandible, or over large flaps.

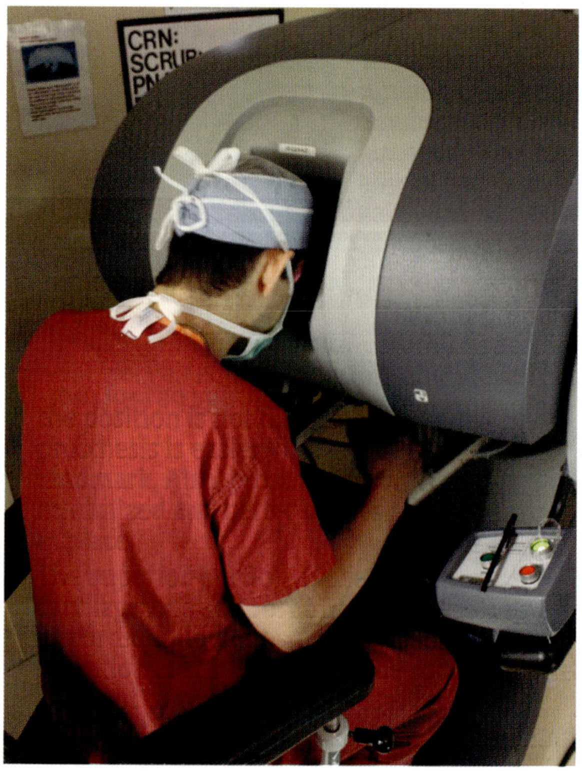


**Fig. 16.3** Surgeon controlling operative robot. Positioning is ergonomic and allows a magnified view of robotic arms that can operate within a confined space.

### Smooth Patient Recovery

For patients, the results of robotic-assisted surgery, by virtue of its minimally invasive nature, include decreased postoperative pain, less risk of infection, and less blood loss, in addition to a potentially shorter hospital stay, faster recovery, and quicker return to normal daily activities. The complications particular to mandibulotomy, such as fistula, malunion, nonunion, infected or exposed hardware, and osteoradionecrosis from periosteal stripping, can be minimized.

## ■ TORRS Disadvantages

### General Limitations of Robotic Surgery

Although rapidly developing, TOR*R*S technology has not achieved its full potential due to a few limitations of the general robotic platform, including, among other technical constraints, lack of haptics (force feedback), size of the devices, instrumentation limitations (both size and variety), and lack of flexibility of certain energy devices.

### Limitations to Acquiring Robotic Skills

Despite technological advancement, surgical training curricula have stayed more or less the same for more than a century. Residents and fellows have always learned surgery through supervised "on the job training." This method makes training completely dependent on the case load, might even prolong surgical training in some cases, and compromises patients' safety. Such an approach cannot be extended to robotics, as current case loads in everything but urology are very limited, drawing out the learning curve for robotics. In this regard, simulation centers might be a better medium for acquisition of robotic surgical skills. In such settings, trainees can use surgical robots to practice operations on three-dimensional, virtual-reality visual simulations and soft tissue models that recreate the textures of human tissues through force feedback (haptics).[38,39] Furthermore, trainees can be supervised through telementoring. Finally, standardized evaluation and competency-based training, which are valuable in every area, would be particularly useful in robotic skill acquisition. This approach has the potential to considerably improve the learning curve of robotic surgery, allowing trainees to acquire robotic skills in a relatively shorter period while minimizing surgical errors and thus enhancing patient safety.

### Cost

Cost represents an obstacle for the dissemination of robotic surgical techniques. The current price of the da Vinci system is $2.2 million, and annual maintenance is $138,000. It is important to recognize that this fixed cost is an investment on the part of the hospital in the hopes of increasing patient volume and is not the variable cost of using the device. Use of the device itself involves the additional costs of the extra OR time and the disposable (sterile drape) and semi-disposable instruments (designed for 10 uses, so cost must be spread out over those cases). These variable costs are actually not substantial, so, although at first glance cost seems to be a major obstacle in reconstructive surgery, when considering the advantages offered, robotic-assisted procedures might compare favorably to traditional approaches.[40] Prospective studies are needed to critically evaluate the cost-effectiveness of this new technology in terms of operative time, recovery period, hospital length of stay, and morbidity rates.

## ■ Conclusion

Robotic technology is expected to play an increasingly important role in the future of reconstructive surgery. We have seen growing applications for various reconstructive procedures.[40,41,42] Adapting the robotic platform for the resection (TORS) and reconstruction (TOR*R*S) of head and neck malignancies appears to have advantages in terms of oncologic and functional outcomes, as well as in terms of increased patient safety, decreased complication rates, and reduced hospital length of stay. Widespread application of this technology is dependent on minimizing cost and implementing competency-based training programs.

## ■ Case Examples

### Case 1

A 74-year-old male had a T2 N1 M0 right tonsillar squamous cell carcinoma that was treated with primary radiation therapy in the distant past. He subsequently developed a T2 N0 M0 squamous cell carcinoma of the left tonsil (**Fig. 16.4**). He underwent transoral robotic resection of the tumor. His defect included the posterior tonsillar pillar, a portion of the soft palate, and a portion of the posterior pharynx. Although the defect was small, the carotid sheath was exposed and there was concern about velopharyngeal incompetence. A left-sided, inferiorly based facial artery musculomucosal (FAMM) flap

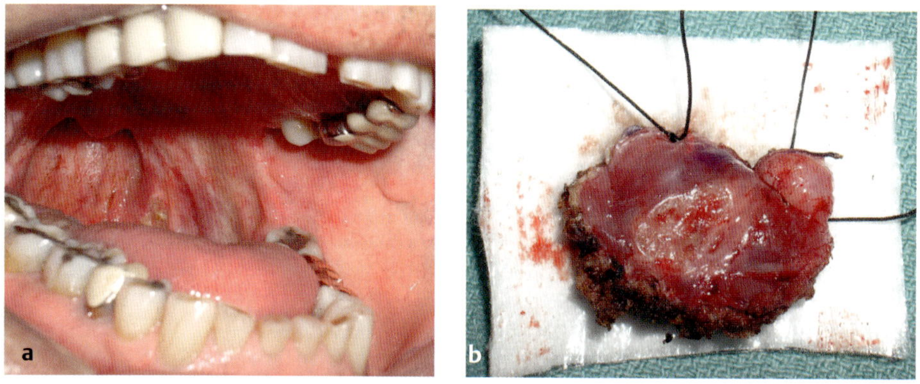

**Fig. 16.4** **(a)** Left tonsillar cancer and **(b)** surgical specimen resected robotically.

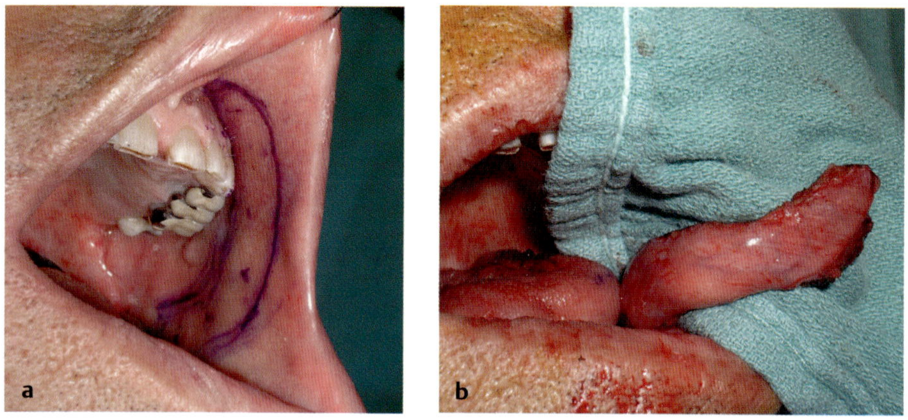

**Fig. 16.5** **(a)** Left facial artery musculomucosal (FAMM) flap for reconstruction following removal of a tonsillar cancer. **(b)** The use of a robot allows improved visualization and dexterity during flap inset.

was planned. The flap extended from the ipsilateral retromolar trigone to the frenulum of the gingivobuccal sulcus. The flap was passed over the third molar and into the defect to reconstruct the posterior tonsillar pillar **(Fig. 16.5)**. A Dingman retractor was used to create an interdental opening and to retract the cheeks and tongue. Inset of the flap was performed robotically using absorbable sutures. A bite block was placed to protect the pedicle.

## Case 2

A 62-year-old man presented with a history of recurrent T3 N1 M0 squamous cell carcinoma of the left posterolateral pharynx following failed radiation treatment in the past **(Fig. 16.6)**. He underwent a combination transoral robotic resection with the addition of a small lateral pharyngotomy, and a left neck dissection. Although the pharyngotomy was small (~ 15 $cm^2$), a large portion of the pharynx (~ 50 $cm^2$) was resected from the epiglottis to the soft palate. A 6 × 9 cm radial forearm flap was harvested **(Fig. 16.7)**. The upper pharyngeal component was inset robotically. The remainder of the inset was completed through the pharyngotomy. The patient side cart, which was already in position from the robotic resection and inset, was adjusted, and the robotic arterial anastomosis was successfully completed **(Fig. 16.8)**. The venous anastomosis was then coupled under loupe magnification. The patient was decannulated, was discharged within a week, and passed a modified barium swallow study 3 weeks postoperatively **(Fig. 16.9)**. His speech and swallowing are normal, and he is tolerating a regular diet independent of tube feeds **(Fig. 16.10)**.

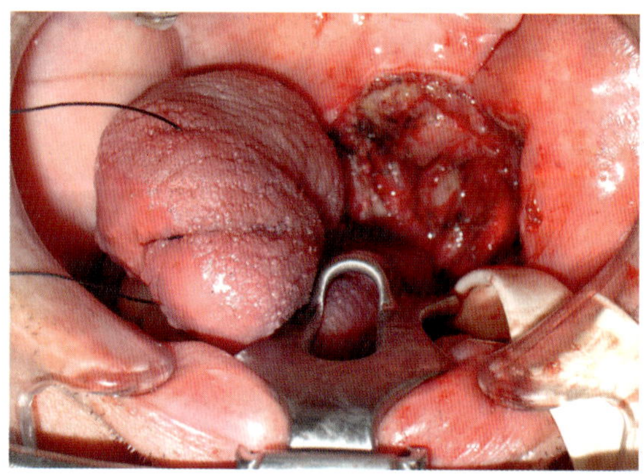

**Fig. 16.6** Surgical defect following salvage resection of a recurrent left pharyngeal cancer.

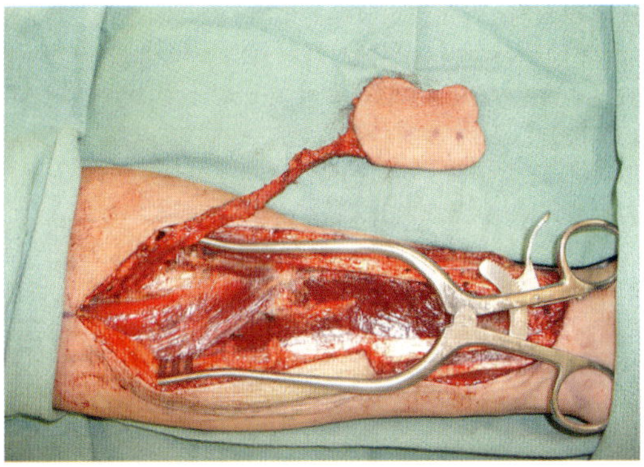

**Fig. 16.7** A radial forearm fasciocutaneous free flap was harvested in preparation for robot-assisted inset.

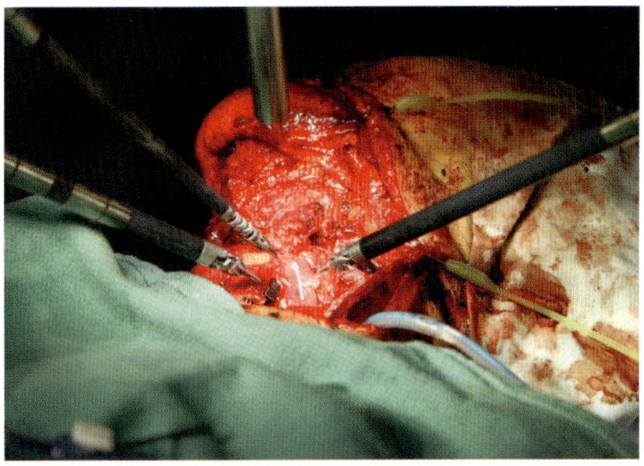

**Fig. 16.8** Robotic microvascular anastomosis of the radial artery to the left facial artery.

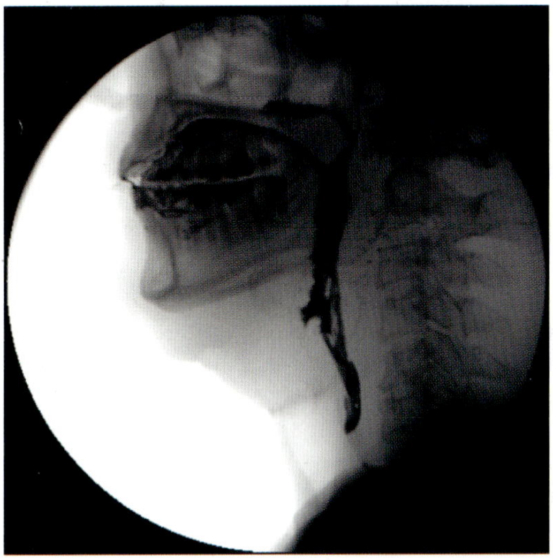

**Fig. 16.9** Modified barium swallow following robot-assisted reconstruction of the oropharynx with a radial forearm free flap demonstrating no leakage of barium and no aspiration.

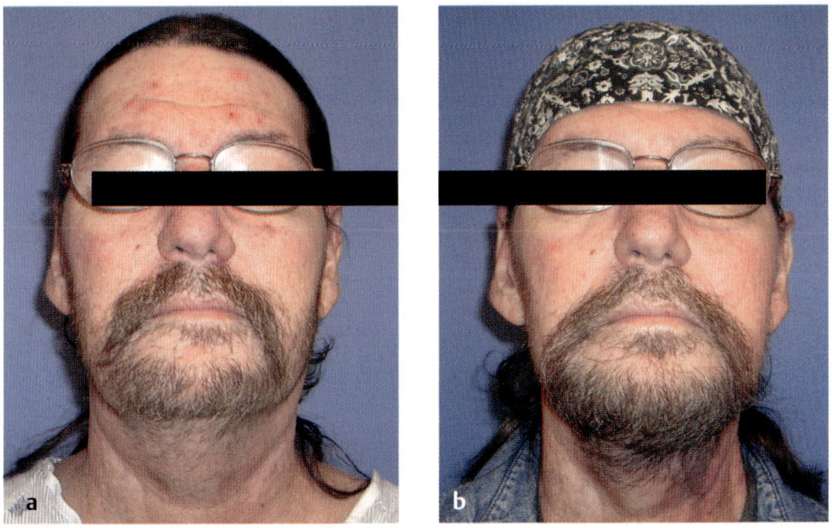

**Fig. 16.10** **(a)** Pre- and **(b)** postoperative appearance following resection and reconstruction of a left oropharnygeal cancer in which use of an operative robot provided improved visualization and surgical manipulation so that a lip- and mandible-splitting approach could be avoided.

## References


1. Machtay M, Moughan J, Trotti A, et al. Factors associated with severe late toxicity after concurrent chemoradiation for locally advanced head and neck cancer: an RTOG analysis. J Clin Oncol 2008;26(21):3582–3589
2. Walvekar RR, Li RJ, Gooding WE, et al. Role of surgery in limited (T1-2, N0-1) cancers of the oropharynx. Laryngoscope 2008;118(12):2129–2134
3. Nguyen NP, Vos P, Smith HJ, et al. Concurrent chemoradiation for locally advanced oropharyngeal cancer. Am J Otolaryngol 2007;28(1):3–8
4. Bhayani MK, Holsinger FC, Lai SY. A shifting paradigm for patients with head and neck cancer: transoral robotic surgery (TORS). Oncology (Williston Park) 2010;24(11):1010–1015
5. Genden EM, Kotz T, Tong CCL, et al. Transoral robotic resection and reconstruction for head and neck cancer. Laryngoscope 2011;121(8):1668–1674
6. Bonawitz SC, Duvvuri U. Robotic-assisted FAMM flap for soft palate reconstruction. Laryngoscope 2013;123(4):870–874
7. Mendenhall WM, Amdur RJ, Stringer SP, Villaret DB, Cassisi NJ. Radiation therapy for squamous cell carcinoma of the tonsillar region: a preferred alternative to surgery? J Clin Oncol 2000;18(11):2219–2225
8. Parsons JT, Mendenhall WM, Stringer SP, et al. Squamous cell carcinoma of the oropharynx: surgery, radiation therapy, or both. Cancer 2002;94(11):2967–2980
9. Amdur RJ, Parsons JT, Mendenhall WM, Million RR, Stringer SP, Cassisi NJ. Postoperative irradiation for squamous cell carcinoma of the head and neck: an analysis of treatment results and complications. Int J Radiat Oncol Biol Phys 1989;16(1):25–36
10. Fein DA, Lee WR, Amos WR, et al. Oropharyngeal carcinoma treated with radiotherapy: a 30-year experience. Int J Radiat Oncol Biol Phys 1996;34(2):289–296
11. Lee NY, de Arruda FF, Puri DR, et al. A comparison of intensity-modulated radiation therapy and concomitant boost radiotherapy in the setting of concurrent chemotherapy for locally advanced oropharyngeal carcinoma. Int J Radiat Oncol Biol Phys 2006;66(4):966–974
12. Adelstein DJ, Moon J, Hanna E, et al. Docetaxel, cisplatin, and fluorouracil induction chemotherapy followed by accelerated fractionation/concomitant boost radiation and concurrent cisplatin in patients with advanced squamous cell head and neck cancer: A Southwest Oncology Group phase II trial (S0216). Head Neck 2010;32(2):221–228
13. Vokes EE, Stenson K, Rosen FR, et al. Weekly carboplatin and paclitaxel followed by concomitant paclitaxel, fluorouracil, and hydroxyurea chemoradiotherapy: curative and organ-preserving therapy for advanced head and neck cancer. J Clin Oncol 2003;21(2):320–326
14. Adelstein DJ, Saxton JP, Lavertu P, et al. Maximizing local control and organ preservation in stage IV squamous cell head and neck cancer With hyperfractionated radiation and concurrent chemotherapy. J Clin Oncol 2002;20(5):1405–1410
15. Brizel DM, Albers ME, Fisher SR, et al. Hyperfractionated irradiation with or without concurrent chemotherapy for locally advanced head and neck cancer. N Engl J Med 1998;338(25):1798–1804
16. Denis F, Garaud P, Bardet E, et al. Final results of the 94-01 French Head and Neck Oncology and Radiotherapy Group randomized trial comparing radiotherapy alone with concomitant radiochemotherapy in advanced-stage oropharynx carcinoma. J Clin Oncol 2004;22(1):69–76
17. Longfield EA, Holsinger FC, Selber JC. Reconstruction after robotic head and neck surgery: when and why. J Reconstr Microsurg 2012;28(7):445–450
18. Iseli TA, Kulbersh BD, Iseli CE, Carroll WR, Rosenthal EL, Magnuson JS. Functional outcomes after transoral robotic surgery for head and neck cancer. Otolaryngol Head Neck Surg 2009;141(2):166–171
19. Cohen MA, Weinstein GS, O'Malley BW Jr, Feldman M, Quon H. Transoral robotic surgery and human papillomavirus status: oncologic results. Head Neck 2011;33(4):573–580
20. Ibrahim AE, Sarhane KA, Baroud JS, Atiyeh BS. Robotics in plastic surgery, a review. Eur J Plast Surg 2012;35(8):571–578
21. Song HG, Yun IS, Lee WJ, Lew DH, Rah DK. Robot-assisted free flap in head and neck reconstruction. Arch Plast Surg 2013;40(4):353–358
22. de Almeida JR, Park RCW, Genden EM. Reconstruction of transoral robotic surgery defects: principles and techniques. J Reconstr Microsurg 2012;28(7):465–472
23. Selber JC. Transoral robotic reconstruction of oropharyngeal defects: a case series. Plast Reconstr Surg 2010;126(6):1978–1987
24. Selber J. Discussion: robotic-assisted FAMM flap for soft palate reconstruction. Laryngoscope 2014; In press
25. Selber JC, Robb G, Serletti JM, Weinstein G, Weber R, Holsinger FC. Transoral robotic free flap reconstruction of oropharyngeal defects: a preclinical investigation. Plast Reconstr Surg 2010;125(3):896–900
26. Holsinger FC, McWhorter AJ, Ménard M, Garcia D, Laccourreye O. Transoral lateral oropharyngectomy for squamous cell carcinoma of the tonsillar region: I. Technique, complications, and functional results. Arch Otolaryngol Head Neck Surg 2005;131(7):583–591
27. Laccourreye O, Hans S, Ménard M, Garcia D, Brasnu D, Holsinger FC. Transoral lateral oropharyngectomy for squamous cell carcinoma of the tonsillar region: II. An analysis of the incidence, related variables, and consequences of local recurrence. Arch Otolaryngol Head Neck Surg 2005;131(7):592–599
28. Rieger J, Bohle Iii G, Huryn J, Tang JL, Harris J, Seikaly H. Surgical reconstruction versus prosthetic obturation of extensive soft palate defects: a comparison of speech outcomes. Int J Prosthodont 2009;22(6):566–572
29. Marsh JL, Wray RC. Speech prosthesis versus pharyngeal flap: a randomized evaluation of the management of velopharyngeal incompetency. Plast Reconstr Surg 1980;65(5):592–594
30. Mukhija VK, Sung C-K, Desai SC, Wanna G, Genden EM. Transoral robotic assisted free flap reconstruction. Otolaryngol Head Neck Surg 2009;140(1):124–125
31. Atiyeh B, Sarhane K. Overweight and obesity: a true global epidemic. In: Atiyeh BS, ed. Body Contouring

Following Bariatric Surgery and Massive Weight Loss Post-Bariatric Body Contouring. Bentham Science Publishers; 2012:3–11

32. Sarhane KA, Flores JM, Cooney CM, et al. Preoperative anemia and postoperative outcomes in immediate breast reconstructive surgery: a critical analysis of 10,958 patients from the ACS-NSQIP database. Plast Reconstr Surg Glob Open 2013;1(5):e30

33. Hill JB, Patel A, Del Corral GA, et al. Preoperative anemia predicts thrombosis and free flap failure in microvascular reconstruction. Ann Plast Surg 2012;69(4):364–367

34. Sarhane K, Kobeissy F. Anesthetic management in body countouring surgery. J Anesth Clin Res 2012;3(8): 1000e106

35. O'Malley BW Jr, Weinstein GS, Snyder W, Hockstein NG. Transoral robotic surgery (TORS) for base of tongue neoplasms. Laryngoscope 2006;116(8):1465–1472

36. Camarillo DB, Krummel TM, Salisbury JK Jr. Robotic technology in surgery: past, present, and future. Am J Surg 2004; 188(4A, Suppl):2S–15S

37. Kim VB, Chapman WHH, Albrecht RJ, et al. Early experience with telemanipulative robot-assisted laparoscopic cholecystectomy using da Vinci. Surg Laparosc Endosc Percutan Tech 2002;12(1):33–40

38. Satava RM. Virtual reality, telesurgery, and the new world order of medicine. J Image Guid Surg 1995;1(1): 12–16

39. Suzuki S, Suzuki N, Hayashibe M, et al. Tele-surgical simulation system for training in the use of da Vinci surgery. Stud Health Technol Inform 2005;111:543–548

40. Selber J, Pederson J. Robotic muscle harvest. In: Liverneaux PA, Berner SH, Bednar MS, Parekattil S, Ruggiero GM, Selber JC, eds. Telemicrosurgery: Robot Assisted Microsurgery. Paris: Springer-Verlag; 2012

41. Selber JC. Robotic latissimus dorsi muscle harvest. Plast Reconstr Surg 2011;128(2):88e–90e

42. Patel NV, Pedersen JC. Robotic harvest of the rectus abdominis muscle: a preclinical investigation and case report. J Reconstr Microsurg 2012;28(7):477–480

# 17 Composite Tissue Allotransplantation of the Face

*Ericka M. Bueno, Ryan Michael Gobble, and Bohdan Pomahac*

## Introduction

The face provides a range of complex functions that include oral competence, speech, airway, swallowing, blinking, facial expression, and communication. In addition, the face plays a major role in social interaction. Facial disfigurement and dysfunction lead to impairments in self-expression and sense of identity. Individuals with severely disfigured faces often suffer from prejudice, stereotyping, social isolation, difficulties finding employment, and depression.[1] The reduction in quality of life experienced by these individuals as a result of their facial disfigurement has been deemed comparable to that with end-stage renal disease or human immunodeficiency virus infection.[2]

Facial reconstructive surgery aims to restore functions lost or affected by trauma, burns, malignancy, and/or congenital or infectious disease, as well as to restore as normal an appearance as possible. However, severe injuries to the face are a very difficult challenge for reconstructive surgeons. The anatomy and sensorimotor functions of the face are highly complex, and restoration of both function and appearance in cases of extensive facial defects is nearly impossible. In general, the complexity of reconstruction is related to the size of the defect and the level of engagement of the underlying soft and hard tissues. When we have to resort to tissues of unrelated origin and function for replacement of highly specialized facial parts, results are increasingly compromised as larger defects are treated. No other tissues in the body can replicate the appearance, function, and anatomy of the facial tissues. Furthermore, for full facial defects to be reconstructed, multiple donor sites would be required, thus increasing donor-site morbidity. Lastly, restoring the complex sensorimotor system of the face and neck is not possible with conventional reconstruction, and thus the results are frequently static and provide limited function. Reconstruction is multi-staged, requiring frequent revisions to address scarring and to improve appearance. Even after multiple reconstructions, the results remain suboptimal. The structures of the central face (i.e., lips, nose, and eyelids) have the worst outcomes.

## Regional Anatomy

The blood supply to the face is among the most robust in the entire human body; this has direct implications in facial allotransplantation. Arterial blood is supplied by a multitude of vessels from the internal and external carotid arterial systems. The internal carotid artery (ICA) enters the skull via the carotid canal. Blood supply is provided to the brain via the middle cerebral artery and the anterior cerebral artery in the circle of Willis. The ophthalmic artery, the first branch of the ICA after the cavernous sinus, ultimately enters the orbit before dividing into multiple branches, including the supraorbital and supratrochlear arteries. These arteries emerge from the superior orbital rim via their respective notches and give blood supply to the medial periorbital and anterior forehead regions. The anterior ethmoidal artery, which supplies the lateral wall and septum of the nose, and the dorsal nasal artery, which ultimately anastomoses with the angular artery, giving blood supply to the nose, both arise from the ophthalmic artery as well.[3]

The external carotid artery (ECA) provides the remainder of the arterial inflow to the face via multiple branches before terminating in the superficial temporal artery (STA) and the internal maxillary artery (IMA). The STA provides blood to the lateral forehead as well as to the orbit before anastomosing with branches of the supratrochlear and supraorbital arteries. Important branches from the IMA include the inferior alveolar artery, which provides blood to the lower gingiva and lower lip and chin via the mental artery, and the inferior orbital artery, which supplies the midface and nasal dorsum. Other important branches of the ECA prior to the terminal branches include the lingual artery and its branches, which supply blood to the tongue, and the external maxillary artery, which provides blood to the nose via the angular and lateral nasal arteries. The facial artery provides blood to the upper lip, columella, alar rim, and membranous septum via the superior labial artery, as well as supplying the lower lip and chin via the inferior labial artery. The facial artery continues as the angular artery, which supplies the nasal dorsum and medial cheek before anastomosing with branches of the ICA.[4] Arterial blood supply to the scalp is provided via the above-mentioned supratrochlear, supraorbital, and superficial temporal arteries, as well as the posterior auricular artery and the occipital artery, all branches of the ECA.

Venous outflow from the face and scalp, for the most part, mirrors that of arterial inflow. Supraorbital and supratrochlear veins drain into the superior and inferior orbital veins before ultimately draining into the cavernous sinus. Therefore, there is the possibility for intracranial spread from facial or scalp infections. The superior and inferior labial veins and the submental vein join the angular vein before becoming the anterior facial vein and ultimately the common facial vein. The superficial temporal vein follows the course of the artery and becomes the retromandibular vein, which along with the common facial vein, drain into the internal and external jugular vein in a variable pattern.

Lymphatic drainage of the face and scalp may play a significant role in facial transplantation given the immunological interactions between the donor and the recipient; the regions of the forehead, frontal, lateral temporal, and periorbital regions drain into the periparotid and intraparotid lymph nodes and ultimately into the upper jugular nodes. The midface, including the glabella, nose, medial cheek, and upper lip, drain into submandibular nodes, while the lower lip and mentum drain into submental nodes. Both submandibular and submental nodes eventually drain into the jugular lymph node system. In all of our face transplant cases where the allograft contained neck tissues, we observed marked enlargement of these lymph nodes within weeks after the transplant, with resolution in ~ 6 weeks, corresponding to presumed reconnection of the lymphatic channels.

Sensory innervation to the face is provided via the trigeminal nerve and its branches, including the ophthalmic branch ($V_1$), the maxillary branch ($V_2$), and the mandibular branch ($V_3$). The ophthalmic branch provides sensory innervation to the skin of the forehead, vertex of the scalp, and periorbital regions via the supraorbital and supratrochlear nerves, the upper lateral lid via the lacrimal branch, and the glabella and nasal dorsum via the nasociliary branch. The maxillary branch provides sensory innervation to the midface skin via zygomaticofacial and zygomaticotemporal nerves, which supply the lateral canthal regions and zygoma. The infraorbital nerve provides sensory innervation to the upper alveolus, gingiva, palate, and nasal floor, as well as the cheek, lower eyelid, upper lip, and nasal vestibule. The mandibular branch provides sensory innervation to the buccal mucosa and lateral cheek via the buccal nerve, preauricular skin and temporal scalp via the auriculotemporal nerve, to the lower alveolus via the inferior alveolar nerve, and finally to the chin and lower lip via the mental nerve. Posterior and lateral scalp sensation is provided via the greater and lesser occipital nerves, respectively, both of which are branches of cervical nerves and thus not supplied by the trigeminal nerve.

Motor innervation to the face is provided via the facial nerve. Motor recovery after facial allotransplantation proceeds more slowly than sensory recovery, and recovery is to a lesser extent, which is unfortunate, as motor recovery is more important in resulting in a functionally useful and aesthetic face. The facial nerve gives off five major branches (frontal, zygomatic, buccal, marginal mandibular, and cervical), which are responsible for providing animation to the face as well as protecting the globe and maintaining oral competence. The posterior auricular nerve, which provides motor input to muscles of the scalp around the ear, is an early branch of the facial nerve after it exits the stylomastoid foramen. The frontal branch of the facial nerve provides motor innervation to the frontalis, orbicularis oculi, and corrugator supercilii, while also serving as the efferent limb of the corneal reflex. The zygomatic branch supplies the orbicularis oculi, while the buccal branch provides motor innervation to the risorius, buccinators, levator labii superioris, levator anguli oris, levator labii superioris alaeque nasi, nasalis, and orbicularis oris, which are important in facial animation and in maintaining oral competence. The marginal mandibular branch supplies the depressor labii inferioris, depressor anguli oris, and mentalis, which function to depress and pucker the lower lip. The cervical branch supplies the platysma as well as the depressor anguli oris.

The facial muscles described above, along with their motor innervation, are important in facial allotransplantation because the muscles are moved as part of a larger tissue group, including skin, subcutaneous tissue, nerves, arteries, veins, and osseous components, if osteomyocutaneous transplantation is to be performed. The muscles included depend upon which particular part of the face that requires reconstruction.

### Reconstructive Options

Skin grafts, local flaps, distant pedicled flaps, and free flaps are multiple modalities available for the reconstruction of face and neck defects.[5] Free flaps are increasingly viewed as the primary modality for reconstructing major head and neck defects. The most extensive facial defects can be addressed with multiple free and pedicled flaps. The limitations of free flaps are similar to those of other reconstructive options: color and texture mismatch, static reconstruction without function, and contractures.

The more specialized units of the face are particularly not amenable for reconstruction. Full-thickness lip defects, where up to 80% of the lips are missing, can be repaired using local flaps, but often result in microstomia and need multiple procedures.[6] If more than 80% of the lips are missing, reconstruction is not possible. The nose cannot be reconstructed satisfactorily using a single-stage free flap reconstruction. A multistage approach involving cartilage grafts in combination with local and free flaps yields a better aesthetic appearance, but the mean time of reconstruction is over 2 years.[7]

In general, three-dimensional defects of the face involving endo-, ecto-, and mesoderm are extremely difficult if not impossible to reconstruct with conventional techniques. The goal of reconstruction is often diminished to mere wound control.

## ■ Algorithm

Our decision-making algorithm is depicted in **Fig. 17.1**. The decision-making process leading to facial transplantation relies on a thorough, individualized analysis of the risk-to-benefit ratio. At this time, the American Society for Reconstructive Transplantation (ASRT) guidelines for determination of the medical necessity for face transplantation[8] state that the procedure is indicated in patients with defects that comprise 25% or more of the facial surface area and/or that involve one or more central subunits of the face; that is, the eyelids, lips, and/or nose. Transplantation of the underlying bones or even the tongue is indicated as needed for the defects described above. Clinical criteria that must be met include:

1. Comprehensive medical history and physical examination performed by a plastic and reconstructive surgeon, and/or by a craniofacial surgeon, to evaluate the current impact of the defect and the potential risks and restorative benefits of transplantation.
2. Comprehensive medical history and physical examination performed by a transplant physician or surgeon to evaluate whether the patient can safely and effectively receive the necessary immune suppression treatment to manage the transplant.
3. Comprehensive psychosocial evaluation performed to evaluate the motivation, understanding, and coping ability of the patient to manage the facial transplant.
4. Determination that the patient suffers from functional complications, with evidence of loss of quality of life as a result of the facial defect, and from psychological effects as determined by the psychological evaluation.
5. Determination that the results of conventional reconstructive options are inadequate or unsatisfactory.
6. A surgical treatment plan for the facial transplantation, with prognosis for specific functional and aesthetic gains.

Our team at Brigham and Women's Hospital currently follows the ASRT guidelines. In addition, we have previously stated that face transplants are contraindicated in cases of pregnancy and when adequate follow-up care and immunosuppression cannot be guaranteed due to a history of poor compliance and/or lack of third-party coverage. There is controversy among centers that provide face transplantation services about the inclusion of patients who are blind, or present with concomitant bilateral upper extremity amputation, malignancy, self-induced injuries, or human immunodeficiency virus (HIV)-positive status.[9] For our team, HIV-positive status is an absolute contraindication. We consider active psychiatric illness, malignancy, and other potential barriers to face transplantation on a case-by-case basis and using a multidisciplinary approach. With regard to the clinical criteria presented above, we place special emphasis on the prognosis for functional and aesthetic gains from facial transplantation. Eligibility is contingent upon the projected gains being significant, and upon our ability to identify a safe back-up plan for reconstruction (in case of allograft failure) that would allow the patient to return to a state close to the preoperative state, and not significantly worse.

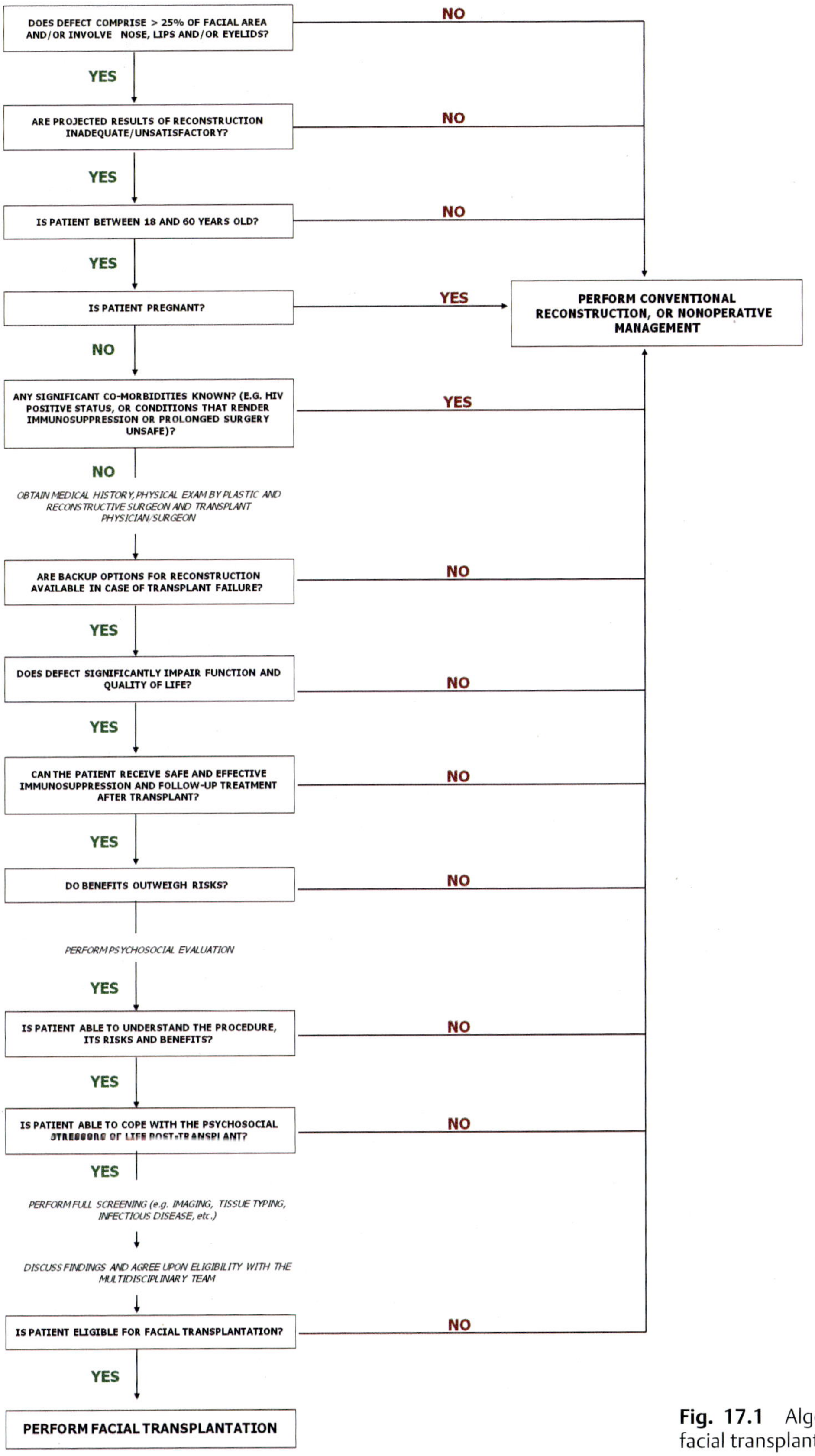


**Fig. 17.1** Algorithm for decision making in facial transplantation.

## Complications

- Surgical
  - Vascular: Vascular complications can be avoided with proper planning (preoperative imaging),[10] efficient communication, selection of large-caliber vessels for anastomoses, proper microsurgical technique, and preoperatively formulated back-up plans for vascular salvage.
- Infectious: The risk for opportunistic infections is always present due to the recipient's immunosuppressed status. Early postoperative infections are typically due to technical problems during surgery.[11] Careful monitoring and tailored infection prophylaxis are critical in management of these complications.
- Immune rejection
  - Acute (**Fig. 17.2**): The risks for acute rejection can be minimized by following the criteria for cross-matching,[12] keeping the ischemia time of the donor allograft short, and minimizing blood loss. The transplant team must closely monitor for, and educate the patient and his/her support network about, signs of rejection. The patient and support team must also be well informed about compliance with immunosuppressant medications.
  - Chronic: The risks for chronic rejection can be minimized with close monitoring, compliance with maintenance immunosuppression, and early treatment of acute rejection episodes.
- Psychological: The risks of psychological complications stem from the recipient's inability to deal with a new/changed appearance, from publicity, and from the complex and intensive medical treatment. We minimize the risks for psychological complications by performing detailed psychosocial evaluation of our face transplant candidates and their support network.

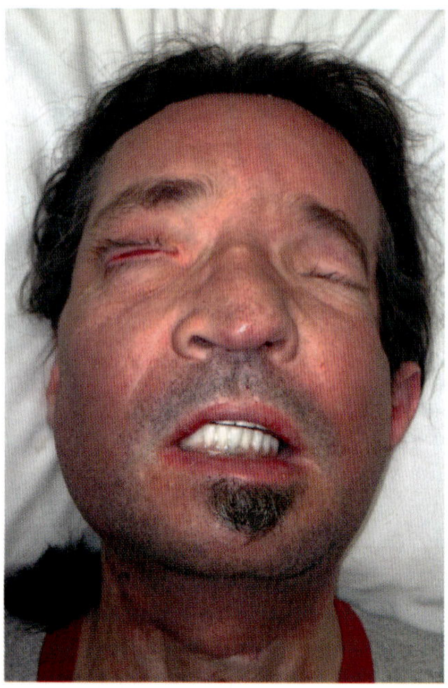

**Fig. 17.2** An episode of acute rejection in a full-face transplant recipient. Rejection-associated changes in the facial allograft are easily appreciated and include redness and swelling.

## Postoperative Care

Immediately following the operation, the patient is transferred to the intensive care unit (ICU) for monitoring of the facial flap (and sentinel monitoring flap, when applicable). The patient remains in the ICU for 24 hours, or more if needed. Doppler ultrasound of the allograft is monitored hourly. The head of the bed must be elevated 45 degrees for aspiration prophylaxis and to facilitate venous outflow. The patient is placed on a nothing-per-mouth diet (with the exception of medications) for at least 24 hours. Typically, the patient will have drains in the neck and no dressings on the face or neck. Antimicrobial coverage is determined based on specific donor and recipient indications, as well as cultures. Common medications during this period include heparin, 5,000 units subcutaneously twice daily; aspirin, MMF 1 g orally twice daily; thymoglobulin 1.5 mg/kg IV daily for the first 4 postoperative days (with premedication of Tylenol 650 mg orally; and Benadryl 25 mg orally), methylprednisolone taper (100, 80, and 60 mg IV twice daily on postoperative days 1, 2 and 3, respectively); prednisone (40 mg orally twice daily on day 4, then 20 mg orally twice a day afterward); tacrolimus 2 mg orally twice daily, then draw blood levels through 12 hours post second dose (goal for trough level is 10 to 15 ng/mL); ganciclovir 5 mg/kg IV twice daily until the patient is able to tolerate oral medications, followed by valganciclovir 900 mg orally once a day if donor or patient is cytomegalovirus-positive. Antiviral prophylaxis is maintained for at least 6 months, or longer if needed. Immunosuppression is gradually reduced, but it must be maintained for life.[11,12]

From the second postoperative day onward, the flap continues to be monitored, with a gradual decrease in frequency (but still every 3 hours during the acute postoperative phase); the patient is typically out of the ICU by day 2, and nutrition can be started via oral nutrition or tube feeding. Some patients may require tube feeding throughout their hospital stay. Oral care, nasal lubrication, and incision line treatment are determined on a case-by-case basis. The patient receives psychiatric and/or social work support daily or as needed. Because the transplanted face is initially insensate and paralyzed, the speech-language pathologist, physical therapist, occupational therapist, and swallowing therapist are all consulted and their plans followed. Speech and swallowing therapy are provided to implement safe oral feeding, swallowing maneuvers, and communication compensation strategies as needed. Physical and occupational therapy are provided to optimize respiration, ambulation, posture, tone, motor function, and symmetry of the face, and to minimize hypertrophic scarring and synkinesis of the facial muscles. Therapy is daily during hospitalization, typically starting by postoperative day 3 as cleared by the surgical team. Afterward, frequency and duration of therapy depend on the specific needs of each patient but can typically range from 2 to 5 times per week during the first few postoperative months, with gradual weaning. Sensory function typically returns gradually, so that by 3 months there is protective sensation in most of the flap, while motor function takes longer, but the first signs are typically appreciated by the sixth month.

The estimated hospital stay is ~ 7 to 14 days and depends upon stable blood levels of immunosuppressive medications. The patient visits the transplant clinic twice weekly during the first month after discharge for assessment of the flap and for monitoring of immunosuppression, infectious disease surveillance, and management of medications. For patients without complications, imaging with MRI or CT is typically done at 6 months. Biopsies of the skin are taken weekly for the first month after transplant, 1, 2, and 4 weeks following discharge, and then 3, 6, and 12 months postoperatively, and also at times of suspected rejection or during rejection treatment. Biopsies are processed for histology and graded according to the Banff system.[13] Rejection is usually treated with temporary adjustment of immunosuppressive medications on an outpatient basis, although in some instances, boluses of steroid or antibodies need to be administered on an inpatient basis. At least one episode of acute rejection should be expected in the first year following facial transplantation, with two or more episodes possible. To date, all rejection episodes have been managed successfully at our institution.

## Case Examples

### Case 1

This case has been described previously.[9,14,15] A 59-year-old male of Native American and Japanese background had a complex defect of the midface involving bone and soft tissues. The patient had suffered a high-voltage electrical burn injury 2 years previously. He had been treated with an anterolateral fasciocutaneous free flap to separate the oral and nasal cavities. In spite of multiple conventional reconstruction attempts, he had unsatisfactory aesthetic and functional results **(Fig. 17.3)**. He suffered from oral incompetence and bilateral epiphora, he had to breathe through a tracheostomy, and his speech was slurred. After a full screening, our team found that the patient's indication for facial transplantation was strong, owing to a central defect involving over 25% of the facial area and including the nose, upper lip, and maxilla. A partial facial transplant was expected to restore oral competence and nasal breathing and to improve speech and social interactions. The patient was placed on the waiting list with the local organ-processing organization, and in April of 2009 he was matched with a brain-dead donor compatible for gender, blood type, and

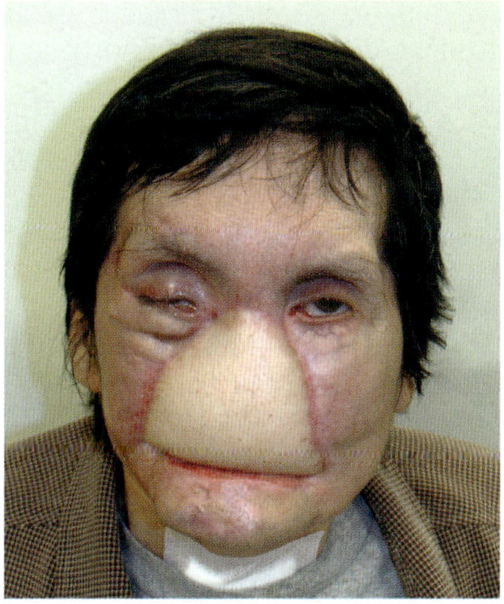

**Fig. 17.3** A 59-year-old male patient who had suffered high-voltage electrical burn injury 2 years earlier and had received an anterolateral fasciocutaneous free flap to separate the oral and nasal cavities. The aesthetic and functional results were unsatisfactory.

skin color/texture. The operation involved transfer of an allograft comprising the nasal, oral, and maxillary sinus mucosa; zygomatic, nasal, and maxillary bones with teeth; nasal cartilage; muscles of facial animation; nerves; and skin. Revascularization of the allograft was accomplished in 75 minutes. Neurorrhaphy was performed on five facial nerve branches on the right and six on the left side of the face, immediately anterior to the parotid gland. Buccal and infraorbital nerves were reconnected. A radial sentinel forearm flap was placed on the right hand, where it also released a web-space contraction. The patient received 500 mg methylprednisolone, 1000 mg MMF, and rabbit antithymocyte globulin (1.5 mg/kg) prior to the operation. Maintenance immunosuppression was performed with MMF 1000 mg twice per day, tacrolimus was adjusted to a trough level of 10 to 15 ng/mL, and steroid was tapered to 20 mg on postoperative day 5. The patient received antiviral and antibacterial prophylaxis of cefazolin, trimethoprim-sulfamethoxasole, and valganciclovir for 6 months up to a year.

In the initial postoperative period, the patient healed well. Speech was immediately improved due to restoration of the hard palate. A functional nasal airway was also immediately established. Facial edema resolved by day 21. The patient was discharged from the hospital on day 15. On day 17, there was redness of the allograft and the sentinel flap. Mild acute rejection was diagnosed and was treated with a methylprednisolone bolus (500 mg × 3). From then until month 6, subsequent biopsies showed minimal or mild rejection. Steroid bolus treatments were administered on days 74 and 107 to treat suspected acute rejection, along with topical clobetazol cream on days 27 to 35 and 37 to 45, and tacrolimus cream on days 107 to 113. The redness persisted, and this therapeutic failure prompted further investigation into the cause for the facial redness and cutaneous lymphocytic infiltrates. A history of rosacea in the donor was identified; the patient was subsequently treated for rosacea with metronidazole cream, and the facial redness disappeared effectively.

The patient suffered left parotitis in months 5 and 35, subcutaneous dermatophytosis of the right foot in month 6, and cytomegalovirus viremia in month 15. All were successfully treated. Sensation was gained gradually, so that by 6 months, the patient had light sensation throughout the entire facial allograft. Motor function improved gradually during the second half of the first postoperative year. At 1 year, the patient was highly satisfied with the results. He was able to smile symmetrically and gained control of the transplanted upper lip. He reintegrated into society. As a side effect of immunosuppression, the patient developed insulin-dependent diabetes (the patient had preoperative glucose intolerance). He underwent small revision procedures over the first 3 years after transplant. He received a local flap for closure of a right medial canthal fistula, revisions of redundant skin, extraction of donor teeth due to decay, insertion of a chin implant, musculomucosal flaps to lower lip, and implant placements for future dental prostheses. Three years after face transplantation, the aesthetic results are excellent **(Fig. 17.4)**. The patient has achieved normal sensation in ~ 92% of the allograft, excluding the bulb of the nose and the bilateral nasal alae, which recovered only diminished protective sensation. He has near-normal sensory discrimination and normal thermal sensation in all of the allograft, he can recognize the texture of food, and he can identify if his mouth is empty or full. Motor function is intact in some muscles (zygomaticus, risorius), while some muscles contract weakly (left levator anguli oris), and others are difficult to identify in contraction or contraction may be absent **(Fig. 17.5)**. Immunologic, infectious, and metabolic complications have been minimal. The patient's immunosuppressive therapy at 3 years consisted of tacrolimus (trough levels 3 to 5 ng/mL) and MMF 180 mg twice per day. At 2 years and 9 months, he suffered an acute rejection episode, which was successfully treated with a temporary increase of tacrolimus to trough levels of 8 to 10 ng/mL and MMF 360 mg twice per day.

## Case 2

This case has been described in detail previously.[9,16] A 24-year-old Caucasian male presented to our clinic to consult regarding face transplanta-

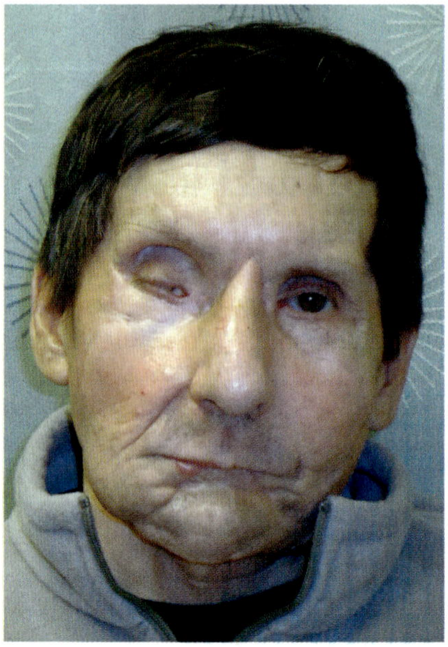

**Fig. 17.4** Aesthetic restoration of a partial face transplant recipient, 3 years after the transplant.

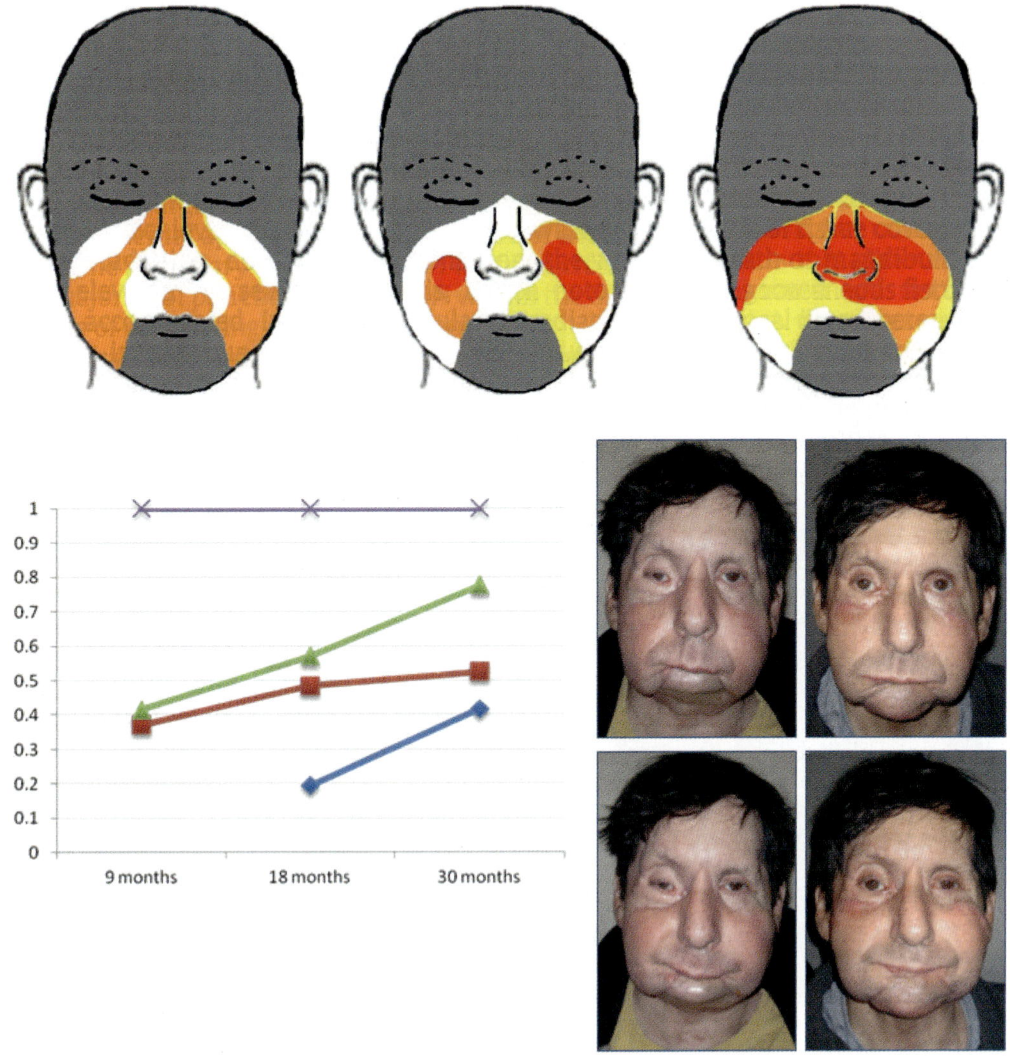


**Fig. 17.5** Territories of accurate perception of two-point discrimination sensation at 15 mm (yellow), 10 mm (orange), and 5 mm (red) resolution are demonstrated at 9, 18, and 30 months (5 mm resolution two-point discrimination testing was not performed at 9 months) in the patient described in Case 1. Proportion of facial allograft skin with gross touch sensation and two-point discrimination at 10 mm resolution is illustrated in graph form. Return of motor function is illustrated at right, with the patient in neutral and smiling position at 10 and 20 months after surgery.

tion. Fourteen months prior to his presentation, he had suffered high-voltage electrical burn injuries to the entire face, extending into the scalp and the left hip. His left eye had been enucleated and his right eye, although present under a reconstructive muscle flap, had no light perception. The patient had lost all the soft tissues of the face to the level of bone. He had no nose, lips, or teeth and had a palatal fistula **(Fig. 17.6)**. His face had been covered with bilateral latissimus dorsi/serratus flaps and skin grafts. He had normal tongue mobility, but his oral opening was only ~ 2 cm. Therefore, he suffered from oral incompetence, could not breathe through his nose, and was incapable of facial expression. He had no sensation or motor function in the reconstructed face. He was socially isolated.

We performed full screening procedures on this remarkable patient. In spite of his visual impairment and all his injuries, the patient had a positive outlook on life and a very supportive family network.

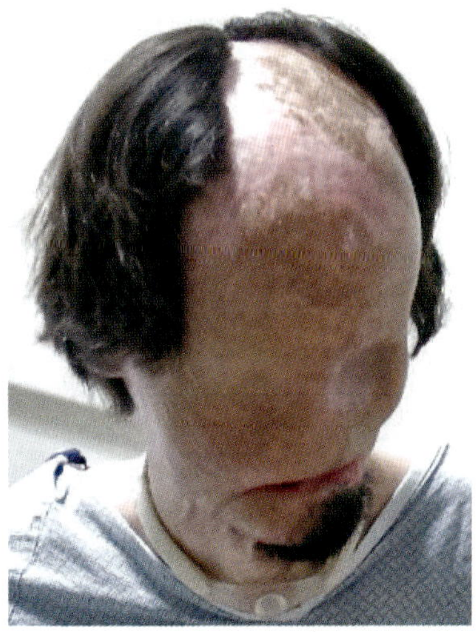

**Fig. 17.6** Extent of loss of facial tissues in a young man presenting for evaluation for facial transplantation. The left eye had been enucleated. All the soft tissues of the face were lost to the level of bone. The patient had no nose, lips, teeth, or palatal fistula.

Our team expected that full-face transplantation could provide him with remarkable improvement in all facial functions, which would in turn improve his quality of life and social interactions. We predicted challenges in the postoperative period related to his being visually impaired; specifically, we predicted his rehabilitation, self-monitoring, and daily medication intake to be affected. Therefore, we scrutinized his support network and found it fully committed to assisting the patient with these challenges. We therefore placed the patient on the waiting list with the local organ-processing organization to wait for a compatible brain-dead facial allograft donor. Five months later, in March of 2011, a donor matched for gender, blood type, and skin color/texture was identified.

The full-face allograft recovered from the donor included all soft tissues of the face and neck and a portion of the scalp, eyelids, nose, lips, orbicularis oris, intraoral mucosa, and the left parotid gland to provide bulk **(Fig. 17.7)**. The main trunk of the facial nerve was found to have been cut and clipped on the left side in the patient, with only the upper and lower divisions available for reconnection. We preserved the lining of the patient's perioral region to serve as adequate sewing surface; we also preserved the grafted surfaces over the patient's orbits. Due to orbital exenteration, we could not locate the infraorbital nerves on the patient's left side. After anastomosis, full revascularization took between 5 and 10 minutes. Nerve grafts were used to bridge distances during neurorrhaphies.

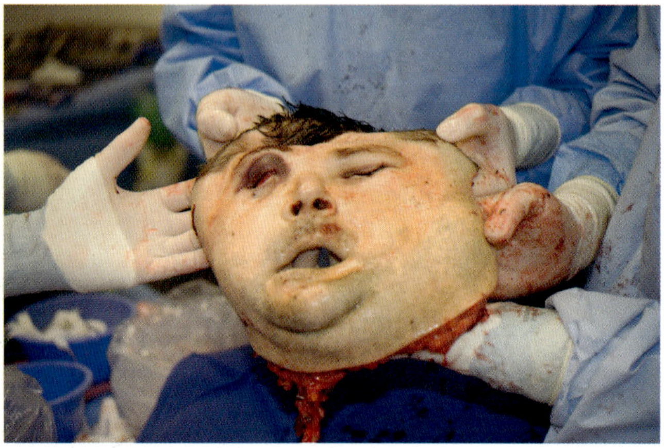

**Fig. 17.7** Full facial allograft to restore all the soft tissues of the face, as well as the nose, in the young man presented in Case 2. Photograph of the facial allograft immediately after procurement from the donor.

Perioperatively, the patient received 24 units of packed erythrocytes and 17 units of blood (Cell Saver, Haemonetics). The face transplant operation lasted 17 hours. The patient received a full-face allograft and a sentinel skin flap placed in an inconspicuous area of the body to be used for monitoring for rejection. The patient recovered well in the immediate postoperative period. He reported return of olfaction on day 3. He was discharged from the intensive care unit on day 4. Shortly after, he was treated for *Candida albicans* and *Pseudomonas aeruginosa* infections detected on the suture lines, and he suffered a recurrent submental collection identified as sterile saliva and treated with botulinum toxin injection to the donor's submandibular glands, as well as antimicrobial treatment. The donor submental lymph nodes enlarged. On day 13, the patient was discharged from the hospital to a nearby residential facility. On week 4 he was re-admitted to our hospital and was treated for a fever of unknown origin. During the postoperative second month, he was again admitted due to elevated creatinine levels and dehydration. He underwent resections of redundant neck skin postoperatively on several occasions, and he received eye and dental implants.

The patient received 500 mg methylprednisolone, 1000 mg MMF, and rabbit antithymocyte globulin (1.5 mg/kg) prior to the operation. Maintenance immunosuppression was performed with MMF 1000 mg twice per day, tacrolimus adjusted to trough level of 10 to 15 ng/mL, and steroid taper to 20 mg on postoperative day 5. He received antiviral and antibacterial prophylaxis of cefazolin, trimethoprim-sulfamethoxasole, and valganciclovir for 6 months to a year. Corticosteroids were withdrawn on day 55. Although the patient did not present any episodes of acute rejection during the first year, 22 months after facial transplantation, he presented with upper respiratory symptoms and general malaise that were treated with over-the-counter medications with limited improvement. He developed progressively worsening facial erythema without pain or pruritus. We obtained biopsies of the facial and sentinel allografts, and they were consistent with grade III acute rejection according to the Banff classification.[13] We provided treatment with 6 doses of methylprednisolone pulse (500 mg/day), prednisone taper (initially 80 mg/day), ATG (88 mg/day/kg), and increased tacrolimus (from 1 to 4 mg twice a day) and MMF (from 500 to 1000 mg twice a day), with limited improvement. After 2 weeks, there were bleeding ulcerations and lichenoid changes in the oral mucosa and upper and lower lips, which were mildly painful. These were treated with dexamethasone rinse and tacro-

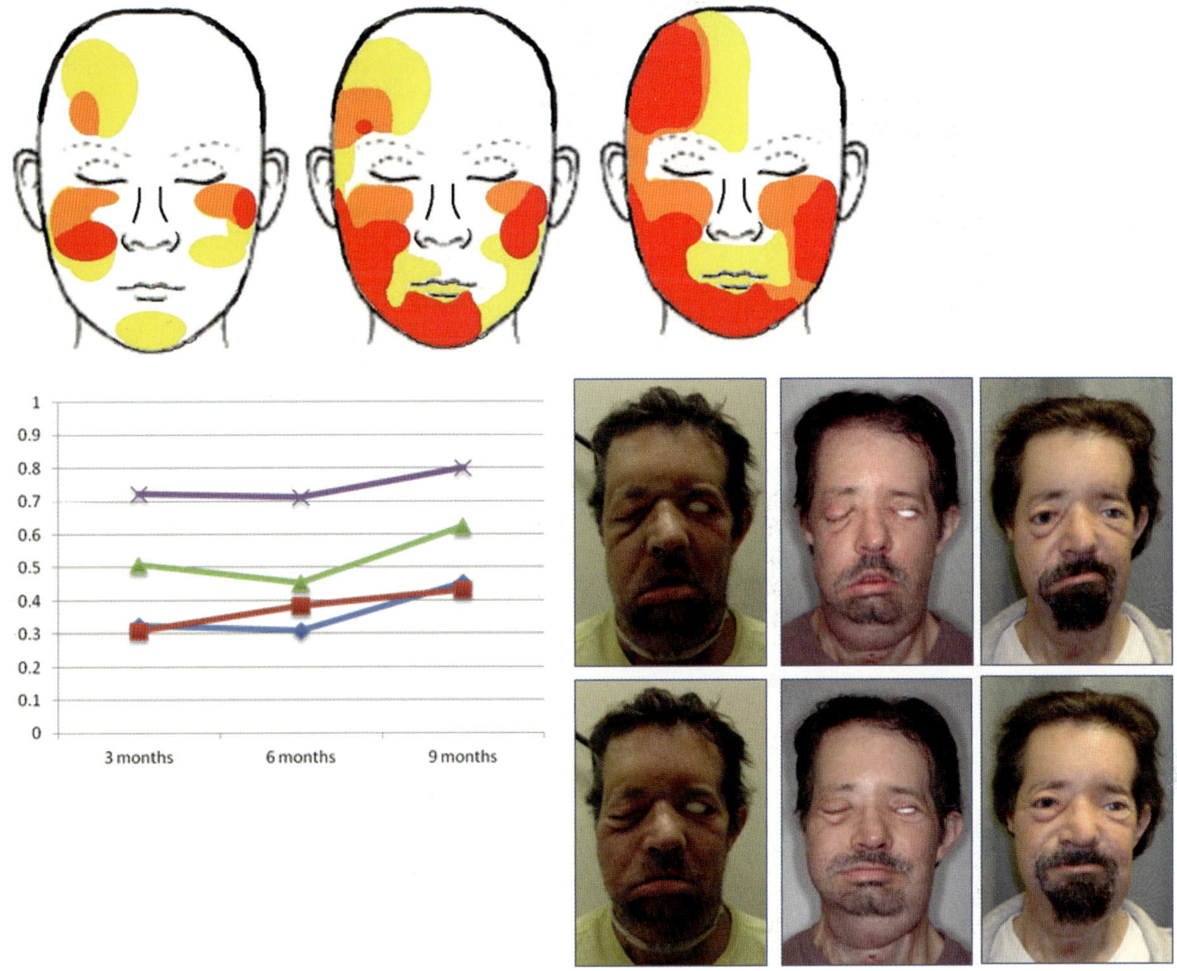


**Fig. 17.8** Territories of accurate perception of two-point discrimination sensation at 15 mm (yellow), 10 mm (orange), and 5 mm (red) resolution are demonstrated at 3, 6, and 9 months for the patient described in Case 2. The proportion of facial allograft skin with gross touch sensation and two-point discrimination at 10 mm resolution is illustrated in graph form. Return of motor function is illustrated at right, with the patient in neutral (top) and smiling (bottom) positions at 3, 6, and 9 months after surgery. Of note, left supra- and infraorbital nerves were not coapted due to existing patient anatomy.

limus ointment (0.1%) to lips and oral mucosa, and they rapidly improved. The facial erythema and histopathological diagnosis of acute rejection resolved more gradually.

At 4 months, sensation and motion of muscles in the right side of the allograft were detected. Sensation had not yet returned on the left side, where sensory nerves were not connected. By 6 months, the patient had recovered 15-mm two-point discrimination in ≥ 40% and 5-mm discrimination in ≥ 20% of the allograft's area, and he continued to gain gross motion of the muscles in the allograft. He presented with residual synkinesis on the left side likely associated with proximal facial nerve coaptation; only the recipient's upper and lower subdivisions were utilizable during the operation **(Fig. 17.8)**. The aesthetic restoration at 18 months after transplantation is depicted in **Fig. 17.9**. The improvements in the patient's quality of life have been remarkable.

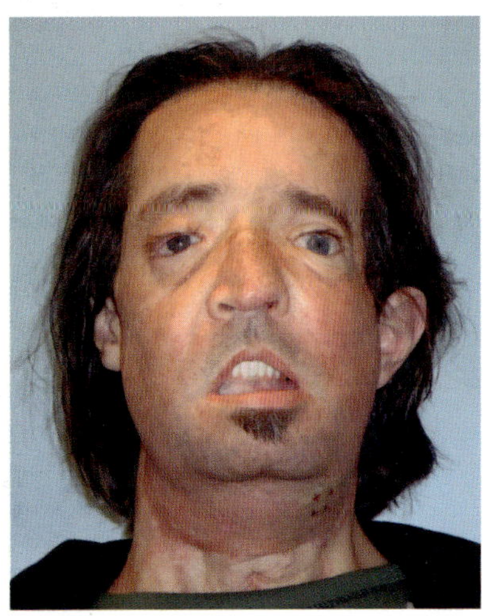

**Fig. 17.9** Aesthetic restoration of the patient in Case 2, 18 months after full facial transplantation. Please note that the eyes are prostheses.

## Pearls and Pitfalls

### Pearls

- Facial allograft recovery
  - Harvest from scalp to neck and lateral to medial directions
  - Two surgeons working together are more efficient if one is on each side
  - Significant resistance can be expected during allograft perfusion with University of Wisconsin solution
- Inset
  - Perform in opposite direction to recovery (neck to scalp; medial to lateral)
  - Skin inset under slight tension with proximal pull and a tight neck inset

### Pitfalls

- Submandibular gland sialocele (inadequately tied-off duct) is treated by injecting botulinum toxin in the gland at the time of inset.
- Loose, droopy face when swelling resolves that can be prevented by performing proximal inset under moderate tension.

## References


1. Furr LA, Wiggins O, Cunningham M, et al. Psychosocial implications of disfigurement and the future of human face transplantation. Plast Reconstr Surg 2007;120(2):559–565
2. Sinno HH, Thibaudeau S, Duggal A, Lessard L. Utility scores for facial disfigurement requiring facial transplantation [outcomes article]. Plast Reconstr Surg 2010;126(2):443–449
3. Gray H, Williams PL, Bannister LH. Gray's Anatomy: The Anatomical Basis of Medicine and Surgery. 38th ed. New York, NY: Churchill Livingstone; 1995
4. Bentsianov B, Blitzer A. Facial anatomy. Clin Dermatol 2004;22(1):3–13
5. Liu R, Gullane P, Brown D, Irish J. Pectoralis major myocutaneous pedicled flap in head and neck reconstruction: retrospective review of indications and results in 244 consecutive cases at the Toronto General Hospital. J Otolaryngol 2001;30(1):34–40
6. Kroll SS. Staged sequential flap reconstruction for large lower lip defects. Plast Reconstr Surg 1991;88(4):620–625, discussion 626–627
7. Burget GC, Walton RL. Optimal use of microvascular free flaps, cartilage grafts, and a paramedian forehead flap for aesthetic reconstruction of the nose and adjacent facial units. Plast Reconstr Surg 2007;120(5):1171–1207, discussion 1208–1216
8. About Us. Chicago, IL. Accessed March 20 at http://www.a-s-r-t.com/aboutus3.html
9. Pomahac B, Diaz-Siso JR, Bueno EM. Evolution of indications for facial transplantation. J Plast Reconstr Aesthet Surg 2011;64(11):1410–1416
10. Soga S, Mitsouras D, Schultz K, et al. Pre-operative CT and MR angiography protocols for composite tissue allotransplantation of the face. (Received 2010 Certificate of Merit.) Paper presented at: Proceedings of the Radiological Society of North America 2010
11. Knoll BM, Hammond SP, Koo S, et al. Infections following facial composite tissue allotransplantation—single center experience and review of the literature. Am J Transplant 2013;13(3):770–779
12. Pomahac B, Nowinski D, Diaz-Siso JR, et al. Face transplantation. Curr Probl Surg 2011;48(5):293–357
13. Cendales LC, Kanitakis J, Schneeberger S, et al. The Banff 2007 working classification of skin-containing composite tissue allograft pathology. Am J Transplant 2008;8(7):1396–1400
14. Pomahac B, Pribaz J, Eriksson E, et al. Restoration of facial form and function after severe disfigurement from burn injury by a composite facial allograft. Am J Transplant 2011;11(2):386–393
15. Pomahac B, Lengele B, Ridgway EB, et al. Vascular considerations in composite midfacial allotransplantation. Plast Reconstr Surg 2010;125(2):517–522
16. Pomahac B, Pribaz J, Eriksson E, et al. Three patients with full facial transplantation. N Engl J Med 2012;366(8):715–722

# 18 Imaging and Computer Modeling in Head and Neck Reconstruction

*Matthew M. Hanasono and Roman J. Skoracki*

## ■ Introduction

In recent years, surgeons have taken advantage of various technologies to aid in microvascular free flap reconstructions. In this chapter, we discuss virtual surgical planning using computer-assisted design (CAD) software and rapid prototype modeling (also known as medical modeling) to assist with performing more efficient and accurate head and neck reconstructions involving vascularized and nonvascularized bone. We have combined this technology in select cases with intraoperative stereotactic navigation to assist with accurate flap positioning and inset when surgical exposure is limited and to facilitate flap inset through more minimal access incisions. We also explain how computed tomography angiography (CTA) can be useful not only for confirming blood vessel patency preoperatively but also for localizing perforator blood vessels to aid flap design. Finally, we examine the uses and limitations of intraoperative indocyanine green angiography as a method for identifying perforator location and for assessing tissue perfusion.

## ■ Virtual Surgical Planning and Rapid Prototype Modeling

Three-dimensional reformatting of sequential two-dimensional images, such as those acquired by computed tomography (CT), has become routine practice to assist in the visualization of various traumatic and neoplastic lesions that affect the bony structures of the head and neck. In addition to producing three-dimensional computer representations of the facial skeleton, CAD software can be used to manipulate the images to perform virtual resections and reconstructions prior to performance of the actual surgery.[1,2] Medical CAD software, which was initially engineered for applications in neurosurgery and radiation therapy, is now commercially available for various applications in congenital craniofacial surgery, orthognathic surgery, dental implant surgery, and head and neck reconstructive surgery.[3] While the applications for computer simulation of reconstructive surgeries continue to expand, they are currently most widely used for bony reconstruction of mandibular, maxillary, and other craniofacial defects **(Fig. 18.1)**.

Concurrent with advances in software, the introduction of rapid prototype modeling (one of the technologies known as computer-aided manufacturing, or CAM) via three-dimensional printers for reconstructive surgery has led to the use of physical models from CAD computer data that not only are helpful in allowing the surgeon to visualize the patient's actual anatomy but also, more practically, can serve as a template for bending and shaping the hardware used for bone flap, graft, and implant fixation **(Fig. 18.2)**. Computer-generated cutting guides

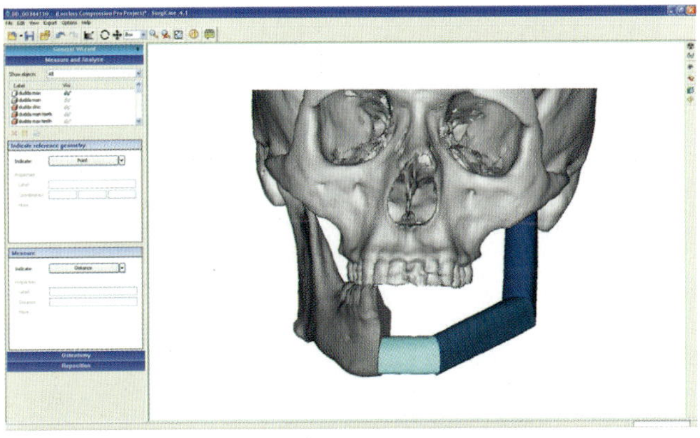

**Fig. 18.1** Computer-assisted design (CAD) virtual reconstruction of the mandible with a fibular free flap. The head can be rotated in any direction to confirm that the planned reconstruction is ideal in terms of restoring the patient's mandibular shape and occlusion.

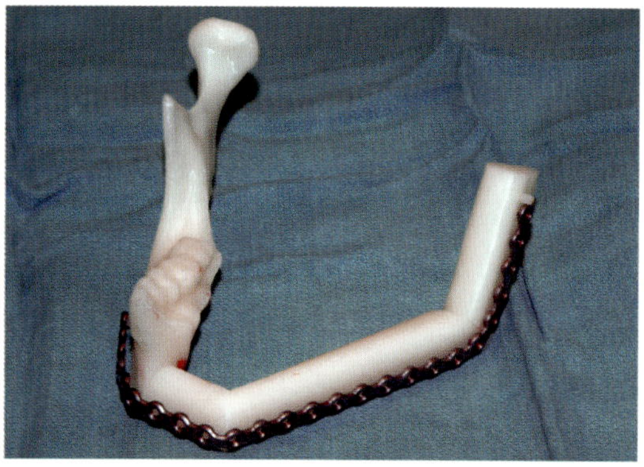

**Fig. 18.2** A three-dimensional rapid prototype model made of acrylic polymer that can be used to guide surgery as well as act as a template for bending titanium hardware, which can be done preoperatively to save time, and that then can be sterilized in preparation for surgery.

can also be manufactured using the same three-dimensional printing process to assist with making osteotomies at the precise lengths and angles needed to replicate the planned reconstruction **(Fig. 18.3)**.

Three-dimensional printing typically involves laying down successive thin layers of material that are bound or hardened by glue, light, or heat until the desired object has been manufactured. Three-dimensional printing processes are available for polymers, ceramics, glass, and metals. Because the process does not involve molds or dies, three-dimensional printing is substantially faster and less expensive than conventional manufacturing processes. The term stereolithography specifically refers to manufacture of three-dimensional models using ultraviolet light-cured acrylic polymer resins. An ultraviolet laser traces an area on the surface of a vat of liquid resin, curing or polymerizing only where it traces.

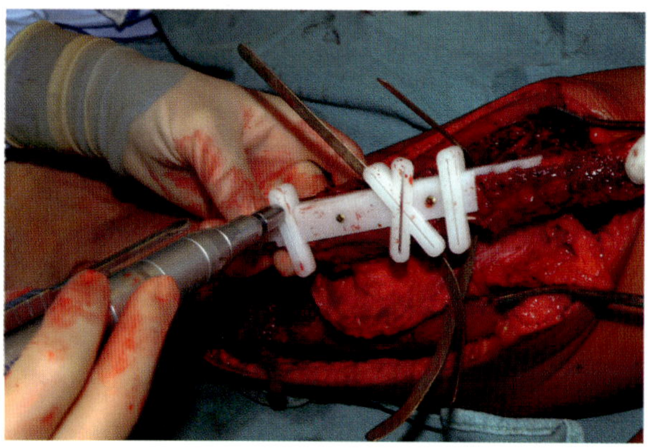

**Fig. 18.3** Computer-generated cutting guides can also be manufactured to simplify osteotomies, making it easier to cut the fibula at the precise lengths and angles needed to duplicate the virtual plan.

The single layer, ranging from ~ 0.05 to 0.2 mm in thickness, is then hardened and "dipped" into the liquid vat to coat it with a new liquid layer. Subsequent scanning of the laser on the new layer solidifies the new layer and adheres it to the layer below. Post-processing is performed to remove excess liquid resin and fully cure the resultant parts. Stereolithographic models can be gas sterilized for use during surgery.

For head and neck reconstruction, a fine cut (1.5 mm or less) axial head and neck CT scan with 0° of gantry tilt is obtained. The data are saved to computer disk in a generic format (Digital Imaging and Communications in Medicine, DICOM). DICOM files are then converted to a stereolithographic file format (STL), which is utilized by CAD software to create a virtual three-dimensional model of the facial skeleton that can be rotated in any direction. A CT scan of the bony free flap donor site is obtained so that it can be manipulated using the software to create an idealized reconstruction. The fibula is among the most commonly used source for bony free flap reconstruction in most practices, but virtually any site (e.g., scapula or iliac crest) can be imaged and imported into the CAD platform (see case example, below). If a donor site CT scan is not obtained, outcomes using generic donor site data are usually acceptable.

Virtual resection osteotomies are then planned on the mandible or maxilla in consultation with the resecting surgeon, if different from the reconstructive surgeon. Next, the desired fibula, left or right according to the desired pedicle orientation and skin island location if applicable, is selected, and virtual osteotomies are performed as needed to reconstruct the missing mandible or maxilla. The original mandible or maxilla can be visualized as a partial transparency or "ghost" to help guide the shaping of the fibular reconstruction. When the existing mandible is misaligned due to displaced fracture or prior resection, the remaining mandibular remnants can be repositioned on the CAD platform into their optimal position. When parts of the facial skeleton are severely distorted or misaligned, such as by tumor, trauma, or prior surgery, CAD software can "erase" these parts and replace them with idealized parts by creating a mirror image of the normal side. It is even possible to import an age, sex, ethnically and size matched dataset template of another individual and superimpose this as a surgical guide for the patient at hand. The planned fibular reconstruction is checked from multiple angles prior to finalizing the plan.

Once the virtual plan is finalized, a model of the reconstructed mandible or maxilla is constructed using three-dimensional printing technology. Cutting guides are made for the maxilla or mandible that fit along the existing bony contours as well as for the fibula or other free flap donor site, utilizing the unique surface characteristics of the given area as a match, not unlike a puzzle piece. During surgery, the cutting guides are temporarily fixated to the mandible or maxilla and to the fibula with titanium screws, and a reciprocating saw blade is inserted into the cutting guide slots. Newer-generation cutting guides feature metal inserts that snap into the slots, to minimize saw blade play and increase the accuracy of osteotomies. The mandible or maxilla model is used to bend the titanium hardware, either prior to the case or by an assistant during the surgery, to save operative time.

In our experience, use of virtual computer planning and three-dimensional medical models with cutting guides saves operative time and increases reconstructive accuracy **(Fig. 18.4)**.[2] Prebending hardware, as well as using the cutting guides to simplify osteotomies, saves operative time, particularly when multiple osteotomies are needed. The preoperative planning that occurs may also increase operative efficiency by improving surgical decision making and reducing trial and error during flap harvest and shaping, since the virtual planning session serves as a kind of rehearsal for the actual surgery. We have shown increased accuracy compared with traditional methods of template bending along the native contours of the maxilla or mandible, and "eyeballing" the reconstruction when necessary, as well as a close correlation between the final reconstruction and the computer-assisted virtual plan. It has been suggested that virtual planning and medical modeling make bony head and neck reconstruction more accessible to less-experienced osteocutaneous free flap surgeons.[3]

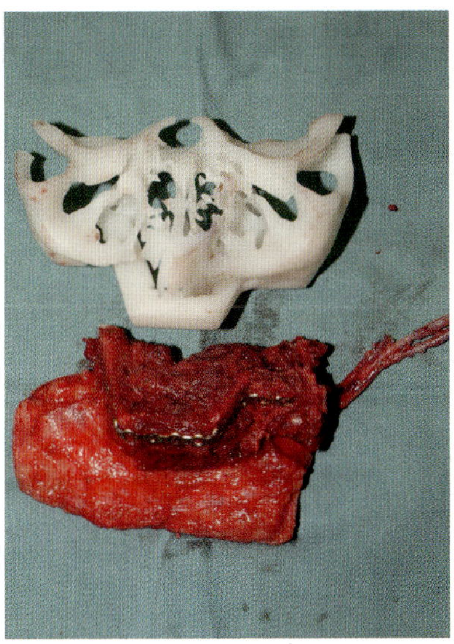

**Fig. 18.4** A three-dimensional rapid prototype model (above) compared with an actual fibular osteocutaneous free flap (below) created using custom cutting guides and fixated with a titanium reconstruction plate bent according to the model.

Even in experienced hands, however, computer planning and three-dimensional models are beneficial for patients in whom the original architecture of the mandible or maxilla is not easily identifiable, including patients with large exophytic tumors, displaced or comminuted pathologic fractures, and prior resections with or without prior reconstructions. In these patients, creating a template for shaping the reconstruction along the native contours of the mandible or maxilla is often difficult or impossible.

A negative of utilizing these technologies includes costs for engineering and manufacturing the models, which are arguably offset by operative time saving and increased accuracy. Virtual planning also requires anywhere from 30 to 60 minutes and is usually performed by the surgeon and a software engineer via Web conference. Time is also needed to print and ship the models. While this usually only takes a day or two with express shipping, it makes the technique unfeasible when the initial consultation with the patient is performed just prior to surgery or intraoperatively. Perhaps the greatest limitation is that the benefits of virtual planning and medical modeling are reduced when the operative plan changes, for example, due to tumor growth. To limit the potential for change in the resection and needed reconstruction, recent imaging is recommended, as is close communication between the resecting and reconstructive surgeons.

Rapid prototyping and CAD software continue to evolve. Such technologies are already commonly used by oral surgeons to guide endosteal implant placement in the native mandible and maxilla.[4] Levine et al[5] have explored performing immediate implant placement at the time of free flap reconstruction, utilizing computer planning and custom drill guides to precisely place implants between hardware screws. Immediate implant placement takes advantage of the increased accuracy of bony reconstruction, since implants are rendered unusable if placed inaccurately at the wrong angulation. Another step that may substantially contribute to increased accuracy is the creation of patient-specific titanium hardware that is not pre-bent, but is milled from a solid block of titanium, since this results in greater strength. Such patient-specific hardware allows the surgeon to select individual screw hole placement in the number, location, and angulation that are most optimal for a specific defect **(Fig. 18.5)**. This also allows for unique plate designs that may optimize hardware use according to preselected parameters, such as force distribution, surface design requirements, and minimized stress shielding.

In addition to mandibular and maxillary reconstruction, virtual surgical planning and medical models have also been useful for orbital reconstruction.[6] Very precise restoration of the orbital cavity is necessary to avoid enophthalmos, exophthalmos, or

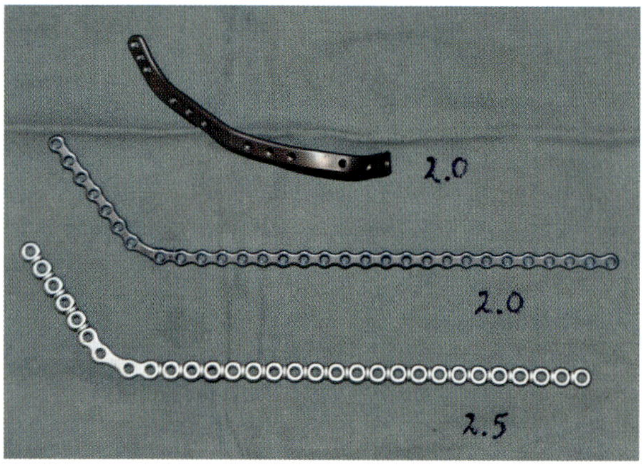


**Fig. 18.5** A 2.0 mm thick custom-made titanium plate based on computer-assisted design plans for fibular free flap reconstruction (top) compared with standard 2.0 mm and 2.5 mm titanium reconstruction plates (middle and bottom, respectively). The plate is created using a computer-guided milling process, rather than by printing, for increased strength. The screw hole placement and angulation are defined by the surgeon during computer planning (photo courtesy of Patrick Garvey, MD).

vertical dystopia (eyes at different heights). Bony free flaps can be designed for orbital reconstruction virtually just as for the mandible and maxilla. More commonly in our practice, titanium mesh or bone grafts are used for orbital reconstruction and are supported by soft tissue flaps. In these cases, we find that using a three-dimensional model as a template for shaping bone grafts and mesh implants is easier than using the patient's actual orbit, because surgical exposure is often limited and retraction of the eye can result in injury to the globe, traction on the optic nerve, or bradycardia due to the oculocardiac reflex. Hardware or mesh is bent along the contours of a rapid prototype model **(Fig. 18.6)** so that accurate restoration

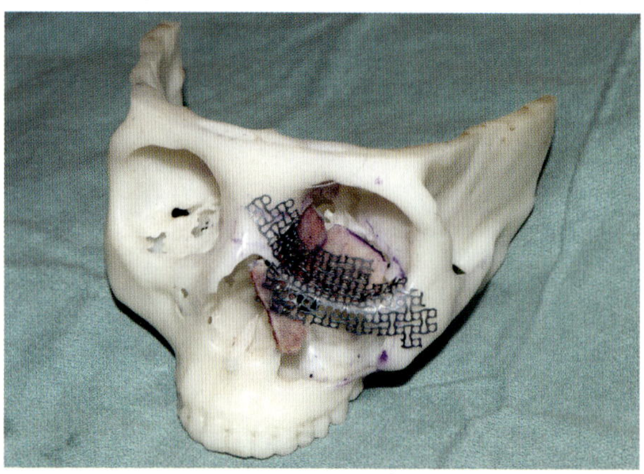

**Fig. 18.6** A three-dimensional model used to guide orbital reconstruction with titanium mesh and bone graft for accurate restoration of the orbital floor, which is critical to prevent enophthalmos, exophthalmos, and/or orbital dystopia.

of the orbit is achieved. In cases where the original anatomy is distorted or absent, such as by tumor or trauma, a virtual template for reconstructing the bony contours of the orbit can be created by mirroring the unaffected side onto the affected side on the CAD platform and printed using CAM.[7]

Other uses of CAD software in reconstructive surgery include creation of patient-specific implants. Patient-specific implants have been commercially made of titanium, acrylics, ceramics or polyetheretherketone (PEEK), a thermoplastic, for the replacement of craniofacial bones, most commonly, of the calvaria.[8] These implants are most useful when the exact dimensions of the defect are already known and have been imaged, since intraoperative contouring, while still possible, takes away from the time-savings associated with customization. Thus, they are mostly used for delayed reconstruction. Additionally, preformed titanium mesh plates have been created using CAD software from a composite of normal orbital data (Synthes, Paoli, Pennsylvania).

## Intraoperative Stereotactic Navigation

Image-guided intraoperative stereotactic navigation has a long history of use in neurologic and sinus surgery. More recently, stereotactic navigation has been used in craniofacial surgery to verify correct positioning of the reconstructed orbital wall after surgery for trauma and in oncologic surgery to verify that the resection in patients with maxillofacial fibrous dysplasia results in symmetry with the normal contralateral side. In reconstructive surgery, the same stereotactic navigation systems used for neurologic and sinonasal surgery can be used to assist with insetting of free flap constructs, particularly when access is limited and accurate positioning is crucial.[9–12]

All stereotactic navigation systems incorporate a computer to track the location of instruments and the patient in three-dimensional space. Several different tracking systems have been developed, including optical, electromagnetic, electromechanical, and ultrasonographic.[9] Optical tracking systems are currently the most commonly used and include active and passive designs. Active tracking systems use infrared light-emitting diodes (LEDs) attached to the patient and the surgical instruments. As long as the LEDs stay within the line of sight of a digital camera, the location of the instrument and the patient can be accurately presented on the computer monitor. In passive tracking systems, reflective spheres rather than LEDs bounce infrared light back from an emission source to a receiver. Both the emitter and the receiver are located within the camera unit.

All navigation systems require performing a registration process to accurately define the location of the patient. Prior to the start of surgery, fiducial markers placed on various points of the patient's face are identified with a navigation probe, allowing the system to integrate *x*, *y*, and *z* coordinates on the patient with *x*´, *y*´, and *z*´ coordinates on the images loaded into the navigation system workstation. These images are from preoperative scans (either CT or MRI) obtained with the patient wearing the same fiducial markers prior to the surgery. During this registration process, either a headset or a navigation array replaces the fiducial markers **(Fig. 18.7)**. Headsets are convenient and noninvasive, but limit access to the midface and orbits. The navigation array allows free movement of the head during surgery without the need for repeating the registration process, which is desirable for free flap reconstruction, but must be rigidly fixed to the patient's head by means of small incisions and screw placement into the calvarium. Accuracy following registration is usually within ~ 1 mm.

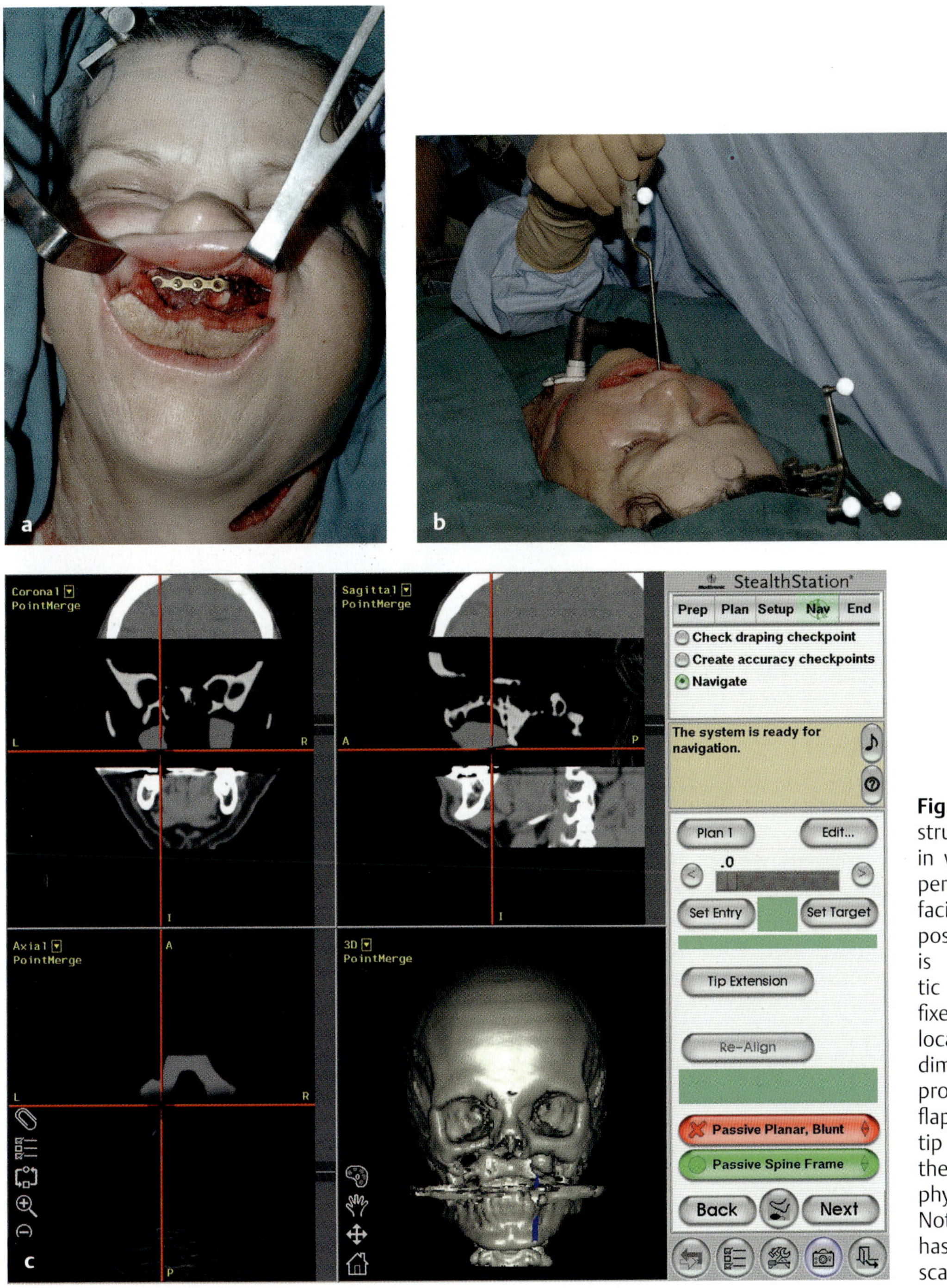


**Fig. 18.7** **(a)** Midfacial reconstruction with a fibular free flap in which the inset of the flap is performed transorally, without facial incisions. **(b)** Correct flap positioning prior to rigid fixation is confirmed using stereotactic navigation, which requires a fixed array so that the system can locate the facial skeleton in three-dimensional space. **(c)** A handheld probe is used to confirm that the flap is in the planned position. The tip of the probe can be located on the patient's computed tomography (CT) scan in multiple planes. Note that the virtual fibular flap has been superimposed on the CT scan images.

During surgery, the probe is used to verify the correct positioning of the free flap in three dimensions. Some CAD programs (e.g., Surgi Case CMF, Materialise, Leuven, Belgium) allow conversion of the virtually altered images back to DICOM format files. These files can then be combined with, or superimposed on, the preoperative CT data and uploaded into the navigation system. During surgery, the location of the real-world reconstruction can be compared with the planned position of the virtual reconstruction. This allows the surgeon to verify that the position of the free flap construct matches the planned position. In facial reconstructions, malposition of a vascularized bone flap by as little as a few millimeters can result in malocclusion or orbital malposition, as well as distortion of facial landmarks, although this can be camouflaged to some extent by soft tissues or later contouring.

## Computed Tomography Angiography

Computed tomography angiography (CTA) using multidetector row CT scanners is an imaging modality that can be used to evaluate recipient, pedicle, and perforator blood vessels. Because of its less invasive nature, CTA has become more popular than digital subtraction angiography, which involves additional risks of arterial puncture, pseudoaneurysm, and bleeding. CTA not only provides high-resolution images of both the arterial and venous systems, but also permits simultaneous examination of the surrounding bony and soft tissue architecture. In addition to verifying the patency of major blood vessels in settings like vascular disease, prior surgery, trauma, and congenital anomalies, CTA can be used in reconstructive surgery to map perforators in deep inferior epigastric perforator (DIEP), anterolateral thigh, and fibula free flaps as well as other flaps used for head and neck reconstructive surgery. The disadvantages of CTA include modest radiation exposure, cost, and risk for allergic reactions to intravenous contrast.

The DIEP flap is often preferred to the rectus abdominis myocutaneous free flap because of potentially lower donor-site morbidity and equal reliability. In head and neck soft tissue reconstruction, the DIEP flap may also be preferred when less bulk is desired. Successful DIEP harvest is dependent on having adequate (typically medium- to large-sized) perforators to supply the skin paddle of the flap, which may not always be present and may be quite time-consuming to locate and dissect. Furthermore, donor-site morbidity becomes equivalent to myocutaneous free flap dissection when extensive interruption of the rectus abdominis muscle and its innervation is necessary to harvest a DIEP flap with tortuous, mostly intramuscular, perforators, lessening the theoretic advantage of this flap.

CTA has been used for localizing the best cutaneous perforators preoperatively for DIEP flap harvest by several investigators (**Fig. 18.8**). In theory, this results in a time-savings during surgery by allowing the surgeon to focus only on the dominant perforator (or perforators) while ligating smaller, inessential perforators. It also allows the surgeon to pick the side of the abdomen with better perforators. CTA is also useful in preoperatively visualizing the branching pattern and course, particularly intramuscular, of the vascular pedicle to determine whether it is amenable to straightforward dissection without substantial destruction of the rectus abdominis muscle. In cases where the branching pattern requires the surgeon to sacrifice a large amount of muscle to capture the desired perforator(s), plans for a DIEP flap are abandoned and a standard or muscle-sparing rectus abdominis myocutaneous flap is harvested instead.

Patients undergo multidetector helical CT scans with 100 to 150 mL of contrast injected at a rate of 4 to 6 mL per second via a peripheral IV. Axial planar CT data are used to create sagittal and coronal images as well as a three-dimensional image of the abdominal wall vasculature that can be rotated horizontally and vertically. The branching patterns of the flap pedicle vessels and perforators are determined, as is whether they travel through a short or an extensive intramuscular course or take a septocutaneous path. Perforators as small as 0.3 mm can be visualized by CTA.

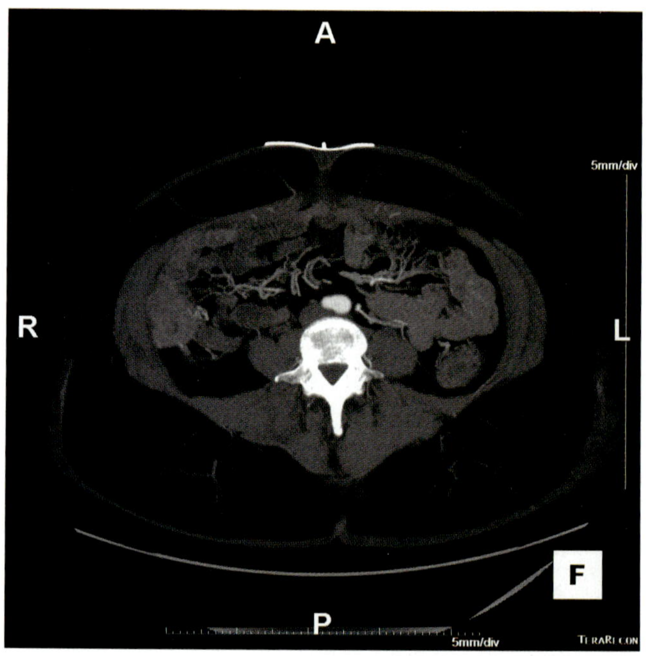


**Fig. 18.8** A computed tomography angiogram (CTA) of the abdomen used for preoperative planning prior to deep inferior epigastric perforator flap harvest. Several perforators can be seen within the subcutaneous fat emanating from the deep inferior epigastric arteries bilaterally.

Rozen et al[14] performed a study of 42 patients undergoing DIEP flap surgery in which they mapped all perforators larger than 1 mm. CTA identified 280 major perforators in 42 patients, with 1 false-positive and 1 false-negative, resulting in a sensitivity of 99.6% and positive predictive value of 99.6%. Casey et al[15] performed a retrospective review of DIEP and superficial inferior epigastric artery (SIEA) breast reconstruction, comparing operative times in 186 flaps performed with the assistance of handheld Doppler to 100 flaps performed subsequently with CTA. They found a statistically significant decrease in operative times in both unilateral and bilateral cases (370 versus 459 minutes, and 515 versus 657 minutes, respectively; both $p < 0.01$). Smit et al[16] performed a similar study and also found a shorter operative time associated with CTA compared with Doppler (264 versus 354 minutes, $p < 0.001$).

Garvey et al[18] examined the accuracy of CTA in the detection of perforators for ALT free flaps. Among 16 flaps, CTA identified 40 out of 54 perforators confirmed intraoperatively, resulting in a sensitivity of 74%. The perforator location averaged 3.5 mm from the location predicted by CTA. Furthermore, CTA was able to differentiate between septocutaneous and intramuscular perforators 77.5% of the time. As mentioned above, CTA is probably most useful in cases where the subcutaneous fat is ample, since the perforators can be visualized easily in the background of low-density fatty tissues. In individuals with thin thighs, handheld Doppler or possibly ICG angiography (see below) may be more sensitive for identifying perforator location.

In another study, Garvey et al[19] examined the utility of CTA for examining cutaneous perforators in the fibular osteocutaneous free flap (**Fig. 18.9**). In a series of 40 patients, CTA identified 94.9% of cutaneous perforators that were later verified intraoperatively. The perforators were located an average of 8.7 mm from their predicted locations. The slightly lower accuracy in predicting perforator location than when CTA is used in the thigh may be because perforators are best seen between the muscles of the lower leg and not in the scant subcutaneous fat, through which they may change course and reach the skin obliquely. CTA was able to differentiate between a septocutaneous and a musculocutaneous course 93% of the time.

In addition to being used for flap design, CTA may be of great benefit in verifying three-vessel flow to the lower extremity, particularly in patients with equivocal findings by history or physical exam, such as when the dorsalis pedis and posterior tibial arteries are not easily palpable. We, therefore, choose to selectively obtain CTA of the lower leg prior to possible fibular free flap reconstruction only when the vascular supply to the lower extremity is in question or when precise positioning of the skin paddle is desirable. A potential application is to combine CTA with CAD and medical modeling, allowing precise design of the bony reconstruction as well as precise positioning of the skin paddle perforator.

## Indocyanine Green Angiography

Indocyanine green (ICG) is a nontoxic contrast agent that is bound to protein in plasma. Laser-assisted ICG angiography (Spy Elite System, LifeCell Corp., Branchburg, NJ) is an imaging modality that provides real-time imaging of tissue perfusion in which an 806 nm laser light source is used to induce fluorescence of protein-bound ICG dye that is captured on a near-infrared camera with filters that block out ambient and laser light (**Fig. 18.10**). Clinical uses of ICG angiography include assessing vascular perfusion to the skin of locoregional and free flap tissues,

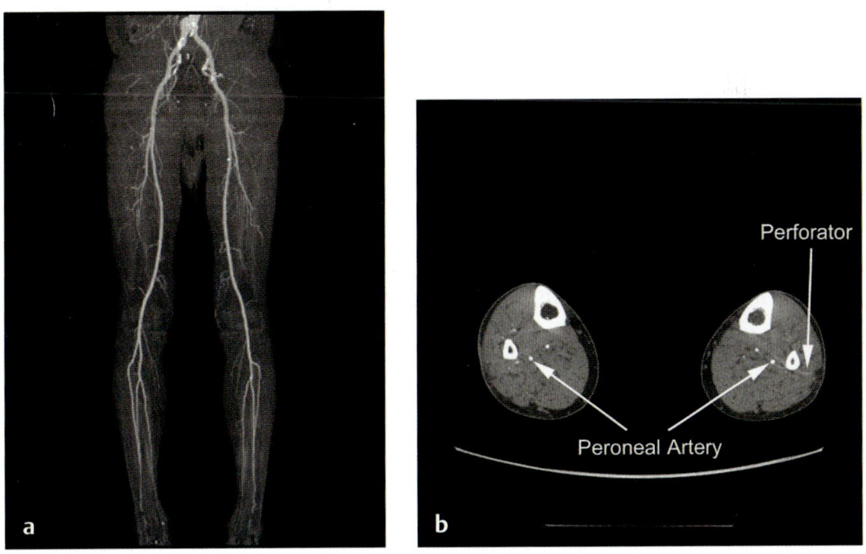


**Fig. 18.9 (a)** A three-dimensional CT angiogram reconstruction of a patient's lower extremities showing patency of the anterior tibial, posterior tibial, and peroneal arteries. **(b)** The course of cutaneous perforators can be observed arising from the peroneal artery in cross-section.

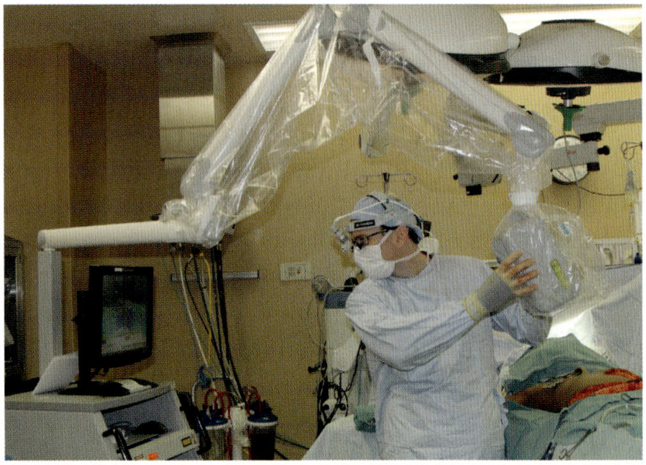

**Fig. 18.10** Indocyanine green (ICG) intraoperative angiography system (Spy Elite System, LifeCell Corp., Branchburg, NJ). A sterile drape allows the surgeon to position the laser light source.

and, possibly, assessing perforator location to aid in the design of perforator flaps. ICG angiography is used in breast reconstruction to assess breast skin viability after mastectomy and could, similarly, be used in head and neck reconstruction to determine whether potentially devascularized local tissues need to be resected and reconstructed along with those removed for oncologic reasons. For example, radiated neck skin may be substantially devascularized and prone to wound-healing problems after tumor resection and might require a second free flap or pedicled flap to ensure safe closure without exposure of the carotid artery and internal jugular vein.

ICG has an excellent safety profile, having been used to measure cardiac output, to assess hepatic function, and for ophthalmic angiography for over 40 years. There is a small risk (0.17%) of adverse drug reaction, including anaphylaxis in patients allergic to iodides, which are present in the injectable solution.[20,21] ICG is excreted by the liver with a half-life of 3 to 5 minutes. Because of the short plasma half-life, multiple evaluations can be performed during the same operative procedure. Performing intraoperative angiography with the Spy Elite System (LifeCell Corporation, Bridgewater, NJ) typically takes 10 to 15 minutes.

Early reports described using ICG angiography to assess first cardiac bypass, and then later free flap anastomoses. ICG angiography is very accurate when used to verify the patency of an anastomosis that is questionable. The dye is injected via a peripheral IV and can rapidly be seen crossing first the arterial anastomosis then the venous anastomosis. Imperfections or blockages along the anastomotic suture line can be readily visualized. For practical purposes, most of the time this is not necessary since signs of anastomotic failure are usually apparent by examination of the flap. However, in cases of partial obstruction due to an accumulating thrombus at the anastomosis or around an intimal tear, ICG angiography may be of benefit in predicting impending flap compromise when clinical signs are equivocal.

More commonly, ICG angiography is used to assess blood flow to the skin paddle of pedicled and free flaps to ensure its adequacy. If ICG dye does not accumulate in a portion of the flap skin paddle, generally within 2 minutes or less after intravenous injection, it suggests that this portion of the skin will ultimately be nonviable. Five to 10 mL of ICG is injected, then the skin is observed on the imaging system monitor, while the camera is focused on the skin flap. Tissue that demonstrates subjectively questionable perfusion on black-and-white imaging is examined clinically for signs of hypoperfusion. In this way, partial flap loss is decreased.

Another related technique is to use ICG angiography to determine which or how many perforators are necessary to avoid partial skin flap loss or fat necrosis. In this case, multiple perforators are dissected then individually temporarily occluded with microvascular clamps, except for the perforator or perforators that the surgeon plans to use. Blood flow to the skin flap is then analyzed by ICG imaging. If the skin flap appears well perfused, then the temporarily occluded perforators can be divided. If the skin flap appears hypoperfused, then additional clamp(s) are released until the entire flap appears adequately perfused. This second technique has mostly been utilized to analyze DIEP flap perforator flow, but has also been reported for various flaps used in head and neck reconstruction, such as the anterolateral thigh and fibula free flaps.[22]

In addition to the black-and-white video image captured by the charge-coupled video camera, the Spy Elite system comes bundled with analysis software (SPY-Q). The software features two options for quantitative measurement of the fluorescence recorded on the video images. The first option is a relative percentage technique, which reports the fluorescence of many areas of the image relative to a user-defined reference point that is designated as 100% perfusion (**Fig. 18.11**). The second method is an absolute measurement that uses a 255-level gray scale and assigns a point value (0–250) to various points on the image based on the gray scale that corresponds to the signal intensity. In this scale, a value of 6.0 is considered the lower limit of acceptable perfusion.[22]

Wu et al[23] reported a 14% false-negative rate (specific area of the flap looked viable by ICG angiography, but resulted in necrosis) and a 9% false-positive rate (specific area of the flap looked nonviable by ICG angiography but did survive). Although they concluded that ICG angiography was not superior to clinical judgment in assessing flap perfusion for most patients, they hypothesized that a good indication for ICG angiography was in assessing flap vascularity in dark-skinned individuals, since clinical assessment is

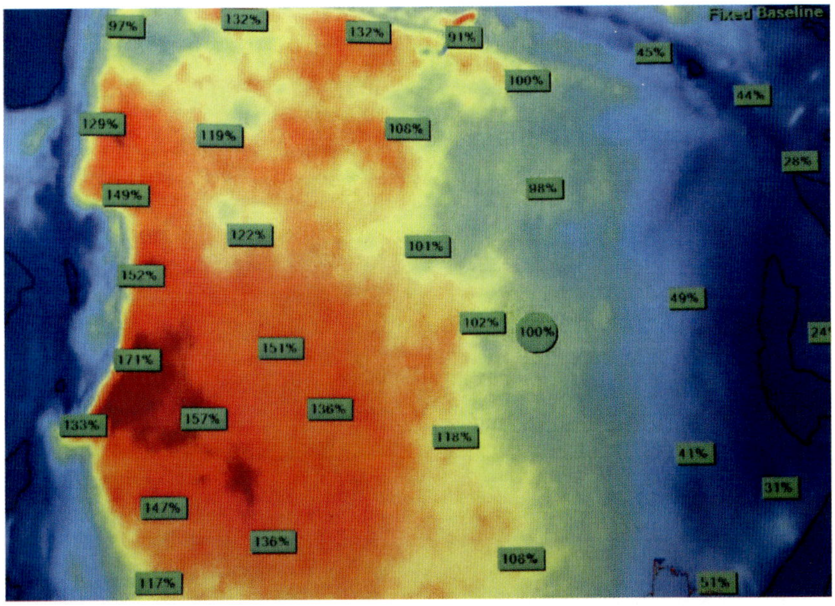


**Fig. 18.11** Image captured using ICG angiography of a left abdominal deep inferior epigastric perforator free flap following dissection. The user assigns a value of "100%" to area that appears to have an optimal perfusion and the software included with the system analyzes the intensity of signal of the rest of the image, assigning relative perfusion values to add a degree of objectivity to the study. Note that some areas were found to have greater signal intensity than the user-defined reference point; consequently, some areas have perfusion values greater than 100%.

more difficult in these patients. A caveat of utilizing ICG to assess flap viability includes the fact that skin perfusion at the time of dye injection can be affected by many variables, including blood pressure, volume status, use of vasopressors, patient temperature, vasospasm secondary to surgical dissection, and other factors that influence resistance in the microcirculation.

Criteria for diagnosing venous congestion have not been defined for ICG angiography. Delayed clearing of fluorescent dye is expected when venous compromise to a flap exists, but no set time points for what should be considered delayed have been established. Expert opinion has suggested re-imaging 5 to 20 minutes after administration of ICG if venous congestion is a concern following flap dissection, transfer, or inset.[24]

ICG angiography has also been used to locate perforators so that cutaneous flaps can be appropriately centered on them prior to making any skin incisions. If accurate, ICG angiography has the potential to eliminate the occasionally unnecessary skin incision when no viable perforator exists, allowing a different donor site to be chosen. An accurate method of pre-incision perforator localization also helps to minimize the size of the incision needed by eliminating the need for a large exploratory incision to look for the perforator, reducing the cosmetic deformity created at the flap donor site.

The accuracy of ICG in assessing perforators is higher in thin flaps, since the depth of visualization is only ~ 1 cm. In thicker flaps, the ICG "blush" becomes very diffuse as it travels farther away from the perforator, where it is carried by smaller and smaller branching blood vessels to the skin. Thus, ICG angiography has been used to help design thin cutaneous perforator flaps, such as the anterolateral thigh flap in non-obese patients. As the amount of subcutaneous fat increases, for example in rectus abdominis myocutaneous flaps of most patients, the accuracy of ICG angiography in locating the position of deep perforators decreases.

Onoda et al[25] compared ICG angiography, using another system available in Japan, called the Photodynamic Eye (Hamamatsu Photonics K.K., Hamamatsu, Japan), to CTA. They found ICG angiography had an 84% positive predictive value and CTA had a 100% positive predictive value in a series of 50 patients undergoing a variety of free and pedicled flaps with a skin paddle component. Perforators were difficult to detect by ICG angiography when the flap thickness was greater than 20 mm, with perforators being identified on only 12 of 50 flaps (24% sensitivity). In contrast, CTA was not very useful in detecting perforators when the flap thickness was less than 8 mm, showing only 30% sensitivity in these patients. Perforators with a long course through subcutaneous fat are most easily visualized by multidetector CT angiography (MDCTA). The authors recommended utilizing ICG angiography in combination with handheld Doppler ultrasound when the flap thickness is ≤ 8 mm and CTA in combination with handheld Doppler ultrasound to localize perforators when the flap thickness is ≥ 20 mm, thereby minimizing time and expense while still maintaining reasonable accuracy.

For flaps with intermediate thickness, they recommended using a combination of all three modalities.

## Conclusions

In recent years, surgeons have harnessed technology to further refine microvascular free flap reconstruction. Diagnostic and planning technologies complement rather than replace good judgment and surgical technique. Used appropriately, they have the potential to increase the reliability, accuracy, and efficiency of reconstruction.

## Case Example

A 48-year-old woman with a history of a right mandibular ameloblastoma was treated with a segmental mandibulectomy and had two failed attempts at reconstruction with fibular osteocutaneous free flaps. Further reconstruction was performed with a titanium reconstruction plate and right pectoralis major muscle flap. She then presented to us with a titanium reconstruction plate that was exposed intraorally **(Fig. 18.12)**. The etiology of her fibula free flap losses was unknown. A CTA of the pelvis was obtained to evaluate the quality of the deep circumflex iliac arteries as part of her work-up **(Fig. 18.13)**. The deep circumflex iliac arteries appeared patent bilaterally and a right iliac crest free flap was planned. The CTA data was exported as DICOM format and utilized to perform CAD planning for right mandibular reconstruction **(Fig. 18.14)**. A computer-generated cutting guide was manufactured to assist with making the flap osteotomies so that the flap would mimic the virtually planned reconstruction **(Fig. 18.15)**. A radial forearm fasciocutaneous free flap was used for intraoral soft tissue reconstruction. Postoperatively, her mandibular symmetry has been restored and she is able to retain a dental prosthesis for restoration of her teeth **(Fig. 18.16)**.

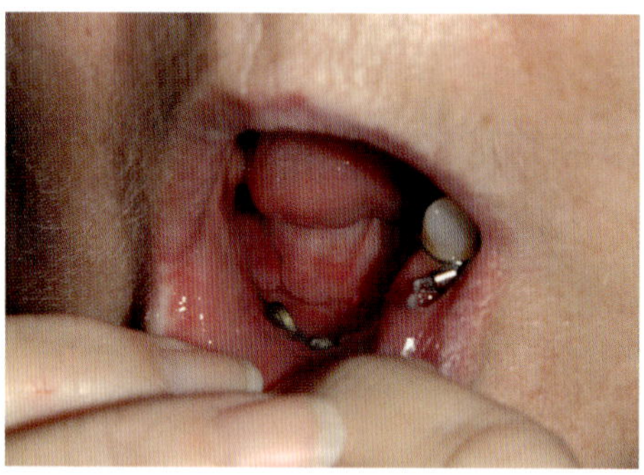

**Fig. 18.12** A patient presented following right hemimandibulectomy and two failed attempts at reconstruction with fibular osteocutaneous free flaps. A titanium plate was used for reconstruction but was now exposed intraorally.

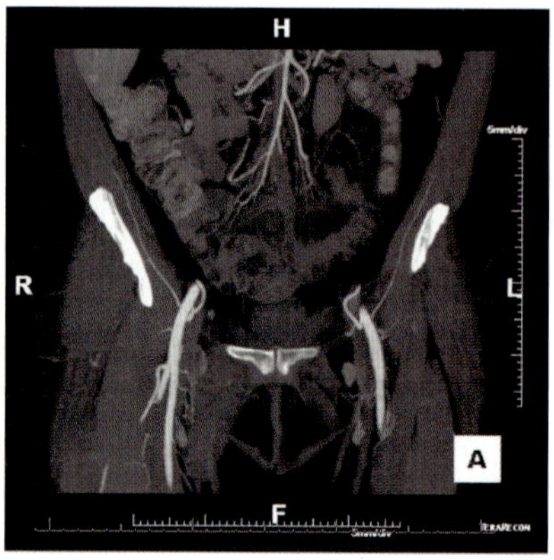


**Fig. 18.13** Because of concern for vascular disease contributing to free flap loss, a CTA of the pelvis was obtained prior to undertaking reconstruction with an iliac crest free flap. The CTA showed patent deep circumflex iliac vessels bilaterally.

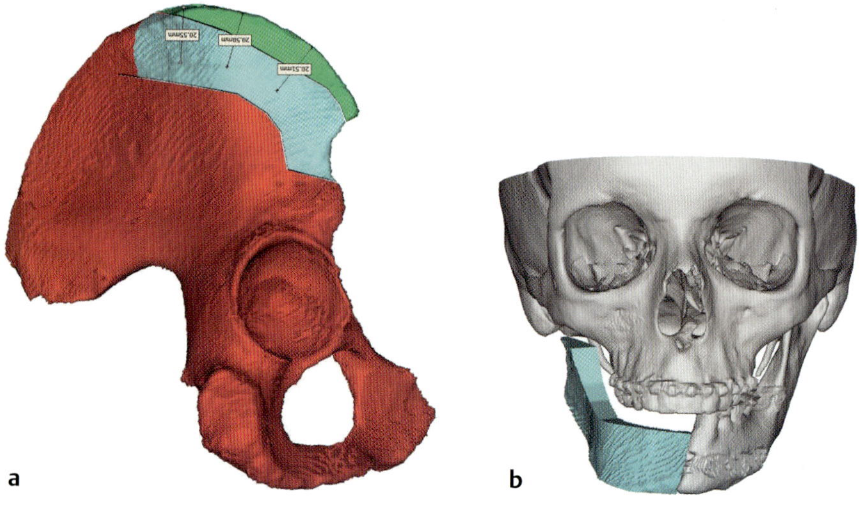

**Fig. 18.14** **(a)** The bony data from the CTA, which was used **(b)** to plan reconstructive surgery using CAD software.

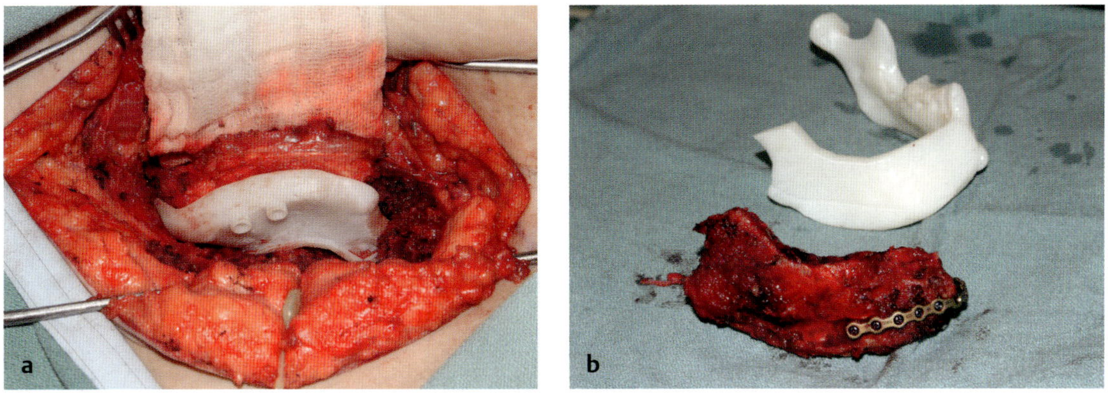

Fig. 18.15 **(a)** A computer-generated cutting guide was used to help make osteotomies so that **(b)** the iliac crest free flap accurately resembled the reconstruction planned on the computer.

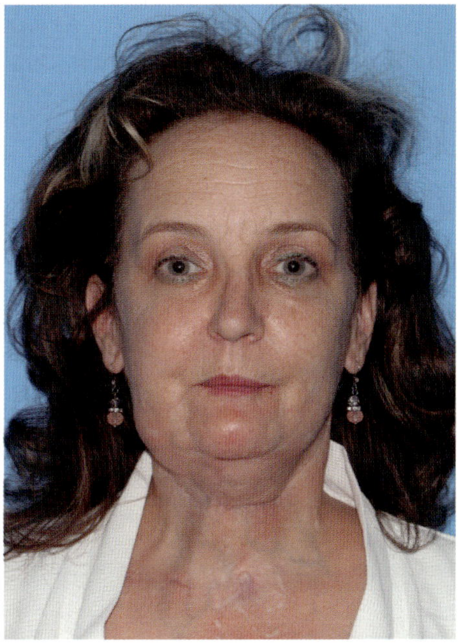

**Fig. 18.16** Postoperative appearance following CAD-planned reconstruction and utilization of a computer-generated mandibular model and iliac crest cutting guide.

## References


1. Levine JP, Patel A, Saadeh PB, Hirsch DL. Computer-aided design and manufacturing in craniomaxillofacial surgery: the new state of the art. J Craniofac Surg 2012;23(1):288–293
2. Hanasono MM, Skoracki RJ. Computer-assisted design and rapid prototype modeling in microvascular mandible reconstruction. Laryngoscope 2013;123(3): 597–604
3. Antony AK, Chen WF, Kolokythas A, Weimer KA, Cohen MN. Use of virtual surgery and stereolithography-guided osteotomy for mandibular reconstruction with the free fibula. Plast Reconstr Surg 2011;128(5):1080–1084
4. Okay DJ, Buchbinder D, Urken M, Jacobson A, Lazarus C, Persky M. Computer-assisted implant rehabilitation of maxillomandibular defects reconstructed with vascularized bone free flaps. JAMA Otolaryngol Head Neck Surg 2013;139(4):371–381
5. Levine JP, Bae JS, Soares M, et al. Jaw in a day: total maxillofacial reconstruction using digital technology. Plast Reconstr Surg 2013;131(6):1386–1391
6. Gellrich NC, Schramm A, Hammer B, et al. Computer-assisted secondary reconstruction of unilateral posttraumatic orbital deformity. Plast Reconstr Surg 2002;110(6):1417–1429
7. Golfinos JG, Fitzpatrick BC, Smith LR, Spetzler RF. Clinical use of a frameless stereotactic arm: results of 325 cases. J Neurosurg 1995;83(2):197–205
8. Hanasono MM, Goel N, DeMonte F. Calvarial reconstruction with polyetheretherketone implants. Ann Plast Surg 2009;62(6):653–655
9. Roessler K, Ungersboeck K, Dietrich W, et al. Frameless stereotactic guided neurosurgery: clinical experience with an infrared based pointer device navigation system. Acta Neurochir (Wien) 1997;139(6):551–559
10. Strong EB, Rafii A, Holhweg-Majert B, Fuller SC, Metzger MC. Comparison of 3 optical navigation systems for computer-aided maxillofacial surgery. Arch Otolaryngol Head Neck Surg 2008;134(10):1080–1084
11. Pham AM, Rafii AA, Metzger MC, Jamali A, Strong EB. Computer modeling and intraoperative navigation in maxillofacial surgery. Otolaryngol Head Neck Surg 2007;137(4):624–631
12. Hanasono MM, Jacob RF, Bidaut L, Robb GL, Skoracki RJ. Midfacial reconstruction using virtual planning, rapid prototype modeling, and stereotactic navigation. Plast Reconstr Surg 2010;126(6):2002–2006
13. Masia J, Clavero JA, Larrañaga JR, Alomar X, Pons G, Serret P. Multidetector-row computed tomography in the planning of abdominal perforator flaps. J Plast Reconstr Aesthet Surg 2006;59(6):594–599
14. Rozen WM, Ashton MW, Stella DL, Phillips TJ, Grinsell D, Taylor GI. The accuracy of computed tomographic angiography for mapping the perforators of the deep inferior epigastric artery: a blinded, prospective cohort study. Plast Reconstr Surg 2008;122(4):1003–1009

15. Casey WJ III, Chew RT, Rebecca AM, Smith AA, Collins JM, Pockaj BA. Advantages of preoperative computed tomography in deep inferior epigastric artery perforator flap breast reconstruction. Plast Reconstr Surg 2009;123(4):1148–1155
16. Smit JM, Dimopoulou A, Liss AG, et al. Preoperative CT angiography reduces surgery time in perforator flap reconstruction. J Plast Reconstr Aesthet Surg 2009;62(9):1112–1117
17. Tong WMY, Dixon R, Ekis H, Halvorson EG. The impact of preoperative CT angiography on breast reconstruction with abdominal perforator flaps. Ann Plast Surg 2012;68(5):525–530
18. Garvey PB, Selber JC, Madewell JE, Bidaut L, Feng L, Yu P. A prospective study of preoperative computed tomographic angiography for head and neck reconstruction with anterolateral thigh flaps. Plast Reconstr Surg 2011;127(4):1505–1514
19. Garvey PB, Chang EI, Selber JC, et al. A prospective study of preoperative computed tomographic angiographic mapping of free fibula osteocutaneous flaps for head and neck reconstruction. Plast Reconstr Surg 2012;130(4):541e–549e
20. Takahashi M, Ishikawa T, Higashidani K, Katoh H. SPY: an innovative intra-operative imaging system to evaluate graft patency during off-pump coronary artery bypass grafting. Interact Cardiovasc Thorac Surg 2004;3(3):479–483
21. Benya R, Quintana J, Brundage B. Adverse reactions to indocyanine green: a case report and a review of the literature. Cathet Cardiovasc Diagn 1989;17(4):231–233
22. Green JM III, Thomas S, Sabino J, et al. Use of intraoperative fluorescent angiography to assess and optimize free tissue transfer in head and neck reconstruction. J Oral Maxillofac Surg 2013;71(8):1439–1449
23. Wu C, Kim S, Halvorson EG. Laser-assisted indocyanine green angiography: a critical appraisal. Ann Plast Surg 2013;70(5):613–619
24. Gurtner GC, Jones GE, Neligan PC, et al. Intraoperative laser angiography using the SPY system: review of the literature and recommendations for use. Ann Surg Innov Res 2013;7(1):1–14
25. Onoda S, Azumi S, Hasegawa K, Kimata Y. Preoperative identification of perforator vessels by combining MDCT, Doppler flowmetry, and ICG fluorescent angiography. Microsurgery 2013;33(4):265–269

# II

# Flap Atlas

# 19 Anterolateral and Anteromedial Thigh Flaps

*Peirong Yu*

## Introduction

The anatomy of the anterolateral thigh (ALT) flap was first described in the Chinese literature.[1,2] The first report in the English literature, by Song et al, appeared in the *British Journal of Plastic Surgery* in 1984.[3] The ALT flap did not gain popularity for more than a decade. The main reason for delayed adaption of this flap was thought to be the rather confusing and inconsistent anatomy of the vascular pedicle. Currently, with better understanding of the vascular anatomy, particularly the perforator anatomy,[4] the ALT flap has become the workhorse flap for soft tissue reconstruction. The anteromedial thigh (AMT) flap is less well known. It was first described by Song et al in 1984 along with the ALT flap.[3] There have been very few reports on the AMT flap, and the descriptions of vascular anatomy in the literature have been confusing. The AMT flap perforator anatomy was further clarified by the author in 2011.[5]

The main advantages of the ALT flap include minimal donor-site morbidity and a long and large vascular pedicle. The main disadvantages include tedious perforator dissection, occasional inconsistent perforator anatomy, and bulkiness in some patients.

## Anatomy

### Vascular Anatomy of the ALT flap

In most cases (96%), the main pedicle artery for the ALT flap is the descending branch of the lateral circumflex femoral artery, which is a direct branch of the profunda femoris artery. The lateral circumflex femoral artery has three terminal branches: the ascending, transverse, and descending branch. The descending branch usually travels in the intermuscular space between the rectus femoris and the vastus lateralis and intermedius muscles. Soon after its take-off from the lateral circumflex femoral artery, it sends out a rectus femoris branch supplying the rectus femoris muscle. The rectus femoris branch also gives off cutaneous perforators supplying the AMT flap. The main descending branch then gives off the vastus intermedius branch and continues to descend along the medial edge of the vastus lateralis muscle. It sends out numerous branches to supply this muscle and one to three cutaneous perforators to supply the ALT flap skin (type I) (**Fig. 19.1a** and **Fig. 19.2**). The diameter of the descending branch is usually between 2 and 2.5 mm immediately below the rectus femoris branch and 2.5 to 3.5 mm above the rectus femoris branch.

In 2% of cases, the cutaneous perforator derives from the transverse branch of the lateral circumflex femoris artery (type II) (**Fig. 19.1b** and **Fig. 19.3**). The perforator travels longitudinally within the vastus lateralis muscle for its entire length before it enters the fasciocutaneous flap and requires tedious intramuscular dissection for a long distance. To obtain a larger pedicle vessel, the transverse branch needs to be included.

In the remaining 2% of cases, the cutaneous perforators pierce the rectus femoris muscle and derive from the rectus femoris branch (type III) (**Fig. 19.1c** and **Fig. 19.4**), essentially a variation of the AMT flap with an unusually lateral location of the perforator.

Two venae comitantes accompany the perforator artery and then travel alongside the descending branch

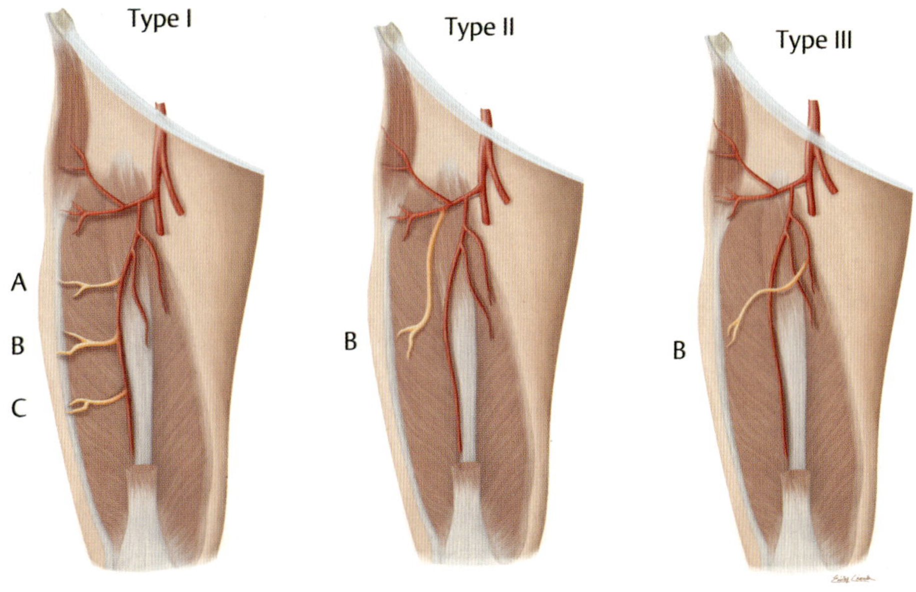


**Fig. 19.1** Types of vascular supply to the anterolateral thigh (ALT) flap. The main blood supply arise from the lateral circumflex femoris artery, which gives off the ascending branch, the transverse branch, and the descending branch. Based on the origin, three types of perforators are identified supplying the ALT flap. Type I: perforators originating from the descending branch. Type II: perforators originating from the transverse branch via the vastus lateralis muscle. Type III: perforators originating from the rectus femoris branch via the rectus femoris muscle. Up to three perforators can be found. Perforator B is located near the midpoint between the anterior superior iliac spine and the supralateral corner of the patella. Perforators A and C are approximately 5 cm proximal and distal to perforator B, respectively.

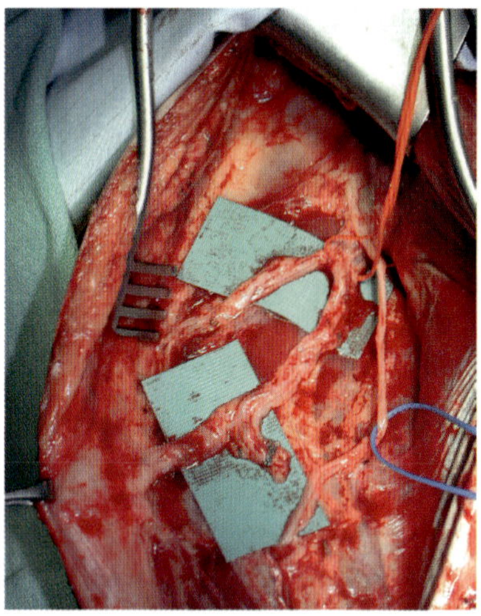

**Fig. 19.2** Type I blood supply to the anterolateral thigh flap, in which the perforators originate from the descending branch.

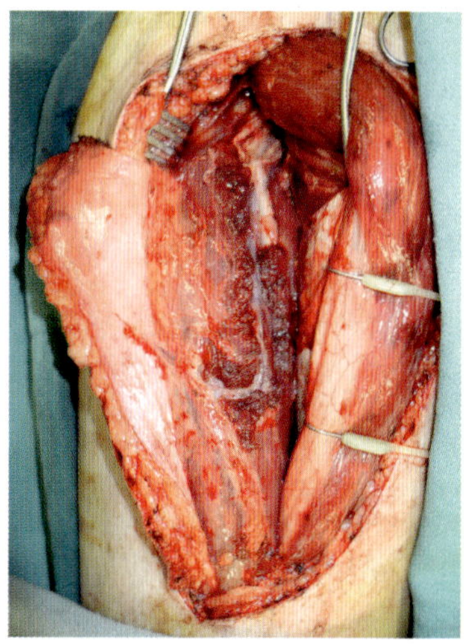

**Fig. 19.3** Type II blood supply to the anterolateral thigh flap, in which the cutaneous perforator originates from the transverse branch and travels within the vastus lateralis muscle for the entire path, making perforator dissection more difficult.

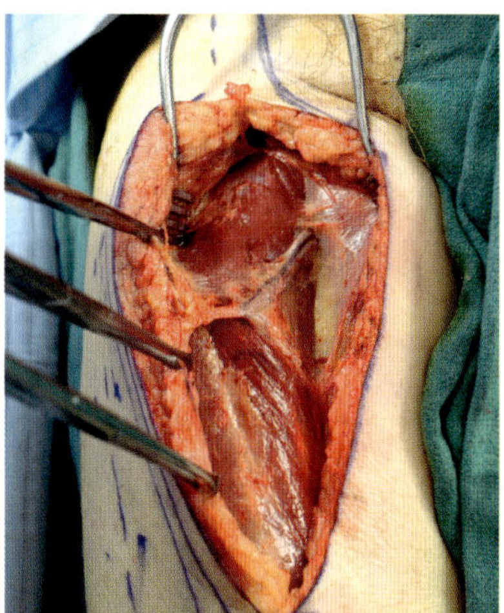

**Fig. 19.4** Type III blood supply to the anterolateral thigh flap, in which the perforator originates from the rectus femoris branch and pierces the rectus femoris muscle.

artery throughout its course. There are numerous H connections between the two venae comitantes; therefore, using either one of them should provide adequate venous drainage. The venae comitantes have a diameter of 2 mm to 3.5 mm. The two venae comitantes usually converge above the rectus femoris branch, forming a common trunk with a diameter of 3 mm to 5 mm.

## Neural Anatomy

The lateral femoral cutaneous nerve (L2–L3) can be included with the flap for sensory reinnervation. This nerve enters the thigh through the lateral end of the inguinal ligament and travels in the plane immediately above the deep fascia (**Fig. 19.5**). At ~ 10 cm below the inguinal ligament, the nerve branches into a lateral branch and a medial branch. The former continues to travel along or lateral to the line connecting the anterior superior iliac spine (ASIS) and the supralateral corner of the patella (AP line), while the latter turns medially and descends ~ 2 to 3 cm medial to the AP line. The lateral branch is within the ALT flap and can be taken for sensory reinnervation while the medial one can be left intact. The diameter of the femoral cutaneous nerve in the proximal thigh before the bifurcation is usually between 1.5 mm and 2 mm.

Various amounts of, or even the entire, vastus lateralis muscle can be included in the ALT flap when indicated. The main motor nerve for the vastus lateralis muscle travels closely with the vascular pedicle. Proximal in the thigh, the motor nerve travels lateral to the descending branch vessels (**Fig. 19.2**). Before the descending branch vessels enter the vastus lateralis muscle, the motor nerve takes a turn underneath (sometimes above) the descending branch and travels medially along the descending branch vessels. The nerve then sends out numerous small branches that accompany the vascular branches to supply the vastus lateralis muscle.

## Perforator Anatomy: The Surface Location of Cutaneous Perforators—The "ABC System"

The surface location of the ALT perforators appears to follow a pattern. The perforator that is most consistently present is located around the midpoint between the line connecting the ASIS and the supralateral corner of the patella (the AP line). Approximately 5 cm more proximal and 5 cm more distal to that, second and third perforators may be found. Based on this pattern, the location of the cutaneous perforators is classified as Perforator A (most proximal), Perforator B (middle), and Perforator C (most distal), thus, forming the basis for what is now commonly referred to as the "ABC system."[4] The average distances (longitudinally) measured from the ASIS to perforators A, B, and C in a Western population are 18.4 ± 2.2 cm, 23.5 ± 2.0 cm, and 28.6 ± 2.3 cm, respectively. Therefore, these three perforators are separated from each other by ~ 5 cm.

The measured distance between the ASIS and the cutaneous perforators obviously depends on the height of the patient. The relative location of each perforator between the ASIS and supralateral patella can be determined, with the ASIS being point 0, the supralateral patella being point 1.0, and the midpoint being point 0.5. The location, number, size, and types of perforators are summarized in **Table 19.1** and **Fig. 19.6**. Horizontally, the cutaneous perforators are located, on average, 1.5 cm lateral to the AP line. Twenty-six percent of flaps had a single perforator, most commonly perforator B, 49% had two perforators, and 25% had three perforators.

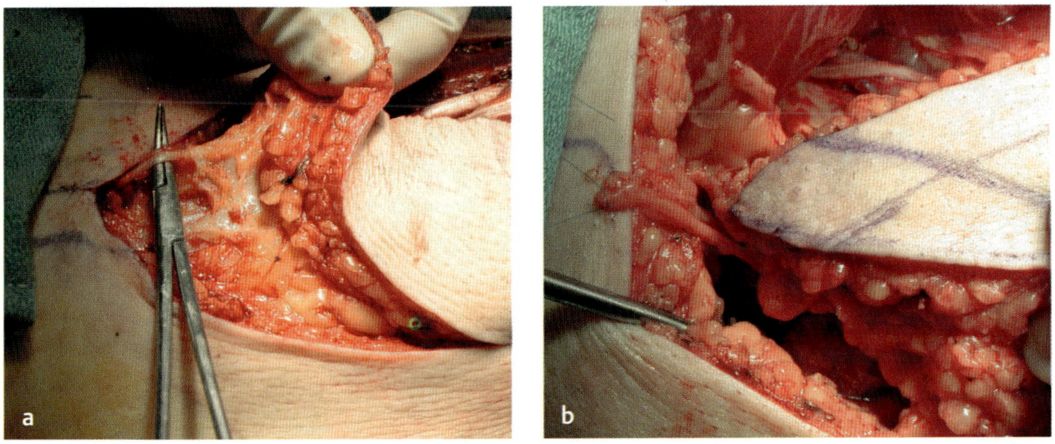


**Fig. 19.5** The lateral femoral cutaneous nerve, a sensory nerve to the anterolateral thigh flap, can be included for sensory innervation. **(a)** The nerve can be found deep to the subcutaneous tissue immediately above the deep fascia along the line connecting the anterior superior iliac spine and the supralateral corner of the patella through the superior incision. **(b)** An additional 5 cm nerve length can be obtained via proximal subcutaneous dissection.

**Table 19.1** Anterolateral thigh flap perforator anatomy

| Perforators | A | B | C |
|---|---|---|---|
| Presence | 53% | 87% | 59% |
| Septocutaneous | 46% | 19% | 12% |
| y-axis | 18.4 ± 2.2 cm<br>point 0.4* | 23.5 ± 2.0 cm<br>point 0.5* | 28.6 ± 2.3 cm<br>point 0.6* |
| x-axis | 1.4 ± 0.6 cm | 1.4 ± 0.7 cm | 1.5 ± 0.6 cm |
| Size: small (< 0.5 mm) | 18% | 17% | 72% |
| Size: medium (0.5–1 mm) | 27% | 37% | 19% |
| Size: large (> 1 mm) | 55% | 46% | 9% |

* Distance from the ASIS (cm) or relative location (point) between the ASIS and supralateral corner of the patella.

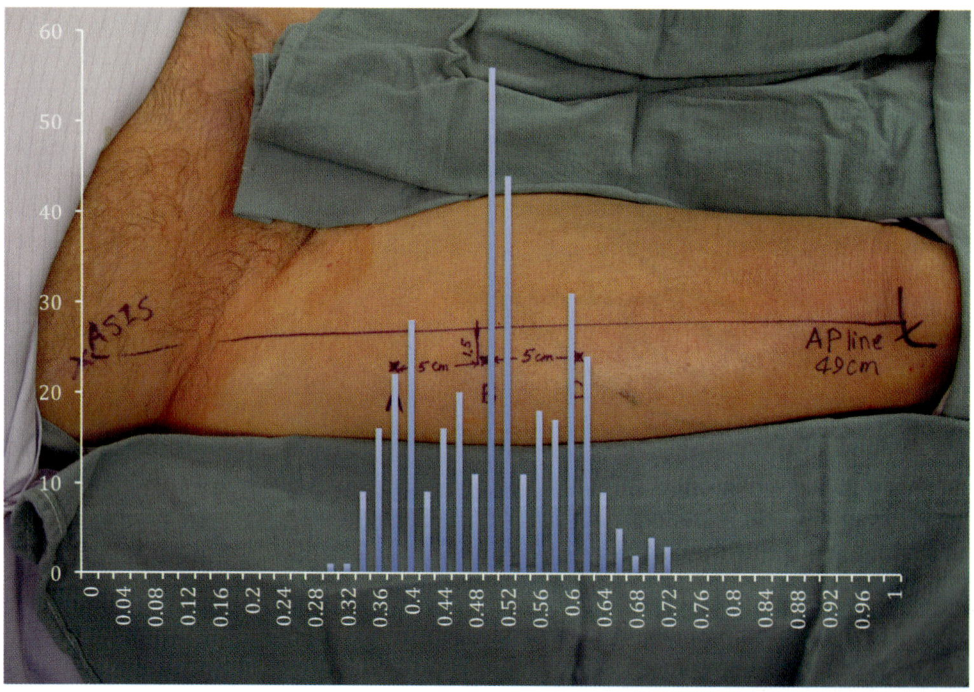


**Fig. 19.6** Surface locations of the cutaneous perforators of the anterolateral thigh flap. Based on the locations, the cutaneous perforators are classified as perforators A, B, and C. Perforator B is located near the midpoint of the line connecting the anterior superior iliac spine (ASIS) and the supralateral corner of the patella (AP line).

## Vascular Anatomy of the AMT Flap

The main vascular pedicle of the AMT flap is the rectus femoris branch, which arises from the descending branch (**Fig. 19.7a**). It travels along the medial edge of the rectus femoris muscle or within the muscle itself and sends out perforators to the skin (**Fig. 19.7b**). The AMT perforators are, however, present in only 51% of the cases (43% had a single perforator, 8% had two perforators, and 49% had no perforators). The majority of perforators were concentrated near the midpoint of the AP line, with fewer perforators located more proximal and distal to the midpoint—an "ABC system" similar to that with the ALT perforators.[5] The locations of the perforators on the y- and x-axis are summarized in **Table 19.2**.

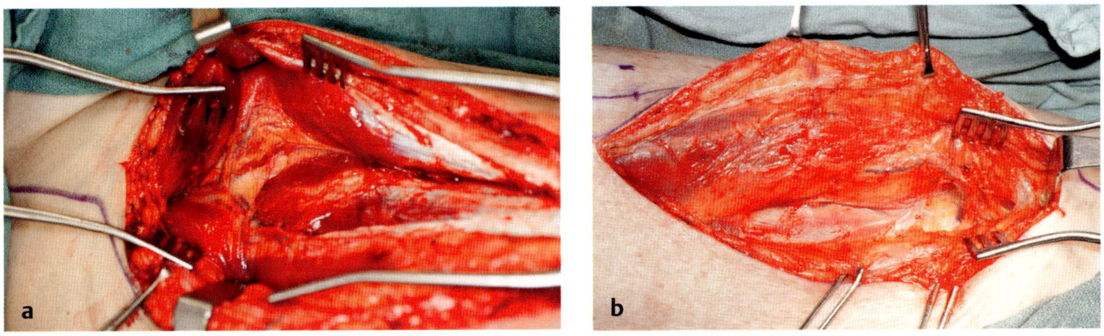

**Fig. 19.7** **(a)** The descending branch gives rise to the rectus femoris branch that supplies the rectus femoris muscle and **(b)** gives off perforators to the anteromedial thigh flap.

**Table 19.2** Anteromedial thigh flap perforator anatomy (based on 100 thighs explored)

| Perforator | Number present | y-axis* | x-axis** | Perforator Size*** |
|---|---|---|---|---|
| A | 12 | 18.4 ± 1.5<br>0.40 ± 0.01 | 3.3 ± 1.4 | 17% small, 42% medium, 42% large |
| B | 33 | 23.2 ± 2.3<br>0.50 ± 0.04 | 3.2 ± 1.6 | 12% small, 55% medium, 33% large |
| C | 14 | 27.8 ± 3.3<br>0.60 ± 0.06 | 3.2 ± 1.7 | 43% small, 50% medium, 7% large |

* Distance from the ASIS (cm) or relative location (point) between the ASIS and supralateral corner of the patella.
** Distance (cm) medial to the AP line.
*** Small, < 0.5 mm; medium, 0.5–1 mm; large, > 1 mm.

## Relationships of ALT and AMT Perforators

There is an inverse relationship between ALT and AMT perforator numbers and sizes.[6] Most patients without ALT perforators have one or more AMT perforators, while most patients with three ALT perforators have no AMT perforators **(Table 19.3)**.

**Table 19.3** Relationship between number of perforators in anterolateral thigh (ALT) flap and number in anteromedial thigh (AMT) flap

| Perforators in ALT flap (N) | Perforators in AMT flap (N) | | |
|---|---|---|---|
| | 2 | 1 | 0 |
| 3 | 0 (0%) | 5 (24%) | 16 (76%) |
| 2 | 2 (4%) | 24 (49%) | 23 (47%) |
| 1 | 2 (11%) | 12 (63%) | 5 (26%) |
| 0 | 3 (60%) | 1 (20%) | 1 (20%) |

Therefore, when unfavorable perforator anatomy is encountered in the ALT flap territory, one should explore the AMT flap through the same incision. The chances are quite good that a single or double skin island flap can be harvested using AMT perforators.

# ■ Preoperative Considerations

The only contraindication to the ALT flap may be severe peripheral vascular disease. The profundus artery can be a source of collateral blood supply to the lower extremity when the superficial femoral artery is occluded. Therefore, harvesting the ALT flap by taking the descending branch and ligating the vastus intermedius branch and possibly the rectus femoris branch may compromise the circulation to the leg in patients with severe peripheral vascular disease, although direct evidence for this is lacking.

Preoperative imaging studies are usually not necessary. CT angiography (CTA) may help identify the perforators and determine which thigh is preferable based on the perforator anatomy.

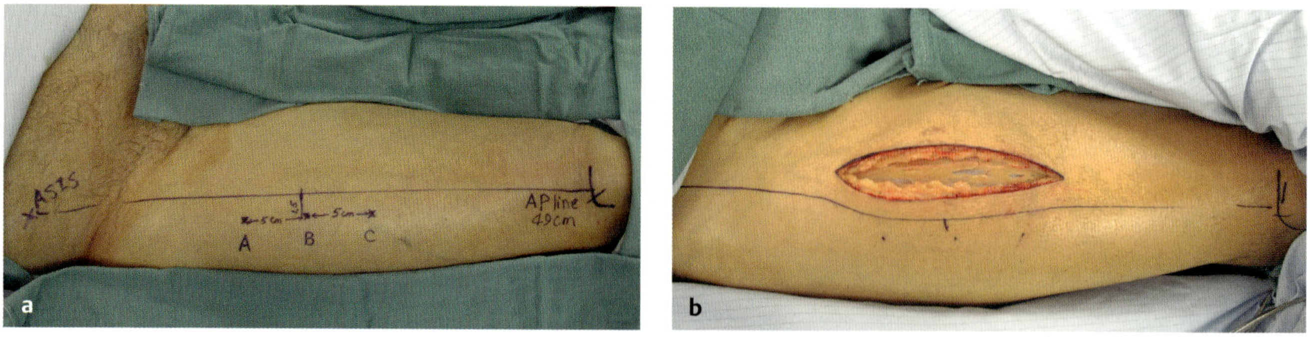


**Fig. 19.8** **(a)** Marking the locations of the three cutaneous perforators based on the "ABC" system, with perforator B near the midpoint but 1.5 cm lateral to the AP line. Perforators A and C are marked 5 cm proximal and distal to perforator B, respectively. **(b)** Only the anterior incision is made initially over the rectus femoris muscle, and it is made long enough to cover all three perforators.

## ■ Patient Positioning and Skin Marking

The patient is placed in a supine position, with the leg in a neutral position without supination. This is particularly important in obese patients. Circumferential skin preparation is unnecessary.

The key landmarks are the supralateral corner of the patella and the most prominent point of the ASIS. A line is drawn to connect these two landmarks (AP line). The midpoint of the line is marked. The presumed location of perforator B is marked 1.5 cm lateral to the AP line near its midpoint **(Fig. 19.8)**. The presumed locations of perforators A and C are marked 5 cm proximal and distal to the presumed perforator B, respectively. A hand-held Doppler device can be used to attempt to detect perforator B, which may be helpful for beginners and teaching, although the accuracy is low, particularly in obese patients. The estimated flap dimension is then outlined centering on perforator B, bearing in mind that the flap design may need to be recentered based on the actual perforator locations.

## ■ Operative Technique—ALT Flap

An anterior incision ~ 15 cm long, spanning across all three presumed perforators, is made first down to the fascia over the rectus femoris muscle. For a flap width of 7 to 10 cm, the anterior incision is usually at 1.5 to 2.0 cm medial to the AP line, approximately along the anterior midline of the thigh. The fascia is incised and subfascial dissection proceeds laterally. Subfascial dissection is easier for beginners because the "septum" between the vastus lateralis and rectus femoris muscles can be easily identified in the subfascial plane. The fascia is retracted laterally with three Allis clamps, with each one positioned at the perforator location **(Fig. 19.9)**. The septum appears as a layer of light brown fatty tissue through which the intermuscular space can be entered by bluntly separating the two muscle groups. The rectus femoris muscle is retracted medially, exposing the descending branch. Septocutaneous perforators can be seen running in this intermuscular space and can be traced back to the descending branch. Otherwise, dissection is continued laterally until musculocutaneous perforators piecing the vastus lateralis muscle are seen. The surface locations of the visualized perforators are marked with a 5–0 Prolene suture on the skin surface and the flap is re-centered as needed.

Next, the descending branch running along the medial edge of the vastus lateralis muscle is dissected out. Dissection of the septocutaneous perforators is straightforward. There may be numerous small branches off the perforators supplying the vastus lateralis muscle. These branches are clipped and divided to free the perforators. Small motor nerves

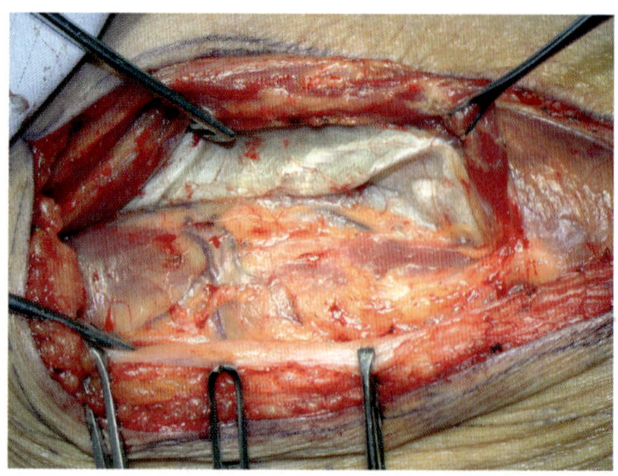

**Fig. 19.9** Three Allis clamps are placed on the fascia to retract it laterally during subfascial dissection. Each clamp corresponds to each perforator location. The intermuscular space (septum) between the rectus femoris and vastus lateralis muscles is entered and the rectus femoris muscle is retracted medially to expose the descending branch.

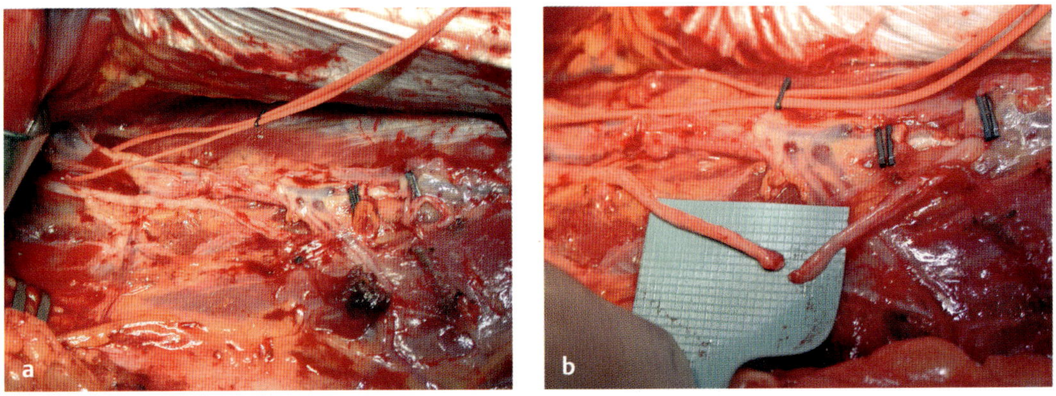

Fig. 19.10 **(a)** The motor nerve that supply the vastus lateralis muscle may travel between two perforators. **(b)** The nerve is divided to release the perforators and is re-anastomosed.

may also be seen accompanying the perforators. If possible, these nerves should be spared. All perforators are then traced back to the descending branch. The descending branch vessels distal to the last perforator are ligated and divided **(Fig. 19.10)**. Care should be taken to identify and separate the motor nerve that travels closely with the descending branch before its division. Occasionally, a motor nerve may travel between two perforators. If both perforators need to be included, the nerve is divided to release the perforators and is repaired. Once the vessels are dissected out and the motor nerve has been separated, the flap dissection is essentially complete. All these dissections can be performed through the anterior incision only.

For musculocutaneous perforators, intramuscular dissection begins at the fascial level where the perforators exit the muscle in a retrograde fashion. With loupe magnification, the muscle fibers are carefully separated with a pair of fine tenotomy scissors along the fiber direction. The dissection continues by following the direction of the perforators toward the main vessel. Tiny muscular branches off the perforators should be carefully cauterized using fine bipolar tips. Larger branches are clipped. In most cases, there is only a small, thin layer of muscle (2 to 3 cm wide and less than 1 cm thick) covering the perforator. The small muscle can be simply divided to free the perforator. It is of great importance not to island the flap before identifying and dissecting out the perforators. In the event no suitable cutaneous perforators are found, an alternative flap, such as the AMT flap, may be harvested.

Flap design is finalized according to the dimensions of the final defect and exact locations of the perforators. When a sensate flap is needed, the lateral femoral cutaneous nerve is identified through the proximal incision. An additional 5 cm of nerve is harvested via proximal subcutaneous dissection. After the recipient vessels are prepared, the vascular pedicle is divided either below or above the rectus femoris branch, depending on the needs. A 19-French Blake drain is placed in the thigh wound. The majority of the donor sites can be closed primarily.

## ■ Operative Technique—AMT Flap

Since the AMT perforators are present in only half of patients, an AMT flap should not be planned as the primary flap. The planned flap should still be the ALT flap. When no suitable perforators are found in the ALT flap territory, subfascial dissection is performed medially through the same incision **(Fig. 19.11)**. The dissection proceeds over the rectus femoris muscle to the intermuscular space between the rectus femoris and the sartorius muscles to explore the cutaneous perforators in the AMT flap territory. The main vascular pedicle, the rectus femoris branch, can be easily identified along the medial edge of the rectus

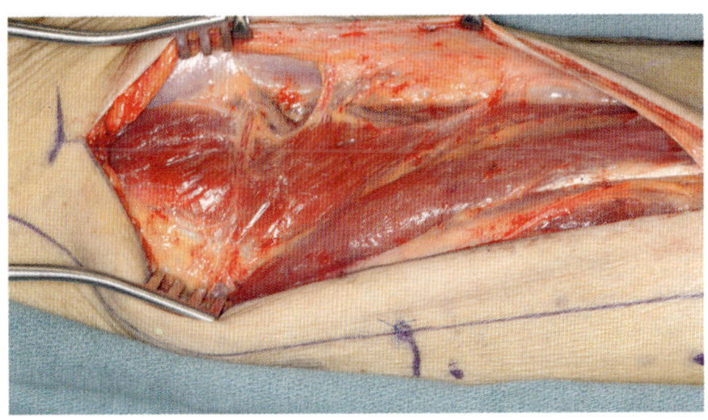

**Fig. 19.11** When no suitable perforators are found in the ALT flap territory, subfascial dissection is performed medially through the same incision over the rectus femoris muscle to the intermuscular space between the rectus femoris and the sartorius muscles, to explore the cutaneous perforators in the AMT flap territory.

femoris muscle and dissected out proximally to its origin from the descending branch. Various amounts of the rectus femoris muscle can be included in the flap, depending on the needs. Once the final defect dimensions are known, the medial border of the AMT flap is incised. Since the rectus femoris branch arises from the descending branch, it is possible to create multiple components/combinations, such as one skin paddle from each ALT and AMT, with or without the vastus lateralis or the rectus femoris muscle (**Fig. 19.12**).

## Donor-Site Care

In most patients, the donor site can be closed primarily over a drain. The entire leg is wrapped with an elastic wrap from the toes to the groin for several days. Patients are encouraged to ambulate with full weight bearing as tolerated, starting postoperative day 1. Drains can usually be removed within a week once the drainage is less than 30 mL/24 hours. When skin grafts are used, knee immobilization is applied until the skin graft dressing is removed on day 6. Patients are advised to keep the knee immobilizer on for ambulation until the graft has completely healed.

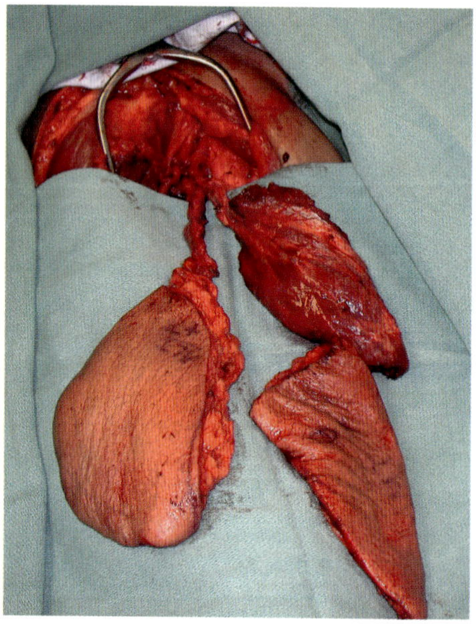

**Fig. 19.12** Chimeric flap with both the anterolateral thigh and anteromedial thigh flaps and a segment of the rectus femoris muscle based on the same vascular pedicle.

In our experience, no significant clinical donor-site morbidity, other than a small area of numbness, has been observed after harvesting the ALT flap with or without a portion of the vastus lateralis muscle, and with or without skin grafting to the donor site. All patients regain their preoperative level of activity. When the entire vastus lateralis muscle is taken, 25% of patients have leg weakness. Taking a cuff to half of the vastus lateralis muscle does not increase the rate of leg weakness. Skin grafting the donor site and dividing one or more of the motor nerve branches also does not produce an increase of weakness.[7]

### Pearls and Pitfalls

- The ALT flap perforators lie slightly lateral to an imaginary line connecting the anterior superior iliac spine and the supralateral corner of the patella (AP line).
- The most commonly occurring perforator (perforator B) occurs at the midpoint of the AP line in the vertical dimension and ~ 1.5 cm lateral to the line in the horizontal dimension.
- The perforators to the ALT are usually found traveling between the vastus lateralis and rectus femoris muscles, while the perforators to the AMT are usually found traveling between the rectus femoris and vastus medialis muscles. Both may occasionally take an intramuscular, rather than septocutaneous, course.
- The blood supply to the AMT flap usually arises from a proximal branch of the descending branch of the lateral circumflex femoral artery.
- When no satisfactory ALT perforators can be located, the surgeon may be able to find a satisfactory AMT perforator rather than explore another flap donor site.
- AMT perforators are found only 51% of the time.
- The lateral femoral cutaneous nerve can be included with the flap for sensory reinnervation. It travels in a plane immediately superficial to the deep fascia.
- The ALT flap can be harvested as a cutaneous perforator flap or as a myocutaneous flap by inclusion of some or all of the vastus lateralis muscle.
- Most ALT and AMT donor sites, up to ~ 10 cm in width, can be closed primarily.

## References


1. Zhou CM, Zhong SZ, Liu MZ. Anatomy of the anterolateral leg flap. Chin J Appl Anat 1983;1:97
2. Xu DC, Zhong SZ, Kong JM, Lou LS, Gao GH. Anatomy of the anterolateral thigh flap. Chin J Appl Anat 1984;2:158–160
3. Song YG, Chen GZ, Song YL. The free thigh flap: a new free flap concept based on the septocutaneous artery. Br J Plast Surg 1984;37(2):149–159
4. Yu P. Characteristics of the anterolateral thigh flap in a Western population and its application in head and neck reconstruction. Head Neck 2004;26(9):759–769
5. Yu P, Selber J. Perforator patterns of the anteromedial thigh flap. Plast Reconstr Surg 2011;128(3):151e–157e
6. Yu P, Selber J, Liu J. Reciprocal dominance of the anterolateral and anteromedial thigh flap perforator anatomy. Ann Plast Surg 2013;70(6):714–716
7. Hanasono MM, Skoracki RJ, Yu P. A prospective study of donor-site morbidity after anterolateral thigh fasciocutaneous and myocutaneous free flap harvest in 220 patients. Plast Reconstr Surg 2010;125(1):209–214

# 20 Radial Forearm Free Flap

*Edward I. Chang and Matthew M. Hanasono*

## Introduction

The forearm free flap was first described by Yang et al[1] as a fasciocutaneous flap that can be used for coverage of a variety of defects. Consequently, the initial description of the flap earned it the colloquial designation of the "Chinese forearm flap," but it is now commonly known as the radial forearm free flap. Since its description, it has become one of the workhorse flaps in head and neck reconstruction, particularly when a thin, pliable flap is needed. Advantages of the radial forearm free flap also include ease of dissection, a long vascular pedicle, minimal donor-site morbidity, and a location that often allows for a two-team approach to donor-site preparation and flap harvest. The radial forearm flap can include a portion of the radius if an osteocutaneous free flap is needed, and the flap can also be neurotized to create a sensate flap by incorporating the lateral antebrachial cutaneous nerve.

## Indications

The radial forearm fasciocutaneous free flap is a versatile flap that is often the flap of choice when a thin, pliable flap is needed. The flap is ideally suited for reconstruction of intraoral mucosal defects, such as the floor of mouth and buccal mucosa, and it is also the flap of choice for reconstruction of partial and hemiglossectomy defects. In these cases, the radial forearm fasciocutaneous free flap is preferred over a skin graft when bone is exposed or when graft contracture will impair functional results, such as tethering of the tongue or restriction of jaw movement. The radial forearm flap has also been utilized in reconstructing defects involving the pharynx, cervical esophagus, and trachea. Further, it can also used for coverage and resurfacing of cutaneous defects of the face and scalp. Finally, the radial forearm free flap is also used for reconstruction of nasal defects to restore the nasal lining while the paramedian forehead flap is used for external cover due to its superior color and texture match to the native nose.

The radial forearm flap can also be harvested as an osteocutaneous flap incorporating a portion of the distal radius. Perfusion of the osseous component requires preservation of osseous perforators that either arise directly from the radial artery or pass through the flexor pollicis longus muscle to supply the periosteum of the bone. To minimize the potential risk of an iatrogenic radial fracture, the bony component should not exceed 50% of the diameter of the radius, and, therefore the bony defect to be reconstructed should be small.[2] Although some authors have reported using the radial bone to harbor osseointegrated implants for maxillary and mandibular reconstruction, we feel that the bone stock provided is usually inadequate for this purpose. For these reasons, the indications for the radial forearm osteocutaneous free flap are very few in our practice, primarily for non-weight-bearing regions of the craniofacial skeleton to give the soft tissue shape and definition.

When a sensate flap is desirable, such as for tongue reconstruction, the radial forearm flap can be harvested with the lateral antebrachial cutaneous nerve. A subsequent epineural neurorrhaphy can then be performed with a recipient nerve to innervate the radial forearm flap thereby providing a sensate reconstruction.

## Anatomy

The arterial supply of the radial forearm flap arises from perforators from the radial artery, which is a terminal branch of the brachial artery along with the ulnar artery. The venous drainage of the flap is predominantly the associated venae comitantes; the cephalic vein can be used as an alternate venous outflow for the flap. We prefer to use the venae comitantes as long as their caliber is satisfactory for the microvascular anastomosis.[3,4] Typically, a vein that is at least 2 mm large is sufficient to allow adequate venous drainage of the flap. The venae comitantes usually converge with the cephalic vein near the antecubital fossa as the profundus cubitalis, which has a generous diameter sufficient for the microvascular anastomosis.[4,5]

The radial vessels lie between the pronator teres and brachioradialis muscles in the proximal third of the forearm. As the pedicle proceeds distally toward the wrist, it comes to lie between the muscle bellies of the brachioradialis and flexor carpi radialis muscles (**Fig. 20.1**). Distally, the radial vessels are very superficial, and the radial artery can easily be palpated as it lies in the lateral intermuscular septum between the fascia of the brachioradialis muscle laterally and the flexor carpi radialis tendon medially.

The lateral antebrachial cutaneous nerve is a branch of the musculocutaneous branch of the brachial plexus that provides sensation to the lateral volar aspect of the forearm. It divides into a volar and a dorsal branch, and the volar branch is included with the skin paddle to create a sensate flap. The nerve travels superficially just medial to the cephalic vein and ends in the thenar area, where it communicates with the radial sensory nerves. While the radial sensory nerves can be preserved, the lateral antebrachial cutaneous nerve is sacrificed during flap elevation.

The radial blood supply can reliably perfuse almost the whole circumference of the forearm except for a posterior strip of the ulnar border. Lengthwise, the flap may extend from the wrist crease to the elbow crease. In most circumstances, the flap is limited to the distal half or third of the forearm, where the skin is thinnest and the perforators are most numerous. As the radial vessels penetrate deep to the muscle bellies more proximally, the cutaneous perforators arising from the radial artery require tedious intramuscular dissection. We prefer to design the flap so that it stops well short of the wrist crease distally and the donor site does not interfere with wrist movement or wristwatch and jewelry wearing. We also try to center the flap eccentrically over the radial artery such that its boundaries are confined to the volar forearm, to better hide the donor-site scar and avoid skin grafting over the radial sensory nerves. Also, by keeping the flap on the volar surface of the distal forearm, the cephalic vein can be preserved for intravenous (IV) access (or use as a vein graft).

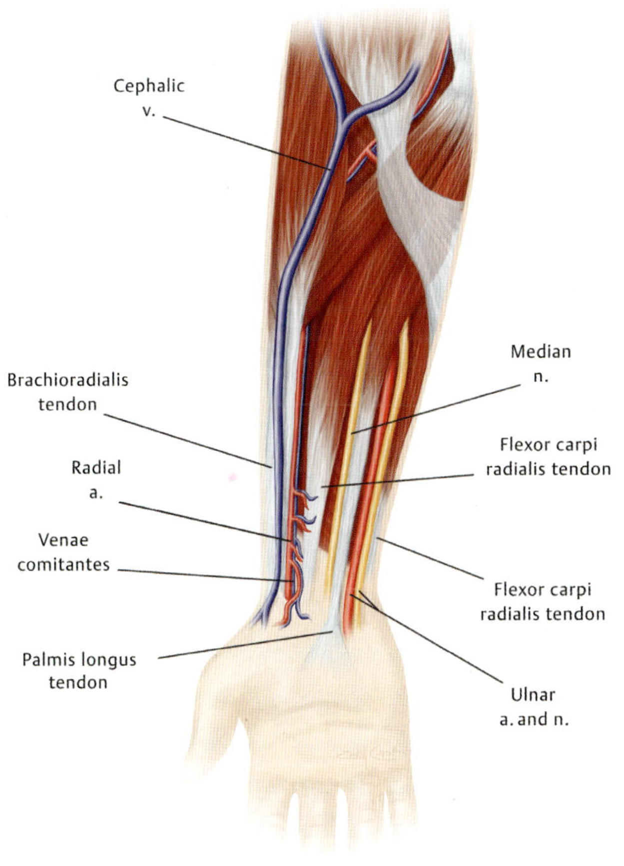


**Fig. 20.1** Anatomy of the radial forearm fasciocutaneous and osteocutaneous free flaps.

## Preoperative Considerations

Harvesting a radial forearm flap requires sacrifice of one of the terminal branches of the brachial artery that provides perfusion to the forearm and hand, namely the radial artery. While its sensitivity and specificity are a subject of debate, an Allen test should be performed to document adequate perfusion through an intact palmar arch prior to flap harvest, in order to maintain the vascular supply to the hand. The patient's handedness should also be documented, and ideally the flap should be harvested from the patient's nondominant arm to maximize the patient's function while the donor site heals. Additionally, communication with the nursing staff, phlebotomy team, and anesthesiologists is critical to avoid IVs, arterial lines, and blood draws in the donor arm to minimize trauma to the pedicle vessels. If the patient has sustained prior injury to the extremity or has already had a flap harvested from the nondominant arm, then the dominant arm may be utilized. If vascular perfusion through either the radial or ulnar artery is in question, then an angiogram may be warranted.

## Patient Positioning and Skin Markings

The patient is placed in the supine position, and typically a hand table or two arm boards positioned side by side are placed to allow the donor arm to be abducted for flap dissection. The entire upper extremity should be prepped from the fingers to the shoulder circumferentially to allow for a sterile tourniquet to be applied. Alternatively, the flap can also be elevated without a tourniquet based on surgeon preference.

Often, a template of the defect is helpful that can be transferred to the forearm. As mentioned, we prefer to keep the boundaries of the flap on the volar surface of the forearm, even if it means positioning the radial artery blood supply eccentrically on the flap, and to avoid the wrist crease **(Fig. 20.2)**. The path of the radial vessels can be marked based on palpation of the pulse distally while the artery is superficial, but as it penetrates deep to the muscle more proximally in the forearm, the pulse is more difficult to appreciate. Doppler ultrasound can be used in this circumstance, or the brachial pulse can be palpated in the antecubital fossa. A line connecting the brachial pulse to the proximal extent of the radial pulse is a close approximation of the trajectory of the vessels. This will also enable an estimate of the pedicle length, allowing the surgeon to design a more distally located flap or to plan for vein grafts if necessary.

## Operative Technique

We find that a tourniquet is helpful during elevation of a radial forearm flap. An Esmarch to exsanguinate the extremity is not necessary and, in fact, can make small perforators more difficult to visualize. Instead, elevating the arm for a brief period prior to inflation of the tourniquet is adequate. Most of the dissection can be performed sharply under loupe magnification, paying careful attention to ligate or cauterize small vessels with bipolar cautery.

The distal border of the flap is incised first **(Fig. 20.3)**. Small subcutaneous veins will be encountered and they should be ligated. The radial artery and venae comitantes should be exposed. If the venae comitantes are at least 1 mm distally, we assume that they will be of satisfactory caliber proximally for reliable microvascular anastomosis. If not, we redesign our flap to include the cephalic vein as the primary outflow by shifting incisions more laterally. At this point, the radial artery and venae comitantes are ligated and divided. The remaining skin incisions are made around the entire skin paddle of the flap.

We prefer a suprafascial harvest for the radial forearm flap, to minimize donor-site morbidity by improving graft take and minimizing tendon exposure, while not decreasing flap reliability in any way.[6,7] Dissection is carried down to the fascia overlying the flexors and is continued in a suprafascial plane up to and including the flexor carpi radialis tendon on the medial (ulnar) side and the brachioradialis tendon on the lateral (radial) side **(Fig. 20.4)**.

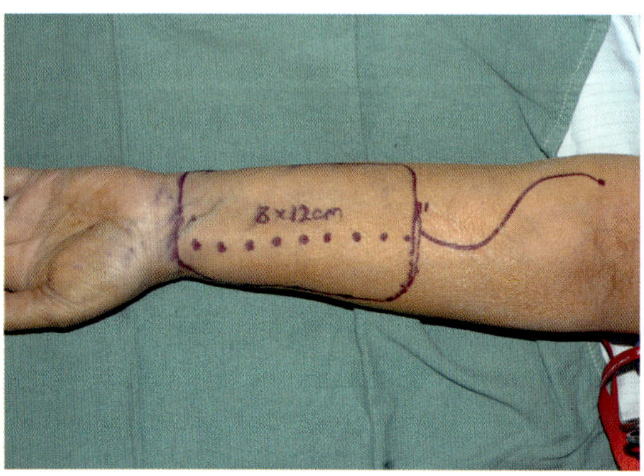


**Fig. 20.2** Skin marking for a radial forearm free flap. A "lazy S" incision was chosen for the dissection of the pedicle to prevent postoperative scar contracture.

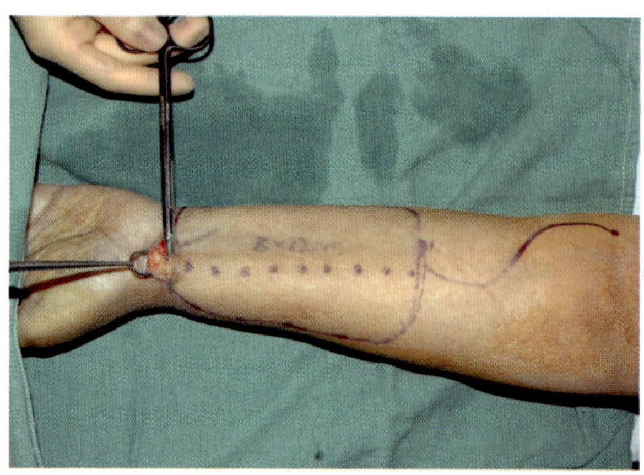

**Fig. 20.3** The distal pedicle is explored first. The radial artery and venae comitantes are ligated and divided. If the venae comitantes are less than 1 mm in diameter, the surgeon may wish to explore the proximal pedicle to ensure that the proximal veins are of reasonable caliber for microvascular anastomosis or to redesign the skin paddle to include the cephalic vein.

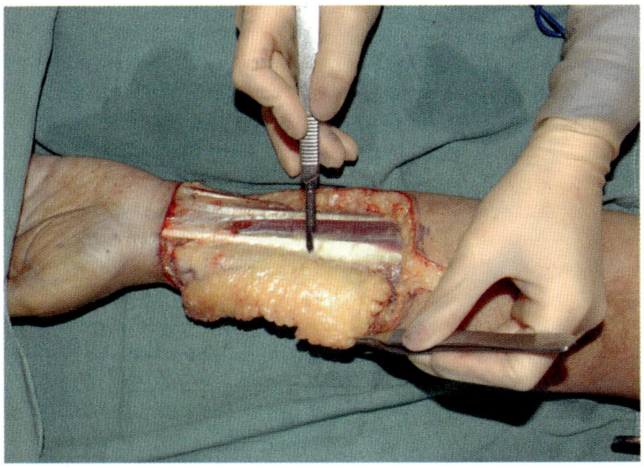

**Fig. 20.4** The skin paddle is elevated in the suprafascial plane from the medial and lateral borders. At the lateral border of the flexor carpi radialis tendon and the medial border of the brachioradialis tendon, the fascia is incised sharply and the plane deepened to include the vascular pedicle and its small perforators that nourish the skin paddle.

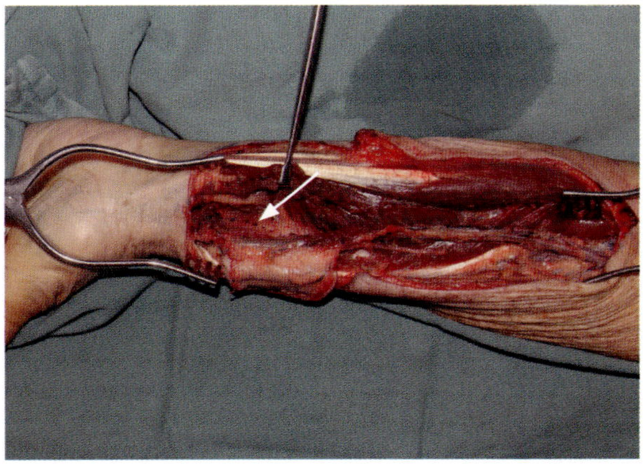

**Fig. 20.5** In the osteocutaneous free flap variant, a partial-thickness keel-shaped wedge of radial bone (outlined in blue with a marker and indicated by the *arrow*) is harvested with the flap, taking care to maintain the periosteal connection to the radial blood vessels.

Care should be taken to preserve the fascia overlying the muscles and the peritenon enveloping the tendons. Further, careful attention should be paid to preserving the sensory branches of the radial nerve while dissecting the radial side of the flap. These nerves usually emerge through the brachioradialis tendon, in contrast to the lateral antebrachial cutaneous nerve, which must be divided distally.

The fascia is incised on the medial border of the brachioradialis and the lateral border of the flexor carpi radialis, and dissection proceeds in a subfascial plane to incorporate the radial vessels and their cutaneous perforators with the flap. At this time, the radial artery and venae comitantes are dissected free from between the brachioradialis and flexor carpi radialis tendons, taking care to carefully ligate and divide all side branches going to the surrounding muscles and radial bone. The dissection proceeds from a distal to proximal direction until the entire flap is elevated.

If an osteocutaneous flap is planned, perforators arising from the radial artery traveling within a fascial septum to the underlying radius are preserved, along with a cuff of the flexor pollicis longus muscle to maximize the periosteal perfusion to the bone. Available bone extends from the insertion of the pronator teres to the distal styloid, where there is no muscle attachment on the radial border. No more than 10 cm of bone length, encompassing no more than 50% of the thickness of the radius, should be harvested, to minimize the risk of a postoperative fracture. Osteotomies are made with powered saws. The bone is harvested by making "boat-shaped" osteotomies, rather than by making osteotomies at right angles to the bone, to avoid overcutting and weakening the remaining radius **(Fig. 20.5)**. Some surgeons advocate prophylactic titanium plate reinforcement of the radius to minimize donor-site fractures following osteocutaneous free flap harvest, but we have not performed this routinely.

A curvilinear "lazy-S" incision is made in the volar forearm along the anticipated trajectory of the radial vessels and dissection proceeds to the flexor muscles. The muscle bellies of the brachioradialis and flexor carpi radialis are separated to gain access to the radial vessels **(Fig. 20.6)**. During this proximal dissection the lateral antebrachial cutaneous nerve should be dissected free of the subcutaneous soft tissues if an innervated flap is needed. Otherwise, the nerve is divided. The radial vessels are then dissected as proximally as necessary to maximize pedicle length and caliber. The maximal length of the artery is dictated by the branching of the brachial artery to the radial and ulnar arteries. However, the veins can be dissected more proximally to the profundus cubitalis vein, where the two venae comitantes converge into a single vein.

The tourniquet is then released to assess for perfusion and viability of the flap. Additionally, the surgeon should also examine the entire hand to confirm the hand is well perfused, with normal capillary refill. Should there be any concern about devascularization of the hand, reconstruction of the radial artery is indicated with a reversed vein graft.

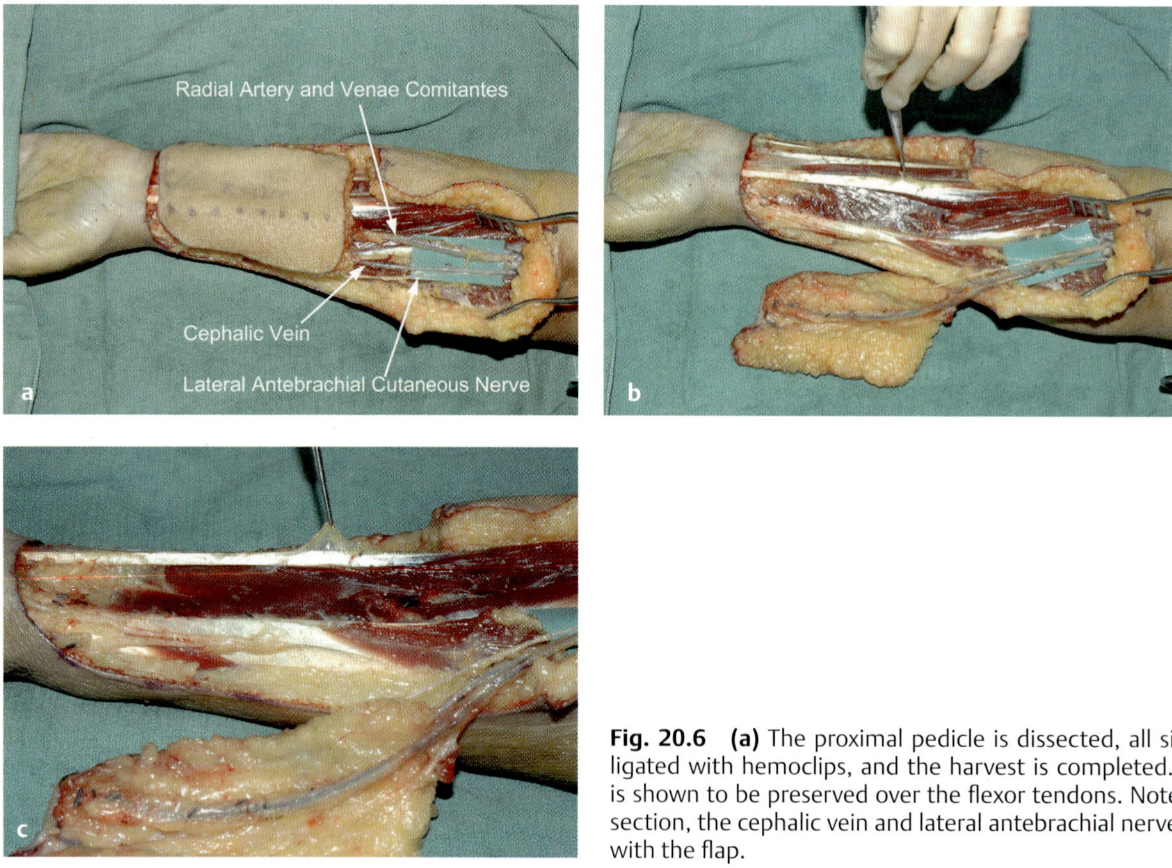


**Fig. 20.6** **(a)** The proximal pedicle is dissected, all side branches are ligated with hemoclips, and the harvest is completed. **(b,c)** The fascia is shown to be preserved over the flexor tendons. Note that in this dissection, the cephalic vein and lateral antebrachial nerve were harvested with the flap.

## Donor-Site Care

Harvesting a radial forearm flap results in an open wound in the volar forearm, with exposure of muscle bellies, tendons, and, in some cases, the radial sensory nerves. The proximal forearm incision used for dissection of the main pedicle is closed primarily in layers over a small drain. The distal flap donor site can then be purse-stringed to reduce the size of the donor site and, consequently, the skin graft needed to resurface the donor site. A thick split-thickness (>0.012 inch) skin graft or a full-thickness skin graft is applied and secured with absorbable suture, then dressed with a bolster of the surgeon's choosing for 5 to 7 days (**Fig. 20.7**). During this time, a volar forearm splint is applied with the fingers free to the metacarpalphalangeal joints and the wrist in gentle extension. Once the dressing is removed, the patient may begin mobilization and range-of-motion exercises. The skin graft is dressed with petroleum gauze, an absorbent pad, and a light compression wrap. Dressings are changed daily until the graft is healed, typically 7 more days. After that point, the patient may stop all dressings except for over-the-counter moisturizers with no other restrictions (**Fig. 20.8**).

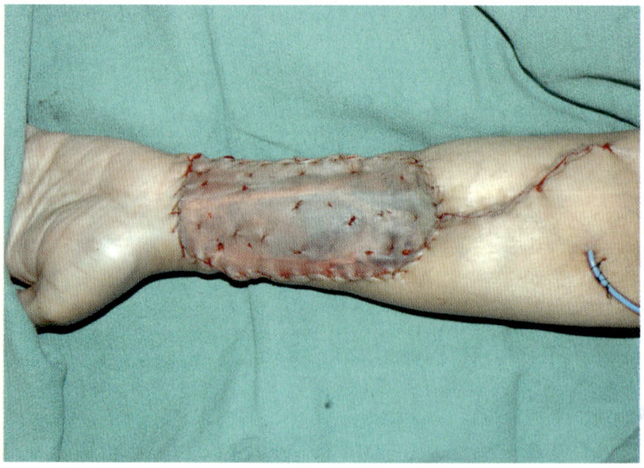

**Fig. 20.7** Either a full-thickness skin graft or a thick (> 0.012 inch) split-thickness skin graft is used to reconstruct the donor site. A 10-French closed suction drain is used to drain the deep portions of the wound.

Small areas of nonhealing graft are not uncommon. In our experience, almost all of these wounds heal spontaneously without long-term sequelae, such as tendon adhesions. If there is delayed healing of the graft, typically, local wound care with antibiotic ointment and daily petroleum-impregnated gauze is adequate until the would heals secondarily.

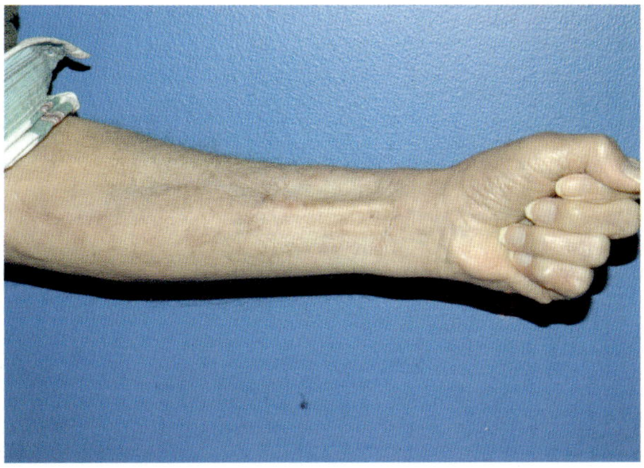

**Fig. 20.8** Postoperative appearance of the suprafascial radial forearm fasciocutaneous free flap donor site following reconstruction with a thick split-thickness skin graft.

## Case Example 1

A 45-year-old male presented with a left buccal mucosa squamous cell carcinoma. Following a wide local excision and neck dissection, a radial forearm fasciocutaneous free flap was used for reconstruction. The radial forearm fasciocutaneous free flap was selected over a skin graft to avoid graft contracture, which could result in trismus. A suprafascial harvest was employed **(Fig. 20.9)**. The radial artery and venae comitantes in the pedicle to the flap were dissected proximally to their origin to maximize vessel diameter, facilitating microvascular anastomosis. However, because of this, the pedicle was very long, and careful attention had to be paid to avoid any kinking or twisting that could

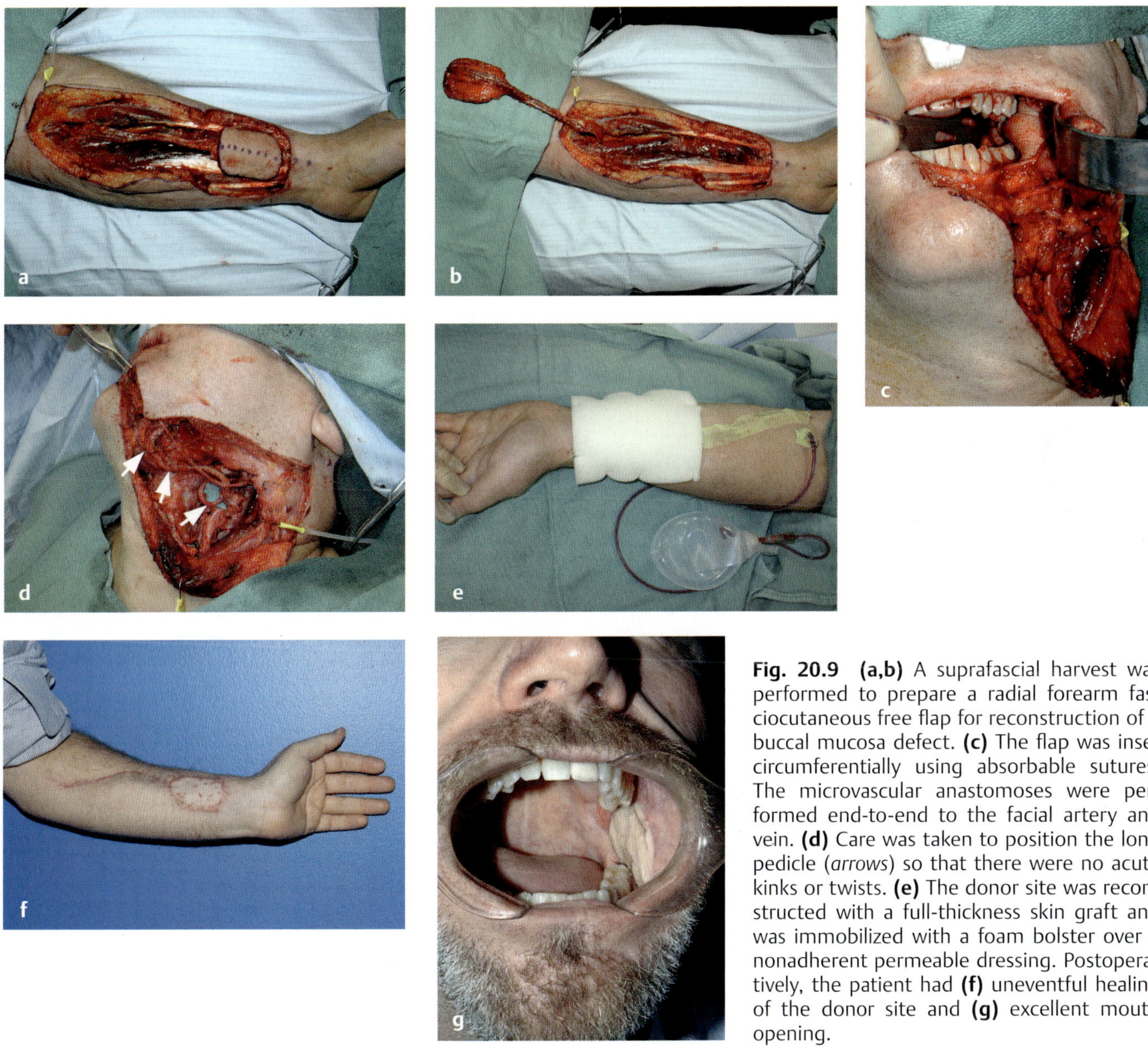

**Fig. 20.9** **(a,b)** A suprafascial harvest was performed to prepare a radial forearm fasciocutaneous free flap for reconstruction of a buccal mucosa defect. **(c)** The flap was inset circumferentially using absorbable sutures. The microvascular anastomoses were performed end-to-end to the facial artery and vein. **(d)** Care was taken to position the long pedicle (*arrows*) so that there were no acute kinks or twists. **(e)** The donor site was reconstructed with a full-thickness skin graft and was immobilized with a foam bolster over a nonadherent permeable dressing. Postoperatively, the patient had **(f)** uneventful healing of the donor site and **(g)** excellent mouth opening.

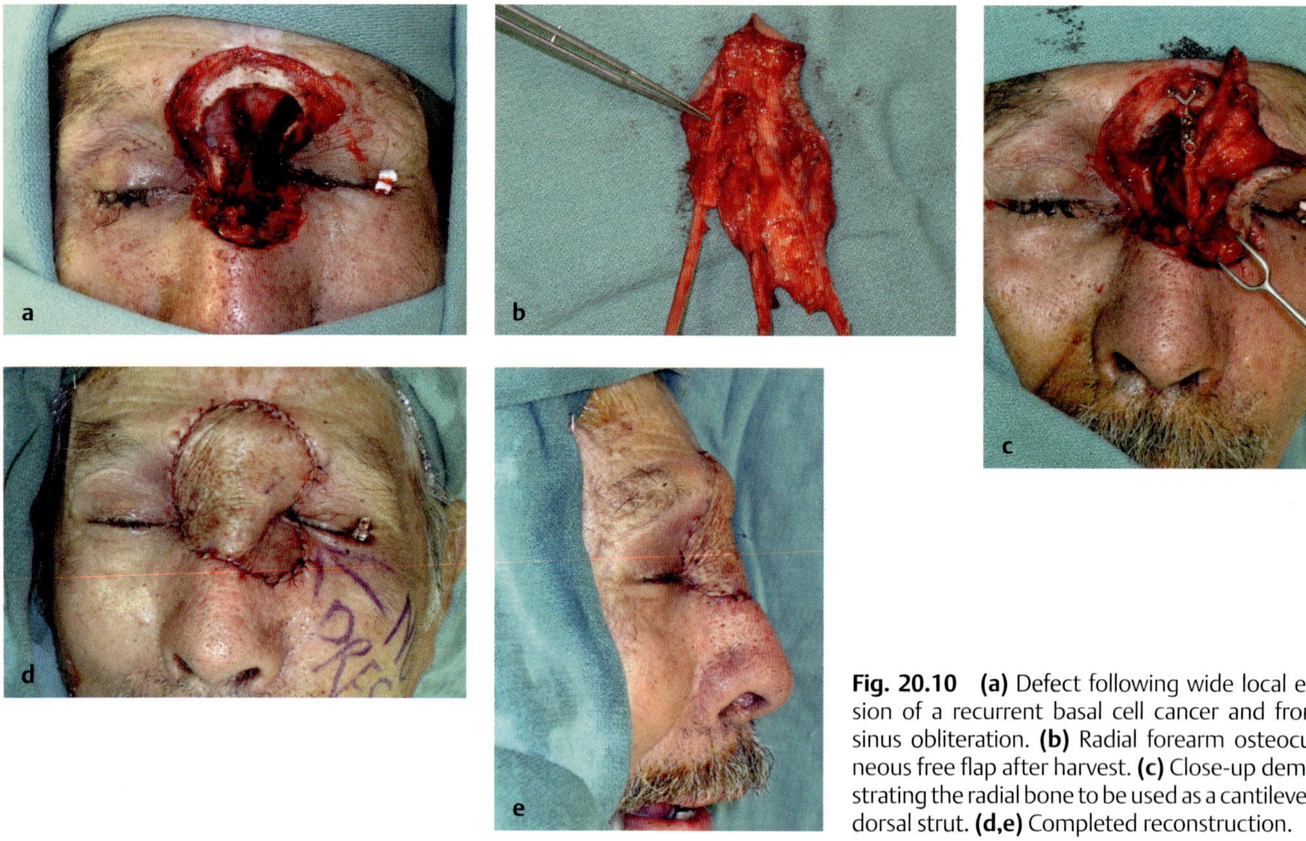

**Fig. 20.10** **(a)** Defect following wide local excision of a recurrent basal cell cancer and frontal sinus obliteration. **(b)** Radial forearm osteocutaneous free flap after harvest. **(c)** Close-up demonstrating the radial bone to be used as a cantilevered dorsal strut. **(d,e)** Completed reconstruction.

lead to thrombosis and flap loss. A lip-splitting incision was used for the resection, but such resections are also often performed without division of the lip, which improves postoperative cosmesis. The donor site was closed with a full-thickness skin graft and bolstered for 5 days postoperatively with a foam bolster over a nonadherent permeable dressing. Postoperatively, the patient did well and had excellent mouth opening.

## Case Example 2

A 79-year-old man presented with a recurrent fungating basal cell carcinoma of the glabella. Imaging demonstrated invasion of the underlying nasal bone cortex, with erosion into the frontal sinus. The patient underwent wide local excision and obliteration of the frontal sinus and reconstruction with a radial forearm osteocutaneous free flap harvested from the nondominant upper extremity **(Fig. 20.10)**. The radius was utilized as a dorsal strut and the cutaneous component was used for soft tissue resurfacing.

## Pearls and Pitfalls

- The radial forearm fasciocutaneous free flap is usually the flap of choice when a thin, pliable flap with a long pedicle is indicated.
- The flap can be made sensate by connecting the lateral antebrachial cutaneous nerve to a recipient-site nerve stump, most commonly the lingual nerve, when performing tongue reconstruction.
- We incise the distal border of the flap first to explore the radial artery and its venae comitantes. If the venae comitantes are at least 1 mm in diameter, we assume that they will be sufficient to serve as the sole venous drainage of the flap proximally.
- While nearly the entire forearm can be harvested as a skin paddle based on the radial artery blood supply, we try to design flaps that are well away from the wrist crease and are confined to the volar surface of the forearm, leaving the radial sensory nerves as well as the cephalic vein undisturbed, to minimize donor-site morbidity.
- Performing a suprafascial harvest minimizes donor-site morbidity by improving skin graft take and minimizing tendon exposure and desiccation, even if the skin graft take is incomplete.
- An osteocutaneous free flap can be harvested by preserving the osseous branches of the radial artery in the region between the pronator teres and the radial styloid, including a cuff of flexor pollicis longus muscle.
- A thick split-thickness skin graft or a full-thickness skin graft helps to improve the cosmetic appearance of the donor site postoperatively.

## References


1. Yang GF, Chen PJ, Gao YZ, et al. Forearm free skin flap transplantation: a report of 56 cases. 1981. Br J Plast Surg 1997;50(3):162–165
2. Cormack GC, Duncan MJ, Lamberty BG. The blood supply of the bone component of the compound osteocutaneous radial artery forearm flap—an anatomical study. Br J Plast Surg 1986;39(2):173–175
3. Demirkan F, Wei FC, Lutz BS, Cher TS, Chen IH. Reliability of the venae comitantes in venous drainage of the free radial forearm flaps. Plast Reconstr Surg 1998;102(5):1544–1548
4. Selber JC, Sanders E, Lin H, Yu P. Venous drainage of the radial forearm flap: comparison of the deep and superficial systems. Ann Plast Surg 2011;66(4):347–350
5. Gottlieb LJ, Tachmes L, Pielet RW. Improved venous drainage of the radial artery forearm free flap: use of the profundus cubitalis vein. J Reconstr Microsurg 1993;9(4):281–284, discussion 284–285
6. Chang SC, Miller G, Halbert CF, Yang KH, Chao WC, Wei FC. Limiting donor site morbidity by suprafascial dissection of the radial forearm flap. Microsurgery 1996;17(3):136–140
7. Lutz BS, Wei FC, Chang SC, Yang KH, Chen IH. Donor site morbidity after suprafascial elevation of the radial forearm flap: a prospective study in 95 consecutive cases. Plast Reconstr Surg 1999;103(1):132–137

# 21 Ulnar Artery Perforator Flap

*Peirong Yu*

## Introduction

The radial forearm flap is a time-honored flap with many advantages, including robust blood supply, ease of dissection, thin and pliable skin, long vascular pedicle, and potential for sensory reinnervation. It has some disadvantages, however, including sacrifice of a major artery supplying the hand, the need for skin grafting to the forearm donor site, frequent partial loss of skin grafts and tendon exposure, tendon adhesion and stiffness, sensory loss in the thenar eminence, possible injury to the radial sensory nerve, hairiness in some patients, and conspicuous scar on the forearm. An alternative flap in the forearm is the ulnar artery (or ulnar forearm) flap. The ulnar artery flap never gained popularity because of the traditional belief that hand perfusion is ulnar artery dominant.

The ulnar artery flap was first described by Lovie et al in 1984.[1] The second report was published by Koshima in 1987.[2] Since then, there have been few reports in the English literature of the use of the ulnar artery flap. Previous reports have described the flap elevation as essentially a forearm flap similar to the radial forearm flap, not a true perforator flap, in that the distal margin of the flap is designed near the wrist crease. Many of the problems associated with the radial forearm flap, such as skin graft loss, tendon exposure, and tendon adhesions, are the result of harvesting the flap in the distal forearm down to the wrist crease. In the more proximal forearm, especially on the ulnar side, harvesting the skin flap will result in no, or minimal, tendon exposure. This flap design and the perforator anatomy of a true ulnar artery perforator (UAP) flap were reported by the author in 2012.[3]

Compared with the radial forearm flap, the advantages of the ulnar artery flap include: (1) inconspicuous scar in the forearm, (2) usually no sensory deficit distal to the flap, (3) less hair on the skin, (4) the possibility of closing some donor sites primarily, (5) less or no tendon exposure, and (6) generally better donor-site skin graft take than the radial forearm donor site. Some disadvantages of the ulnar artery flap include: (1) flap elevation is more difficult because it is a true perforator flap; (2) the ulnar nerve travels closely with the vascular pedicle, and is thus at risk for injury; and (3) there is a shorter vascular pedicle, which may not be a disadvantage in most head and neck reconstruction since the recipient vessels are usually close by. In fact, the radial forearm flap vascular pedicle often needs to be looped around due to its length. Obviously, the UAP flap is not a good option when a long pedicle is needed.

## Anatomy

The blood supply of the ulnar artery flap is the ulnar artery distal to the take-off of the common interosseous artery. At the elbow level, the brachial artery divides into the radial and ulnar arteries. The ulnar artery at this level is significantly larger than the radial artery (4.3 mm versus 3.5 mm).[4] The ulnar artery then gives rise to the common interosseous artery, which further divides into the anterior and posterior interosseous arteries, which supply the muscles and bones in the forearm **(Fig. 21.1)**. The main ulnar artery continues to travel in the ulnar aspect of the forearm to the hand, with few collateral branches. After giving off the common interosseous artery, the ulnar artery is smaller than the radial artery at this level (3.0 mm versus 3.5 mm). At the wrist level, the ulnar artery measures 2.6 mm, whereas the radial artery measures 3.3 mm. In the proximal forearm, the ulnar artery travels between the flexor digitorum superficialis (FDS) and flexor digitorum profundus (FDP) muscles **(Fig. 21.2)** and consistently gives off a branch to supply the flexor carpi ulnaris (FCU) muscle at 3 to 4 cm distal to the common interosseous artery take-off. The ulnar artery then travels more medially between the tendons of the FDP and the FCU in the distal half of the forearm and is closely associated with the ulnar nerve **(Fig. 21.3)**.

Based on perforator mapping from 20 clinical patients,[3] 60% of the patients had three perforators in

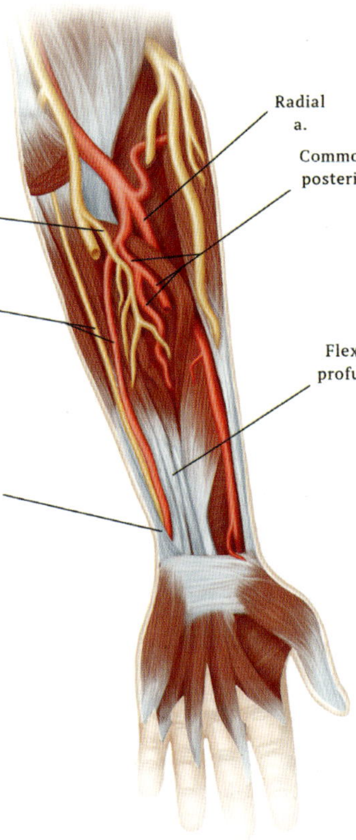


**Fig. 21.1** Anatomy of the ulnar artery. The ulnar artery perforator flap is based on the ulnar artery distal to the origin of the common interosseous artery.

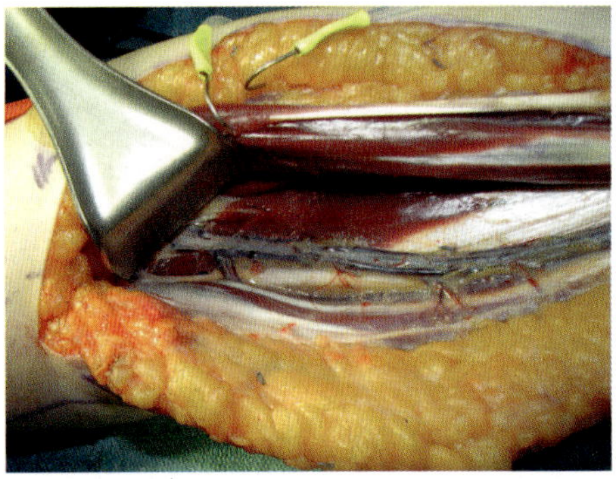

**Fig. 21.2** In the proximal forearm, the ulnar artery travels between the flexor digitorum superficialis (FDS) and flexor digitorum profundus (FDP) muscles. It gives off a branch to supply the flexor carpi ulnaris (FCU).

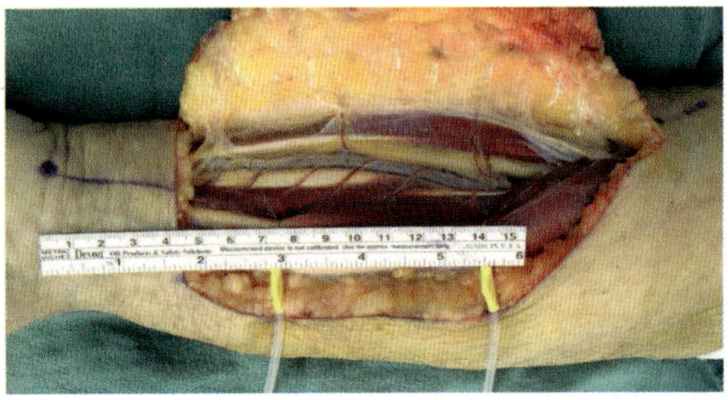

**Fig. 21.3** In the distal forearm, the ulnar artery travels between the tendons of the flexor digitorum profundus (FDP) and flexor carpi ulnaris (FCU) and is closely associated with the ulnar nerve.

the UAP flap territory, named A, B, and C from distal to proximal. The main landmarks are the pisiform and the medial epicondyle of the humerus. The average distance between these two landmarks, i.e., the wrist-elbow (WE) line, is 25.8 ± 2.1 cm. The average distance of perforators A, B, and C from the pisiform is 7.4 ± 1.0 cm, 11.8 ± 1.0 cm, and 16. 3 ± 1.6 cm, respectively (**Fig. 21.3**), or at points 0.29, 0.46, and 0.64 of the WE line, respectively, when the pisiform is defined as point 0 and the medial epicondyle is defined as point 1.0. These perforators are 6 mm, 9.7 mm, and 11 mm medial (ulnar) to the WE line. The average distances between perforators A and B and perforators B and C are 4.5 ± 0.9 cm and 4.5 ± 1.6 cm, respectively. All perforators are septocutaneous perforators. The sizes of the perforators are defined as small (< 0.5 mm), medium (0.5–1.0 mm), and large (> 1 mm). Most perforators are either small (51%) or medium (41%). Only 7% of perforators are large. The diameter of the ulnar artery immediately below the origin of the common interosseous artery is between 2.0 and 2.5 mm. In half of the cases, the two similarly sized venae comitantes do not join to form a common trunk, but there are numerous "H-shaped" connections between them (**Fig. 21.2**). Therefore, using either one of the veins will provide adequate drainage. In some cases, one venae comitantes is significantly smaller than the other. The average distance of the common interosseous artery origin, below which the ulnar artery is divided, from the antebrachial crease is 5.3 ± 1.0 cm, and the average pedicle length is 5 cm (**Fig. 21.4**).

The nerve supply to the skin of the ulnar forearm is the medial antebrachial cutaneous nerve, which can be included for sensory reinnervation.

## Surgical Technique

A straight line is drawn on the skin between the easily palpated pisiform at the wrist and the medial epicondyle of the humerus (the WE line). The locations of the three cutaneous perforators A, B, and C are marked on the skin slightly medial to the WE line at 7 cm, 12 cm, and 16 (or 17) cm from the pisiform, respectively (**Fig. 21.5**). The perforator locations are adjusted according to the length of the arm. The distal end of the flap is usually 5 cm above the wrist crease and the width of the flap is centered on the WE line.

Flap dissection is performed under tourniquet control. Only the lateral (radial) and half of the distal incisions of the flap are made first. Suprafascial dissection

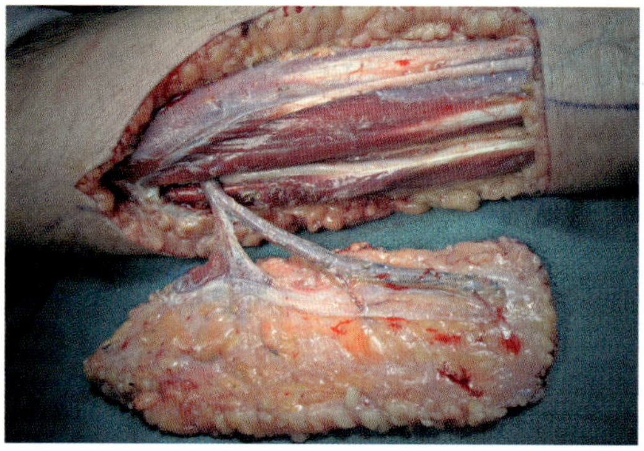

**Fig. 21.4** The average distance of the common interosseous artery origin from the antebrachial crease is 5.3 ± 1.0 cm, and the average pedicle length is 5 cm.

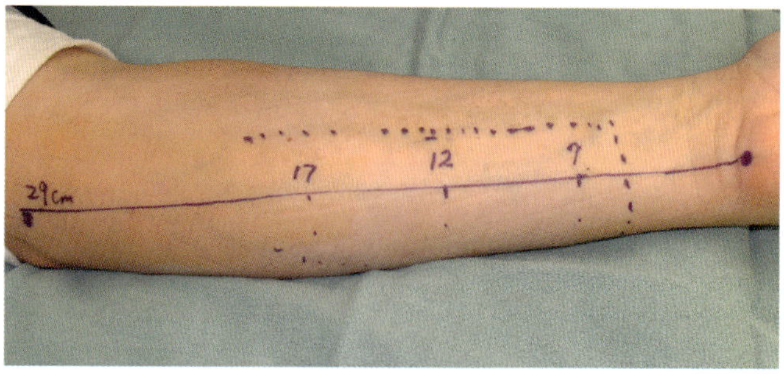


**Fig. 21.5** A straight line is drawn between the pisiform and the medial epicondyle of the humerus (the WE line). The locations of the three cutaneous perforators A, B, and C are marked on the skin slightly medial to the WE line at 7 cm, 12 cm, and 16–17 cm from the pisiform, respectively.

proceeds ulnarly until perforators are seen between the FDS and FCU (**Fig. 21.6**). The fascia radial to the perforators is then incised and the FDS muscle and tendon are retracted radially, revealing the ulnar neurovascular bundle (**Fig. 21.7**). At the distal end of the flap, the ulnar artery and veins are dissected out, ligated, and divided. The vascular pedicle is then carefully separated from the ulnar nerve and small vascular branches to the neighboring muscles are divided. Proximally, the vascular pedicle turns radially away from the ulnar nerve and travels between the FDS and FDP muscles (**Fig. 21.3**). After retraction of the FDS muscle, the vascular pedicle is traced toward the bifurcation with the common interosseous artery, where the anterior interosseous nerve overlying the FDP and the median nerve should be protected (**Fig. 21.8**).

Once the vascular pedicle is dissected out, the posterior incision is made and subfascial dissection is performed toward the septum between the FCU and FDP. Great care should be taken to protect the perforators during the posterior dissection. The perforators are carefully dissected off the FCU muscle (**Fig. 21.9**). The flap is then completely islanded on the vascular pedicle. The basilic vein is usually located on the posterior edge of the flap or outside the flap and thus is not included. However, it can be used as the draining vein if the flap is more posteriorly positioned. A segment of the FCU muscle can be included in the flap if indicated (**Fig. 21.10**). The flap can also be divided into two skin islands based on separate perforators (**Fig. 21.11**).

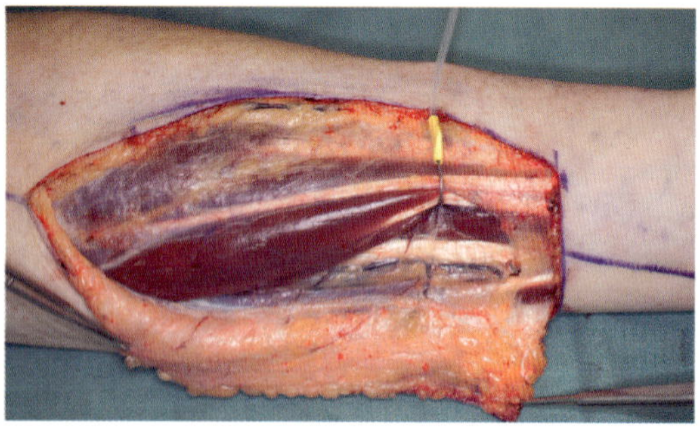

**Fig. 21.6** Suprafascial dissection proceeds ulnarly until perforators are seen between the flexor digitorum superficialis (FDS) and flexor carpi ulnaris (FCU).

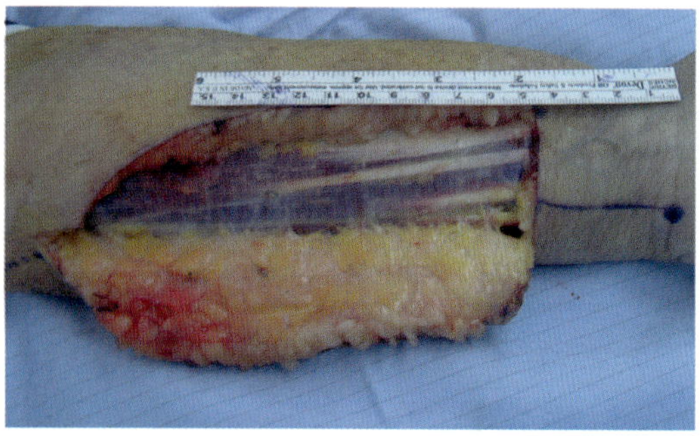

**Fig. 21.7** The fascia radial to the perforators is incised and the FDS muscle and tendon are retracted radially, revealing the ulnar neurovascular bundle.

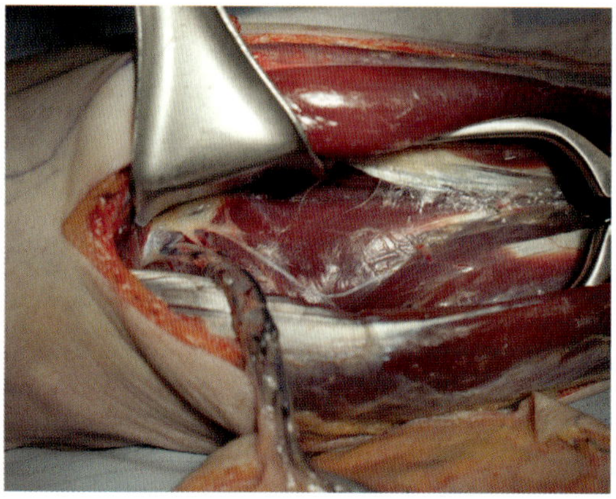

**Fig. 21.8** By retracting the FDS muscle, the vascular pedicle is traced toward the bifurcation with the common interosseous artery, where the anterior interosseous nerve overlying the FDP and the median nerve can be seen.

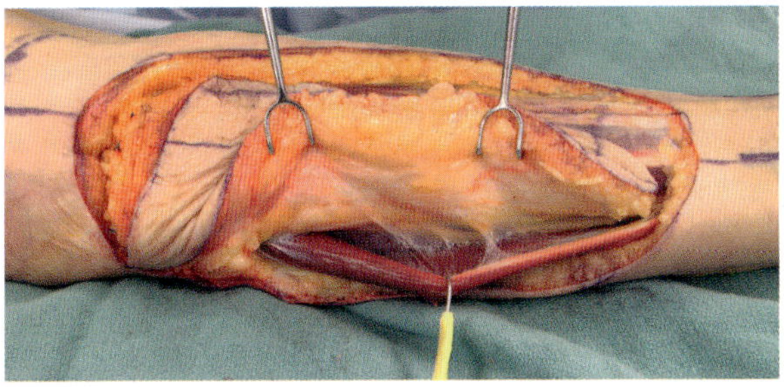

**Fig. 21.9** The posterior incision is made last and subfascial dissection is performed toward the septum between the flexor digitorum profundus (FDP) and flexor carpi ulnaris (FCU). The perforators are carefully dissected off the FCU.

## Donor-Site Care and Morbidity

Either a full-thickness or a split-thickness skin graft is used to cover the forearm donor site. The wrist is immobilized with a short volar forearm splint. The splint and skin graft dressing are taken down on postoperative day 6 when range of motion therapy is started. Small donor-site defects may be closed primarily, particularly in older patients with substantial skin laxity (**Fig. 21.12**).

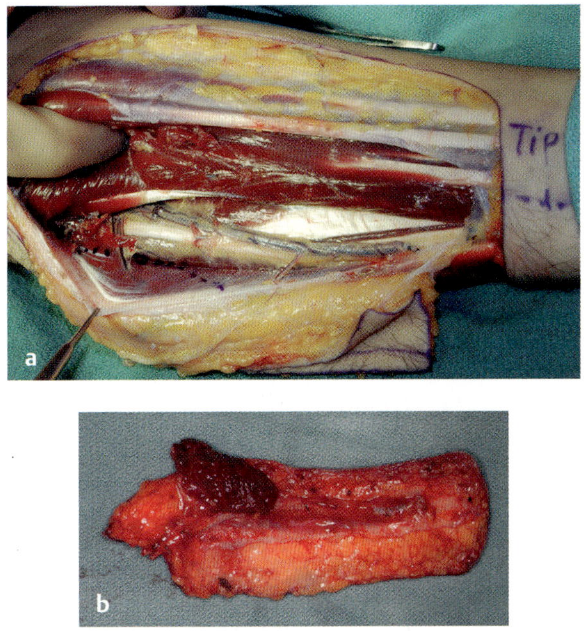


**Fig. 21.10** A segment of the flexor carpi ulnaris (FCU) muscle can be included in the ulnar artery perforator (UAP) flap based on a muscular branch. **(a)** A muscle branch from the ulnar artery can be seen entering the FCU muscle. The amount of muscle to be included in the flap was outlined. **(b)** A small amount of the FCU muscle was harvested along with the UAP flap.

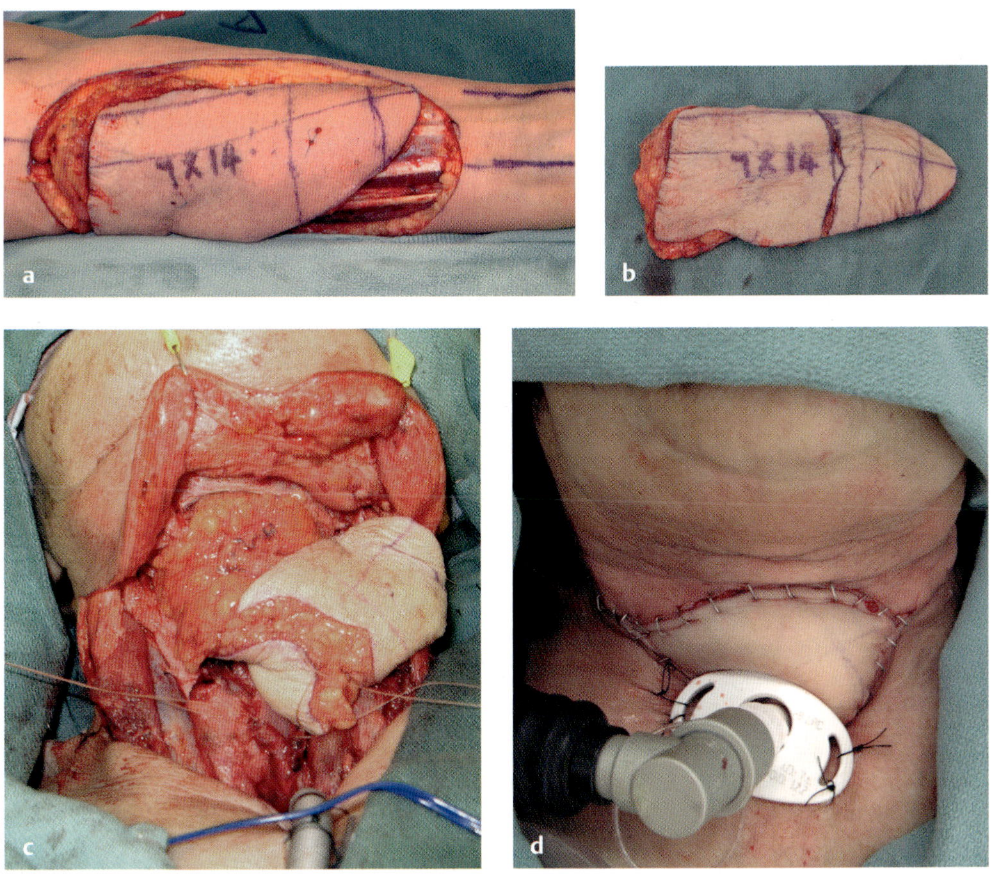


**Fig. 21.11** **(a,b)** The flap can be divided into two skin islands based on separate perforators. **(c,d)** For example, the second skin paddle can be used for neck resurfacing, while the main skin paddle is used to reconstruct the pharyngoesophageal defect.

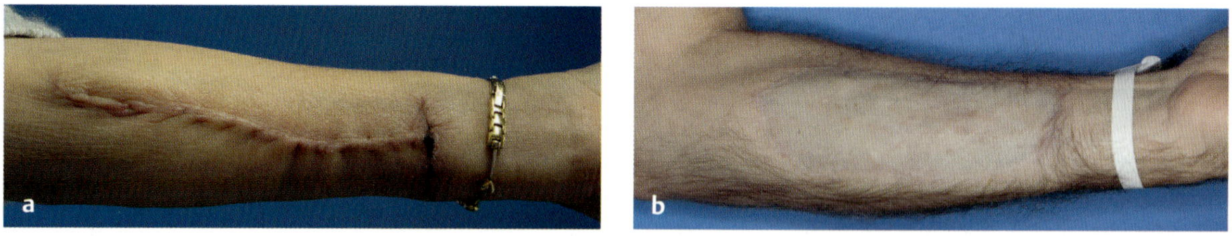


**Fig. 21.12** Postoperative photographs of the ulnar artery perforator (UAP) flap donor site. **(a)** After harvesting a small UAP flap from the proximal forearm, the donor site can be closed primarily. **(b)** Harvesting a large flap necessitates skin grafting to the forearm donor site. Because of the abundance of muscle in the ulnar side of the forearm without tendon exposure, skin grafts heal very well.

Skin graft loss and tendon exposure are rare. Mild transient weakness of the hand and forearm usually recovers within weeks.[3] Although traditionally the ulnar artery is considered the dominant blood supply to the hand, more recent studies have shown that the radial artery is equally important or even dominant in some patients.[4,5,6] The ulnar artery flap can be safely harvested without jeopardizing hand perfusion. Hand ischemia after harvesting the ulnar artery has not been reported.

## Pearls and Pitfalls

- Although traditionally the ulnar artery is considered the dominant blood supply to the hand, more recent studies have shown that the radial artery is equally important or even dominant in some patients.
- Compared with the radial forearm flap, the advantages of the UAP flap include: (1) inconspicuous scar in the forearm, (2) usually no sensory deficit distal to the flap, (3) less hair on the skin, (4) the possibility of closing some donor sites primarily, (5) less or no tendon exposure, and (6) generally better donor-site skin graft take than with the radial forearm donor site.
- Some disadvantages of the ulnar artery flap include: (1) flap elevation is more difficult, because it is a true perforator flap; (2) the ulnar nerve travels closely with the vascular pedicle and thus is at risk of injury; and (3) there is a shorter vascular pedicle.
- The UAP flap is indicated when a thin, pliable fasciocutaneous flap is needed, such as for hemiglossectomy or floor of mouth reconstruction, and a very lengthy pedicle is not required.
- In the distal forearm, the ulnar artery can be located between the tendons of the FDP and the FCU muscles, closely associated with the ulnar nerve.
- Ulnar artery perforators are usually found just medial to an imaginary line connecting the pisiform and the medial epicondyle (wrist-elbow or WE line).
- Perforators are usually found 7.4, 11.8, and 16.3 cm proximal to the pisiform along the WE line.
- The nerve supply to the skin of the ulnar forearm is the medial antebrachial cutaneous nerve, which can be included for sensory reinnervation.

## References

1. Lovie MJ, Duncan GM, Glasson DW. The ulnar artery forearm free flap. Br J Plast Surg 1984;37(4):486–492
2. Koshima I, Iino T, Fukuda H, Soeda S. The free ulnar forearm flap. Ann Plast Surg 1987;18(1):24–29
3. Yu P, Chang EI, Selber JC, Hanasono MM. Perforator patterns of the ulnar artery perforator flap. Plast Reconstr Surg 2012;129(1):213–220
4. Haerle M, Häfner HM, Dietz K, Schaller HE, Brunelli F. Vascular dominance in the forearm. Plast Reconstr Surg 2003;111(6):1891–1898
5. Tonks AM, Lawrence J, Lovie MJ. Comparison of ulnar and radial arterial blood-flow at the wrist. J Hand Surg [Br] 1995;20(2):240–242
6. Dumanian GA, Segalman K, Buehner JW, Koontz CL, Hendrickson MF, Wilgis EF. Analysis of digital pulse-volume recordings with radial and ulnar artery compression. Plast Reconstr Surg 1998;102(6):1993–1998

# 22 Rectus Abdominis Flap

*Geoffrey L. Robb*

## Introduction

Historically, head and neck reconstruction was accomplished with flaps of skin and subcutaneous tissue elevated either from a side adjacent to the wound or from a nearby site. Because the vascular supply of these random flaps was limited, the tissue was at risk of not surviving completely and, particularly in the head and neck, at risk of bacterial contamination, causing an infected wound and potentially partial or complete flap loss. Over time, particularly in surgery of the head and neck, certain vascular pedicles were identified in regional anatomical areas that were relatively superficial in the soft tissues. Because it was recognized that these flaps could be elevated and satisfactorily perfused by the vascular pedicles, reconstruction came to involve flaps with larger dimensions than were possible with random pattern designs. These so-called axial pattern flaps were identified in the chest, back, forehead, scalp, and temporal areas, among others. The axial flaps were a significant advance in terms of the ability to reconstruct head and neck defects with better reliability and larger flap size; however, their fixed arc of rotation and specific anatomical location limited their use. In the middle of the twentieth century, the realization that muscle tissue could be used as a flap revolutionized wound coverage and defect reconstruction.

Muscles are generally available in almost all anatomical areas, so as the particular vascular pedicles to the individual muscles were localized, it became possible to separate the muscle origin or insertion, or both, and move the muscle to the reconstructive site while maintaining satisfactory muscle circulation.[1] As muscle flaps were used more commonly, the ability of muscle flap circulation to carry overlying skin yielded a new reconstructive application. It became clear that muscle groups superficially provided perforating vessels to the overlying soft tissue and skin, so this allowed for the generation of composite flaps of muscle and skin.[2] The next surgical advancement of microvascular free tissue transfer, composite myocutaneous flaps, again revolutionized head and neck surgery. The operating microscope, first built by Zeiss in 1951, provided suitable magnification and lighting for microsurgical reconstruction. This allowed distant flaps, such as the rectus abdominis myocutaneous flap, to be used in remote reconstructive sites, such as the head and neck.

It became evident that the primary attribute of the composite muscle flaps used in head and neck reconstruction was the superb blood supply from readily available sites, which allowed improved perfusion to all the flap components. The arc of rotation limitation with local or regional flaps was soon displaced by the complete application of remote free tissue transfer, which included composite muscle, skin, and bone flaps, to the head and neck defects, particularly those necessarily of larger dimensions or that were three-dimensionally more difficult to repair (**Fig. 22.1**). The potential immediate use of larger flaps, such as the rectus abdominis myocutaneous free flap, allowed the resecting surgeon to be aggressive in the ablation of any head and neck tumor. Fortunately, a variety of composite flaps can be utilized in a larger design to accommodate extensive extirpative defects.[3]

## Indications, Advantages, and Disadvantages

The use of the rectus abdominis muscle as a free tissue transfer satisfies the requirements for any head and neck reconstruction that would require an immediate, versatile, reliable, and single-stage type of flap application. There are several specific advantages to the use of the rectus abdominis flap as a free tissue transfer reconstruction, particularly

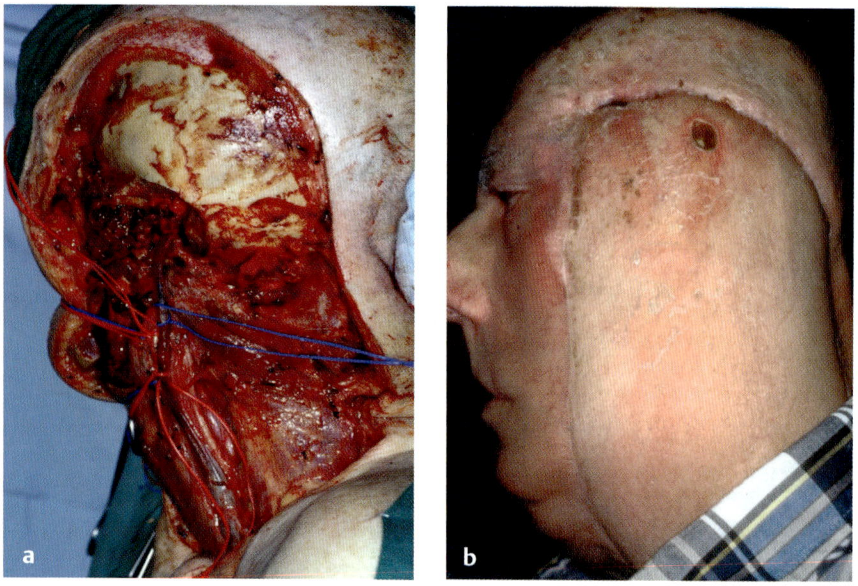

Fig. 22.1 **(a)** A lateral face and neck squamous cell carcinoma was widely excised, leaving a sizeable cutaneous defect. **(b)** A rectus abdominis myocutaneous free flap with a transversely oriented skin paddle (TRAM) was selected for reconstruction because of the wide and long skin paddle that could be harvested while still achieving primary donor-site skin closure.

considering the relatively large size of the deep inferior epigastric vessels that supply the flap. These vessels consistently are roughly 2.5 to 3.0 mm in diameter, which makes the microsurgery all the easier. In addition, the deep inferior epigastric vascular pedicle that supplies the flap can be dissected for a longer length down to the iliac vessels, or up to or within the muscle itself, which facilitates insetting the flap much further from available recipient vessels without interposition vein grafting. In addition, the presence of multiple cutaneous perforators from the rectus abdominis muscle allows for multiple skin paddles, increasing the versatility of the flap and allowing it to be used for closing complex multisurface wounds.[4] The rectus abdominis flap can provide predictable muscular bulk with or without skin coverage that is ideal for many complex internal head and neck defects, such as those of the skull base **(Fig. 22.2)**, total glossectomy, posterior mandible with or without reconstruction plates **(Fig. 22.3)**, and multidimensional maxillary and pharyngeal reconstructions, as well as external defects, such as cheek **(Fig. 22.4)**, orbit, and lateral temporal and scalp reconstruction.

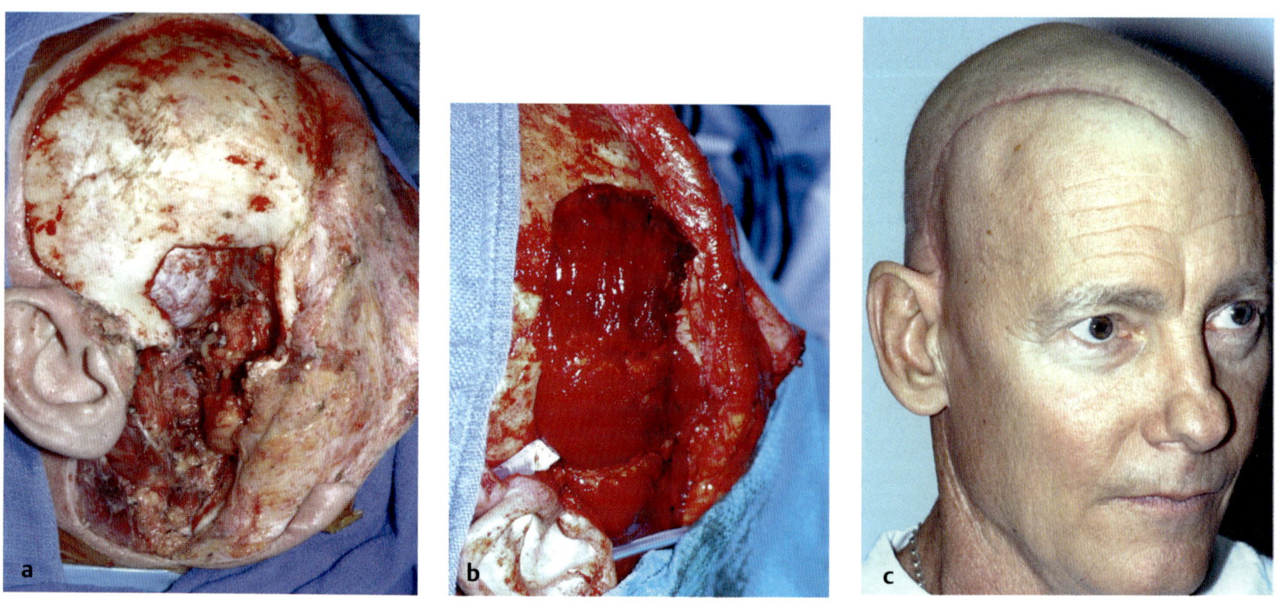

Fig. 22.2 **(a)** Resection of a synovial cell sarcoma arising in the lateral cranial base leaves a bony defect with exposed dura but no skin defect. **(b)** A rectus abdominis muscle free flap is used to protect the dura and provide soft tissue bulk that **(c)** prevents a contour deformity.

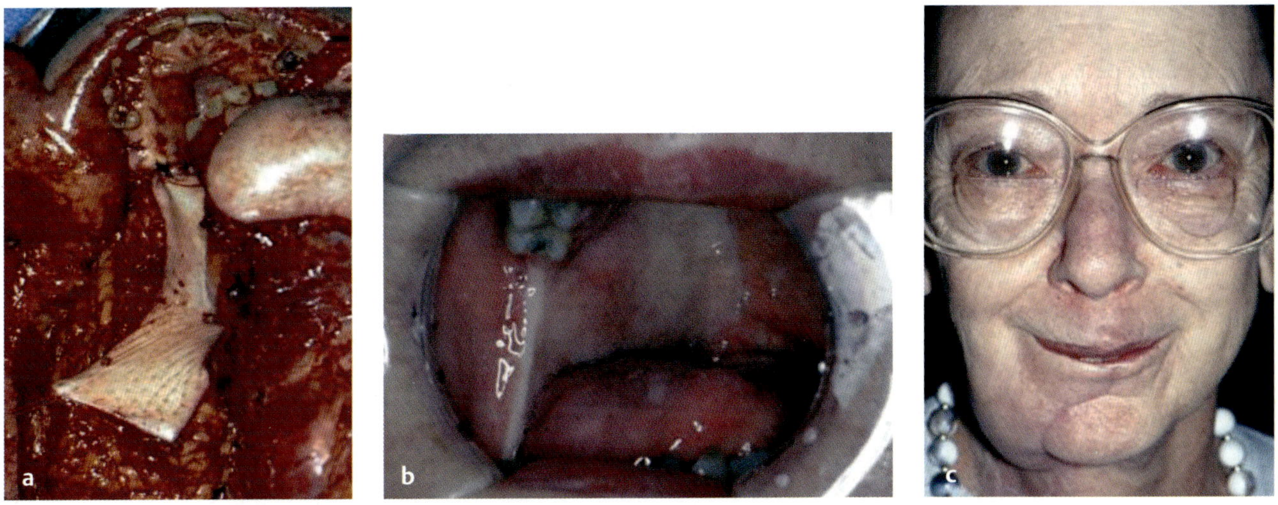

**Fig. 22.3** **(a)** A lateral segmental mandibular defect was reconstructed with soft tissue alone using a rectus abdominis myocutaneous free flap. **(b)** This preserved mouth opening without trismus by providing stable intraoral wound closure with the free flap skin paddle as well as **(c)** an acceptable aesthetic result by providing bulk to minimize contour deformity and mandibular deviation toward the side of the resection.

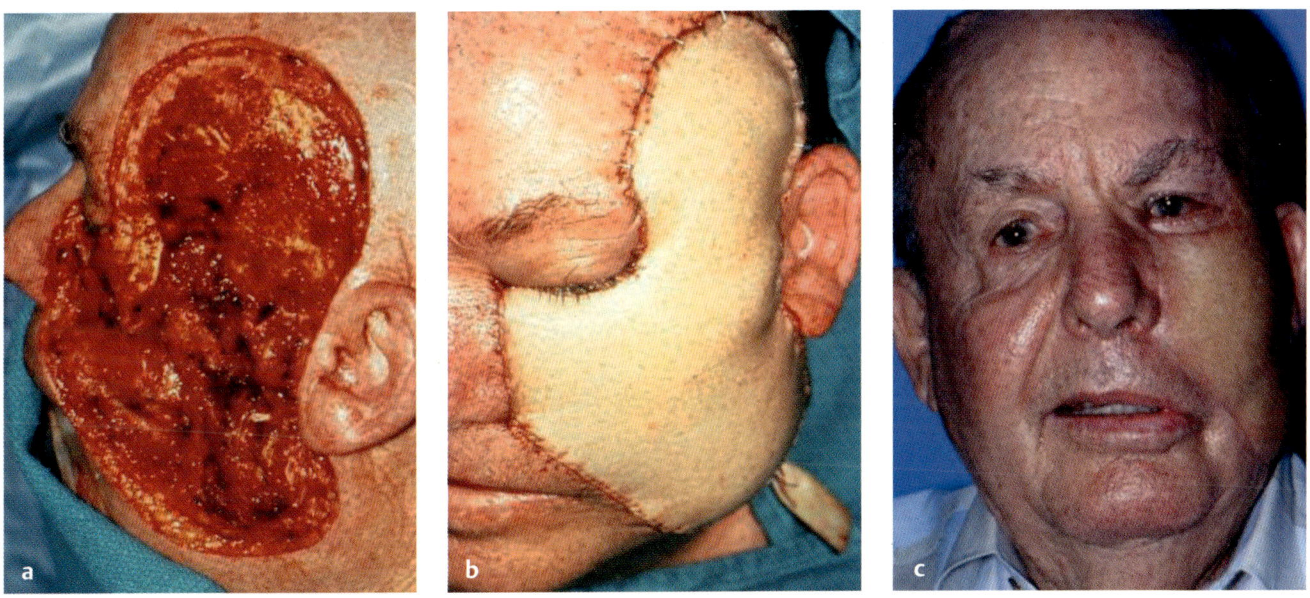

**Fig. 22.4** **(a)** An aggressive recurrent basal cell carcinoma was widely excised, leaving a large left facial soft tissue and zygomatic bony defect. **(b)** The large composite defect was reconstructed with a rectus abdominis myocutaneous free flap. **(c)** The postoperative result following radiation therapy is shown.

In general, with regard to necessary flap dimensions for the purposes of head and neck microsurgical reconstruction, a more vertically oriented skin island over the vertical extent of the muscle may be the most useful application for a particular defect, such as a total glossectomy, with the skin island being as long as the entire extent of the abdominal wall. The extended deep inferior epigastric flap can also be designed obliquely over the costal margin to provide an abundance of well-vascularized, pliable skin. On the other hand, the horizontal application of the skin island over the vertical extent of the muscle, known as the TRAM (transverse rectus abdominis myocutaneous) flap can provide extensive skin coverage useful for external defects, such as lateral facial, temporal, neck, and even more extensive scalp applications **(Fig. 22.5)**.

The most likely shortcoming of the rectus abdominis flap is in obese patients, in whom the bulkiness of the flap may be a disadvantage in intraoral

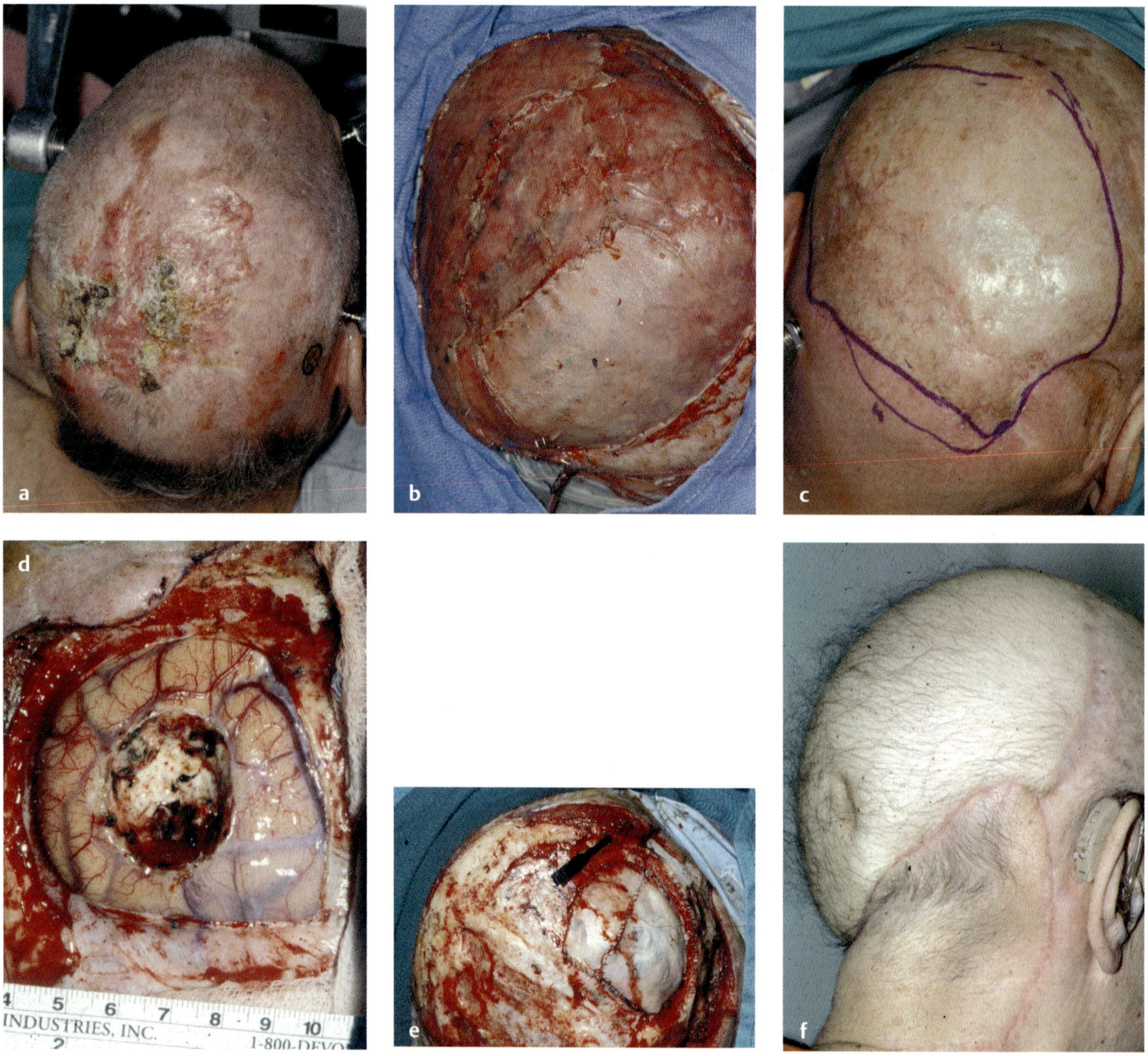


**Fig. 22.5** **(a)** A multiple recurrent squamous cell carcinoma of the posterior scalp was widely excised and **(b)** was reconstructed with a latissimus dorsi muscle free flap covered with an unmeshed split-thickness skin graft. **(c)** The initial result was excellent. Unfortunately, the cancer recurred in the calvaria and **(d)** a composite calvarial and free flap resection was performed, **(e)** resulting in exposed dura. **(f)** A rectus abdominis myocutaneous free flap to the cut pedicle of the earlier latissimus dorsi muscle free flap.

or intrapharyngeal placement. The flap will likely require thinning at a later stage for optimal function. The bulk of the flap in the higher body mass index (BMI) patient, even with an external inset in the temporal, neck, and lateral facial areas, may still be problematic and aesthetically challenging, but because of the ease of obtaining a single flap with a large surface area that can cover large defects, the rectus abdominis flap may still be a viable option despite its excess flap thickness, especially when postoperative radiation therapy may be required, which the flap tolerates well.[5]

An option in patients with thicker subcutaneous tissues includes simply skin grafting the rectus muscle **(Fig. 22.6)**. In 1991, Koshima et al[6] reported on the use of thinner flaps in which no muscle was included with the skin in harvesting paraumbilical tissues perfused by musculocutaneous perforators arising from the deep inferior epigastric vessels; their paper was the original description of the deep inferior epigastric perforator (DIEP) flap. Urken[7] described taking advantage of the rectus anatomy in thicker subcutaneous tissues by using anterior rectus sheath above the arcuate line as inner oral lining,

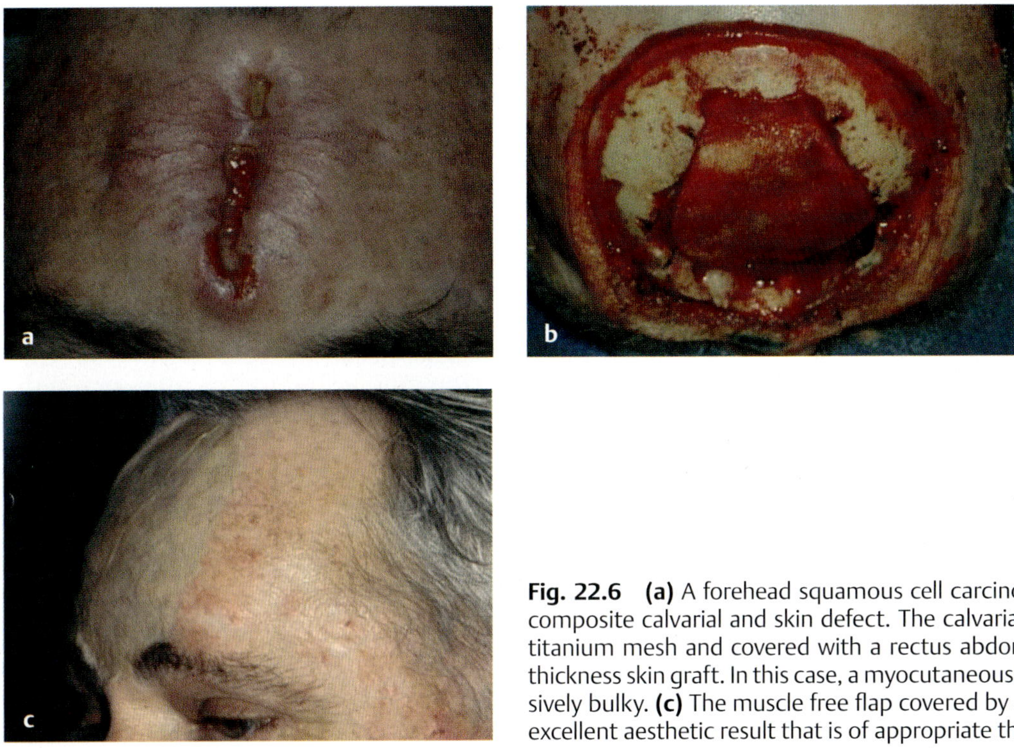

**Fig. 22.6** **(a)** A forehead squamous cell carcinoma was removed, **(b)** leaving a composite calvarial and skin defect. The calvarial defect was reconstructed with titanium mesh and covered with a rectus abdominis muscle free flap and split-thickness skin graft. In this case, a myocutaneous free flap would have been excessively bulky. **(c)** The muscle free flap covered by an unmeshed skin graft gives an excellent aesthetic result that is of appropriate thickness without revision.

folding the muscle in through-and-through cheek defects.

The use of the rectus abdominis flap can result in the development of an abdominal donor-site bulge or hernia that may be symptomatic and require a secondary repair. Moreover, in circumstances in which patients with head and neck malignancies have additional comorbidities, such as compromised pulmonary function, the use of an abdominal donor site, such as for the rectus abdominis flap, can create higher intra-abdominal pressures that may adversely affect overall pulmonary function and complicate the patient's surgical recovery.[8] Using the flap in its muscle-sparing format or as a DIEP flap when feasible may help avert many donor-site issues.[9]

On the other hand, the success rate of the rectus abdominis flap used as a microvascular transfer is among the highest of all the flaps used for head and neck reconstruction, as reflected in many free tissue transfer head and neck databases.[10] In general, both the difficulty of the flap harvest and the dissection time for the flap are less than for many comparable head and neck reconstructive flaps. The rectus abdominis flap now competes primarily with the anterolateral thigh flap.

## Anatomy

The rectus abdominis muscle is a long, flat muscle traversed by multiple tendinous intersections. It is enveloped by the anterior and posterior rectus sheath. The anterior rectus sheath extends the entire length of the anterior abdominal wall from the level of the medial lower ribs down to the level of the pubic bones, while the posterior rectus sheath is absent inferiorly, about one-third the distance from the pubic symphysis to the umbilicus.

### Origin

The muscle has two heads of origin: the lateral head from the pubic crest and the medial head from the symphysis pubis.

### Insertion

Three slips of the muscle attach to the costal cartilage of the fifth, sixth, and seventh ribs; these particular muscle slips are at a deeper level to the pectoralis major muscle. The nerve supply to the rectus abdominis muscle is segmental, with motor branches from the seventh through the twelfth intercostal nerves activating the muscle from laterally to its deep surface.

## Function

The rectus abdominis muscle creates flexion of the vertebral column, tightening the abdominal wall. The muscle is considered relatively nonessential because its function is duplicated by other muscles.

## Blood Supply

The rectus abdominis muscle is supplied by two major vascular pedicles: one superiorly, close to the insertion, and another inferiorly, close to the origin **(Fig. 22.7)**. Each pedicle tends to support just over one-half of the length of the muscle. The upper pedicle is an extension of the internal mammary artery, and the lower pedicle divides from the external iliac artery. In the upper chest, the internal mammary artery divides into the musculophrenic and superior epigastric arteries in the sixth intercostal space. The superior epigastric artery continues inferiorly to enter the sheath of the rectus abdominis muscle. Distally, the inferior epigastric artery branches off the external iliac artery just inside the inguinal ligament and curves up along the medial wall of the internal inguinal ring through the transversalis fascia and the posterior rectus sheath directly into the muscle. In the central portion of the muscle there are multiple anastomotic connections between the branches of the deep inferior and superior epigastric vessels.[11] Initially, both vessels lie deep to the muscle, between the muscle and the posterior rectus sheath, but they quickly enter the muscle and run parallel within the muscle fibers.

For the composite rectus abdominis myocutaneous flap, which involves the overlying skin and fat of the abdominal wall, there are multiple myocutaneous perforating vessels through the muscle into the overlying skin. There are generally two rows of these perforating vessels below the level of the umbilicus: the medial and lateral rows, which supply regions of the overlying skin over the muscle and can extend perfusion to a variable distance across the midline from the medial perforators and much further laterally in the lateral abdominal skin, even over the lateral oblique muscles to roughly the level of the anterior axillary line. If the flap is dissected without

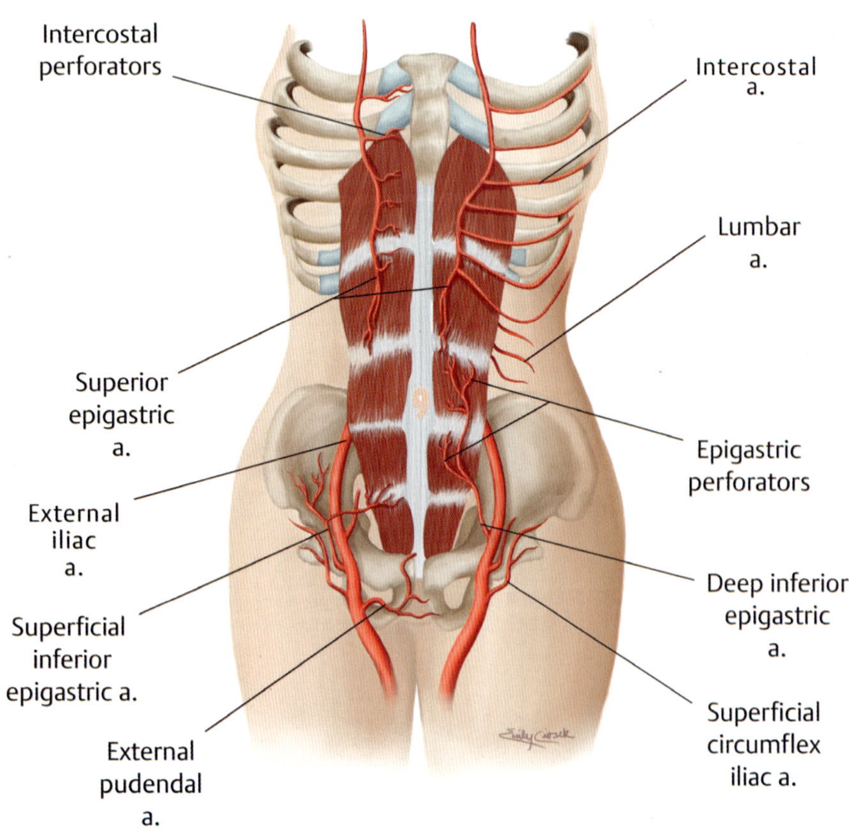


**Fig. 22.7** Vascular anatomy of the rectus abdominis muscle. The muscle is primarily supplied by the deep inferior epigastric artery and the superior epigastric artery. There are minor vascular contributions from the lower six intercostal arteries. The skin over the muscle is supplied by both perforators from the deep inferior epigastric artery and superior epigastric artery and the superficial inferior epigastric artery.

the rectus muscle, isolating the small perforating vessels on the deep inferior epigastric parent vessel through the muscle, the flap is known as the DIEP flap.

## Patient Positioning and Skin Markings

One major advantage is that the rectus abdominis free tissue transfer can be harvested while the patient is in the same supine position that will be used for the head and neck ablative procedure, so there is no need for altering the patient's position. Moreover, the distant location of the flap dissection from the head and neck often allows harvesting of the flap at the same time that the head and neck oncologic procedure is being done. The operating room table may occasionally need to be flexed to some degree to allow for less tension in the abdominal closure when a larger transverse skin island is required.

Skin markings are related to the position of a skin paddle over all or part of the muscle, either vertically over the muscle itself or at 90 degrees to the vertical course of the muscle. The difference in the skin markings for the orientation of the skin relative to the muscle relates to the particular reconstructive recipient-site requirement: for example, the need for more of the vertical aspect of the muscle to accomplish dead space obliteration, or the greater or lesser application of the skin island inset, which may also be utilized as a de-epithelialized buried portion of flap.

## Operative Technique

Once the orientation of the skin paddle over the muscle is determined, if a skin paddle is necessary, a scalpel is used to incise the skin along the lines of the designated boundary of the skin island through the dermal layer. Deeper dissection is typically done with electrocautery to gently separate the subcutaneous tissues, minimize bleeding, and facilitate identification of anatomical structures, such as nerves and perforating vessels coming through the underlying rectus abdominis muscle to the overlying skin paddle. Once the deeper portion of the subcutaneous level of the abdominal adipose tissue is opened completely, the external oblique fascia is identified in the lateral portion of the dissection and the linea alba is identified in the midline. In order to minimize loss of the external oblique fascia, the subcutaneous tissues are elevated off the fascia itself from the medial and lateral sides of the flap until the perforating vessels coming through the rectus muscle are identified. Typically, the lateral perforators are the easiest to identify and the fascia can be opened about a centimeter lateral to the vessels for protection and the underlying rectus muscle thereby exposed. One has the option of taking the entire width of the muscle or the lateral portion of the muscle, which receives collateral blood supply from terminal branches of the intercostal blood vessels and can be spared, or the more medial portion of the muscle taken as the primary flap.

Special care should be taken to identify the deep inferior epigastric vessels making up the vascular pedicle of the muscle and to maintain them with the main body of the flap if the intent is to spare the lateral portion of the muscle. Bipolar electrocautery is extremely helpful in dissecting through the muscle and separating the lateral edge of the muscle from the medial because it significantly limits electrical stimulation and spasm of the muscle. The main focus of the dissection at this point is to continue to follow the main vascular pedicle on the undersurface of the rectus muscle down toward the lateral aspect of the lower portion of the muscle heading toward the external iliac vessels. Throughout the dissection, hemostasis is imperative, with generous use of both bipolar cautery and surgical clips on smaller vessel branches as necessary. Meticulous dissection of the vessels limits small hematomas around the vascular pedicle and also minimizes the vessel spasm that can occur with unclamped vascular side branches of the main pedicle.

Typically, the rectus abdominis muscle is then divided slightly above the highest portion of the skin island part of the flap unless a greater length of muscle is necessary for the reconstruction. On the medial side of the rectus muscle, the muscle split is just outside of the identified medial perforators if further preservation of muscle is desired. The next portion of the procedure involves opening the fascia inferiorly over the vascular pedicle to follow the pedicle to the juncture with the external iliac vessels and to free up the entire vascular pedicle from the surrounding soft tissues while gently separating the artery and two veins at the juncture with the iliac vessels. Careful manipulation of the flap and the pedicle itself protects the free flap elements from excessive traction on the vessels while the flap continues to perfuse in the abdomen. Vessel loops are usually placed across the vascular pedicle itself to help in the dissection of the pedicle from the underlying and surrounding soft tissues, and separate vessel loops can be placed around the vein and artery to facilitate the ultimate vessel ligation and subsequent transfer of the flap for microvascular anastomoses to the recipient vessels.

Following the microvascular anastomosis, the abdominal fascial donor-site repair becomes the priority. Heavy sutures (at the surgeon's preference) are necessary for appropriate repair of the fascia. It is important to include the internal oblique fascia as part of the closure to minimize the risk of abdominal bulge or hernia. Soft tissues external to the fascia are closed with deep sutures to limit the dead space under the skin and also to reduce direct skin tension. Most surgeons place drains at the donor site in the final closure.

The inset of the rectus flap into the head and neck recipient site is then completed with special care to avoid soft tissue tension in the closure as well as to obliterate any dead space within the defect. The closure of the wound is finalized over a drain, and the position of the pedicle is confirmed with regard to tension, compression, and twisting during closure.

## Donor-Site Care

In the immediate postoperative period, patients with a rectus abdominis flap of any type may benefit from slight flexion of the abdomen at the waist to limit tension of the abdomen itself. Simple skin dressings, either antibiotic ointment and petroleum and 3% bismuth tribromophenate gauze (Xeroform gauze; Covidien, Mansfield, MA) supported by an external gauze dressing or simply the use of cyanoacrylate adhesive, are used by surgeon preference. The drains themselves are secured with permanent sutures. If possible, the patient is mobilized after 24 hours as tolerated, with attention to the security of the donor-site drains, which are usually required for about a week. In some cases, an abdominal binder with soft dressing compression over the donor site may be useful for patient comfort during mobilization.

### Pearls and Pitfalls

- The rectus abdominis free flap, based on the deep inferior epigastric artery, has been a workhorse flap in head and neck reconstruction because of its large-caliber pedicle blood vessels and versatility as a myocutaneous, muscle, or perforator skin (also known as DIEP) free flap.
- The rectus abdominis flap and its variants are most useful for reconstruction of defects that require a thick flap, such as total glossectomy, maxillectomy, and temporal bone defects.
- The rectus abdominis free flap can be designed with multiple skin paddles, each supplied by a separate myocutaneous perforator blood vessel.
- A vertically oriented skin paddle has the best perfusion because it captures multiple perforators along its length. A transversely oriented skin paddle may be useful for larger defects owing to the greater volume of skin and adipose tissue that may be harvested with the flap and still achieve primary donor-site closure.
- In obese patients, the bulk of the flap may be a disadvantage and a relative contraindication for use for small defects.
- Donor-site morbidity can be reduced by sparing some or all of the rectus abdominis muscle (DIEP flap) when the defect does not require a substantial muscular component.
- Abdominal wall donor-site closure can be facilitated by minimizing the amount of anterior rectus sheath fascia harvested with the flap. This requires skeletonizing the perforators as they emerge from the anterior rectus sheath, then incising a minimal amount of fascia.

### References


1. Mathes SJ, McCraw JB, Vasconez LO. Muscle transposition flaps for coverage of lower extremity defects: anatomic considerations. Surg Clin North Am 1974;54(6):1337–1354
2. McCraw JB, Fishman JH, Sharzer LA. The versatile gastrocnemius myocutaneous flap. Plast Reconstr Surg 1978;62(1):15–23
3. Boyd JB, Morris S, Rosen IB, Gullane P, Rotstein L, Freeman JL. The through-and-through oromandibular defect: rationale for aggressive reconstruction. Plast Reconstr Surg 1994;93(1):44–53
4. Patel NP, Matros E, Cordeiro PG. The use of the multi-island vertical rectus abdominis myocutaneous flap in head and neck reconstruction. Ann Plast Surg 2012;69(4):403–407
5. Suh JD, Sercarz JA, Abemayor E, et al. Analysis of outcome and complications in 400 cases of microvascular head and neck reconstruction. Arch Otolaryngol Head Neck Surg 2004;130(8):962–966
6. Koshima I, Moriguchi T, Fukuda H, Yoshikawa Y, Soeda S. Free, thinned, paraumbilical perforator-based flaps. J Reconstr Microsurg 1991;7(4):313–316
7. Urken ML. Rectus abdominis. In: Urken ML, Cheney ML, Sullivan MJ, Biller HF, eds. Atlas of Regional and Free Flaps for Head and Neck Reconstruction. New York, NY: Raven Press; 1995:119–138
8. Lo JO, Weber SM, Andersen PE, Gross ND, Gosselin M, Wax MK. Atelectasis after free rectus transfer and abdominal wall reconstruction. Head Neck 2008;30(10):1339–1343
9. Guerra AB, Lyons GD, Dupin CL, Metzinger SE. Advantages of perforator flaps in reconstruction of complex defects of the head and neck. Ear Nose Throat J 2005;84(7):441–447
10. Kroll SS, Schusterman MA, Reece GP, et al. Choice of flap and incidence of free flap success. Plast Reconstr Surg 1996;98(3):459–463
11. Mathes SJ, Nahai F. Rectus abdominis. In: Mathes SJ, Nahai F, eds. Clinical Atlas of Muscle and Musculocutaneous Flaps. St. Louis, MO: The CV Mosby Company; 1979:347–361

# 23 Fibular Flap

*Matthew M. Hanasono*

## Introduction

Many surgeons consider the fibular free flap the preferred free flap for bony mandibular and maxillary reconstruction.[1,2,3,4] Because of its robust blood supply, it tolerates multiple osteotomies, and bony segments as small as 1.5 cm heal reliably, allowing shaping of the flap to mimic the configuration of the original facial architecture. Bony reconstruction with the fibular free flap is particularly indicated when osseointegrated implants for dental restoration are planned. This flap, as well as the iliac crest free flap, has adequate height and thickness for stable osseointegrated implant placement, in contrast to radial and scapular bone flaps, which do not consistently have enough bone stock for implants in all patients, particularly smaller or osteopenic patients.[1]

## Anatomy

The peroneal artery supplies the leg, along with the anterior and posterior tibial arteries **(Fig. 23.1)**. All three blood vessels arise from the popliteal artery. The anterior tibial artery usually arises more proximally, while the peroneal artery and the posterior tibial artery bifurcate from a common tibioperoneal trunk, ~ 5 to 7 cm inferior to the level of the fibular head. After it bifurcates from the posterior tibial artery, the peroneal artery takes a lateral position and runs in very close apposition to the fibula, periodically giving rise to nutrient blood vessels that penetrate the cortex of the bone, as well as periosteal blood vessels and muscular, musculocutaneous, and septocutaneous perforating blood vessels that supply the surrounding leg muscles and skin. Two paired venae comitantes travel with the peroneal artery and join those of the posterior tibial vein at the same level that the peroneal artery bifurcates from the posterior tibial artery.

We and others have studied perforator anatomy of the skin overlying the fibula.[5,6,7,8] The perforators arise from the peroneal artery and veins and travel along the posterior surface of the fibula, ultimately reaching the skin within, or in close apposition to, the posterior intermuscular septum, which separates the lateral and posterior muscular compartments of the leg, in a plane ~ 2 cm posterior to a line connecting the fibular head and the lateral malleolus. These perforators may be septocutaneous or musculocutaneous.

We have observed that a proximal perforator consistently arises ~ 12 cm inferior to the fibular head, or about one-third the distance from the fibular head to the lateral malleolus. The proximal perforator is usually musculocutaneous and, on rare occasion, may arise from the tibioperoneal trunk vessels rather than from the peroneal vessels. A second group of perforators, ranging from one to three in number, arises more distally, ~ 0.5, 0.6, and 0.75 the distance between the fibular head and the lateral malleolus. In a series of 80 fibular free flap dissections, we found that 49% of patients had a single distal perforator, 36% had two distal perforators, and 15% had three distal perforators. The distal perforators were almost always septocutaneous.

## Preoperative Considerations

We usually try to perform fibular free flap harvest concurrent with head and neck oncologic resection, using a separate surgical team to minimize operative time. The location of the fibula far from the head and neck region facilitates the two-team approach, as opposed to most other bony free flap sites, and is another major advantage of utilizing this free flap for head and neck reconstruction.

Preoperatively, both legs should be examined, checking for palpable dorsalis pedis and posterior tibial pulses, as well as other stigmata of vascular insufficiency, such as cool, hairless limbs, as well as

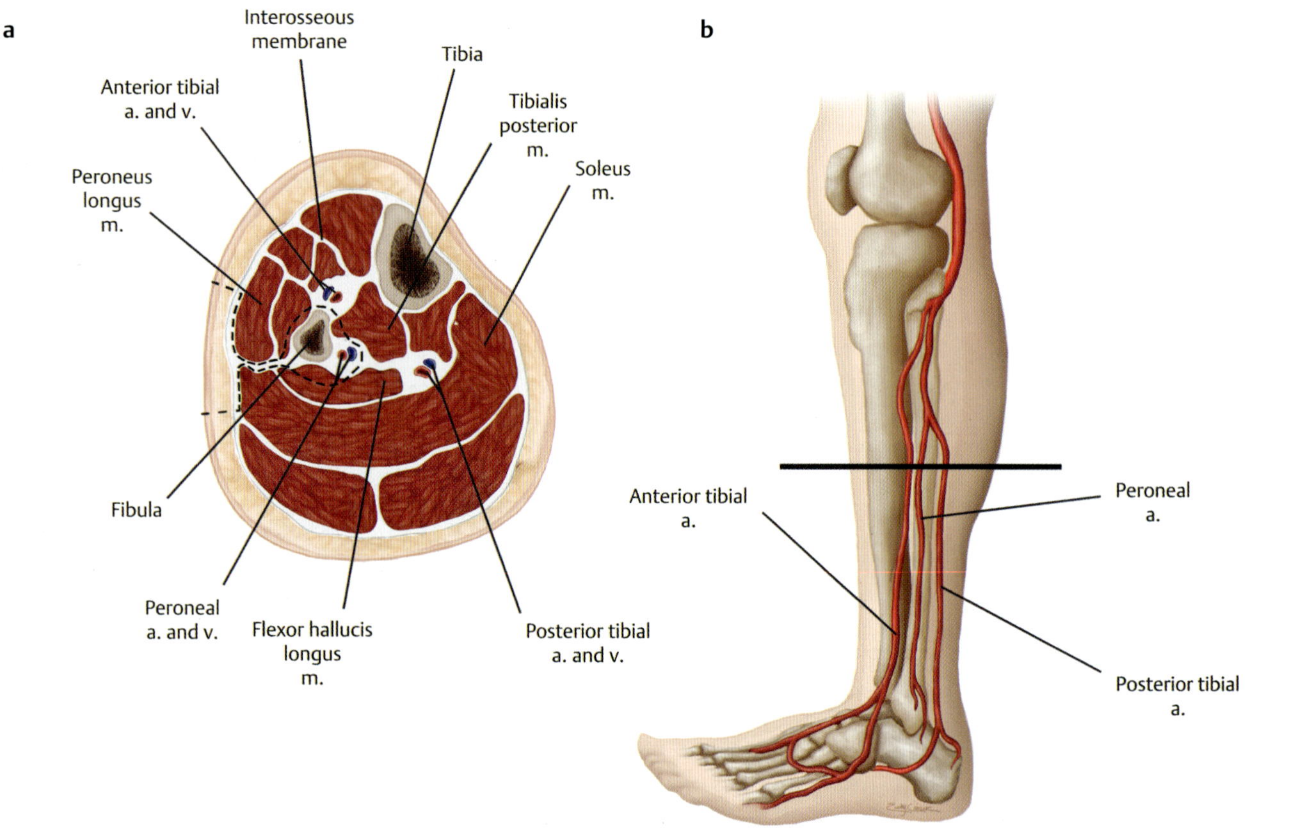


**Fig. 23.1** **(a)** Vascular anatomy of the lower leg in relation to the tibia and fibula and **(b)** cross-sectional anatomy of the lower leg. The fibular osteocutaneous free flap includes the fibula, peroneal artery and vein, and perforating blood vessels to the skin paddle that travel along the posterior surface of the posterior intermuscular septum, as indicated by the dashed lines on cross section.

atrophic or ulcerated skin.[9] The patient should specifically be asked about prior lower limb trauma or surgery, and symptoms, such as claudication, that would suggest peripheral vascular disease. If doubt exists about the vascular status of the lower limbs, angiography should be performed or an alternate flap should be selected. Conventional angiography, magnetic resonance angiography (MRA), and computed tomographic angiography (CTA) are all satisfactory methods of checking the distal flow to the lower leg and foot. We prefer CTA because it can also provide useful data about the location and number of cutaneous perforator blood vessels that can be useful for designing an osteocutaneous flap that includes one or more skin islands.[10]

If both legs have adequate blood supply, we choose the leg contralateral to the side of the mandibular defect for fibular free flap harvest when the ipsilateral recipient blood vessels will be used for microvascular anastomosis. This orientation allows the pedicle to lie on the deep surface of the reconstructed mandible, adjacent to the soft tissues of the tongue, and the lateral fibular bone surface, which is the surface that the titanium reconstruction plate will be fixated to, to lie on the superficial surface of the reconstructed mandible. In this orientation, the skin paddle will naturally lie on the superior surface of the reconstructed mandible, allowing reconstruction of the intraoral mucosal defect. The pedicle will emerge posteriorly, in proximity to the branches of the external carotid artery and internal jugular vein, which are commonly used as recipient blood vessels. If the skin paddle is needed for external cheek or neck reconstruction or if the contralateral neck vessels are chosen as recipient blood vessels, then the fibula from the ipsilateral leg is selected. For maxillary reconstruction, in which the skin paddle is usually used to reconstruct the palatal mucosa, the orientation is also reversed and the fibula from the ipsilateral leg is preferred.

## Patient Positioning and Skin Markings

The fibula is harvested while the patient is in the supine position. A “bump” made of rolled sheets or surgical towels curved into a horseshoe shape is taped to the operative bed beneath the surgical drapes so that it will hold the heel of the leg from the which the fibula is being harvested, thereby keeping the hip and knee both flexed. Some surgeons prefer to harvest the fibula under tourniquet ischemia, allowing dissection in a bloodless field. If a tourniquet is used, ischemic time should be kept to less than 120 minutes.

Once the patient is sterilely prepped and draped, the fibula is outlined with a skin marker **(Fig. 23.2)**. The skin island, if an osteocutaneous free flap is being harvested, is centered over the posterior border of the fibula in the anteroposterior plane, or ~ 2 cm posterior to a line connecting the fibular head to the lateral malleolus, since the cutaneous perforators supplying the skin paddle will emerge from the peroneal blood vessels along this line. The maximal width of the skin paddle that still allows primary closure is usually ~ 4 cm, although this varies from patient to patient and is usually more accurately estimated by pinching the skin to assess its laxity.

The skin paddle should be centered in the superior-inferior plane over the distal-most perforator(s) if pedicle length needs to be maximized. As mentioned, one to three distal perforators are most likely to be present between halfway and three-quarters of the distance between the fibular head and the lateral malleolus. In cases of a double-skin paddle fibular free flap, a second skin paddle can usually be based on the proximal perforator, which is very consistently present about one-third of the distance between the fibular head and the lateral malleoulus. If a bone-only free flap is being harvested, the skin incision is planned directly over the fibula.

Approximately 7 cm of bone superior to the lateral malleolus are spared to preserve ankle stability. We also limit our dissection and make our superior fibular osteotomy ~ 5 cm inferior to the fibular head. This protects the superficial peroneal nerve, which travels across the neck of the fibula, just below the head, while giving exposure to the origin of peroneal blood vessels, where they bifurcate from the posterior tibial blood vessels.

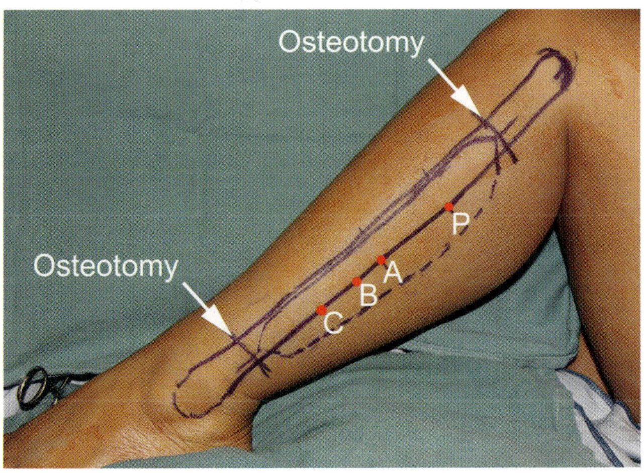


**Fig. 23.2** Skin markings for the fibular osteocutaneous free flap. Osteotomies are planned 5 to 7 cm inferior to the fibular head and 5 to 7 cm superior to the lateral malleolus. The skin paddle is centered on the posterior border of the fibula, ~ 2 cm posterior to an imaginary line connecting the fibular head and the lateral malleolus. While a proximal perforator (marked P) is usually present about one-third of the distance between the fibular head and lateral malleolus, the fibular osteocutaneous free flap skin paddle is usually designed to incorporate one to three distal perforators (marked A, B, and C), most commonly arising ~ 0.5, 0.6, and 0.75 the distance between the fibular head and lateral malleolus, respectively, to maximize pedicle length.

## ■ Operative Technique

The anterior border of the skin island is incised first. The incision is carried through the deep fascia covering the muscles of the lateral compartment of the leg. The skin paddle is elevated from the peroneal muscles in an avascular loose areolar plane until the posterior intermuscular septum is identified. The cutaneous perforators can be seen through the semitransparent posterior intermuscular septum **(Fig. 23.3)**.

The peroneus longus and brevis muscles are then elevated from the fibula **(Fig. 23.4)**. The periosteal blood supply is protected by leaving a small amount of muscle on the fibula. The anterior intermuscular septum is divided carefully, near the fibula, so as not to inadvertently injure the anterior tibial blood vessels as the anterior compartment of the leg is entered. The anterior compartment muscles (extensor digitorum longus and extensor hallucis longus muscles) are dissected away from the bone until the interosseous membrane between the tibia and fibula has been exposed.

A large right-angle dissector is used to dissect around the fibula at the superior and inferior osteotomy sites. Care is taken to "hug" the bone with the

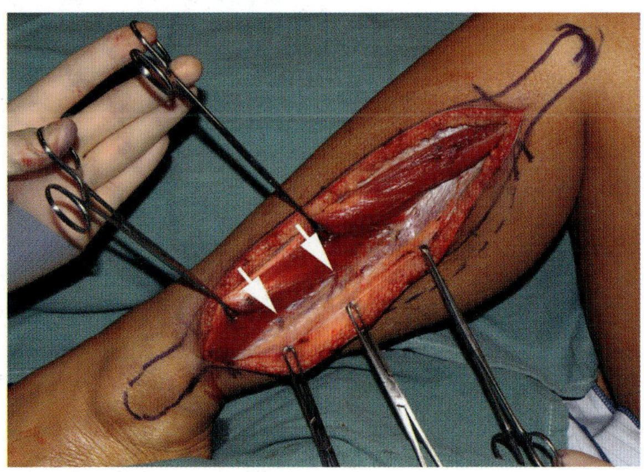

**Fig. 23.3** The anterior border of the skin paddle is incised first and the posterior intermuscular septum is identified. Septocutaneous perforators are seen through the septum (*arrows*).

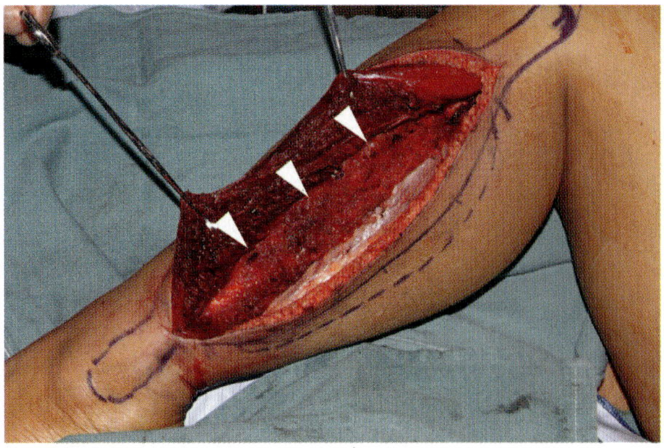

**Fig. 23.4** The peroneus longus and brevis muscles are dissected off the fibula, exposing the anterior intermuscular septum (*arrowheads*).

dissector so as not to injure the peroneal blood vessels, which lie posterior to the interosseous membrane. Thin, malleable retractors are bent into a curved shape and are placed around the fibula, protecting the peroneal blood vessels **(Fig. 23.5)**. The osteotomies are performed with an oscillating saw or a Gigli saw. Bone clamps are then used to retract the fibula laterally while the interosseous membrane is divided, taking care not to injure the peroneal blood vessels, which are beneath (posterior to) the interosseous membrane and the tibialis posterior muscle **(Fig. 23.6)**.

The tibialis posterior muscle is then dissected from the fibula, exposing the peroneal blood vessels beneath a thin layer of translucent fascia. To obtain maximal pedicle length, the peroneal blood vessels are dissected up to their bifurcation from the posterior tibial blood vessels. There are usually large arterial and venous branches from the peroneal blood vessels that supply the soleus muscle within a few centimeters of the bifurcation; they are either ligated or they are preserved if a chimeric flap with a hemisoleus muscle component is desired.

Next, the posterior border of the skin paddle is incised. The incision is carried through the deep crural fascia and the skin paddle is reflected anteriorly, exposing the cutaneous perforators on the posterior surface of the posterior intermuscular septum. Some surgeons prefer to take a cuff of soleus and flexor hallucis muscle around the perforators to avoid injury to these blood vessels. We prefer to dissect the perforators individually. Delicate technique is needed, since the perforators can be adherent to the posterior compartment muscles, and numerous small muscular branches of the blood vessels usually need to be carefully ligated. Some of the muscular branches can cause a septocutaneous perforator to be mistaken for a musculocutaneous perforator. When a muscular branch is observed, further dissection is performed until a clear view of the proximal septocutaneous perforator in the septum is obtained, allowing safe ligation and division of the muscular branch.

Once the perforators have been dissected, the posterior intermuscular septum is easily liberated from the posterior compartment muscles in an avascular plane of loose areolar tissue. At this point the harvest is complete **(Fig. 23.7)**. If a tourniquet has been used, the pressure is released at this point and meticulous hemostasis is achieved by cautery or vessel ligation.

The amount of fibula required for reconstruction is measured, and the pedicle is dissected from the bone up to that point. Additional osteotomies to trim the bone to a smaller length, as well as one or more closing wedge osteotomies to shape the fibula,

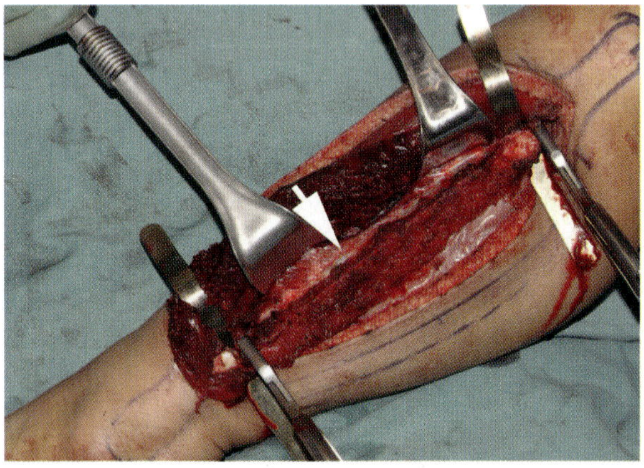

**Fig. 23.5** After the anterior intermuscular septum is incised, the extensor digitorum longus and extensor hallucis longus muscles are dissected off the fibula, exposing the interosseous membrane (*arrow*). Malleable retractors are placed around the fibula in the locations of the planned superior and inferior osteotomies. The anterior tibial blood vessels are partially seen between the two large retractors holding the lateral and anterior compartment muscles.

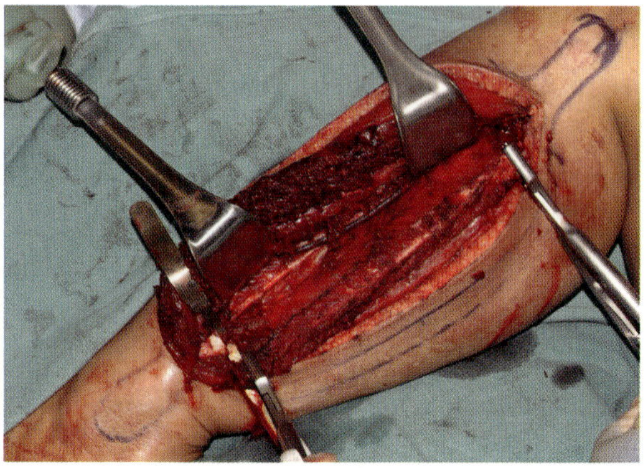

**Fig. 23.6** After superior and inferior osteotomies are made, lateral traction is provided with bone clamps and the interosseous membrane is incised longitudinally. The tibialis posterior muscle is dissected from the fibula, exposing peroneal blood vessels. The distal peroneal blood vessels are ligated and divided.

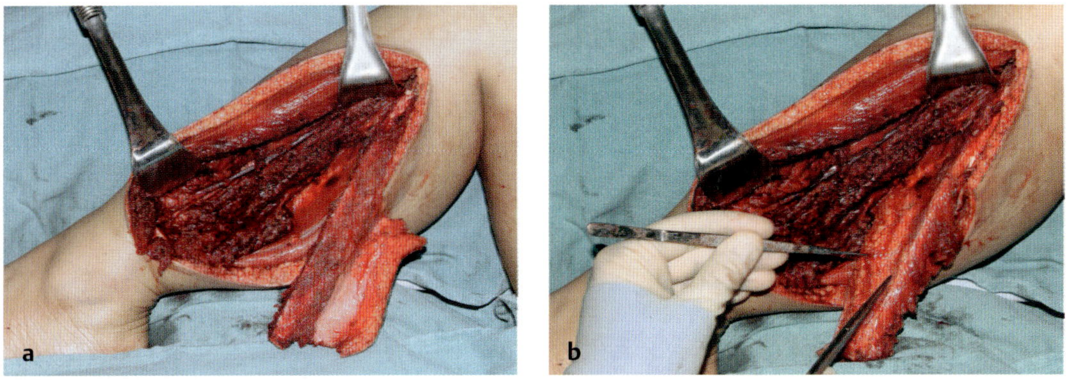


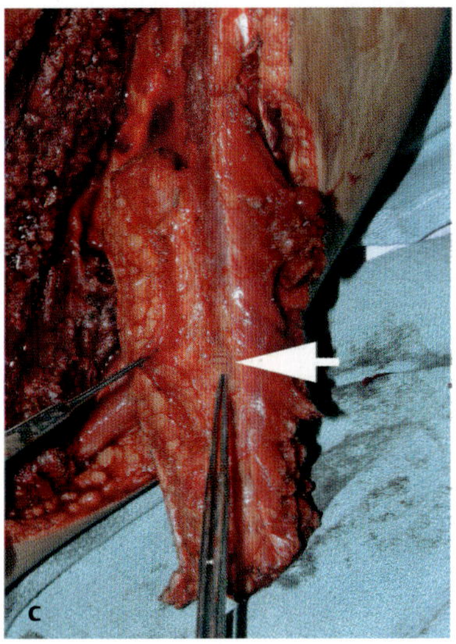


**Fig. 23.7** **(a)** Completed dissection. The posterior tibial blood vessels are visible within the wound bed, medial to the cut edge of the flexor hallucis longus muscle. **(b)** The cutaneous perforating blood vessels are visible on the posterior surface of the posterior intermuscular septum, indicated by the tip of the forceps on the right (**c**, arrow), more easily seen in the close-up view.

can be performed while the fibula is still connected to the leg by the peroneal blood vessels, on a separate operating table after the proximal pedicle has been ligated and divided, or after revascularization by microvascular anastomosis to the recipient blood vessels. Performing the osteotomies while the flap is supplied by an intact blood supply limits ischemia time, but it risks placing tension on the pedicle, which can result in intimal tears that may result in thrombosis if care is not taken.

## ■ Donor-Site Care

If wound tension is substantial, the donor-site wound is closed with a split- or full-thickness skin graft onto the peroneal muscles (**Fig. 23.8**). Regardless of the method of closure, a closed suction drain is placed in the deep portion of the wound and is left in place until the output is below 30 mL per 24 hours. Skin grafts are covered with a bolster or negative-pressure wound dressing that is left in place for 5 days. During this time, a posterior splint is applied with the ankle in 90 degrees of dorsiflexion and sufficient padding applied to the heel. The splint and bolster

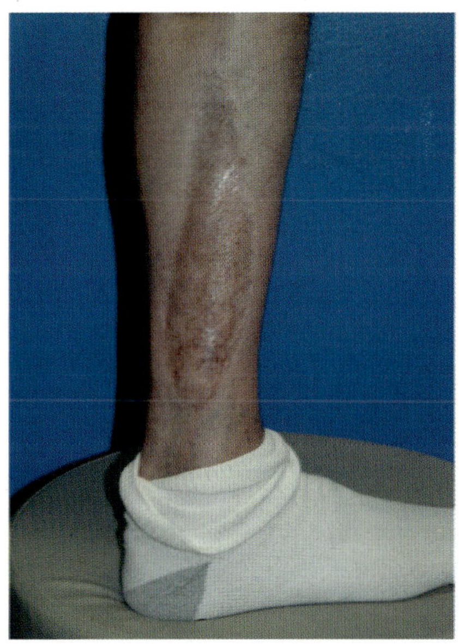

**Fig. 23.8** Donor-site appearance after osteocutaneous free flap harvest and donor-site reconstruction with a split-thickness skin graft.

are removed on postoperative day 5. After bolster removal, antibiotic ointment is applied to the skin graft, which is then covered with nonadherent petroleum gauze and an absorbent dressing wrapped in an elastic compression bandage. Dressings are changed daily until the wound is fully healed. Even when primary closure is performed, a splint may be utilized for a few days for comfort, but it is not necessary. In any case, the toes should be visible to allow for vascular checks, which should be performed after flap harvest, after bolster and splint placement (if used), and every 1 to 2 hours after surgery for the first several days. After complete healing of the incision and skin graft (if performed), compression stockings are recommended until lower leg edema resolves.

Following surgery, the donor leg is kept elevated at all times, whether in bed or in a chair. Ambulation is begun as soon as is practical, generally 2 to 3 days after surgery if the wound is closed primarily and 5 days if it is closed with a skin graft, following bolster and splint removal. We allow patients to ambulate with full weight bearing as tolerated and we involve physical and occupational therapy during the first several days of rehabilitation. Ambulation and dangling are restricted to 15 to 20 minutes three to four times per day initially, and the patient is instructed to keep the donor leg elevated at all other times. Ambulatory time and frequency are gradually increased over several weeks, as dictated by the amount of lower extremity edema present. If there is minimal edema and the patient tolerates exercising the leg well, then mobilization is allowed to take place more rapidly. If the leg is edematous and/or there is concern for delayed wound healing, then increases in ambulatory duration and frequency are more conservative.

The rate of donor-site complications is not insignificant and has been reported to be as high as 38%. In a series of 157 consecutive patients, we observed donor-site complications following fibular free flap harvest in 31%, including skin graft loss (15%), cellulitis (10%), wound dehiscence (8%), and abscess (1%), and some patients had more than one complication.[11] There were no significant differences in the complication rates observed between patients who underwent donor-site repair by primary closure and those who had skin grafting. The timing of ambulation, whether the donor wound was closed primarily or skin grafted, did not appear to have a significant effect on the development of perioperative complications, which is our rationale for relatively early mobilization. Long-term morbidities occurred in 17% of patients and included leg weakness (8%), ankle instability (4%), great toe flexion contracture (9%), and decreased ankle mobility (12%). All patients eventually returned to their preoperative level of ambulatory activity, with the majority achieving normal mobility within 3 to 6 months after surgery.

## Pearls and Pitfalls

- Before a fibular free flap is harvested, angiography should be obtained to confirm adequate blood supply to the distal leg and foot when pedal pulses are not palpable, the leg appears cool and lacks hair, or there are any other signs or symptoms that suggest vascular insufficiency.
- As much as 5% of the population is believed to have variant anatomy in which the peroneal artery is the dominant or only blood supply to the foot, and this is an absolute contraindication to fibular free flap harvest.
- Osteotomies are made 5 cm below the fibular head and 7 cm above the lateral malleolus to protect the superficial peroneal nerve and preserve ankle stability, respectively.
- The bifurcation of the peroneal artery and the posterior tibial artery occurs ~ 5 to 7 cm inferior to the level of the fibular head.
- Pedicle length can be maximized by dissection of the peroneal artery and venae comitantes all the way to the bifurcation from the posterior tibial blood vessels and use of the distal fibula, incorporating the most distal cutaneous perforating blood vessels if a skin paddle is to be included with the flap.
- The skin paddle for an osteocutaneous fibular free flap is usually designed around one to three septocutaneous perforating blood vessels that travel within the posterior intermuscular septum and occur between the midpoint and the three-quarters down the length of a line that connects the fibular head and the lateral malleolus.
- A proximal skin perforator consistently occurs about one-third of the distance down the length of a line that connects the fibular head and the lateral malleolus. This perforator may be useful in designing a second skin paddle for the fibular flap.
- The proximal skin perforator often follows a musculocutaneous course and occasionally arises directly from the tibioperoneal trunk.
- Skin paddles are centered on the posterior border of the fibula, or ~ 2 cm posterior to the midline of the fibula along its vertical axis to best capture the supplying perforating blood vessels.
- Skin paddles more than 3 to 4 cm in width will usually necessitate that a skin graft be used to close the donor site.

## References


1. Chen ZW, Yan W. The study and clinical application of the osteocutaneous flap of fibula. Microsurgery 1983;4:11–16
2. Hidalgo DA. Fibula free flap: a new method of mandible reconstruction. Plast Reconstr Surg 1989;84(1):71–79
3. Wei FC, Seah CS, Tsai YC, Liu SJ, Tsai MS. Fibula osteoseptoctaneous flap for reconstruction of composite mandibular defects. Plast Reconstr Surg 1994;93:294–304
4. Hidalgo DA, Rekow A. A review of 60 consecutive fibula free flap mandible reconstructions. Plast Reconstr Surg 1995;96:585–596
5. Taylor GI, Miller GD, Ham FJ. The free vascularized bone graft. A clinical extension of microvascular techniques. Plsat Reconstr Surg. 1975;55:533–544
6. Wei FC, Chen HC, Chuang CC, Noordhoff MS. Fibular osteoseptocutaneous flap: anatomic study and clinical application. Plast Reconstr Surg 1986;78(2):191–200
7. Schusterman MA, Reece GP, Miller MJ, Harris S. The osteoseptocutaneous free fibula flap: Is the skin paddle reliable? Plast Reconstr Surg 1992;90:787–793
8. Yu P, Chang EI, Hanasono MM. Design of a reliable skin paddle for the fibula osteocutaneous flap: perforator anatomy revisited. Plast Reconstr Surg 2011;128(2):440–446
9. Disa JJ, Cordeiro PG. The current role of preoperative arteriography in fibula free flaps. Plast Reconstr Surg 1998;102;1083–1088
10. Garvey PB, Chang EI, Selber JC, et al. A prospective study of preoperative computed tomographic angiographic mapping of free fibula osteocutaneous flaps for head and neck reconstruction. Plast Reconstr Surg 2012;130(4):542e-–550e
11. Momoh AO, Yu P, Skoracki RJ, Liu S, Feng L, Hanasono MM. A prospective cohort stud of fibula free flap donor-site morbidity in 157 consecutive patients. Plast Reconstr Surg 2011;128(3):714–720

# 24 Iliac Crest Flap

*Peirong Yu and Geoffrey L. Robb*

## Introduction

The iliac crest flap, or deep circumflex iliac artery (DCIA) flap with iliac crest bone, has been one of the commonly used flaps for mandibular reconstruction, although its popularity has significantly decreased since the introduction of the fibular flap. The vascular anatomy of this flap was first described by Taylor et al[1,2] in 1979. The iliac crest flap provides a large segment of vascularized bone that is similar to the shape of the hemimandible.

The traditional iliac crest flap includes bone, muscle, and skin. There are three main disadvantages to the traditional iliac crest flap: (1) the inclusion of an "obligatory muscle cuff" makes the soft tissue component of the flap very bulky in most cases, (2) the skin paddle has a reputation for being unreliable when separated from the muscle, and (3) the detachment of abdominal muscles and thigh muscles from the iliac crest may cause gait disturbance and abdominal wall weakness. Therefore, several refinements have been developed since the 1990s to overcome these problems. In 1997, Safak et al[3] proposed a new design of the iliac crest flap without including the "obligatory" muscle to reduce the bulk of the soft tissue. This design was later further popularized by Kimata et al[4] as the deep circumflex iliac perforator flap. In addition, further refinement was made to preserve the thigh muscle attachment to the iliac bone to minimize donor-site morbidity. In 1992, Shenaq et al[5] described the use of the inner cortex of the iliac crest, so that the thigh muscle attachment to the outer cortex of the iliac crest could be preserved. More recently, perforator anatomy of the DCIA was further studied to make the skin paddle more reliable without including the muscle component.[6]

## Anatomy

### Vascular Anatomy

In most cases, the DCIA arises from the posterolateral side of the external iliac artery at the level of the inguinal ligament where the inferior epigastric artery branches medially **(Fig. 24.1)**. It can also arise slightly below the inguinal ligament from the femoral artery. In 65% of cases, the DCIA gives off a single ascending muscular branch ~ 1 mm in diameter at a level

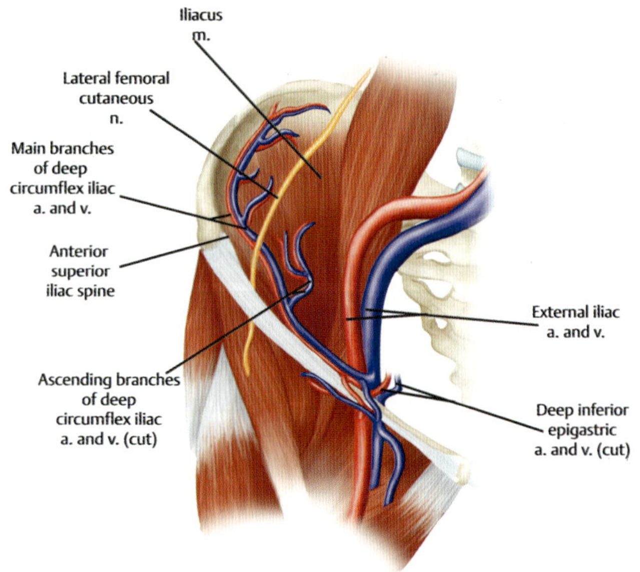


**Fig. 24.1** Anatomy of the deep circumflex iliac artery (DCIA). The DCIA travels ~ 2 cm above the inguinal ligament, and the lateral femoral cutaneous nerve crosses the DCIA anterior to the anterior superior iliac spine (ASIS).

within 1 cm of the anterior superior iliac spine (ASIS). This vessel pierces the transversus abdominis and the internal oblique muscles. In other cases, the ascending branch is replaced by several small branches. After piercing the transversus abdominis muscle and transversalis fascia, the ascending branch ends on the undersurface of the internal oblique muscle. Various amounts of the internal oblique muscle can be included based on the ascending branch.

The main DCIA (the transverse branch of DCIA) continues to travel laterally along the iliac crest, between the insertion of the transversus abdominis and the internal oblique muscles. The artery lies close to the iliac bone within a fibro-osseous tunnel along the inner (deep) surface of the iliac bone, several centimeters inferior to the bony rim. Multiple small perforators enter the medial surface of ilium as the artery travels within this fibro-osseous tunnel. In addition, the artery gives off several branches to supply the abdominal wall muscles and the iliacus muscles. Following the gentle curve of the ilium, the DCIA eventually pierces the transversus abdominis muscle and supplies a cutaneous territory of 12 × 18 cm over the iliac crest.

There are some anatomical variations of the DCIA and its ascending branch. The DCIA may be duplicated. Also, the ascending branch may originate from the main trunk of the external iliac artery, may be multiple in number, and may serve as the dominant vessel to the iliac bone with only a minor contribution from the DCIA.

The DCIA is accompanied by two deep circumflex iliac veins that join to form a single vein 2 to 3 cm lateral to the external iliac artery. The vein either crosses in front of, or travels behind, the external iliac artery to reach the iliac vein. The vein usually has a diameter of 2 to 3 mm, in comparison to the smaller DCIA, which is usually 1.0 to 1.5 mm in diameter. Pedicle length is limited to 4 to 5 cm.

Harvesting the DCIA flap by including only the bone and skin without the muscle bulk can potentially increase its use for oromandibular reconstruction and overcome the limitations of being too bulky when placed intraorally. Although the macroscopic vascular anatomy of the DCIA and its contribution to the skin overlying the iliac crest have been well established, current anatomical descriptions of its cutaneous perforators are conflicting. Taylor et al[1] found an average of six cutaneous perforators above the iliac crest, and Safak[2] found a series of musculocutaneous perforators in 70% of dissections and a single dominant perforator in 30%. A recent study by Bergeron et al[6] found that the DCIA cutaneous perforators were present in 92% of the specimens with an average number of 1.6 (range, 0 to 5 perforators). The perforators are located 5 to 10.5 cm (average 7.4 cm) lateral to the ASIS and 0.1 to 3.5 cm (average 0.8 cm) above the iliac crest bone. It should be noted that there are numerous other perforators in this region in addition to those arising from the DCIA, such as those from the intercostal artery, lumbar artery, superficial circumflex iliac artery, and iliolumbar artery. These perforators should be distinguished from the DCIA perforators during surgical dissection.

## Nerve Anatomy

Important sensory nerves in the groin region should be preserved during flap elevation. The lateral femoral cutaneous nerve and the ilioinguinal nerve travel in the territory of the flap and should be carefully identified. In the groin between the external iliac vessels and the ASIS, the lateral femoral cutaneous nerve lies lateral to the ilioinguinal nerve **(Fig. 24.2)**. The lateral femoral cutaneous nerve (L2, L3) travels through the inguinal ligament ~ 1 cm lateral to the ASIS. This nerve further descends along the line connecting the ASIS and the superolateral corner of the patella to supply sensation to the anterior lateral aspect of the thigh. Entrapment of this nerve may cause severe pain of the thigh and groin. Division of the nerve will result in permanent numbness in the thigh.

The ilioinguinal nerve originates from the L1 ventral ramus. It pierces the transversus abdominis and the internal oblique muscles and then traverses the inguinal canal below the spermatic cord in males or the round ligament in females. The nerve emerges with the spermatic cord from the superficial inguinal ring to supply the proximal medial skin of the thigh and the skin over the root of the penis and upper part of the scrotum in males or the skin covering the mons pubis and the adjoining labium majus in females. Entrapment of the nerve during surgery may cause recurrent pain in this distribution.

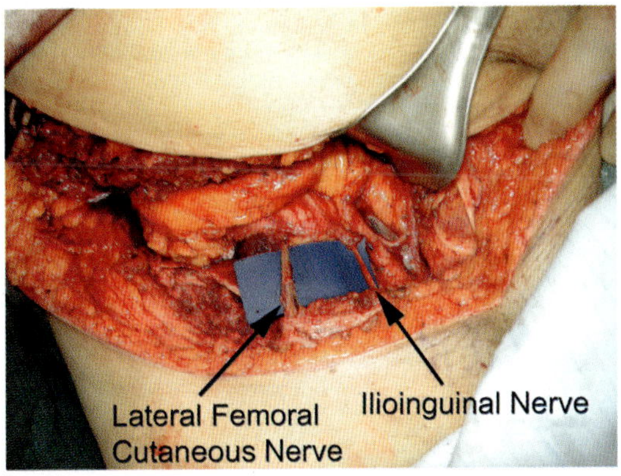


**Fig. 24.2** The lateral femoral cutaneous nerve travels immediately medial to the ASIS, whereas the ilioinguinal nerve travels more medial to the lateral femoral cutaneous nerve before entering the inguinal canal. These nerves should be preserved during surgery.

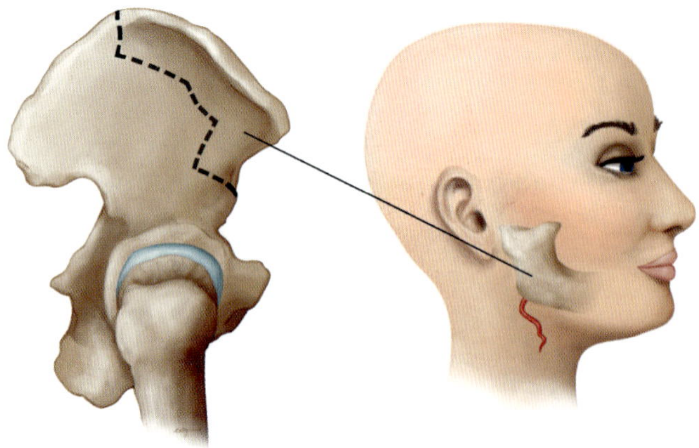

Fig. 24.3 The ipsilateral iliac crest should be chosen for mandibular reconstruction. The ASIS will be the angle of the new mandible and the iliac crest itself will become the body of the new mandible. The flap is flipped over vertically, so that the inner cortex and its vascular pedicle will face intraorally and the titanium plate will be fixed onto the outer surface of the bone flap.

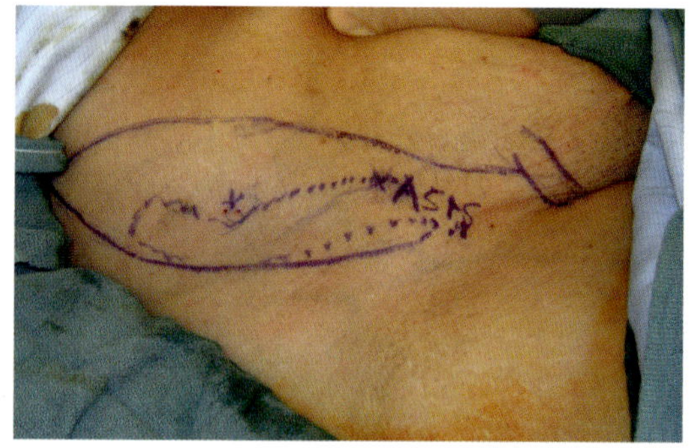

Fig. 24.4 A skin paddle is outlined over the iliac crest lateral to the ASIS.

## Operative Approach

### Choosing the Side of the Iliac Crest Flap

For posterior mandibulectomy defects including the condyle, ramus, and posterior body, the ipsilateral iliac crest flap should be chosen. The outer surface of the bone flap opposite to the vessels should face extraorally and the reconstructive plate is fixed to this surface. The inner surface of the bone flap should face intraorally. The ASIS becomes the angle of the mandible and the anterior inferior iliac spine becomes the condyle of the mandible facing the temporomandibular joint. The iliac crest itself should be used to reconstruct the body of the mandible. The vascular pedicle will be situated behind the new angle of the mandible (**Fig. 24.3**).

### Harvesting the Traditional Iliac Crest Flap

The skin paddle is marked two-thirds above and one-third below the line of the anterior iliac crest (**Fig. 24.4**). The medial skin incision is made 1 cm above the inguinal ligament and extends laterally along the superior border of the outlined flap. The spermatic cord or round ligament is retracted upward and medially to expose the inguinal floor. The external iliac vessels and the origin of the deep circumflex iliac vessels are then exposed (**Fig. 24.5**). If the vessels are followed later-

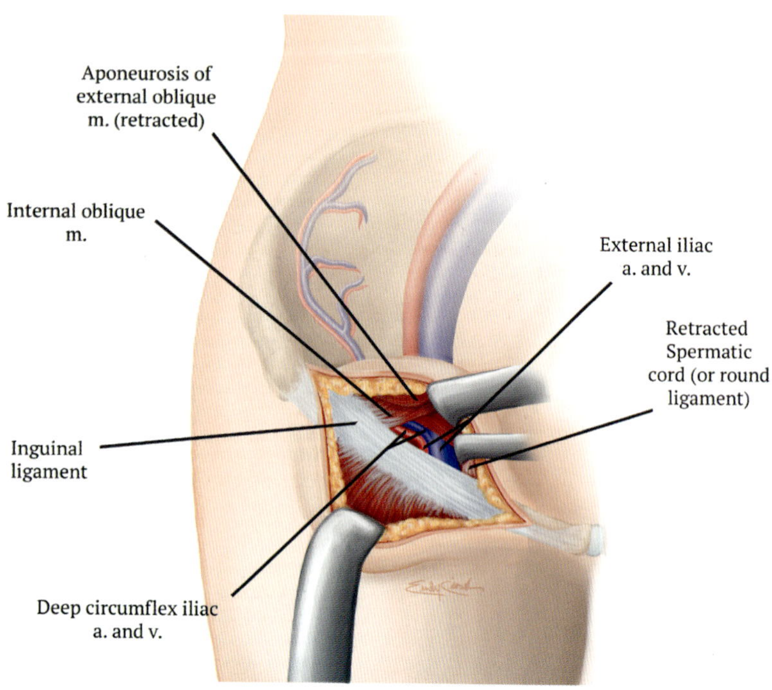


Fig. 24.5 Once the skin incision is made, the spermatic cord in male patients or the round ligament in female patients is mobilized and retracted upward and medially to expose the inguinal floor and the origin of the DCIA.

ally, the internal oblique and the transversus muscles are divided from the inguinal ligament. Near the ASIS, the ascending branch and the lateral femoral cutaneous nerve should be identified. The ascending branch is divided if the internal oblique muscle is not needed. The three layers of the abdominal wall muscles are divided, exposing the vascular pedicle between the overhanging transversus muscle and the iliacus muscle. The iliacus muscle is then divided below the vessels **(Fig. 24.6)**. The DCIA along the inner cortex is palpable or a Doppler device can be used to identify the vessel.

Next, the lower lateral incision is made to separate the thigh muscle attachment to the iliac crest. Care should be taken to preserve some of the muscle/tendon attachment to the iliac crest to minimize functional disturbance. The inguinal ligament is detached from the ASIS. The lateral femoral cutaneous nerve and the ilioinguinal nerve should be identified and preserved. Using an oscillating saw, the outer cortex of the iliac crest is cut, followed by the inner cortex through the already divided iliacus muscle. The cut should be ~ 2 cm below the palpable vascular pedicle.

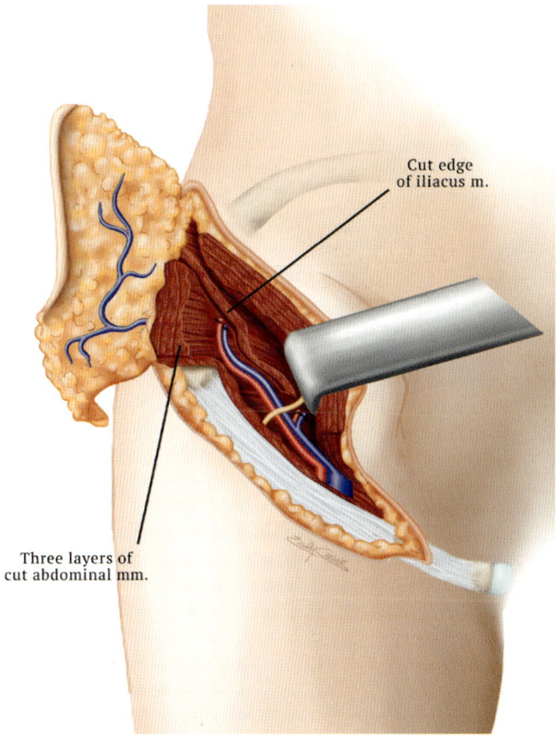


**Fig. 24.6** The three layers of abdominal wall muscles are incised above the vascular pedicle, and the iliacus muscle below the vascular pedicle is also divided to expose the inner cortex. Osteotomy is then performed with an oscillating saw 2 cm below the vascular pedicle.

## Modification of the Iliac Crest Flap–The Inner Cortex Iliac Crest Flap

Because a full-thickness iliac crest harvest creates a disruption of the abdominal wall muscle and thigh muscle attachment, the disruption may result in abdominal hernia formation and gait disturbance. To minimize these complications, the inner cortex can be harvested along with the superior rim of the iliac crest without detaching the thigh muscles. After the lower lateral skin incision is made, the periosteum of the outer rim of the iliac crest is stripped down for only 1 cm without detaching the thigh muscle and tendon attachments. The outer cortex is cut using an oscillating saw perpendicular it. The inner cortex is then cut 2 to 3 cm below the vascular pedicle. The posterior osteotomy is performed. The bone is then split between the inner and outer cortices with a large periosteal elevator. The inner cortex alone is a thin bone, ~ 5 mm in thickness. The 1 cm full-thickness rim of the iliac crest provides additional strength to the bone flap.

## Deep Circumflex Iliac Artery Perforator Flap

One of the main disadvantages of the traditional iliac crest flap is the obligatory inclusion of the full-thickness abdominal wall musculature if the skin paddle is needed. The resulting soft tissue bulk is usually too large to be placed intraorally and will obstruct tongue motility and interfere with oral function. Understanding of the perforator anatomy of the DCIA allows the harvest of the iliac crest flap with a perforator skin paddle without the muscle bulk. In addition, the skin paddle based on a perforator is not tethered with the bone, providing more freedom for flap insetting.

A 4 × 6 cm rectangle is drawn 5 cm posterior to the ASIS on the superior aspect of the iliac crest **(Fig. 24.7)**. The perforators are usually located within this rectangle. They may be detected with a hand-held Doppler device, although the Doppler is not always accurate. With a tentative skin paddle design centered on the perforators, the superior border of the skin paddle is incised to extend medially above the inguinal ligament. Suprafascial dissection proceeds inferiorly toward the iliac crest until the cutaneous perforators are identified **(Fig. 24.8)**. The perforators are marked on the skin surface with a 5–0 polypropylene suture **(Fig. 24.9)** and the flap design is recentered if necessary.

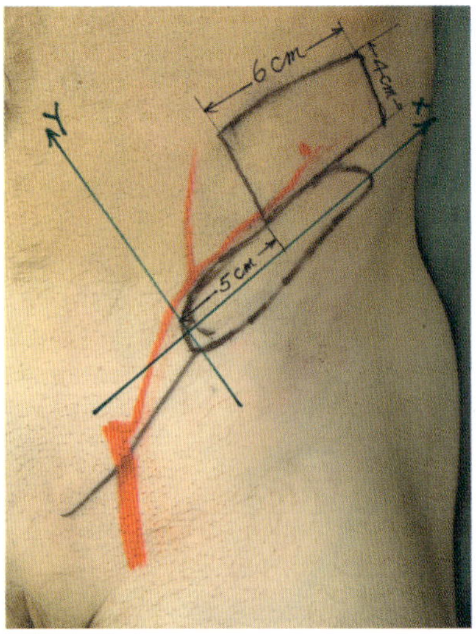


**Fig. 24.7** Design of the DCIA perforator flap skin paddle. The perforators are located in a rectangular area 5 cm lateral to the ASIS.

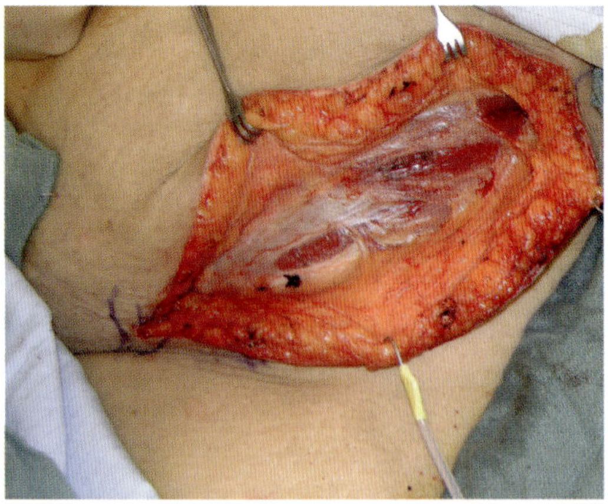

**Fig. 24.8** Only the superior skin incision is made initially, and suprafascial dissection proceeds inferiorly to identify the cutaneous perforators.

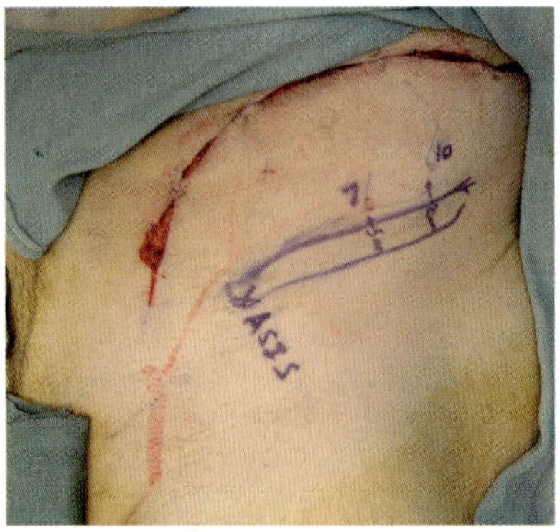


**Fig. 24.9** The exact locations of the cutaneous perforators are marked on the flap skin surface with 5–0 Prolene sutures.

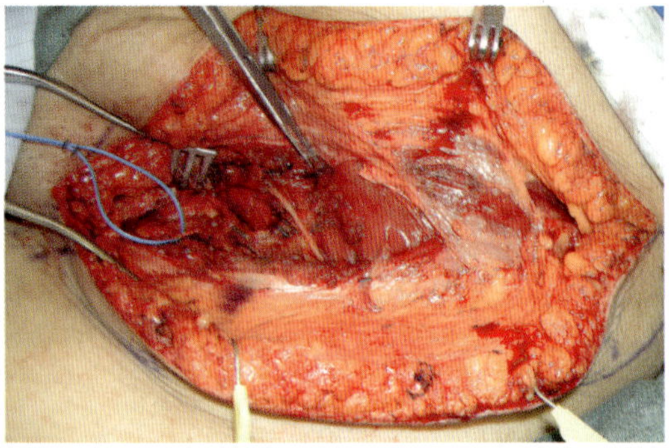

**Fig. 24.10** Once the perforators are identified, the external oblique fascia is incised to further expose the perforators, and intramuscular dissection is performed to trace each perforator to its origin. The ascending branch is divided.

The external oblique fascia is then incised around the perforators, and intramuscular dissection is performed to trace the perforator back to its main pedicle. The ascending branch is divided **(Fig. 24.10)**. There are, however, several perforators in the region that may arise from other arteries, such as the intercostal, lumbar, and iliolumbar arteries. The DCIA perforators can be distinguished from the intercostal and lumbar perforators, as they do not have an accompanying nerve. Distinction between the DCIA and iliolumbar perforators can be made by spreading the external oblique muscle fibers at the base of the perforator. DCIA perforators have an anterior origin, whereas the iliolumbar perforators have a posterior orientation. Once the correct perforators are identified and traced back to the DCIA, the abdominal muscle and fascia between the skin perforator and external iliac vessels are divided. The iliacus muscle below the vascular pedicle is also divided. The rest of flap harvesting is similar to the conventional or inner cortex iliac flap. The DCIA perforator flap has minimal soft tissue bulk and the skin paddle can be inset with ease **(Fig. 24.11)**.

## Donor-Site Care

With the conventional iliac crest flap, removal of the wing of the ilium creates a disruption of the lateral abdominal wall and the thigh muscle attachments. Careful closure is important to prevent abdominal hernia and gait disturbance. It is essential to reattach the transversus muscle to the iliacus or the remaining iliac bone. It may be helpful to drill several holes in the cut edge of the ilium to reattach the transversus muscle. In patients with a weak abdominal wall, mesh reinforcement may be indicated. The

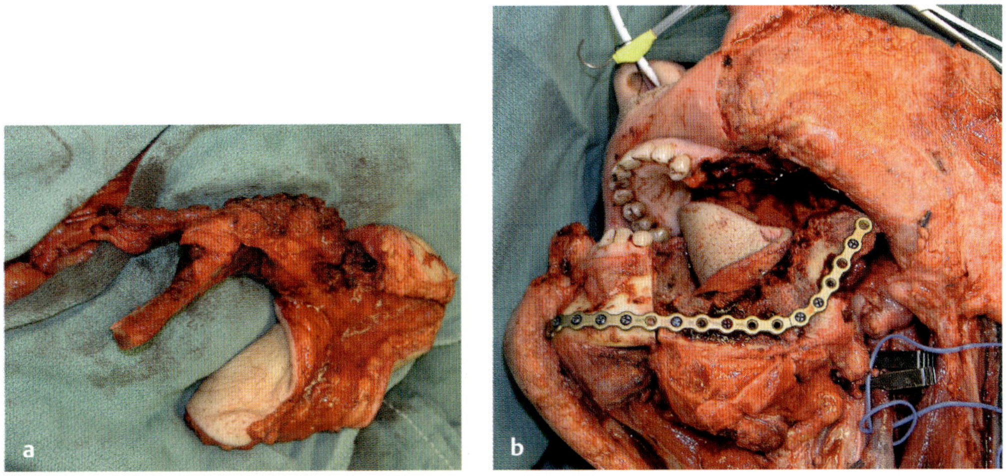


**Fig. 24.11** **(a)** The DCIA perforator flap provides an ample amount of skin without the bulk of abdominal muscles, thus making it more appropriate for intraoral lining. **(b)** Flap inset for a posterior left mandibular reconstruction.

second layer of closure involves suturing the external oblique muscle to the upper thigh muscles and tendons. Flexion of the ipsilateral knee is helpful to relieve tension on the closure. Closure should be done with strong permanent sutures, such as 1–0 polypropylene. With the inner cortex flap, the abdominal muscle and fascia are sewn to the fascia of the thigh muscle attachments and the periosteum. Bone wax is used to control bleeding from the cut edges of the bone. Closed-suction drains are also utilized to prevent fluid accumulation. Early ambulation with assistance is encouraged. However, straining should be avoided.

## References

1. Taylor GI, Townsend P, Corlett R. Superiority of the deep circumflex iliac vessels as the supply for free groin flaps. Plast Reconstr Surg 1979;64(5):595–604
2. Taylor GI, Townsend P, Corlett R. Superiority of the deep circumflex iliac vessels as the supply for free groin flaps. Clinical work. Plast Reconstr Surg 1979;64(6):745–759
3. Safak T, Klebuc MJ, Mavili E, Shenaq SM. A new design of the iliac crest microsurgical free flap without including the "obligatory" muscle cuff. Plast Reconstr Surg 1997;100(7):1703–1709
4. Kimata Y, Uchiyama K, Sakuraba M, et al. Deep circumflex iliac perforator flap with iliac crest for mandibular reconstruction. Br J Plast Surg 2001;54(6):487–490
5. Shenaq SM. Refinements in mandibular reconstruction. Clin Plast Surg 1992;19(4):809–817
6. Bergeron L, Tang M, Morris SF. The anatomical basis of the deep circumflex iliac artery perforator flap with iliac crest. Plast Reconstr Surg 2007;120(1):252–258

## Pearls and Pitfalls

- Dissection of the skin paddle perforator rather than including a cuff of abdominal wall muscle can greatly decrease the bulkiness of the soft tissue component of the osteocutaneous iliac crest free flap.
- Most patients have multiple cutaneous perforators arising from the DCIA, which are usually found 5 to 10.5 cm lateral to the ASIS and 0.8 cm superior to the iliac crest bone.
- Harvest of the iliac crest as a split inner cortical bone flap minimizes donor-site morbidity, including decreasing the risk for hernia formation and gait disturbance.
- The ascending branch of the DCIA is found ~ 1 cm anterior to the ASIS and can be used to supply blood to an internal oblique muscle component, which may be useful to close oral mucosal defects, especially in obese patients, who would otherwise have an unacceptably bulky skin paddle.
- Obesity is a relative contraindication to performing an iliac crest free flap, as exposure can be extremely challenging.
- Care should be taken not to entrap the lateral femoral cutaneous nerve (arising within 1 cm of the ASIS, below or through the inguinal ligament) or the ilioinguinal nerve (traveling alongside the spermatic cord as it exits the superficial inguinal ring), which can be painful.
- Bone wax should be used to control bleeding of the remaining bone at the donor site, because hematoma formation is not uncommon.
- Careful attention needs to be paid to meticulous multilayer donor-site repair to prevent hernia formation.

# 25 Latissimus Dorsi Flap/Thoracodorsal Artery Perforator Flap

*Goo-Hyun Mun*

The muscular portion of the classic latissimus dorsi myocutaneous flap can be left in situ and the overlying skin can be harvested alone as a muscle-sparing latissimus dorsi perforator flap, which is now called the thoracodorsal artery perforator (TDAP) flap. The TDAP flap was first described by Angrigiani et al, who originally used the name latissimus dorsi musculocutaneous flap without muscle.[3] The TDAP flap has gained great interest since its introduction, and it has become one of the workhorse flaps in various reconstructions.

The TDAP flap is a very appealing flap because it has distinct advantages: a long donor vessel, homogeneous flap thickness, and its large dimension, all of which help maintain the function of the underlying latissimus dorsi muscle. Furthermore, the donor scar is located in a relatively hidden area. Another outstanding point of the TDAP flap is the versatility of tissue options provided by the thoracodorsal pedicle and the subscapular vascular tree. A compound flap can be elevated with a segment of latissimus dorsi muscle as one component, and serratus anterior muscle, dorsal thoracic fascia, scapular bone, and/or scapular or parascapular skin flap. The multiplicity of perforators derived from descending and transverse branches of the thoracodorsal artery also provide a separate dual paddle design for complex reconstructions.

Difficulty in finding a reliable perforator and tedious perforator dissection are the main disadvantages of the TDAP flap. Improper perforator selection with respect to perforator size, number, or location within the flap may cause suboptimal perfusion, resulting in partial or tip necrosis. The crowded surgical field caused by the proximity of the donor site to the head and neck region makes a two-team approach difficult.

In the head and neck region, the TDAP flap is useful for resurfacing scalp, forehead, cheek, and neck defects resulting from tumor ablation, traumatic injury, and corrective surgery of secondary deformity (**Fig. 25.1**). When the skin is de-epithelialized, a dermo-adiposal paddle can be used to augment the soft tissue contour of the facial region, such as in progressive hemifacial atrophy. Functional neuromuscular transfer of segmental latissimus dorsi

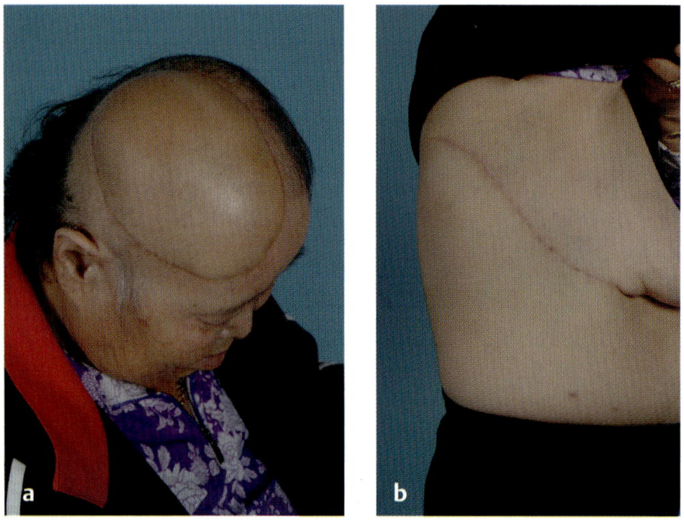

**Fig. 25.1** **(a)** A 72-year-old woman suffering from angiosarcoma of the scalp underwent ablative surgery followed by reconstruction using a free thoracodorsal artery perforator (TDAP) flap. **(b)** The donor-site scar after the harvest of the TDAP flap. In spite of the considerable size of the flap, the donor site was closed primarily and an acceptable linear scar was left.

muscle with thoracodorsal nerve can be combined with a TDAP flap as a chimeric approach for the correction of contour deformity simultaneously with facial reanimation.

## Anatomy

The latissimus dorsi muscle acts as an extender, adductor, and medial (internal) rotator of the humerus. The aponeurotic origin extends from the seventh thoracic vertebra to the middle outer rim of the iliac crest, and the muscle spirals around the tendon of the teres major muscle to insert onto the medial lip of the intertubercular groove of the humerus.

The latissimus dorsi muscle is a Class V muscle, having a dominant blood supply from the thoracodorsal system and a segmental blood supply from the posterior intercostal perforators **(Fig. 25.2)**.

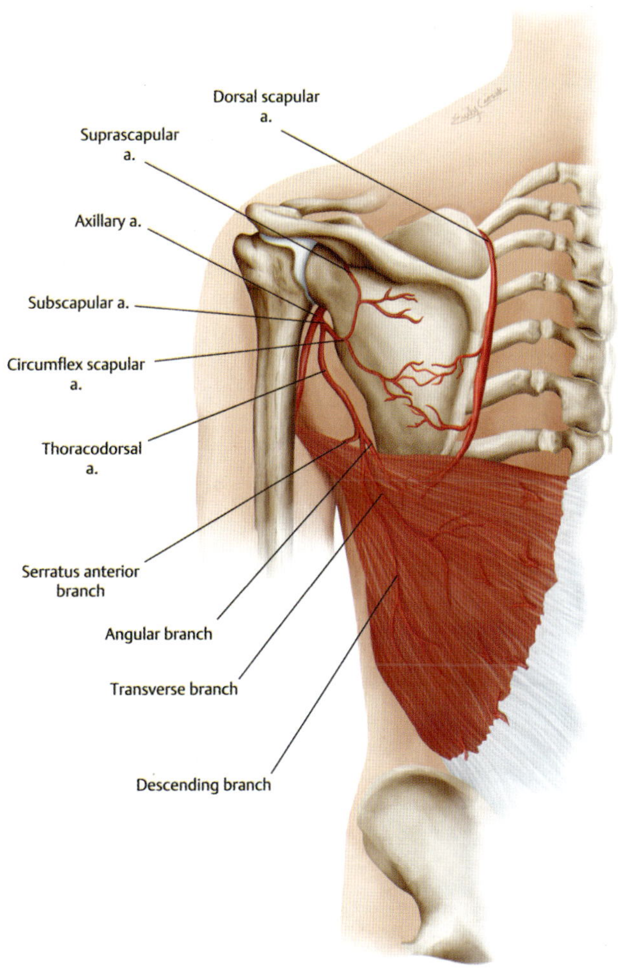


**Fig. 25.2** The latissimus dorsi muscle is a Mathes-Nahai Type V muscle, supplied dominantly from the thoracodorsal system and segmentally from a series of posterior intercostal perforators.

The main pedicle of the latissimus dorsi muscle, the thoracodorsal artery and vein, derive from the subscapular vessels, which are branches of the third segment of the axillary artery and vein. During their course in a cephalocaudal direction, the thoracodorsal vessels give off an angular branch to the tip of the scapula and branches to the subscapularis, teres major, and serratus anterior muscles. The thoracodorsal artery and vein enter the deep surface of the latissimus dorsi muscle at the neurovascular hilus, where the pedicle bifurcates into a descending (lateral) branch and a transverse (medial) branch. The descending branch courses parallel to the lateral border of the muscle at a variable distance from it. The transverse branch runs similarly parallel to the medial (upper) muscle border. In less than 10% of cases, the thoracodorsal vessels divide into three or four major intramuscular branches.

The thoracodorsal nerve, which comes from the posterior cord of the brachial plexus, supplies motor innervation to the latissimus dorsi muscle and runs with the thoracodorsal vessel to a neurovascular hilus. The nerve then divides into intramuscular branches in parallel with the vascular branching pattern.

On the whole, two to seven thoracodorsal artery perforators originate either from the descending (lateral) branch or the transverse (medial) branch of the thoracodorsal artery.[4] Typically, the most proximal perforator from the descending branch is selected for the pedicle of the TDAP flap, and its location has been reported as 8 to 10 cm below the posterior axillary fold and 2 to 3 cm posterior to the lateral border of the muscle, but, due to a wide range of variation in its location (up to 10 cm vertically), the above-mentioned distances are not always helpful. More distally, additional perforators from the same intramuscular branch can be found. The transverse branch of the thoracodorsal artery also provides reliable perforators, and sometimes the largest perforator comes from this branch. The mean location of the first perforator from the transverse branch is 11.5 cm from the posterior axillary fold on the tangential line to the medial muscle border and 1.5 cm inferior to this line. The axial level of the angular tip of the scapula is a helpful landmark for location of perforators from either branch centered at this level **(Fig. 25.3)**.

The perforators located anterior to the free lateral border of the latissimus dorsi muscle derive from different source vessels. In the proximal region, a perforator from a direct cutaneous branch of the thoracodorsal artery can be found in up to 60% of patients, but the size and quality of this perforator are inferior to those of true musculocutaneous perforators. Perforators can also arise from the serratus anterior branch of the thoracodorsal artery and from the lateral intercostal artery. In rare circumstances, these perforators course through the lateral portion

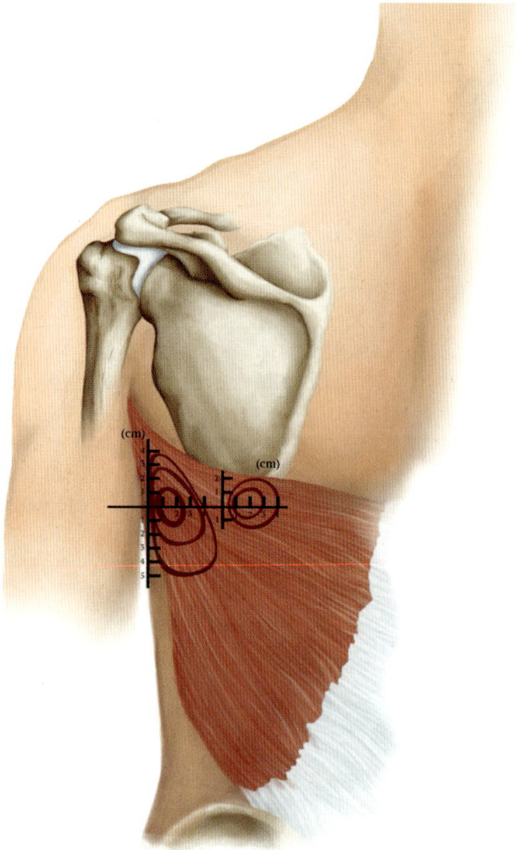


**Fig. 25.3** Map of the thoracodorsal artery perforators. The small center circle indicates the area in which the perforators are encountered most frequently. The axial level of the scapular tip can be used as a landmark in addition to the traditional scheme, namely, 8 to 10 cm below the posterior axillary fold, and 2 to 3 cm posterior to the lateral border of the muscle.

of the latissimus dorsi muscle to mimic musculocutaneus thoracodorsal artery perforators.

The dorsal intercostal artery perforator is distinguished by its location on the posterior, more distal portion of the latissimus dorsi muscle and the posteroinferior direction of muscle penetration by the perforator.

Two venae comitantes accompany the thoracodorsal artery perforator and usually merge to one vein when they meet venae comitantes of the serratus anterior branch of the thoracodorsal artery. Anterior to the lateral muscle border, the lateral thoracic vein courses longitudinally in a deep subcutaneous plane and drains the lateral thoracic region. This superficial vein is not needed for the TDAP flap because the paddle is mostly designed more posteriorly and the venae comitantes of a reliable perforator always drain the paddle territory adequately.

Sensory innervation of the TDAP flap territory comes from the posterior divisions of the lateral cutaneous branches of the intercostal nerves. They sprout between interdigitating slips of serratus anterior and external oblique muscles anterior to the lateral border of the latissimus dorsi muscle and course posteriorly in the transverse direction in a suprafascial plane. Frequently, the nerve branches hitchhike with perforators to enter the subcutaneous tissue. One to three nerve branches can be included to create a sensate TDAP flap, depending on the size and design of the paddle.

The dimensions of the latissimus dorsi muscle flap are up to 35 cm long and 20 cm wide on average, and the limit of safe dimensions for the TDAP flap based on a single perforator are 25 cm long and 15 cm wide.[5]

## ■ Preoperative Considerations

Since the thoracodorsal vessels have reliable and predictable anatomy, no special workup is necessary preoperatively for the latissimus dorsi muscle flap. However, mapping of thoracodorsal artery perforators with tools like acoustic handheld Doppler, color Doppler sonography, and computed tomographic angiography can be requested preoperatively. Because of the perforators' wide topographic variations, preoperative perforator mapping can be helpful for straightforward execution of the TDAP flap elevation.

A scar in the donor site from a previous surgical procedure, such as posterolateral thoracotomy, may indicate postoperative alteration in the structure of the latissimus dorsi muscle that interrupts the continuity of the thoracodorsal vessels and needs special attention. However, when adequate tissue dimensions still exist in the region proximal to old scar, the muscle flap or TDAP flap can still be harvested. When a muscle flap is planned, potential impairment of shoulder function needs to be considered and discussed with patients, especially those who enjoy vigorous sports activities.

For the TDAP flap, a "pinch test" is performed in the expected donor site to determine the subcutaneous thickness and maximal width of flap design that can be closed primarily. Compared with a vertical orientation of the long axis of the flap, a transverse design of the flap parallel to the rib, which the author favors, yields less tension when the same skin width is pinched.

## ■ Patient Positioning and Skin Markings

Harvest of the muscle or perforator flap is usually performed with the patient in the lateral decubitus position. The ipsilateral arm is positioned in shoulder flexion ~ 90 to 100 degrees. It is preferable to have the arm positioned so it can be moved during flap harvest, and the arm can be placed on a draped stand for support. The donor side is chosen by the laterality of the recipient site and recipient vessel to minimize the number of intraoperative patient repositionings required. When limited dimensions of muscle need to be harvested or when a perforator flap has a vertical design along the lateral border of the latissimus dorsi muscle, the patient can be placed in a supine position with the arm in abduction and a padding roll placed under the ipsilateral back for slight elevation.

The lateral margin of the latissimus dorsi muscle, represented by the posterior axillary line, is palpated and marked, and the superior margin of the latissimus dorsi muscle, represented by the inferior angle of the scapula, is also marked. Skin incision design varies considerably depending on the size and location of muscle to be harvested. Typically, a lazy-S type incision is designed on the center of the muscle and extends to the axilla. When segmental harvest of muscle is planned, a transversely designed incision is a good modification to create a more aesthetic donor-site scar. If a skin paddle is being harvested with muscle, the skin paddle needs to be placed so as to capture the thoracodorsal artery perforators in the proximal portion of the muscle. Intraoperatively, the thoracodorsal artery perforators are localized with pencil-type handheld Doppler. A reference point for a perforator derived from the descending branch of the thoracodorsal artery is marked 8 to 10 cm inferior to the posterior axillary fold and 2 to 4 cm posterior to the free lateral border of the muscle. Because of wide variation in perforator location, the adjacent region also needs to be scanned judiciously. The author uses a zonal approach in sequence from zone I to zone IV to find the best perforator (**Fig. 25.4**). The location providing the loudest sound is selected, and other spots may also be marked as backup options or when a multiple perforator flap is planned.

There are two methods of skin paddle placement for the TDAP flap. A vertically oriented paddle design extending beyond the free lateral muscle border was first proposed by other authors, but a transversely oriented paddle is favored by the present author because of easy donor-site closure and better resultant scar, as mentioned earlier.[6] The skin paddle is designed to include the mapped perforator(s) either centrally or eccentrically. Since the perforators run in and above the muscle fascial layer for a variable distance, a transversely oriented skin paddle is placed a little eccentrically at the axial level so that the marked perforator is located closer to the superior border of the paddle than to the inferior border. This placement ensures capture of the perforator(s) within the subcutaneous tissue of the skin paddle (**Fig. 25.5**).

## Operative Technique

When a skin paddle is being harvested with the muscle, the initial incision starting from the axilla courses inferiorly along the lateral border of the cutaneous component. Through this incision, the lateral leading edge of the latissimus dorsi muscle is identified and any adjustment of skin paddle location is made at this stage. The entire skin paddle border is incised and the surface of the muscle is widely exposed. Dissection then proceeds beneath the latissimus dorsi muscle by

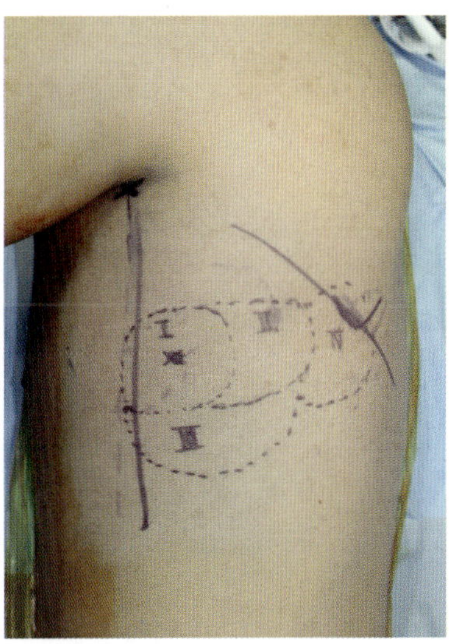

**Fig. 25.4** The zonal approach to finding the most suitable perforators. The number of the zone indicates the author's order for searching for the perforators. If the appropriate perforators cannot be found in zone I, the next zone (zone II) is searched, and so on.

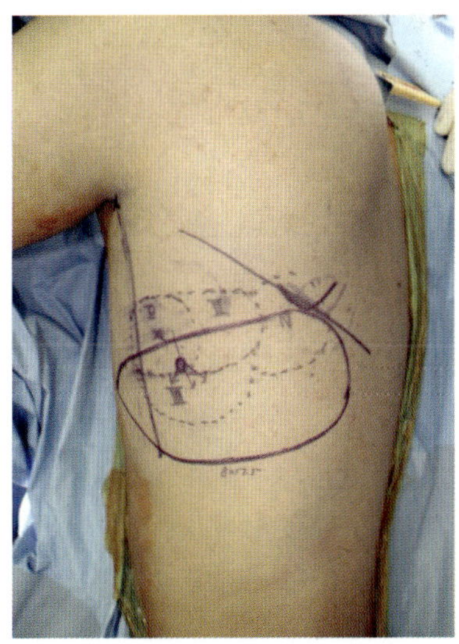

**Fig. 25.5** The preoperative design of the thoracodorsal artery perforator (TDAP) flap. The skin paddle is designed to capture the perforator a little eccentrically, closer to the superior border of the skin paddle than to the inferior border. This design ensures the inclusion of the perforator within the subcutaneous tissue of the flap.

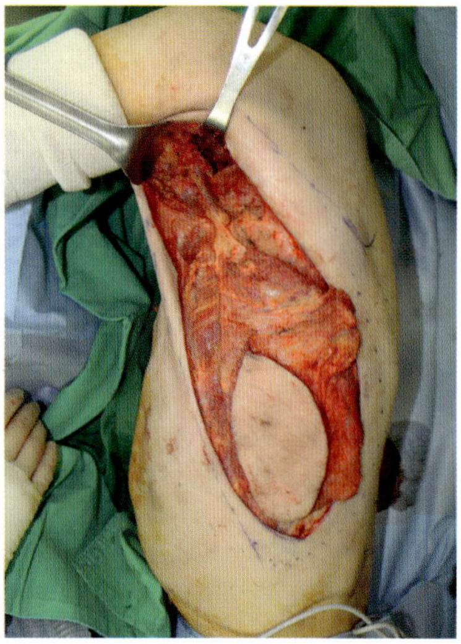

**Fig. 25.6** The latissimus dorsi musculocutaneous flap. To obtain an adequate length of pedicle, the dissection is extended proximally. The humeral insertion of the muscle is cut to facilitate the proximal pedicle dissection.

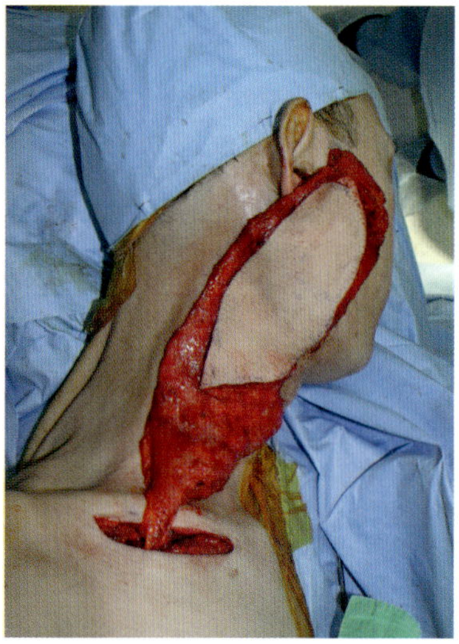

**Fig. 25.7** Transfer of the pedicled latissimus dorsi musculocutaneous flap. When the flap is used as a pedicled flap for the reconstruction of head and neck defects, it is passed from the axilla under the upper chest skin and is transferred over the clavicle, finally reaching the head and neck region.

elevating the lateral border of muscle from the underlying serratus anterior muscle. The muscle is then divided distally with electrocautery, and the muscle flap is elevated from distal to proximal. As the dissection approaches the neurovascular hilus, the bifurcated pedicle is visualized on the undersurface of the muscle, and the main thoracodorsal vessels can be identified within the adipose tissue. The serratus branch is then encountered and divided, and pedicle dissection proceeds until adequate pedicle length is achieved. Cutting the humeral insertion part of the muscle at this stage facilitates proximal pedicle dissection (**Fig. 25.6**). For functional transfer, the length of the thoracodorsal nerve is maximized by following it to the posterior cord of the brachial plexus and including this entire length in the harvest. When this flap is used as a pedicled flap for head and neck reconstruction, the flap is passed from the axilla under the upper chest skin and over the clavicle and into the neck (**Fig. 25.7**).

When a TDAP flap of transverse design is to be harvested, the central portion of the superior border of the flap is incised first and a loose areolar suprafascial plane above the dorsal thoracic fascia is explored. Staying within the loose areolar suprafascial layer during the elevation of the skin paddle is important for easy identification of the perforators (**Fig. 25.8**). The posterior divisions of the lateral cutaneous branches of the intercostal nerves, running posteriorly on top of the muscle, are frequently encountered and can be followed to find perforators because these nerve branches tend to enter the skin together with the perforator. A sensate TDAP flap is possible with harvest of an intercostal nerve branch. To gain length, the nerve is followed anteriorly between the slips of the underlying serratus anterior muscle. When the marked perforator is confirmed, the cutaneous incisions are completed throughout the entire flap boundaries, and, at this time, the surgeon may determine the number of perforators to be included in the flap when multiple perforators are within the skin paddle territory. Although very large flaps based on a single perforator have been reported to be successfully transferred, the author considers the inclusion of multiple perforators when the length of the flap exceeds 20 cm. Safe dimensions for the TDAP flap depend on multiple factors: perforator size, number, and location within the flap, as well as the degree of defatting. When substantial defatting of a large flap is required, the inclusion of additional perforators should be considered, since defatting

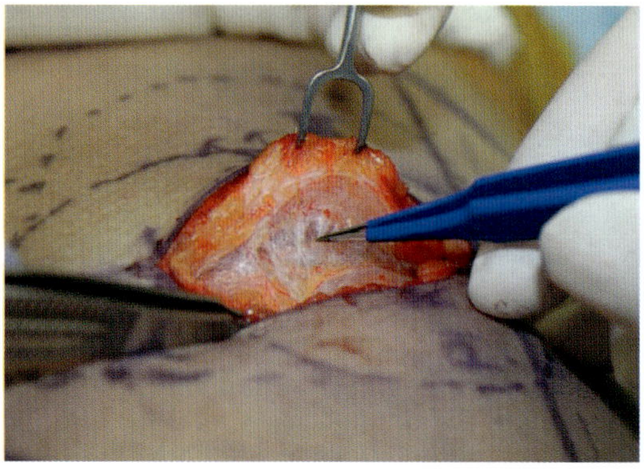

**Fig. 25.8** The loose areolar suprafascial plane above the dorsal thoracic fascia. Staying within this plane during the elevation of the skin paddle is crucial for easy identification of perforators and minimizes unnecessary bleeding.

reduces the safe dimensions of the flap. Occasionally, perforators are found to be smaller than usual, and inclusion of multiple perforators is recommended in this situation to avoid venous congestion.

Full elevation of the paddle from the muscle surface is performed first, and then the intramuscular dissection of the perforator begins **(Fig. 25.9)**. To facilitate pedicle dissection, the proximal subcutaneous tissue overlying the latissimus dorsi muscle superior to the upper flap margin is undermined. Separating muscle fibers around the perforator creates a cleavage space, and intramuscular branches of the thoracodorsal nerve are dissected first away from the perforator. Various dissection tools can be used for intramuscular dissection, but the author favors bipolar electrocautery forceps, which allow delicate dissection and hemostasis simultaneously **(Fig. 25.10)**.

A fully elevated paddle allows adjustment of the paddle position during the pedicle dissection to facilitate the separation of the perforator from the muscle and thoracodorsal nerve branches **(Fig. 25.11)**. When adequate pedicle length has been attained, the pedicle is transected proximally and is retrieved through the muscle cleavage space **(Fig. 25.12)**. The pedicle length can be 8 to 18 cm, depending on the perforator location and the extent of proximal dissection. When multiple perforators are included, an intervening muscle bridge needs to be cut and repaired later.

The TDAP flap can also be combined with functional neurovascular latissimus dorsi segmental transfer if the two components are designed to include different intramuscular thoracodorsal branches **(Fig. 25.13)**.

Flap defatting to decrease thickness can be performed after microvascular anastomosis of the pedicle. To preserve a diameter of several centimeters of fat around the perforator, the deep fat layer and part of the superficial fatty layer are resected with scissors. After hemostasis of the undersurface of the flap, insetting is performed.

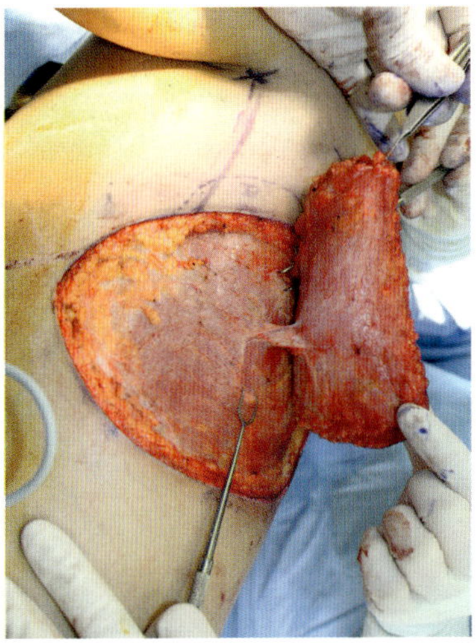

**Fig. 25.9** The appearance of a fully elevated skin paddle from the underlying muscle. Full elevation of the skin paddle before intramuscular dissection allows adjustment of the paddle position and facilitates the intramuscular dissection.

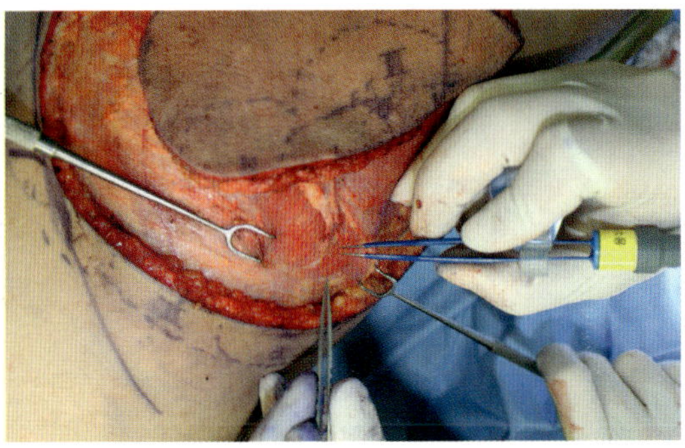

**Fig. 25.10** Intramuscular dissection using bipolar electrocautery forceps, which not only permits delicate dissection but also simultaneous hemostasis.

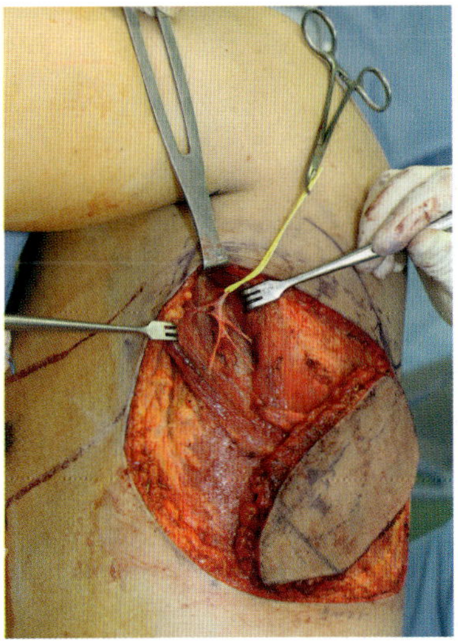

**Fig. 25.11** Separated thoracodorsal nerve branches from the pedicle of the flap. A freely movable skin paddle allows the easy dissection and separation of the pedicle from the adjacent muscle fibers and nerve branches.

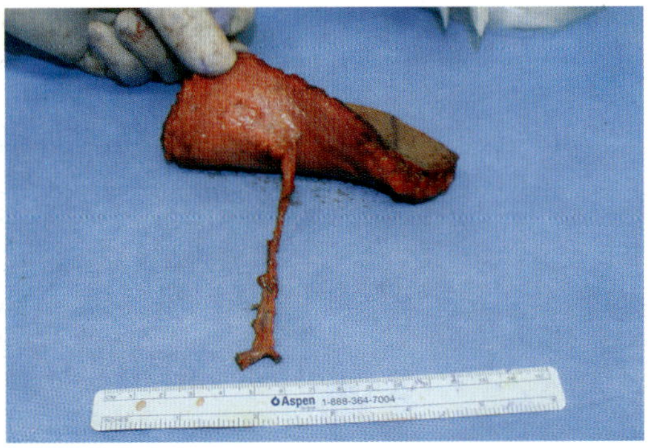

**Fig. 25.12** A harvested free thoracodorsal artery perforator (TDAP) flap.

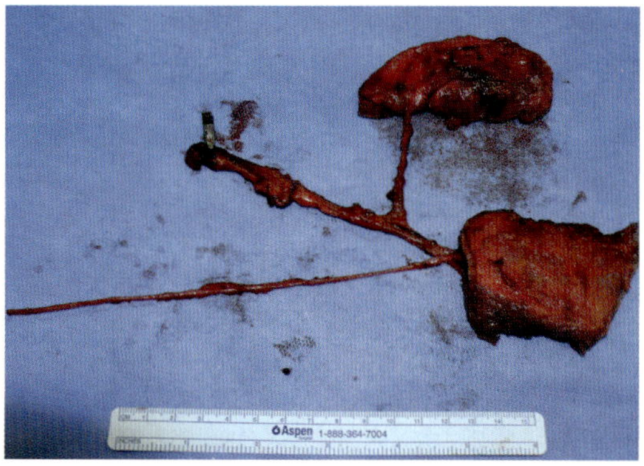

**Fig. 25.13** A latissimus dorsi muscle chimeric thoracodorsal artery perforator (TDAP) flap with thoracodorsal nerve for functional transfer. The muscle component and skin paddle are designed to include different thoracodorsal vascular branches.

## Donor-Site Care

Although there is individual variation, primary closure is usually possible with a skin flap width of up to 12 cm **(Fig. 25.14)**. Drains are usually removed within several days when a perforator flap is harvested, but they need to remain significantly longer when a muscle flap has been elevated. A simple dressing is applied and the shoulder is immobilized for a week or until the drain is removed. After the drain has been removed, shoulder motion is permitted and the shoulder range of motion can be gradually increased over a period of several weeks. Because the muscle and its innervation are preserved in TDAP flap elevation, the recovery is especially fast and patients can ambulate very early in their postoperative course,[7] in contrast to patients whose flap was taken from a lower limb. Latissimus dorsi muscle strength seems to be maintained after TDAP flap harvest.

The latissimus dorsi muscle flap is notorious for donor-site seromas, which frequently develop and require serial aspiration, but seromas are rare when only a skin perforator flap has been harvested. Vertically oriented skin paddle design tends to result in donor-scar widening and hypertrophic change, especially in Asian and pediatric patients. Generally, a transversely oriented paddle design results in a more acceptable scar.

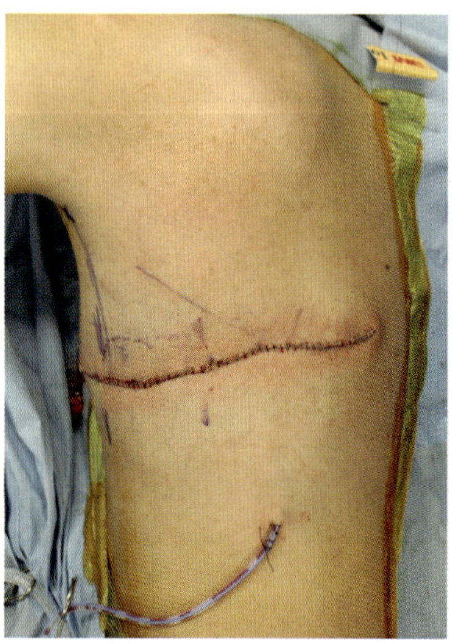

**Fig. 25.14** Donor-site repair following a transversely oriented thoracodorsal artery perforator (TDAP) flap harvest. Primary closure is usually possible with up to ~ 12 cm of skin paddle width. The drain can be removed within a few days.

### Pearls and Pitfalls

- The latissimus dorsi muscle free flap is most typically used for scalp reconstruction. A split-muscle flap can be used for facial reanimation.
- The TDAP flap is useful for cutaneous resurfacing of the scalp, forehead, cheek, and neck defects.
- The thoracodorsal artery divides into a descending and a transverse branch as it enters the deep surface of the latissimus dorsi, allowing harvest of a split-muscle flap that is composed of either the lateral (descending) branch or medial (transverse) branch of the muscle.
- Typically, the most proximal thoracodorsal artery perforators arising from the descending branch are selected to supply the TDAP flap. They are most commonly found 8 to 10 cm below the posterior axillary fold and 2 to 3 cm posterior to the lateral border of the muscle, at the same horizontal level as the tip of the scapula.
- The dimensions of the latissimus dorsi muscle flap are up to 35 cm long and 20 cm wide on average, and the limits of safe dimensions for the TDAP flap based on a single perforator are 25 cm long and 15 cm wide.
- A vertically or transversely oriented latissimus dorsi skin paddle or TDAP flap is possible. The transversely oriented paddle donor site is usually easier to close and results in less scar widening.
- The TDAP flap can be defatted as long as several centimeters of fat are preserved around the perforator.
- The donor site is prone to seroma formation, so closed suction drains should be utilized for extended durations if necessary. We have not found quilting sutures or hemostatic agents to be of significant help in shortening drain duration.

## References

1. Quillen CG. Latissimus dorsi myocutaneous flaps in head and neck reconstruction. Plast Reconstr Surg 1979; 63(5):664–670
2. Harii K, Asato H, Yoshimura K, Sugawara Y, Nakatsuka T, Ueda K. One-stage transfer of the latissimus dorsi muscle for reanimation of a paralyzed face: a new alternative. Plast Reconstr Surg 1998;102(4):941–951
3. Angrigiani C, Grilli D, Siebert J. Latissimus dorsi musculocutaneous flap without muscle. Plast Reconstr Surg 1995;96(7):1608–1614
4. Mun GH, Lee SJ, Jeon BJ. Perforator topography of the thoracodorsal artery perforator flap. Plast Reconstr Surg 2008;121(2):497–504
5. Kim JT. Latissimus dorsi perforator flap. Clin Plast Surg 2003;30(3):403–431
6. Lee SH, Mun GH. Transverse thoracodorsal artery perforator flaps: experience with 31 free flaps. J Plast Reconstr Aesthet Surg 2008;61(4):372–379
7. Hamdi M, Decorte T, Demuynck M, et al. Shoulder function after harvesting a thoracodorsal artery perforator flap. Plast Reconstr Surg 2008;122(4):1111–1117, discussion 1118–1119

# 26 Scapular and Parascapular Flaps

*Sydney Ch'ng and Roman J. Skoracki*

## Introduction

The first anatomical study of the scapular fasciocutaneous flap was published by dos Santos[1] in 1980 based on bilateral dissections of 35 cadavers. Gilbert and Teot[2] published the first clinical series in 1982, using the flap for ankle resurfacing in four patients. Swartz et al[3] introduced the inclusion of a vascularized segment of the lateral scapular bone in 1986, and this osseocutaneous free flap was subsequently modified and improved by Coleman and Sultan.[4] More recently, Seneviratne et al[5] described the scapular tip as a potential variant of the osseous component.

The osseocutaneous scapular free flap is a good alternative for osseous reconstruction of mandibular or maxillary defects where the fibular free flap is contraindicated or unavailable.[5,6,7,8,9] We have also found it useful for reconstruction of composite scalp defects when harvested as a chimeric free flap with the latissimus dorsi muscle.[10]

### Advantages

1. Hidden donor-site scar in most clothes.
2. Long and large-caliber vascular pedicle, especially if the subscapular vessels are included with the pedicle.
3. A large amount of bone can be harvested from the scapula, including the medial border, lateral border, and the scapular tip.
4. Various chimeric flap configurations (including skin, bone, muscle flaps) allow freedom in orientation of the different flap components to tailor for composite defects.
5. Skin portion is non- or minimally hair bearing.

### Disadvantages

1. Poorer quality of bone stock for osseointegration.
2. Risk for restricted shoulder abduction in some patients.

## Anatomy

### Landmarks

The fasciocutaneous flap from this donor site can be oriented horizontally (scapular flap), or vertically (parascapular flap), or both ways if two skin islands are dissected based on the two terminal cutaneous branches of the circumflex scapular artery.

The axis of a scapular flap skin island extends horizontally from the triangular space (bound by the long head of the triceps muscle laterally, the teres major inferiorly, and the teres minor and subscapularis superiorly), which is situated at the lateral border of the scapula two-fifths of the way from the scapular spine to the scapular tip, to the posterior midline. The vertical dimension of the flap spans the distance between the scapular spine and the scapular angle. The parascapular flap skin island is centered vertically or obliquely along a line between the triangular space and the posterior superior iliac spine. Skin flap dimensions of 5 to 7 cm in width and 10 to 15 cm in length can usually allow for easy primary closure.

A vascularized bone segment from the lateral scapular border, which receives blood from the circumflex scapular artery either directly or via its musculoperiosteal branches to the teres minor and major, can be harvested from this region, alone or in combination with a fasciocutaneous flap component. A segment of bone (usually ~ 3 × 11 cm in size) from the scapular angle to within 1 cm of the articular capsule can be harvested. The scapular tip (3 × 20 cm with intrinsic curvature) based on the angular branch is another option when the thoracodorsal pedicle is included. Although it is less commonly used, harvest of the medial scapular border (3 × 12 to 14 cm) has also been described.[6]

## Vascular Anatomy

The subscapular artery (external diameter of 5 to 6 mm) originates from the axillary artery, and after an average course of 2.2 cm, divides into the circumflex scapular artery (external diameter 2.5 to 3.5 mm) and thoracodorsal artery (external diameter 3 to 4 mm) (**Fig. 26.1**).

The circumflex scapular artery passes posteriorly into the triangular space and is 3 to 4 cm long. In the triangular space, the circumflex scapular artery gives off subscapular, infrascapular, and direct muscular branches to the teres major and teres minor muscles. The subscapular branch runs between the subscapularis muscle and the scapula. The infrascapular branch passes between the scapula and the infraspinatus muscle, forming a collateral anastomotic network with the suprascapular artery, a branch of the thyrocervical trunk. Beyond these branches, the artery is called the descending branch of the circumflex scapular artery, and as it emerges from the triangular space, it divides into its terminal branches; the cutaneous scapular artery (traveling horizontally) and the cutaneous parascapular artery (descending vertically).[6]

The vascular supply to the lateral border of the scapula comes from the musculoperiosteal branches off the circumflex scapular artery just before it enters the triangular space. The scapular tip is supplied by the angular branch that generally originates from the thoracodorsal artery (see below). Fasciomusculoperiosteal branches arising from the scapular cutaneous artery as it travels through the infraspinatus muscle supply the medial scapular border.

The thoracodorsal artery travels an average of 8.4 cm before dividing into the serratus anterior and latissimus dorsi branches. The angular artery arises from the latissimus dorsi branch in 51% of cases, from the serratus anterior branch in 25%, as the third branch of a trifurcation of the terminal thoracodorsal vessel in 20%, and as a branch of the thoracodorsal vessels arising proximal to its bifurcation into latissimus and serratus branches in 4%.[5] It travels parallel to, and just deep and inferior to, the cephalad (medial) border of the latissimus dorsi muscle in a layer of fat. As it approaches the tip of the scapula, it divides into two or three branches terminating in the soft tissues attached to the scapula tip (**Fig. 26.2**). At its origin it measures 2 to 2.5 mm in diameter and has an average length of 7 cm.

The venous anatomy parallels the arterial anatomy.

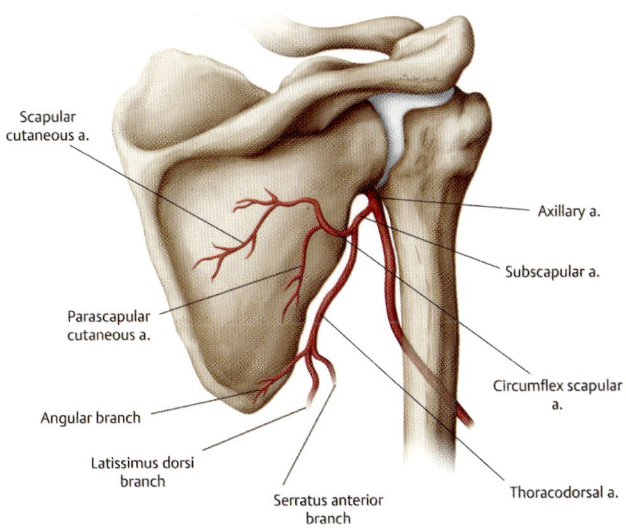


**Fig. 26.1** Vascular anatomy of the subscapular system, showing arteries supplying the scapula, scapular and parascapular skin flaps, and latissimus dorsi and serratus anterior muscles.

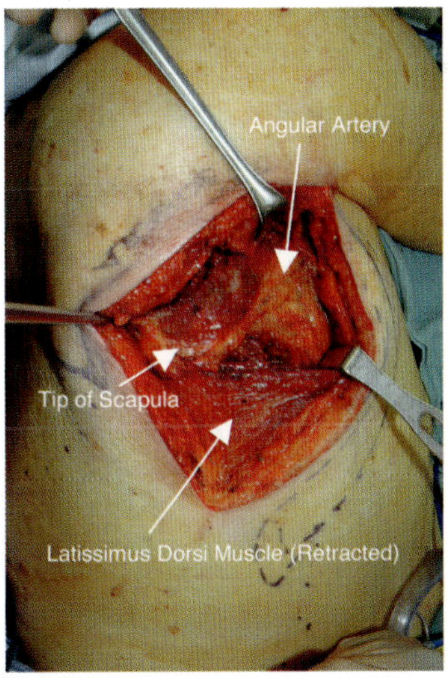


**Fig. 26.2** The angular artery is a branch of the thoracodorsal artery (and vein) and can be found traveling in the fat pad deep to the latissimus dorsi muscle to the tip of the scapula, as can be seen here in this dissection of the patient's right scapula.

## Preoperative Considerations

No significant long-term morbidity has been associated with the scapular flap donor site. Limited shoulder abduction of up to 6 months can be expected following harvest of an osseous component, but thereafter the range of movement should normalize.[7,8]

Specific patient requirements, such as use of a cane on one side, may favor harvest of the contralateral scapula. Similarly, a history of prior axillary surgery, such as axillary lymph node dissection, and prior axillary radiation therapy, or upper limb lymphedema should prompt use of the contralateral scapula. Otherwise, the ipsilateral scapula is generally used for convenience of patient positioning and flap configuration.

### Mandibular Reconstruction

For mandibular reconstruction, the lateral scapula is often favored due to the thicker cortical bone along the lateral border. When the flap is placed with the lateral edge inferiorly, better cosmesis is achieved with the external contour of the jaw. In this orientation, a tapered neo-alveolus results that is suitable for retention of a conventional denture but poor for osseointegration. When the lateral edge is placed superior, the opposite is true. To increase the vertical height of the neomandible it is possible to cut the bone more medially to match the native mandible. Closing wedge osteotomies can be performed if additional bone branches are preserved.

For reconstruction of a bilateral mandibular defect, especially when combined with total glossectomy, the scapular angle is a good reconstructive option. The osseous flap is oriented in a transverse direction so that the angle of the scapula replaces the mentum and the dorsal surface of the scapula is oriented cephalad (**Fig. 26.3**). Grooves 1.0 to 1.5 cm deep are cut into the body of the mandible bilaterally; they should be large enough to precisely accommodate the width of the medial and lateral scapular bone in a tongue-in-groove manner.[9]

### Maxillary Reconstruction

The scapular angle is preferred for maxillary reconstruction due to the longer pedicle length. It is oriented either vertically or horizontally depending on the defect.[9]

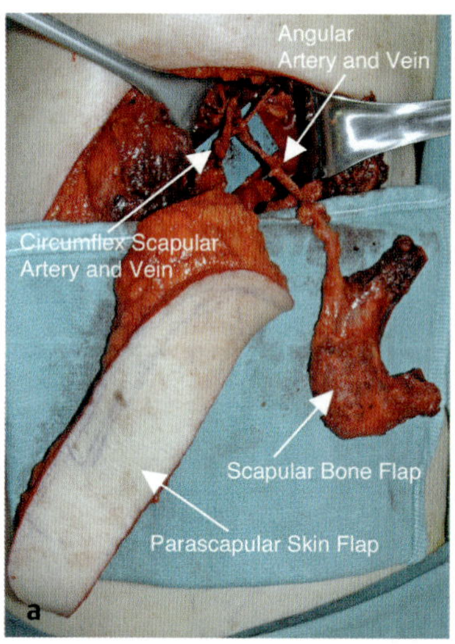


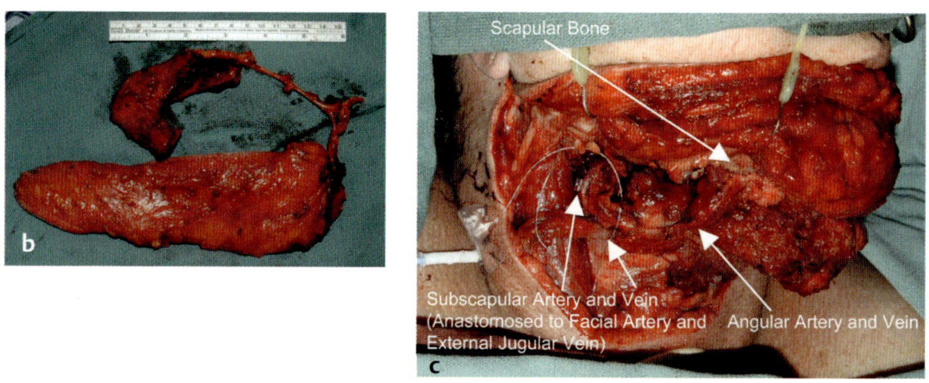


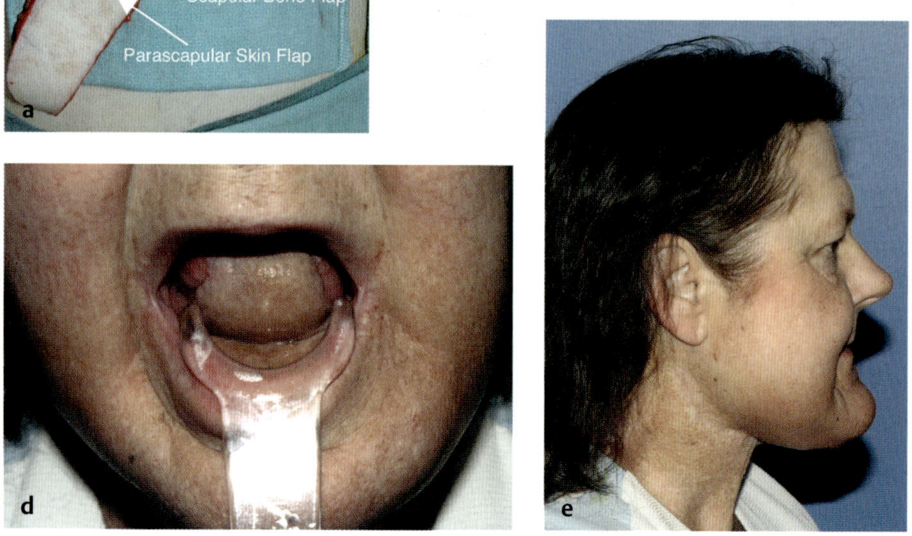


**Fig. 26.3** **(a)** The scapular tip flap, based on the angular branch of the thoracodorsal artery harvested with a parascapular cutaneous flap based on the parascapular cutaneous branch of the circumflex scapular artery. **(b)** After dissection, the chimeric flap based on the subscapular artery and vein is complete. **(c)** An anterior mandibular defect is reconstructed with the scapular tip. **(d)** The parascapular skin flap is used to reconstruct the floor of the mouth and ventral tongue. **(e)** Postoperative result.

When placed horizontally, the scapular angle is ideal for infrastructural defects and can replace the entire palatoalveolar complex without any contouring osteotomies. Unfortunately, the bone quality at the scapular angle and the medial border in this orientation is inadequate for placement of osseointegrated implants without additional bone grafting.

When oriented vertically, the ipsilateral scapular angle flap insets to a hemimaxillectomy defect with its convexity matching that of the alveolus, and with its pedicle entering the angle posteriorly. In this arrangement, the broader lateral edge is oriented inferiorly, with the thicker cortical bone ending up in the incisor to premolar region, which is better for dental implant osseointegration. Maintaining the periosteum and a cuff of muscle on this surface, which is then allowed to remucosalize, will give an immobile surface suitable for a denture. The thinner, more medial scapular bone can be fractured to simulate the zygomaticonasal contour. Soft tissue reconstruction of the palate can be achieved by using teres major or latissimus dorsi oriented horizontally.

### Calvarial Reconstruction

The broad and gently curved bone of the scapula is uniquely similar to the calvaria in thickness. Combined with the latissimus dorsi muscle and an overlying skin graft, the chimeric flap is well suited for reconstruction of full-thickness scalp and cranial defects (**Fig. 26.4**).

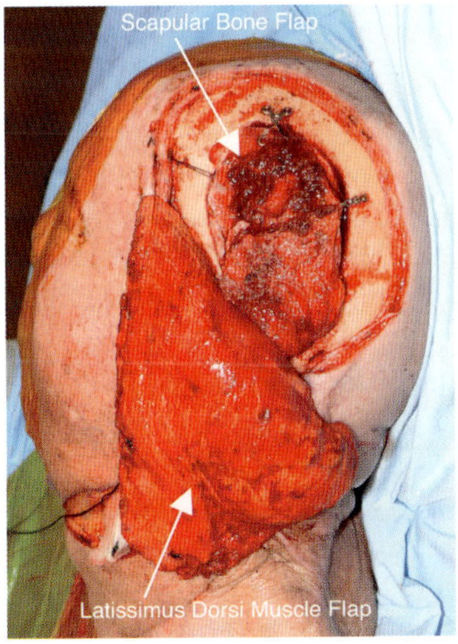


**Fig. 26.4** A chimeric flap, including the lateral scapular bone and latissimus dorsi muscle, to reconstruct a combined scalp and calvarial defect.

## Patient Positioning and Skin Markings

To facilitate transition from ablation to reconstruction, the patient is positioned and prepped at the time of ablation on a beanbag in the lateral decubitus position. The pelvis is securely strapped to the operating table to allow safe rotation intraoperatively.

For the ablative component of the procedure, the operating table is rotated 45°, thus bringing the patient back close to horizontal. The table is then rotated ~ 60° in the opposite direction for the reconstructive phase to allow access for flap harvest, thereby eliminating the need for patient repositioning during the surgery. For access to the flap, the scapular angle needs to be readily palpable. The entire ipsilateral upper limb is prepared to the elbow and is kept in the operating field to allow for flexion and abduction of the shoulder as required.

A practical point for consideration with this method of patient positioning is that it does not allow full access to the horizontal scapular skin flap. The parascapular flap is therefore favored unless a second skin paddle is required.

The triangular space, bounded superiorly by the teres minor muscle, inferiorly by the teres major muscle, and laterally by the long head of the triceps, is palpable in a thin patient. It corresponds to a point two-fifths of the distance between the scapular spine and the scapular angle on the lateral border of the scapula (**Fig. 26.5**). The axis of the scapular flap extends from the triangular space horizontally to the posterior midline, and the axis of the parascapular flap extends from the triangular space along the lateral scapular border to the posterior superior iliac spine. The skin territory of the scapular flap extends from the posterior axillary line laterally to the midline medially, and that of the parascapular flap from just inferior to the triangular space to halfway between the scapular angle and the posterior superior iliac spine. The width of either skin flap is planned to allow for primary closure of the donor site.

## Operative Technique

### Parascapular Skin Paddle

The patient is positioned as described above, and the upper extremity is prepared and draped in the operative field. The triangular space is identified by

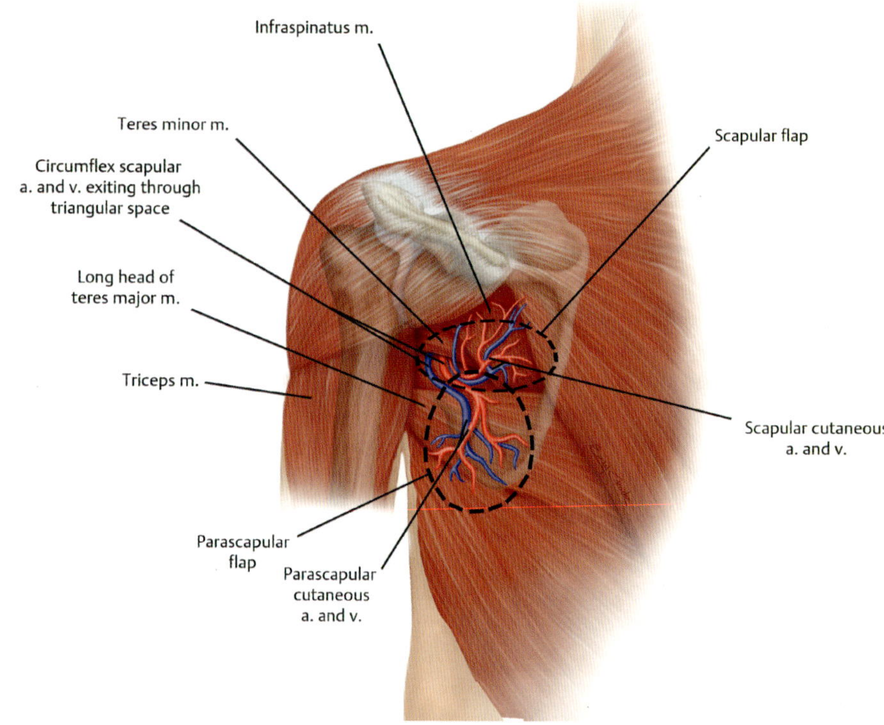


**Fig. 26.5** A transverse skin flap can be elevated over the scapula based on the scapular cutaneous artery and vein, or an oblique skin flap can be elevated along the lateral border of the scapula based on the parascapular cutaneous artery and vein, both terminal branches of the circumflex scapular artery and vein, which can be found in the triangular space.

palpation or by percutaneous Doppler ultrasound examination. A line drawn inferiorly along the lateral border of the scapula from the triangular space represents the course of the parascapular cutaneous vessels. The flap is centered over this line and may be designed to be as long as 30 to 35 cm.

Dissection of the flap may begin with initial pedicle identification. The superolateral incision is performed first, down to the muscular aponeurosis covering the infraspinatus, the teres minor and major, and the long head of the triceps muscles. Superficial to this aponeurotic layer is a loose subfascial areolar plane that allows for a bloodless dissection. The descending branch of the circumflex scapular vessel emerging from the triangular space is identified, and the flap markings may be adjusted as necessary. The medial flap incision is then made, facilitating dissection and muscular retraction beyond this point. The dissection then continues into the triangular space with ligation of the numerous muscular and periosteal branches. Once the infrascapular branch is ligated, the circumflex scapular vessels are reached.

In the alternate approach of distal to proximal flap elevation, careful skin island planning is necessary. Distal skin incisions are made down to the latissimus dorsi. Dissection proceeds deep to the dorsal thoracic fascia until the teres major and minor muscles are encountered, and the circumflex scapular pedicle with its branches is visualized in the triangular space. Proximal skin incisions are then completed to isolate the flap on its vascular pedicle.

Dissection of the proximal trunk of the circumflex scapular vessels to increase the vessel length by an additional 4 to 6 cm is facilitated by shoulder abduction and flexion and may be further improved by an axillary counterincision, allowing better exposure of the axillary vessels.

## Scapular Skin Paddle

A line drawn parallel to the scapular spine from the triangular space to the patient's posterior midline represents the course of the scapular cutaneous vessels. The flap is centered over this line and may extend from the posterior axillary line to the midline.

The superolateral incision is performed as previously described to identify the cutaneous branches of the circumflex scapular vessels emerging from the triangular space. The inferior flap incision is made, facilitating dissection and muscular retraction beyond this point. The dissection then continues into the triangular space with ligation of the numerous muscular and periosteal branches. The remainder of the dissection proceeds as outlined in the previous section.

To minimize flap ischemia, particularly if patient repositioning is necessary, much of the donor site can be closed before the flap vessels are divided. This also allows observation of flap perfusion on the pedicle alone. If the scapular or parascapular flaps are to be combined with additional chimeric flap components, division of the teres major muscle is usually necessary to deliver the skin component with the remaining flap on a single pedicle. The teres minor muscle is repaired during donor-site closure.

## Lateral Scapular Bone Flap

The patient is positioned and is prepared as outlined in the previous sections. Depending on the defect to be reconstructed, a cutaneous island may be included, as described above. As described, the circumflex scapular vessels are exposed as they exit the triangular space. Careful dissection into the triangular space exposes several small muscular and musculoperiosteal branches that enter the musculature originating and inserting on the lateral border of the scapula **(Fig. 26.6)**. These branches are

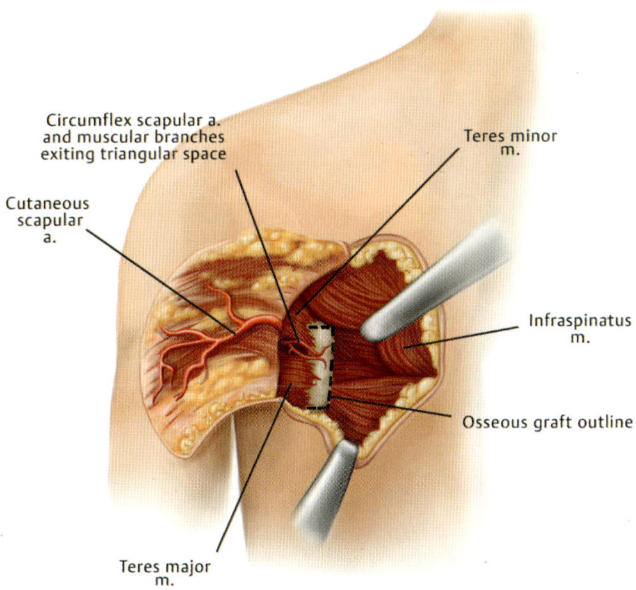


**Fig. 26.6** The vascular supply to the lateral scapular bone flap comes from the musculoperiosteal branches of the circumflex scapular artery arising from the triangular space. A skin paddle based on the scapular cutaneous artery, which is a terminal branch of the circumflex scapular artery, is also shown being dissected.

cautiously preserved. The desired segment of bone is palpated and outlined along the lateral border of the scapula, and as much as 3 cm in width and 11 cm in length is harvested. The infraspinatus muscle can be retracted laterally to better expose this area. The incision is then carried down to the bone, dividing muscle fibers of the teres minor superiorly and teres major inferiorly as well as the underlying periosteum along the desired outline. The scapula tip is not included with this flap. Osteotomies are then performed along this outline using an oscillating or reciprocating saw. Elevation of the scapula by the tip will facilitate the osteotomies. The cephalad osteotomy should be located at least 1 cm below the shoulder joint capsule to avoid inadvertent entry and injury to the joint. The bone segment can then be retracted laterally, exposing the underlying fibers of the subscapularis muscle, which are then divided, leaving a thin stippling of muscle on the bone to avoid damage to the periosteal blood supply. The vascular dissection continues proximally until the desired length of vascular pedicle is achieved. Again, an axillary counterincision may be necessary to facilitate this, as previously discussed.

## Medial Scapular Bone Flap

A scapular or parascapular skin flap is outlined, as previously described, and the lateral incisions are made. The medial portion of the flap, overlying the medial scapular border, is left attached. The pedicle dissection proceeds as previously described. The medial or distal portion of the flap remains attached by its fascial and muscular attachments to the medial scapula, which can be exposed by incising the skin island inferior and superior to this area. The desired bone segment is outlined around these attachments. As much as 3 cm in width and 12 cm in length can be harvested between the scapular spine and the tip. The medial edge of the bone is palpated and identified by detaching the rhomboid muscle. The scapula is lifted off the chest wall, and the serratus anterior muscle is also divided along the medial border of the bone. A tunnel is then created between the infraspinatus muscle and the scapula, 3 to 4 cm lateral to the attachment of the flap to the medial edge of the scapula. The muscle is then incised along this line, exposing the scapular periosteum below **(Fig. 26.7)**. Osteotomies are performed with an oscillating or reciprocating saw, and attachments of the rhomboid major, subscapularis, and serratus anterior muscles are divided, leaving only a thin stippling of muscle on the bone and thereby freeing the bone from its bed.

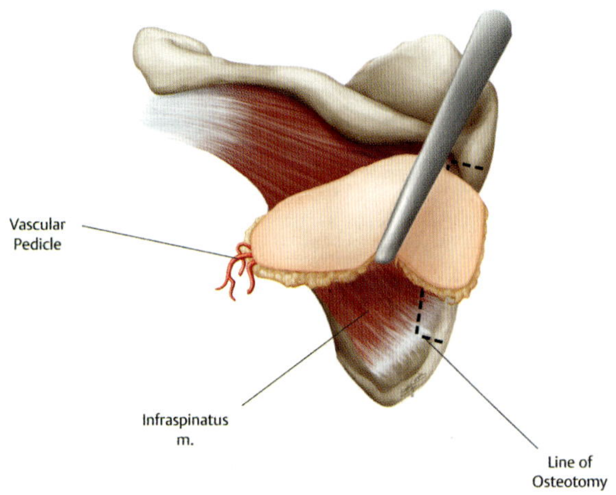


**Fig. 26.7** The scapular cutaneous artery, a terminal branch of the circumflex scapular artery, supplies the medial scapular bone flap. It is shown here being elevated with a transversely oriented skin paddle, but can be elevated as a strictly osseous flap by dissecting the scapular cutaneous artery from the subcutaneous adipose tissue.

### Scapular Tip Bone Flap Based on the Angular Artery

As with the lateral and medial scapular flaps, exposure is obtained through a parascapular cutaneous free flap or the latissimus dorsi myocutaneous free flap harvest incisions. If only a scapular osseous free flap is indicated to reconstruct a given defect, then an incision over the lateral border of the scapula should be made. The angular branch pedicle originates from thoracodorsal vessels and is identified by retracting the latissimus dorsi muscle inferiorly **(Fig. 26.2)**. The teres major muscle is partially released from the lateral border of the scapula, and the rhomboid major muscle is partially released from the medial border of the scapula. The infraspinatus muscle is also partially elevated from the superficial surface of the scapula just enough to expose the amount of bone needed. On completion of osteotomies, the underlying fibers of the subscapularis muscle are divided.

Once the flap harvest is complete for this flap and as well as the lateral and medial scapular flaps, the divided musculature is sutured back to the scapula. Drill holes may facilitate this, although the bone tends to be thin enough to allow direct suturing through the scapula.

## ■ Donor-Site Care

Skin flaps with dimensions as noted above can usually be closed primarily. A "pinch test" is used to confirm the possibility of primary closure, which is preferable given commonly poor skin graft take on the back. As mentioned, muscles that attach to the scapular bone are reattached to the scapular remnant when divided, either through drill holes or by use of a sturdy needle to pierce the thin central bone of the scapula without the need for a drill. Closed suction drains are used. We do not immobilize the shoulder. Within several days after surgery, range of motion exercises are started as long as the wound closure is intact and healing well. Range of motion is generally regained in a month. For poorly compliant patients, a formal consultation with a physical therapist is indicated.

### Pearls and Pitfalls

- The scapular flap is a useful second-line option for mandibular and maxillary reconstruction when the fibular flap is not available. It has also been used as a chimeric flap for composite scalp and calvarial reconstruction.
- The chimeric scapular bone flap combined with scapular or parascapular skin and the latissimus dorsi and/or serratus anterior muscles allow for complex multisurface reconstruction with a single anastomosis, which may be indicated in patients with a recipient vessel-depleted neck.
- The scapular (transverse) or parascapular (oblique) skin paddle is based on the circumflex scapular artery, as is the lateral and medial scapular bone, while the scapular tip is based on the angular branch of the thoracodorsal artery.
- The lateral scapular bone or the scapular tip is usually preferred over the medial bone due to ease of dissection and better blood supply.
- The circumflex scapular artery is located coming through the triangular space formed by the teres major, teres minor, and long head of the triceps, about two-fifths the distance from the scapular spine to the scapular tip.
- The angular branch is found beneath the latissimus dorsi muscle, extending from the thoracodorsal artery to the scapular tip within a pad of fat.
- The curved tip of the scapula can be used to reconstruct the anterior mandible or maxilla when oriented transversely, but it does not provide sufficient bone stock for osseointegrated implants. We fixate the bone in a tongue-in-groove manner to the native mandible for stability.
- Detached muscles, such as the teres major laterally and the rhomboid major medially, should be reattached to the remaining scapula by suturing the muscle to the bone. This can be accomplished by drilling holes in the scapula or by using a heavy needle to pierce the thin central scapular bone.

## References


1. dos Santos LF. The scapular flap: a new microsurgical free flap. Rev Bras Cir 1980;70:133–144
2. Gilbert A, Teot L. The free scapular flap. Plast Reconstr Surg 1982;69(4):601–604
3. Swartz WM, Banis JC, Newton ED, Ramasastry SS, Jones NF, Acland R. The osteocutaneous scapular flap for mandibular and maxillary reconstruction. Plast Reconstr Surg 1986;77(4):530–545
4. Coleman JJ III, Sultan MR. The bipedicled osteocutaneous scapula flap: a new subscapular system free flap. Plast Reconstr Surg 1991;87(4):682–692
5. Seneviratne S, Duong C, Taylor GI. The angular branch of the thoracodorsal artery and its blood supply to the inferior angle of the scapula: an anatomical study. Plast Reconstr Surg 1999;104(1):85–88
6. Urken ML, Bridger AG, Zur KB, Genden EM. The scapular osteofasciocutaneous flap: a 12-year experience. Arch Otolaryngol Head Neck Surg 2001;127(7):862–869
7. Miles BA, Gilbert RW. Maxillary reconstruction with the scapular angle osteomyogenous free flap. Arch Otolaryngol Head Neck Surg 2011;137(11):1130–1135
8. Clark JR, Vesely M, Gilbert R. Scapular angle osteomyogenous flap in postmaxillectomy reconstruction: defect, reconstruction, shoulder function, and harvest technique. Head Neck 2008;30(1):10–20
9. Hanasono MM, Skoracki RJ. The scapular tip osseous free flap as an alternative for anterior mandibular reconstruction. Plast Reconstr Surg 2010;125(4):164e–166e
10. Ch'ng S, Clark JR. The scapular angle adds versatility to the latissimus dorsi free flap in complicated scalp reconstruction. J Plast Reconstr Aesthet Surg 2011;64(9):e248–e249

# 27 Free Jejunal and Supercharged Jejunal Flaps

*Peirong Yu*

## Introduction

In 1947, Longmire[1] modified the Roux technique of pedicled bowel transfer for esophageal reconstruction by anastomosing a mesenteric vessel to the internal mammary artery to augment the blood supply of the distal bowel. Complete revascularization of the intestinal transfers was then conducted in animal experiments. In 1959, Seidenberg[2] reported the first clinical case of the free jejunal flap for esophageal reconstruction. This was the first free flap performed in humans. The free jejunal flap became popular in the early 1980s for pharyngoesophageal reconstruction.[3,4] Due to the segmental blood supply, the use of free jejunal flaps is limited to partial defects in the cervical esophagus. Once the esophageal defect is greater than 20 cm, longer jejunal segments based on multiple mesenteric vessels are necessary, with a "supercharging technique." The supercharged jejunal flap can replace the entire esophagus and pharynx up to the base of the tongue.[5]

### Anatomy

The small intestine is ~ 7 m long. The duodenum transitions into the jejunum at the ligament of Treitz. The jejunum and ileum are suspended from the posterior wall of the abdomen by mesentery, where the mesenteric blood vessels are located. The small intestine receives its blood supply from the superior mesenteric artery (SMA), except for the proximal half of the duodenum, which is supplied by the celiac artery. The SMA originates from the abdominal aorta ~ 1 cm inferior to the takeoff of the celiac artery. It then passes behind the neck of the pancreas and the splenic vein and gives off numerous mesenteric branches to supply the small bowel **(Fig. 27.1)**. The mesenteric branches form a network of arcade vessels with anastomoses with adjacent branches. Veins accompany the mesenteric branches and drain into the superior mesenteric vein, which ultimately joins the splenic vein to empty into the portal system.

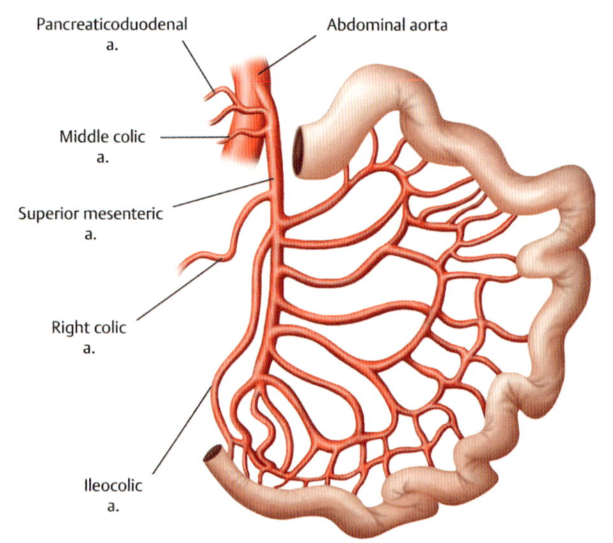


**Fig. 27.1** Vascular anatomy of the small intestine. The small bowel receives segmental blood supply from several mesenteric branches of the superior mesentery artery (SMA).

## Preoperative Considerations

Preoperative assessment includes evaluation of the patient's cardiopulmonary, renal, and nutritional status. Many head and neck cancer patients have concomitant cardiovascular and pulmonary diseases. A thorough medical evaluation, including pulmonary function tests, is often necessary. The patient's cardiopulmonary function should be optimized before surgery. Severe comorbid diseases and previous intra-abdominal surgeries are relative contraindications for jejunal flap harvest. On the day before surgery, the patient should consume only a liquid diet. A mechanical bowel preparation is not routinely per-

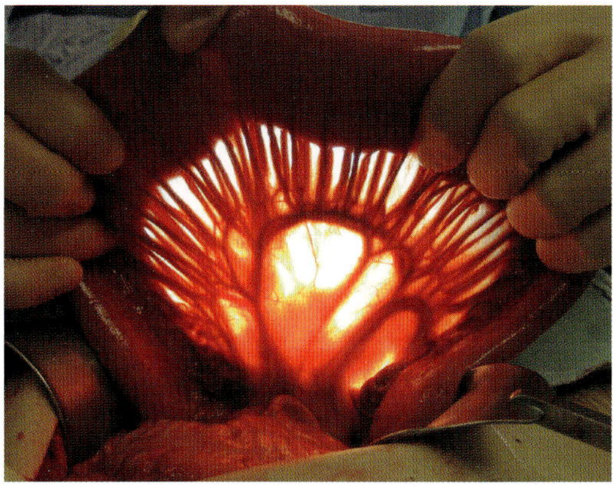

**Fig. 27.2** The anatomy of the mesenteric vessels can be transilluminated with a fiberoptic light as backlighting.

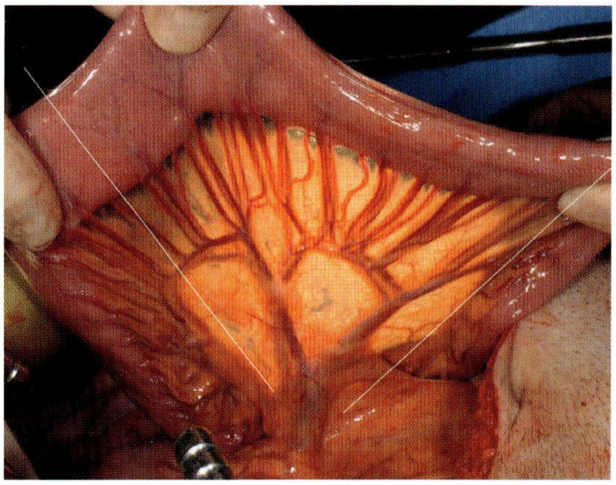

**Fig. 27.3** The length of the jejunal flap is determined based on the main mesenteric branch, usually the second or third.

formed. Three surgical teams are usually involved: the head and neck surgery team, reconstructive surgery team, and the general surgery team. Therefore, appropriate preoperative consultations with other team members should be obtained. A workflow should be established to minimize operative time. Flap harvesting can be performed simultaneously with tumor ablation. Once the ablative surgeons are finished, the reconstructive team may transfer the flap to the head and neck while the general surgery team begins to re-establish small bowel continuity, place gastrointestinal feeding tubes if necessary, and complete the abdominal wound closure.

# Operative Technique

## Free Jejunal Flap

The abdomen is entered through an upper midline incision. The intra-abdominal organs and the entire small bowel are examined before preparing for the jejunal flap. The segment of jejunum chosen is usually 40 cm from the ligament of Treitz over the second (most commonly) or third mesentery branch. The length of the jejunal flap is usually 15 to 20 cm. The mesentery is transilluminated with a sterile fiberoptic light source as backlighting to reveal the mesentery arcades **(Fig. 27.2)**. Once the second or third mesentery vessels are chosen, the segment of the jejunum to be harvested is determined **(Fig. 27.3)**. A window in the mesentery close to the bowel is created between the terminal arcade vessels at each end of the jejunal segment to be taken. Similarly, a larger window is created on each side of the main mesentery branch—the vascular pedicle. The mesentery between the main mesentery branch vessels is rather avascular and can be divided with an electric cautery. The mesentery arcade vessels are then ligated with 3–0 silk ties and are divided all the way to the bowel wall **(Fig. 27.4)**. Meticulous control of crossing vessels is important, as even small vessels can form a significant mesenteric hematoma and threaten the safety of the flap. The main trunk of the vascular pedicle is cleaned of peritoneal lining, lymphatics, and fat for ~ 2 cm. The mesenteric veins are extremely thin and delicate. They should be handled with extreme caution to prevent injury to them.

Once the vascular pedicle is isolated, the fan-shaped mesentery corresponding to the jejunal flap is divided, and the bowel is ready to be divided with a gastrointestinal stapling device **(Fig. 27.5)**. A marking suture is placed at the proximal end of the jejunal flap for orientation purposes. The vascular pedicle is then ligated with 2–0 silk ties and is divided. The flap is taken to a back table. The staple lines on each end of the bowel are cut away to empty the bowel con-

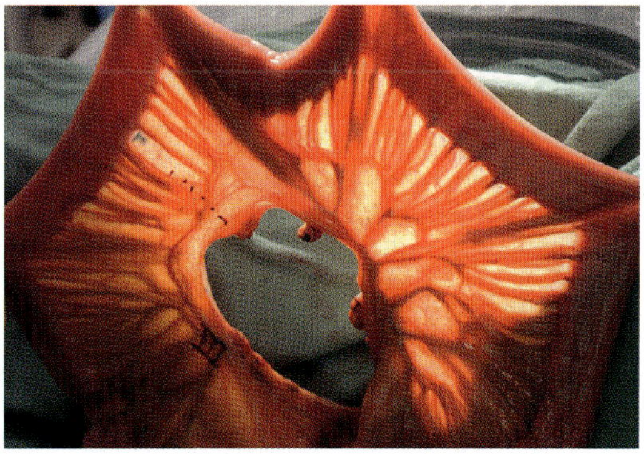

**Fig. 27.4** The mesentery on each side of the mesentery branch is divided. The arcade vessels are ligated with 3–0 silk ties.

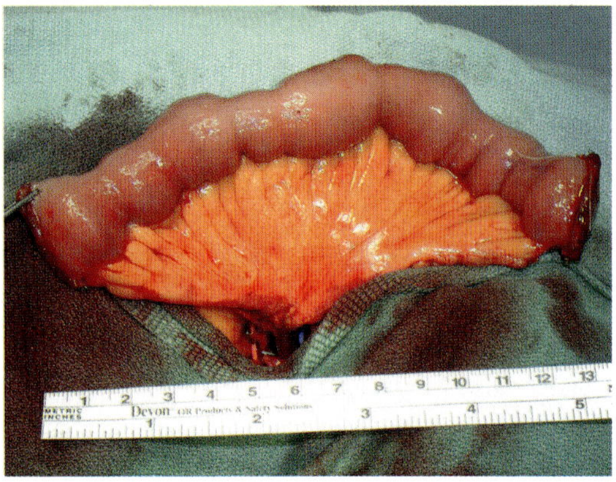

**Fig. 27.5** The jejunal segment is divided with a gastrointestinal stapling device once the vascular pedicle is isolated.

tents. The lumen is then irrigated with cold normal saline until clear. The flap is then ready for transfer. The general surgery team begins bowel anastomosis to restore small bowel continuity, placement of a feeding jejunostomy tube distal to the bowel anastomosis (or a gastrostomy), and abdominal closure while the reconstructive team proceeds with reconstruction in the neck.

## Supercharged Jejunal Flap

### Planning

Total esophageal reconstruction with the supercharged jejunal flap is an extremely complex procedure with significant surgical risks. The patients are often older and have cardiopulmonary comorbidities. Surgery itself involves two major cavities, the peritoneal cavity and the chest cavity, as well as the neck. Significant third spacing and fluid shifts are common after such a lengthy major surgery. Therefore, meticulous operative planning and intraoperative execution are essential. To minimize the operating time, it is important to establish a coordinated flow between the various teams. If a thoracotomy is required, the patient is first placed in a lateral decubitus position and then is switched to supine. While the ablative surgical team is operating in the abdomen, the reconstructive surgeons can start to prepare recipient vessels in the neck. The teams then change positions. The reconstructive surgeons now prepare the jejunal flap while the ablative surgeons expose the proximal esophagus through the neck incision and remove the manubrium and clavicular head if a substernal approach is desired. The jejunal conduit is then passed through the chest and into the neck, and the teams switch positions again. The reconstructive surgeons revascularize the proximal jejunum, complete the esophagojejunal anastomosis in the neck, and fashion the monitoring segment while the other surgical team restores gastrointestinal continuity in the abdomen. When the procedure is properly organized, no time is wasted for all teams involved. Clear communication between surgical teams and anesthesia regarding fluid resuscitation and avoidance of vasopressor medications is imperative, because different disciplines may manage these issues differently.

### Flap Harvesting

Once resection is complete, the length of the esophageal defect is measured to estimate the length of the conduit needed.[5] Typically, the supercharged jejunal flap consists of a pedicled portion, usually based on the fourth mesentery branch, and a supercharged portion based on the second mesentery branch. With backlighting transillumination, the first mesenteric branch beyond the ligament of Treitz is identified and is preserved to maintain blood supply to the distal duodenum and most proximal portion of the jejunum. The second mesenteric branch is dissected out for later supercharging. In the simplest cases, the mesentery between the second and third branches is divided up to the serosal border, allowing the jejunal segment to unfurl **(Fig. 27.6)**. This step helps straighten the natural sinusoidal properties of the small bowel and reduce redundancy. If more length is required, the third mesenteric branch is ligated and divided **(Fig. 27.7)**. Secondary arcade vessels between the third and fourth mesenteric branches are preserved, so that the segment of bowel normally supplied by the third branch is now supplied by the pedicled fourth branch through intact

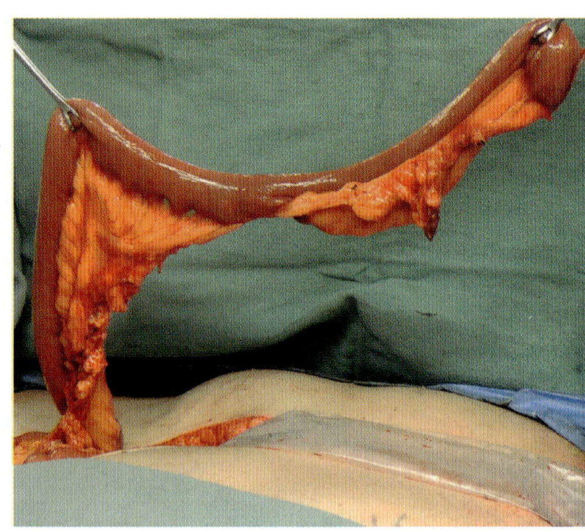

**Fig. 27.6** In preparation of the supercharged jejunal flap, the mesentery between the second and third mesenteric branch vessels is divided up to the serosal border, allowing the jejunal segment to unfurl. The second mesenteric vessels are "supercharged" to the vessels in the neck or the internal mammary vessels. The third mesenteric vessels are left intact to serve as the vascular pedicle for the pedicled portion of the jejunal flap.

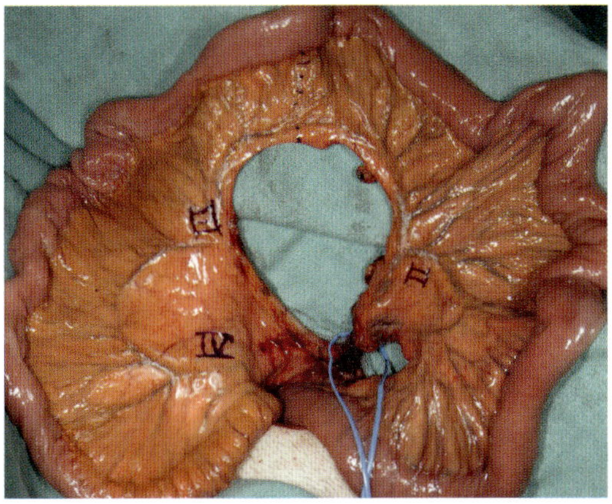

**Fig. 27.7** When more length is needed, the third mesenteric branch is ligated and divided. The mesentery between the second and third mesenteric vessels is divided to the serosal border of the jejunum while the arcade vessels between the third and fourth mesenteric vessels are kept intact so that the small bowel normally perfused by the third branch can be perfused by the pedicled fourth branch via these arcade connections.

arcade vessels. This approach is the most common. If still greater length is required, such as in patients with a very long torso or a concomitant total laryngopharyngectomy, the fourth mesenteric branch can also be ligated and divided. In these cases, only the mesentery between the third and fourth branches is divided to the serosal border, while the arcade connections are preserved between the second and third branches, and between the fourth and fifth branches. The third segment receives perfusion from the supercharged second segment, and the fourth segment receives perfusion from the pedicled fifth branch. Once adequate length is achieved, the jejunum is divided proximally with a linear cutting stapler, typically 30 to 40 cm distal to the ligament of Treitz.

## Flap Transfer

There are two potential routes to deliver the jejunal flap to the neck: retrocardiac, which is the orthotopic route, or substernal, which is the heterotopic route.[5] The former is used for patients undergoing immediate reconstruction. The latter is usually reserved for patients undergoing a delayed reconstruction after previous failed esophageal reconstruction. It can also be used for immediate reconstruction if the use of internal mammary vessels as recipient vessels is desired. In these cases, portions of the manubrium, clavicular head, and first rib are removed to enlarge the thoracic inlet and to avoid constriction on the jejunal conduit. With either route, transfer is accomplished using a sterile laparoscopic camera bag to protect the conduit and to avoid traction injury to the arcade vessels **(Fig. 27.8)**. Once the jejunal flap is

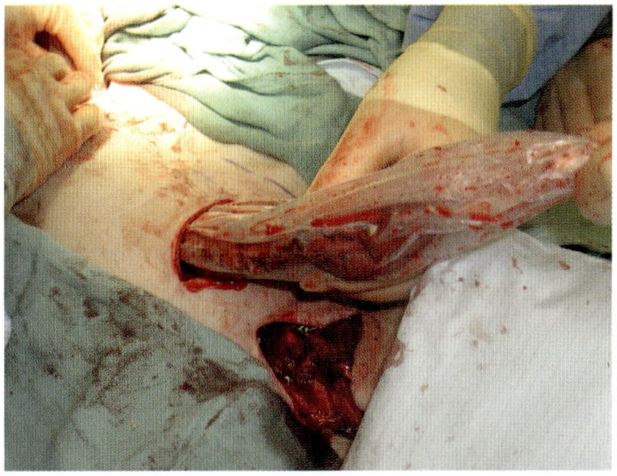

**Fig. 27.8** The small bowel and its mesentery are placed in a plastic bag and are pulled to the neck through the chest. The bag protects the mesentery vessels from evulsion injury.

pulled up to the neck, vascular anastomoses are performed, most commonly to the internal mammary vessels (substernal route) or the transverse cervical vessels (retrocardiac route). Excess length of jejunal conduit is removed to minimize redundancy in the neck. The proximal 3 to 5 cm of jejunum based on one or two terminal arcade vessels is exteriorized as a postperative monitoring segment, as with free jejunal flap reconstruction. Esophagojejunal anastomosis is then performed in the neck using a single layer of 3–0 polyglactin suture in an end-to-end fashion or using a gastrointestinal stapling device. In patients with a concomitant total laryngopharyngectomy, the jejunal flap is sewn to the base of the tongue **(Fig. 27.9)**.

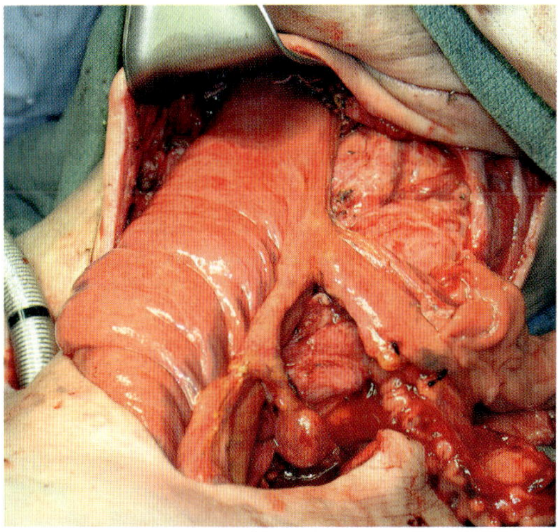

**Fig. 27.9** Once vascular anastomoses are completed, the jejunal flap is sewn to the remaining esophageal stump or the base of the tongue if a concomitant total laryngopharyngectomy is performed.

### Donor-Site Closure

Intestinal continuity is re-established in the abdomen by the thoracic or general surgical team through a gastrojejunal anastomosis using the posterior wall of the stomach, or through a Roux-en-Y jejunojejunal anastomosis if a gastrectomy is performed. A feeding jejunostomy tube is routinely placed distal to the jejunojejunal anastomosis.

## Donor-Site Care

The gastrostomy tube is maintained on intermittent suction until return of active bowel sounds. Jejunostomy feeding may be initiated on the second postoperative day. A modified barium swallow study is performed to confirm healing and to assess swallowing function 7 to 14 days after surgery depending on whether previous radiotherapy was given. If satisfactory healing and function are confirmed, the patient may be started on a liquid diet, which may be advanced to a regular diet within the next several days as tolerated. The feeding tube may be removed when the patient is consistently taking adequate nutrition by mouth, usually several weeks after postoperative radiotherapy, if given.

### References


1. Longmire WP Jr. A modification of the Roux technique for antethoracic esophageal reconstruction. Surgery 1947;22(1):94–100
2. Seidenberg B, Rosenak SS, Hurwitt ES, Som ML. Immediate reconstruction of the cervical esophagus by a revascularized isolated jejunal segment. Ann Surg 1959;149(2):162–171
3. Coleman JJ III, Searles JM Jr, Hester TR, et al. Ten years experience with the free jejunal autograft. Am J Surg 1987;154(4):394–398
4. Reece GP, Schusterman MA, Miller MJ, et al. Morbidity and functional outcome of free jejunal transfer reconstruction for circumferential defects of the pharynx and cervical esophagus. Plast Reconstr Surg 1995;96(6):1307–1316
5. Poh M, Selber JC, Skoracki R, Walsh GL, Yu P. Technical challenges of total esophageal reconstruction using a supercharged jejunal flap. Ann Surg 2011;253(6): 1122–1129


## Pearls and Pitfalls

- The free jejunal flap is our second-line option for pharyngoesophageal reconstruction following tubed fasciocutaneous free flaps, such as the anterolateral thigh flap, while the supercharged jejunum is our preferred method of esophageal reconstruction when direct repair or gastric pull-up is not feasible.
- The free jejunal flap is usually based on the second or third segmental branch of the superior mesenteric artery and its accompanying vein.
- A marking suture is placed at the proximal end of the jejunal flap for orientation, since isoperistaltic insetting of the transferred segment is preferred.
- In the supercharged jejunal flap, the second mesenteric branch is usually anastomosed to recipient vessels in the chest or neck while the third mesenteric branch is ligated and the fourth mesenteric vessels remain intact to act as a pedicle blood supply.
- The arcade blood vessels between the third and fourth mesenteric branches are preserved, while the messentery and the arcade blood vessels are divided between the second and third mesenteric branches to unfurl the jejunum, extending its reach and making the superior part of the flap conduit straighter, which facilitates food bolus transit by gravitational drainage.
- When a longer supercharged jejunal flap is needed, the third and fourth mesenteric branches are ligated and the mesentery is usually divided between them, while the arcade vessels between the second (reanastomosed) and third, as well as the fourth and fifth, mesenteric vessels are preserved.
- The cervical and mediastinal portion of the jejunal conduit should be as straight as possible, to facilitate passage of the food bolus, which is primarily by gravity drainage.
- A 3 to 5 cm segment of distal jejunum supplied by a branch of the vascular arcade can be exteriorized and can be used to monitor the flap. This branch is ligated and divided at the bedside after several days or prior to discharge from the hospital.

# 28 Pectoralis Major Flap

*Matthew M. Hanasono*

## Introduction

The pectoralis major flap was first described for head and neck reconstruction by Ariyan in 1979.[1,2] Shown to be more versatile and reliable than previous techniques, such as random pattern flaps and the deltopectoral flap, the pectoralis major flap revolutionized head and neck reconstructive surgery. Usually harvested as a muscle flap or a myocutaneous flap, it was considered the workhorse flap for the majority of head and neck oncologic defects encountered until microvascular free flaps became commonplace. Today, the pectoralis major flap, which has a reasonable arc of rotation and a straightforward dissection technique, remains an invaluable tool in the reconstructive surgeon's armamentarium.[1]

## Indications

The pectoralis major muscle and myocutaneous pedicled flaps are useful for reconstructing cutaneous defects of the neck and lower face as well as defects of the hypopharynx, floor of mouth, buccal mucosa, posterior mandible, and oropharynx. In some patients, the reach of the pectoralis major muscle is such that it can be used to reconstruct orbitomaxillary and temporal bone defects. For reconstruction of through-and-through defects, the skin paddle of the pectoralis major myocutaneous (PMMC) flap can be used to resurface one defect and a skin graft can be placed over the undersurface of the muscle to resurface the other defect.

In recent years, pectoralis major flaps are often considered secondary options in patients who are not candidates for microvascular free flaps, or in patients who have experienced a complication after free flap reconstruction, such as a wound dehiscence, fistula, or free flap loss. Pectoralis major flaps are also used in combination with free flaps for extensive defects, such as those that are through-and-through, requiring both a mucosal and cutaneous wound closure. Compared with free flaps, pectoralis major flaps are usually faster to perform, but are limited in their reach, and they may be less desirable due to the neck contracture that develops along the pedicle of the flap, a bulky appearance of the neck in the region of the proximal flap, and poor donor-site cosmesis. In addition, although the pectoralis muscle flap is considered extremely reliable, the PMMC flap's skin paddle has been reported to have high rates of partial or total necrosis. The technical points discussed below can help to minimize these negative sequelae.

Variants of the pectoralis major flap include a myo-osseous or an osteomyocutaneous flap by inclusion of the fifth rib or the outer table of the sternum.[3,4] Such a flap can be used for mandibular reconstruction, avoiding the need for free tissue transfer. Less commonly used variants of the myo-osseous or osteomyocutaneous flap are those that include the lateral sternal bone via thoracoacromial connections with the internal mammary artery perforators, or the clavicular head, via the clavicular head of the pectoralis major muscle, supplied by the clavicular branch of the thoracoacromial artery.[5] Myo-osseous and osteomyocutaneous pectoralis major flaps are now rarely performed due to the routine use of osteocutaneous free flaps, but they may still have a place as a secondary option in composite mandibular reconstruction, such as in a patient who is not a candidate for free flap reconstruction.

It is also possible to use the pectoralis major as a muscle or myocutaneous free flap, although, in practice, this is rarely done owing the availability of other free flaps with longer pedicles of larger caliber and donor sites with less morbidity.[6] On occasion, division of the pedicle and anastomosis to recipient vessels at a different site can be used to relocate the pectoralis major flap, such as following a wound dehiscence or distal flap loss. The technique of harvest of the pectoralis major free flap is identical to that of the pedicled flap and is not described separately here.

## Anatomy

The pectoralis major muscle is a thick, fan-shaped muscle that abducts and internally rotates the humerus. It originates on the anterior surface of the medial half of the clavicle, the anterior surface of the lateral half of the manubrium and sternum, costal cartilages from the second to the sixth rib, and the aponeurosis of the external oblique muscle. The pectoralis major converges laterally toward a flat tendon that inserts into the crest of the greater tubercule of the humerus. The pectoralis minor muscle, as well as the intercostal muscles, lie deep to the pectoralis major. The cephalic vein lies external to the lateral portion of the pectoralis major muscle, within the deltopectoral groove, and should be preserved during flap elevation.

The pectoralis major is considered a Mathes and Nahai Type V muscle, with the dominant blood supply coming from the thoracoacromial artery and secondary blood supply arising from the lateral thoracic artery (laterally) and branches of the internal mammary artery (medially) as well as perforating branches of the anterior intercostal arteries **(Fig. 28.1)**.[7] The thoracoacromial artery, which itself arises from the second portion of the axillary artery, pierces the clavipectoral fascia and branches into pectoral, clavicular, acromial, and deltoid branches inferior to the middle third of the clavicle. The pectoral branch is the dominant blood supply to the muscle and lies medial to the pectoralis minor muscle and descends on the deep surface of the sternocostal portion of the pectoralis muscle. The clavicular branch supplies the clavicular head of the pectoralis major muscle. The lateral thoracic artery, which also arises from the second part of the axillary artery, follows the lateral border of the pectoralis minor muscle and supplies the lateral part of the pectoralis major muscle. It is possible to design the pectoralis major flap as two separate flaps; one based on the pectoral branch of the thoracoacromial artery, the traditional blood supply, and one based on the lateral thoracic artery.[8] The venous drainage is via venae comitantes, which accompany the arteries. Venae comitantes of the thoracoacromial and lateral thoracic arteries drain into the axillary vein.

The main blood supply to most of the skin overlying the pectoralis major muscle comes from the perforating branches of the internal mammary artery, in the second through sixth intercostal spaces medially, and the perforating branches of the third through sixth anterior intercostal arteries laterally. The internal mammary artery perforators are the blood supply to the deltopectoral and internal mammary artery perforator flaps. The pectoral branch of the thoracoacromial artery also supplies small perforating branches to the skin overlying its course, although the artery dissipates at about the level of the fourth costal cartilage and rib.

To design a myocutaneous flap with maximal reach of the skin paddle from the origin of the thora-

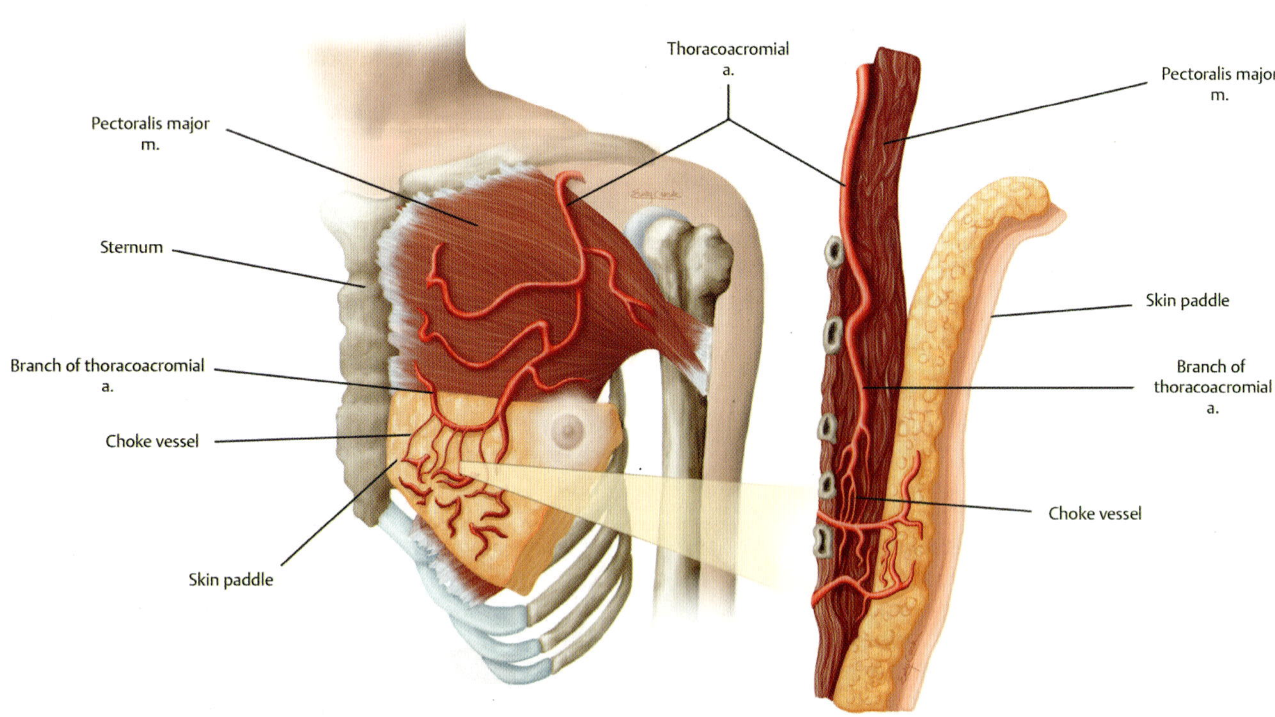


**Fig. 28.1** Vascular anatomy of the pectoralis major muscle and overlying skin.

coacromial artery, the skin paddle is usually centered over the inferior portion of the pectoralis major muscle, outside the vascular territory of the musculocutaneous perforating branches of the thoracoacromial artery. The skin paddle is, therefore, usually supplied by the musculocutaneous perforating branches of the anterior intercostal blood vessels of the fourth, fifth, and sixth costal interspaces, which communicate with the thoracoacromial artery via "choke" vessels, which dilate in response to interruption of the primary blood supply. Skin paddles may also be placed over the medial portion of the pectoralis major muscle, which is primarily supplied by perforating branches of the internal mammary artery, also connected to the thoracoacromial artery via choke vessels.[9,10] Skin below the level of the seventh costal cartilage is supplied by the superior epigastric artery, which is another angiosome (i.e., another vascular territory) further away from the pectoral branch of the thoracoacromial artery and, therefore, usually unreliable if included in the flap.

Anterior cutaneous branches of the second to seventh intercostal nerves supply the skin over the anterior chest wall. The lateral and medial pectoral nerves are the motor nerve supply to the pectoralis major muscle. They are named for their origin from the brachial plexus rather than the anatomical location of the portion of the muscle they supply. The lateral pectoral nerve originates from the lateral cord of the brachial plexus but supplies the clavicular head and anteromedial part of the sternal head of the muscle, while the medial pectoral nerve originates from the medial cord of the brachial plexus but supplies the posterolateral part of the sternal head of the muscle as well as the pectoralis minor muscle. Both enter the pectoralis major muscle on its deep surface ~ 3 cm apart.

## ■ Preoperative Considerations

In obese patients and in women (due to the presence of the breast), a skin paddle may be excessively bulky. Unlike many free flaps, which usually have a more robust skin paddle blood supply, the PMMC flap may not tolerate primary flap thinning or suction lipectomy, although such procedures can safely be performed secondarily, usually a few months later. The blood supply to the skin paddle may not be as reliable in female patients with very ptotic breasts, and harvest of a PMMC flap may also significantly distort the breast architecture, resulting in poor postoperative donor-site appearance. In such cases, consideration should be given to performing a pectoralis muscle flap and covering it with a split- or full-thickness skin graft. An alternative would be to center the skin paddle more superiorly, above the nipple-areolar complex, in the upper half of the breast, where there is usually less parenchyma. Such a skin paddle should be designed to include blood vessels that predominantly arise from the internal mammary artery in the third intercostal space, but are also connected to the thoracoacromial artery by "choke" vessels. The contralateral breast can be treated with a mastopexy for symmetry after the patient has recovered and there is confidence that a second, contralateral flap will not be needed. However, designing the skin paddle in a more proximal location shortens the reach of the flap, limiting its usefulness for many applications.

## ■ Patient Positioning and Skin Markings

Most commonly, the patient is in the supine position for head and neck reconstruction with the pectoralis major flap. The chest is prepared to the costal margin. The course of the thoracoacromial artery can be estimated by drawing a line from the acromion to the xiphoid process. The thoracoacromial artery dissipates as it crosses an imaginary line drawn from the suprasternal notch to the nipple, which is almost perpendicular to its course. If a pectoralis major muscle flap is being elevated, an incision is planned within the inframammary fold in women or along the inferior border of the pectoralis major muscle in men. If a PMMC flap is being elevated, surgical dissection of the muscle is performed through the skin incision.

In addition to the access afforded by an inframammary incision (in the pectoralis muscle flap) or the skin paddle incision (in the PMMC flap), it is often helpful to make a counterincision, just below and parallel to the clavicle. This incision facilitates dissection of a skin tunnel over the clavicle and neck. While a direct vertical or oblique incision could be made over the proximal pectoralis major muscle, a transverse incision is preferable, since it preserves the skin over the second and third intercostal spaces, which could be used for a deltopectoral or internal mammary artery perforator flap.

If a myocutaneous flap is being harvested and the maximal reach of the flap is needed, the skin paddle should be designed over the fourth, fifth, and, if necessary, sixth intercostal spaces (**Fig. 28.2**). The perforating vessels are particularly large in the fourth intercostal space, medial to the nipple, and they are especially important to include in the skin paddle design for maximum skin paddle reliability. The skin paddle may extend 2 to 3 cm lateral to the lateral margin of the pectoralis muscle. Skin below the seventh costal cartilage is not very reliable and its inclusion in the skin paddle should be performed with caution.

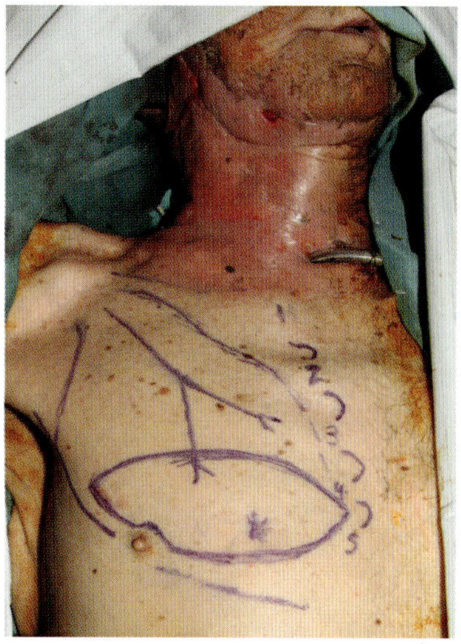

**Fig. 28.2** Skin markings for a pectoralis major myocutaneous pedicled flap.

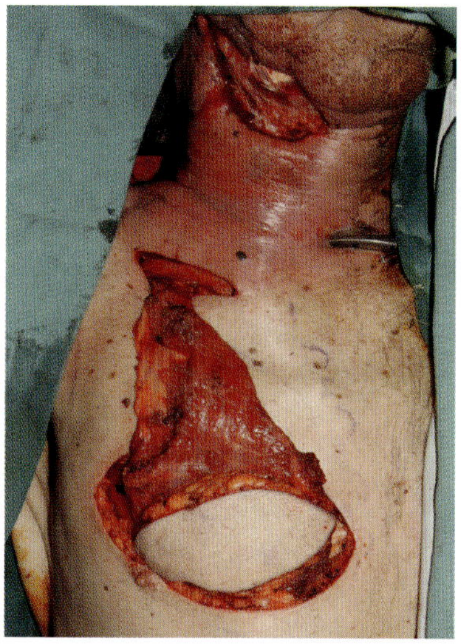

**Fig. 28.3** Elevated pectoralis major myocutaneous pedicled flap. Note that very little proximal muscle is included in the flap to minimize a proximal bulge in the neck.

In female patients with small, nonptotic breasts, the skin paddle for the PMMC is designed within the inframammary fold over the fourth interspace, as in males. In females with larger or ptotic breasts, placement of the skin paddle in this region may not be reliable since the course of the cutaneous perforating blood vessels may not be predictable. In these cases, the skin paddle is designed more superiorly and medially, centered over the third internal mammary perforating blood vessel. Harvesting a small skin paddle medially over the third intercostal perforator with a z-plasty to transfer lax lateral chest skin into the donor-site skin defect may avoid significant distortion of the breast. While a reliable skin paddle could be designed directly over the proximal thoracoacromial artery, such a flap would have a very limited reach.

## Operative Technique

After the incision around the skin island (if any) is made, the rest of the skin is elevated from the underlying muscle. The muscle is then detached and raised from the chest wall. The pectoralis major is easily dissected from the pectoralis minor muscle in an avascular plane. Care is taken to ligate rather than cauterize musculocutaneous perforating blood vessels arising from the intercostal spaces, since these communicate directly with the skin paddle after they course through the thickness of the muscle. The thoracoacromial pedicle should be identified early, on the undersurface of the muscle, and should be protected.

The proximal muscle is divided with electrocautery above the skin island (if any), and the muscle portion of the flap is "narrowed" overlying the pedicle **(Fig. 28.3)**. This detaches the flap from both the humerus laterally and the sternum medially. Proximally, minimal muscle needs to be left over the pedicle, and, in fact, the pedicle can be completely dissected from the muscle with appropriately delicate technique, to minimize bulk in the upper chest and lower neck. The lateral thoracic blood vessels lie lateral to the thoracoacromial vessels and do not need to be included with the flap, if the maximum arc of rotation is required to reach the defect. The medial and lateral pectoral nerves are also divided to maximize the flap arc of rotation.

The skin between the donor-site incisions and the head and neck defect is elevated. Lighted retractors may be of some use here. Caution needs to be used when elevating the neck skin away from the external jugular vein and the subclavian blood vessels to avoid inadvertent vascular injury, especially in the radiated neck. The clavicular head of the pectoralis muscle can be divided along the path of flap rotation to maximize flap reach and minimize proximal bulkiness. Muscle-only flaps and myocutaneous flaps where the skin paddle is used to reconstruct an intraoral or intraluminal pharyngeal defect can be transposed into the defect such that the deep surface of the muscle comes to lie superficially **(Fig. 28.4)**. Myocutaneous flaps are usually rotated medially up to 180 degrees into the head and neck defect if the skin paddle is needed for an external defect **(Fig. 28.5)**. When the myocutaneous flap is used, several tacking sutures are employed to minimize tension on the skin paddle. The proximal flap must be checked for compression by the overlying skin.

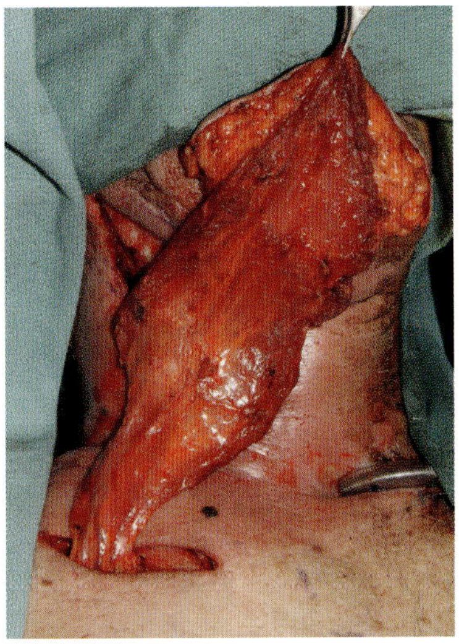

**Fig. 28.4** Rotation of the pectoralis major myocutaneous pedicled flap for an intraoral reconstruction.

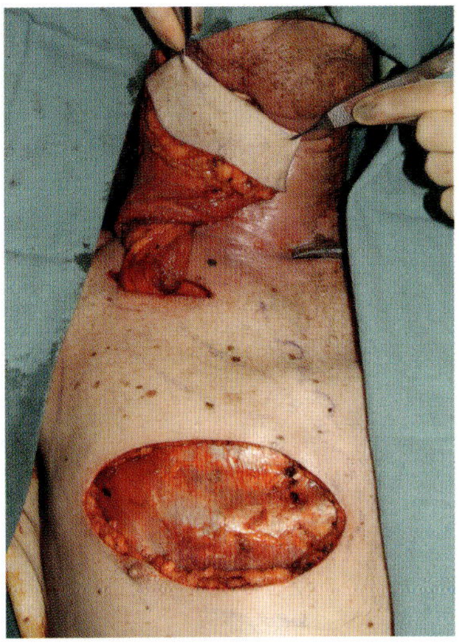

**Fig. 28.5** Rotation of the pectoralis major myocutaneous pedicled flap for a cutaneous neck reconstruction.

## Myo-osseous or Osteomyocutaneous Variants

Both the fifth rib and the outer table of the sternum have been used along with the pectoralis major muscle and overlying skin to reconstruct composite mandibular defects. When using the sternal variant, the skin island is designed along and over the sternum. The pectoralis major muscle attachments to the anterior part of the sternum are preserved. A longitudinal incision through the outer table and the cancellous portion of the sternum is made with a reciprocating saw and osteotome. Preservation of the inner table of the sternum minimizes risk of pneumothorax.

The fifth rib may be included with the pectoralis major flap by similarly preserving all of the pectoralis major muscle attachments. The intercostal muscles are separated from the rib, and the rib periosteum is incised long the rib's superior and inferior borders. A subperiosteal elevation of the rib is performed after making medial and lateral osteotomies. An 18 cm segment of bone may be harvested. Subperiosteal dissection reduces the risk of a pneumothorax. If a small pleural tear occurs, the lungs are insufflated, a small catheter is inserted through the tear and is placed under suction, and a primary repair is attempted as the catheter is withdrawn. For larger tears, a chest tube should be placed. Postoperative respiratory monitoring and chest X-ray are required.

# ■ Donor-Site Care

Substantial undermining is often necessary when a wide skin paddle (> 5 cm) is included with the flap (**Fig. 28.6**). One or more closed suction drains are indicated and may need to be left in more than a week before

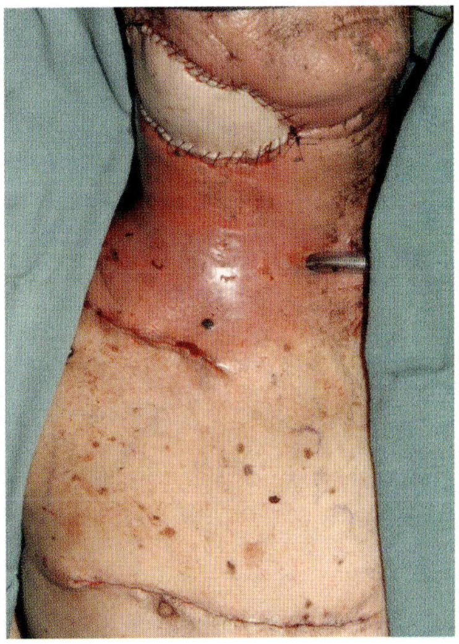

**Fig. 28.6** Completed pectoralis major myocutaneous pedicled flap inset and donor-site closure for a cutaneous neck reconstruction following development of an orocutaneous fistula. The oral mucosa was closed primarily.

drainage decreases to < 30 mL per day. If the donor-site wound cannot be closed primarily, skin grafting of the donor site may be necessary. Skin grafts over the costal cartilages and ribs may take poorly and healing may be prolonged. Tight tracheostomy ties must be avoided to minimize vascular pedicle compression.

## Case Example

A 64-year-old male presented with a left retromolar trigone squamous cell carcinoma, stage T4N0M0. He had a medical history that included coronary artery disease and severe peripheral vascular disease. He had previously undergone an abdominal aortic aneurysm repair, aortobifemoral bypass grafting, and a left carotid endarterectomy. Because of these conditions, we wished to avoid a microvascular free flap procedure. Following a composite mandibular resection and neck dissection, a pectoralis major myocutaneous flap was performed (**Fig. 28.7, Fig. 28.8, Fig. 28.9,** and **Fig. 28.10**). Postoperatively, the patient did well and had good mouth opening (**Fig. 28.11** and **Fig. 28.12**).

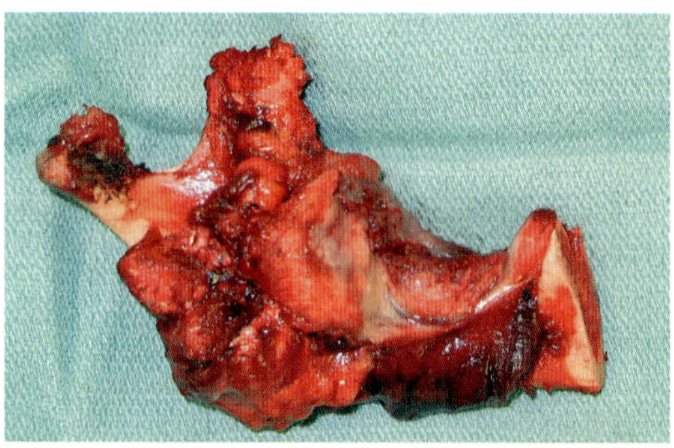

**Fig. 28.7** Specimen from a composite mandibular resection of a retromolar trigone squamous cell carcinoma in a patient deemed not to be a suitable candidate for a microvascular free flap reconstruction.

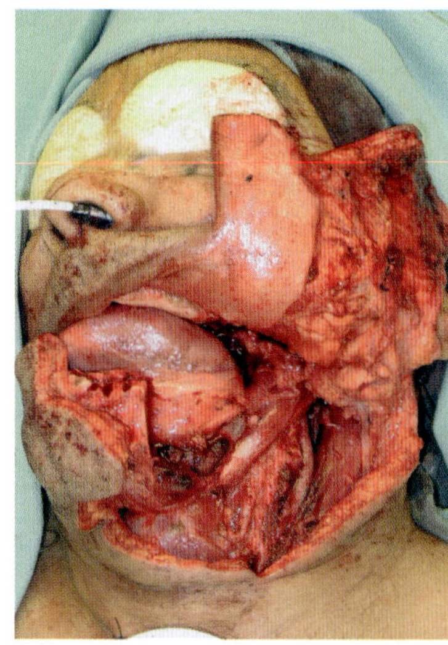

**Fig. 28.8** Oromandibular defect resulting from a composite mandibular resection of a retromolar trigone squamous cell carcinoma in a patient deemed not to be a suitable candidate for a microvascular free flap reconstruction.

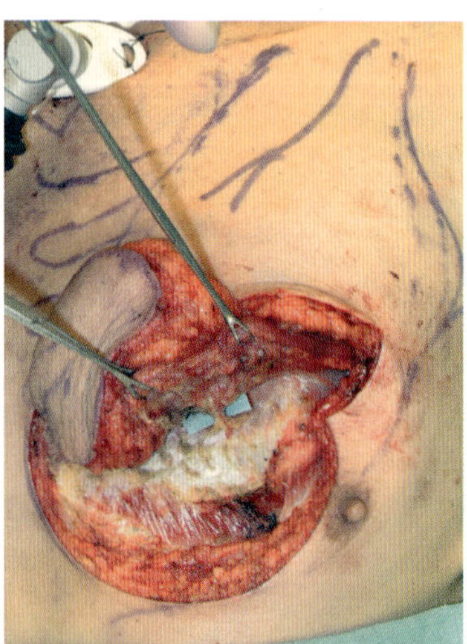

**Fig. 28.9** Elevation of the pectoralis major myocutaneous pedicled flap showing the intercostal perforating blood vessels arising from the interspace between the fourth and fifth ribs, adjacent to the nipple. These vessels should be ligated rather than cauterized to avoid injury to the blood supply to the skin paddle.

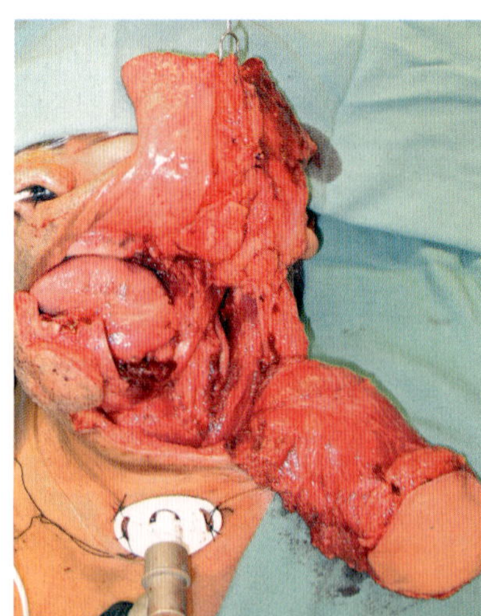

**Fig. 28.10** Rotation of the pectoralis major myocutaneous pedicled flap into the composite mandibulectomy defect. Note the long reach of the flap owing to design of the skin paddle over the fourth intercostal space.

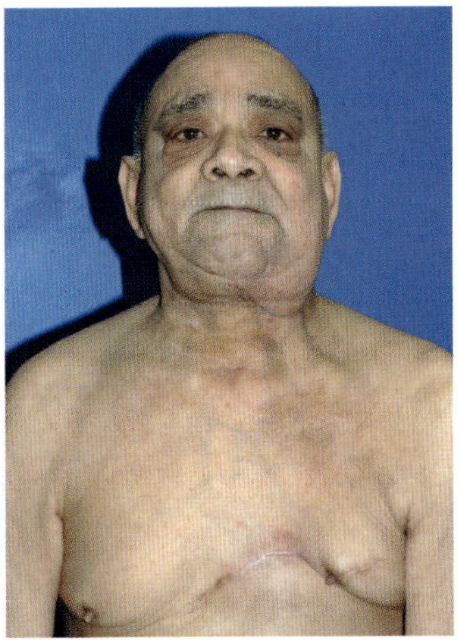

**Fig. 28.11** Postoperative appearance. Bulkiness in the proximal neck is minimized by including only a modest amount of muscle around the proximal pedicle.

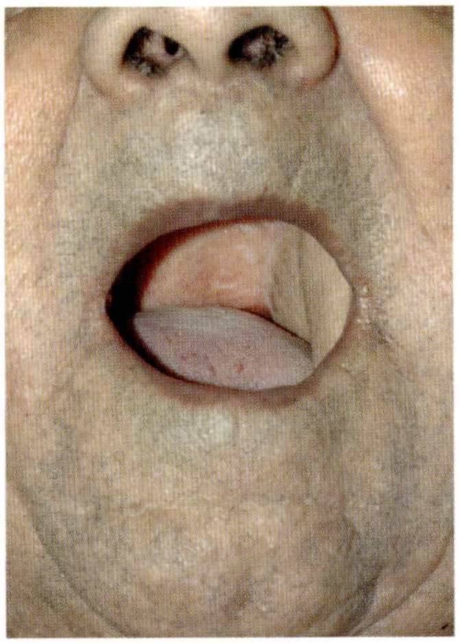

**Fig. 28.12** Intraoral pectoralis major myocutaneous pedicled flap skin paddle showing good healing and adequate mouth opening.

## Pearls and Pitfalls

- For the longest arc of rotation, the skin paddle of the pectoralis major myocutaneous pedicled flap should be centered over the fourth intercostal space, which is where multiple musculocutaneous perforating blood vessels enter the skin. Such length can be advantageous in preventing restriction of neck mobility due to contraction of the muscular portion of the flap postoperatively, a frequent complication associated with this flap.
- In obese patients and female patients with moderate to large breasts, a skin paddle centered medially over the third intercostal perforating branch of the internal mammary artery may allow harvest of a thinner skin paddle without significantly distorting the breast. Otherwise, consideration should be given to performing a pectoralis muscle flap covered with a skin graft instead.
- Perforating blood vessels arising from the anterior intercostal and internal mammary arteries and veins and entering the underside of the pectoralis major muscle should be ligated rather than cauterized, to avoid injury to the blood supply to the skin paddle of the pectoralis major myocutaneous flap.
- Only a small cuff of proximal muscle around the vascular pedicle should be included in the flap design to minimize the bulge in the lower neck as well as later contracture that can limit neck movement.
- In the event of a partial flap loss in which the flap cannot be re-advanced without significant tension, the pedicle may be divided proximally and re-anastomosed to alternate recipient vessels as a microvascular free flap.

## References


1. Ariyan S. The pectoralis major myocutaneous flap. A versatile flap for reconstruction in the head and neck. Plast Reconstr Surg 1979; 63:73–81
2. Ariyan S. Further experiences with the pectoralis major myocutaneous flap for immediate repair of defects from excisions of head and neck cancers. Plast Reconstr Surg 1979; 64:605
3. Green MF, Gibson JR, Bryson JR, Thomson E. A one-stage correction of mandibular defects using a split sternum pectoralis major osteomusculocutaneous transfer. Br J Plast Surg 1981; 34:11–16
4. Lam KH, Wei WI, Siu KF. The pectoralis major costomyocutaneous flap for mandibular reconstruction. Plast Reconstr Surg 1984; 73:904-910
5. Robertson GA. The role of sternum in osteomyocutaneous reconstruction of major mandibular defects. Am J Surg 1986; 152:367-370
6. Yeh JT, Chen HC, Laverty LA, Wei FC, Lin CH. Conversion of pedicled to free flap for salvage of the compromised pectoralis major myocutaneous flap in head and neck reconstruction. Plast Reconstr Surg 2004; 114:152–157
7. Freeman JL, Walker EP, Wilson JSP, Shaw HJ. The vascular anatomy of the pectoralis major myocutaneous flaps. Br J Plast Surg 1981; 34:3–8
8. Yuen APW, Ng, RWM. Surgical techniques and results of lateral thoracic cutaneous, myocutaneous, and conjoint flaps for head and neck reconstruction. Laryngoscope 2007; 117:288–294
9. Rikimaru H, Kiyokawa K, Inoue Y, Tai Y. Three-dimensional anatomical vascular distribution in the pectoralis major myocutaneous flap. Plast Reconstr Surg. 2005; 115:1342–1352
10. Rikimaru H, Kiyokawa K, Watanabe K, Koga N, Nishi Y, Sakamoto A. New method of preparing a pectoralis major myocutaneous flap with a skin paddle that includes the third intercostal perforating branch of the internal thoracic artery. Plast Reconstr Surg 2009; 123:1220–1228

# 29 Supraclavicular Artery Island Flap

*Michael W. Chu and Ernest S. Chiu*

## Introduction

The supraclavicular flap has been successfully used for various challenging facial reconstruction cases, providing acceptable results without requiring microsurgical techniques. In 1949, Kazanjian and Converse first described the fasciocutaneous flap and referred it as the acromial flap.[1] This flap has also been described as the arteria cervicalis superficialis flap, Charretera flap, acromial flap, Dermagasso flap, and the laterally extended cervicohumeral flap. Mathes and Vasconez performed the first anatomical study of a supraclavicular artery-based flap in 1978, and they named it the cervicohumeral flap.[2] They described the vascular territory, flap dimensions, and clinical applications in head and neck reconstruction. In 1983, Lamberty and Cormack named the supraclavicular artery—a vessel cephalad to the clavicular insertion of the trapezius muscle.[3] Use of the flap has been controversial because of the reported incidence of distal flap necrosis.[4] In 1997, Pallua and Noah "rediscovered" this flap by demonstrating its use in postburn mentosternal contractures and by performing detailed anatomical studies examining the vascular territory.[5,6] Their findings were confirmed in clinical and vascular studies by multiple independent surgical units for reconstructing burn contracture and oncologic head and neck defects.[7,8,9,10,11,12,13,14,15,16,17,18] The authors prefer the term *supraclavicular artery island flap* (SCAIF) because it most accurately describes their surgical technique.

Recent efforts in reconstructive surgery to minimize donor-site morbidity and the advent of perforator flaps have increased the popularity of the SCAIF. It is a versatile flap consisting of thin, pliable skin with a large arc of rotation and excellent color match for reconstruction of cervicofacial, scapular, and anterior chest wall defects. Although the SCAIF does not require microsurgical expertise, prolonged operative times, or hospital stays, it does require attention to detail and an understanding of appropriate patient selection criteria. Previous concerns about distal tip ischemia have been addressed with refinement in operative techniques, cadaveric perfusion studies,[14] and radiographic imaging, such as computerized tomographic angiography (CTA).[19]

## Indications

The SCAIF may be considered a nearly ideal regional fasciocutaneous reconstructive choice for head and neck defects calling for a thin and pliable flap, even in obese patients. The skin is a good color match for cervicofacial and anterior chest wall defects. The location of the source artery and the arc of rotation of the flap allow it to reliably reach most neck and lower facial defects as well as the tongue, the floor of the mouth, and hypopharyngeal defects. Although it can be used both as a regional (rotational, transpositional, interpolated) or a microvascular free flap, there are more attractive free flap options in terms of vascular pedicle length and vessel diameter.

## Anatomy

The SCAIF is an axial flap based on the supraclavicular artery, which is a branch of the transverse cervical artery that originates from the thyrocervical trunk **(Fig. 29.1)**. The supraclavicular artery on rare occasions can arise from the suprascapular artery.[8] The supraclavicular artery is a small-diameter vessel that can be reliably found in the supraclavicular triangle, between the clavicle and the sternocleidomastoid and trapezius muscles.

Anatomical studies and characterization of the supraclavicular artery have been performed in detail by several groups.[5,8,10,14] The study by Abe et al,[8]

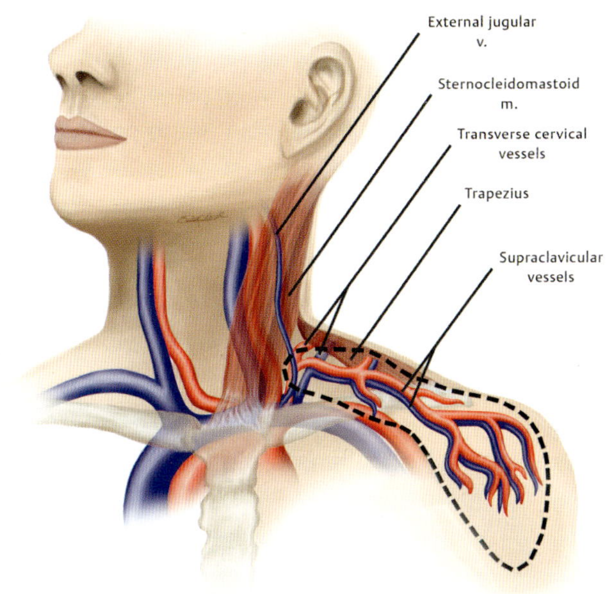


**Fig. 29.1** Anatomy of the supraclavicular artery island flap (SCAIF).

based on 55 cadaver dissections, suggests that the supraclavicular artery is present 80% of the time and has a diameter of 1.1 to 1.5 mm, with a functional pedicle length of 1 to 7 cm. The arc of rotation for the supraclavicular flap, as a pedicled fascial flap or a tunneled island flap, has been reported up to 180 degrees.[7] In a vascular injection study, Chan et al[14] showed a mean perfused paddle length of 24.2 cm and a width of 8.7 cm. Consistent with other studies, the mean diameter of the supraclavicular artery was 1.33 mm, and it was located an average of 3.6 cm above the clavicle and 8.6 cm from the sternoclavicular joint. Their study suggested the skin paddle is perfused beyond the deltoid muscle in 9 out of 10 cadaveric dissections.

Sensory cervical nerves can be harvested with the supraclavicular flap and potentially used to provide sensation to the reconstructed area. The senior author found that 20% of patients in his initial case series reported referred sensation to the shoulder in response to contact with the flap skin paddle. Cadaver studies were performed to investigate this phenomenon. Branches of the supraclavicular nerves, from cervical roots C3 and C4, were found to emerge from the deep fascia at a separate location from the vascular pedicle.[20] The major nerve root exits underneath the sternocleidomastoid muscle near the midpoint of the muscle belly. The nerve branches proximal to the pedicle, with one branch exiting anterior to the flap and another running axially along the length of the flap. In this study, nine out of ten flaps had major cutaneous nerves located 1 to 2 cm anterior to the pedicle, and one out of ten flaps had a major cutaneous nerve located 1 to 2 cm posterior to the pedicle heading toward the trapezius muscle. Smaller cutaneous nerves were also found posterior to the pedicle in a more distal location of the flap. These anatomical findings suggest a potential for using the SCAIF as a sensate flap in head and neck reconstructions.

## Preoperative Considerations

The relative contraindications for the supraclavicular flap are a prior history of neck dissection and neck irradiation, because the supraclavicular artery or its source vessels may have been previously injured or occluded by radiation fibrosis. Potential pitfalls and complications include distal tip ischemia, inadvertent transection of the pedicle during flap harvest, referred shoulder dysesthesia with stimulation of the skin paddle, and donor-site wound dehiscence or scarring.[12] Patients should be informed that a shoulder scar can be visible with certain clothing choices, especially in women who prefer tank tops and strapless tops. However, the scar is usually well tolerated and delayed healing at the donor site is rare.

Routine preoperative radiographic imaging is not done for SCAIF, but if there is a concern, angiography can be done to confirm the length, patency, and diameter of the supraclavicular artery.[19]

## Patient Positioning and Skin Markings

During preoperative assessment, the course of the supraclavicular artery should be identified using a handheld Doppler ultrasound in the office. The vessel is located in the posterior triangle of the neck, whose boundaries are the sternocleidomastoid muscle, trapezius muscle, and the clavicle, and runs toward the acromion. It can be auscultated traveling perpendicular to the transverse cervical artery, which courses posteriorly toward the trapezius muscle **(Fig. 29.1)**. On the day of surgery, prior to the induction of general anesthesia, the pedicle location is confirmed again. A suture can be fixated at the pivot point and the radius of rotation and skin paddle length can be estimated and marked out with a surgical marker. An elliptical skin paddle is then designed according to the defect and also includes an additional 2 to 3 cm of skin medial to the pedicle origin. The widest part of the elliptical skin paddle should be 6 to 8 cm, depending on the skin laxity of the shoulder area, to allow primary closure; the length can extend up to 3 cm distal to the acromion. The size of the SCAIF skin island can be increased by delaying the flap, incising and elevating it but returning it to its original position without rotation for a period of ~ 7 days. The largest reported SCAIF skin island in the literature was in a delayed flap that measured 12 by 35 cm.[7]

On the operating table, the patient is positioned supine, and folded towels are placed under the shoulder to create a bump so the neck is extended to expose the supraclavicular region. The neck, chest, and upper arm (circumferentially to elbow) are prepped and draped sterilely; the hands, forearm, and elbow are wrapped with a stocking and gauze, then the padded arm is tucked to the side.

## Operative Technique

The skin incision is carried down through the skin and subcutaneous tissue through the fascia of the anterior deltoid muscle. The SCAIF is then dissected with monopolar cautery from distal to proximal in a subfascial plane. As the flap is harvested more proximally, the underside of the flap is checked with a sterile handheld Doppler to confirm vascular flow. A vascular signal often can be obtained all the way to the most lateral extent of the flap. Blunt dissection and bipolar cautery are used when the flap harvest is within 2 to 3 cm of the pedicle origin to avoid thermal injury to the vessel. The pedicle can also be visualized in the medial third of the flap by transillumination of the skin. If multiple vessels are perfusing the flap, small vascular clamps can be used to occlude collateral vessels to confirm adequate pedicle blood flow. Collateral blood vessels should not be ligated and divided until adequate distal blood flow from a source vessel is verified.

Proximally, a 1 to 2 cm cuff of soft tissue/fat surrounding the pedicle is preserved to avoid injury to the source vessel. Several sensory nerves are encountered during the dissection and can be incorporated if a sensate flap is desired, but they are often divided to increase the arc of flap rotation. Leaving any attached nerve may result in referred sensation to the shoulder. Once the flap dissection is completed lateral to the pedicle, the remaining medial skin incisions are performed to complete the skin island paddle.

## Donor-Site Care

The surrounding skin of the donor site is widely undermined and can be closed primarily for skin paddles up to 6 to 8 cm in width. If tension is excessive, a split-thickness skin graft can be performed and a negative-pressure wound dressing applied. Drains are not necessary after adequate hemostasis. Tracheostomy ties and pressure around the donor site and vascular pedicle are to be avoided, and dry dressings are used to prevent soilage from tracheostomy secretions.

## Case Example

A 70-year-old man presented with recurrent intraoral squamous cell carcinoma and trismus secondary to radiation fibrosis. He underwent tumor ablation, coronoidectomy, and reconstruction. Following this, the intraoral defect measure 4 × 6 cm, with exposed mandibular bone **(Fig. 29.2)**. A left supraclavicular artery island flap, measuring 28 × 7 cm, was designed. A Doppler signal was noted (lateral to the circle at the flap base). Electrocautery was used to elevate the flap distally, then bipolar cautery and blunt dissection were used to complete the flap harvest near the vascular pedicle.

The flap was tunneled lateral to the mandible to reach the intraoral defect. At 12-month follow-up, the patient was disease free, had a viable skin island, and had improved mouth opening.

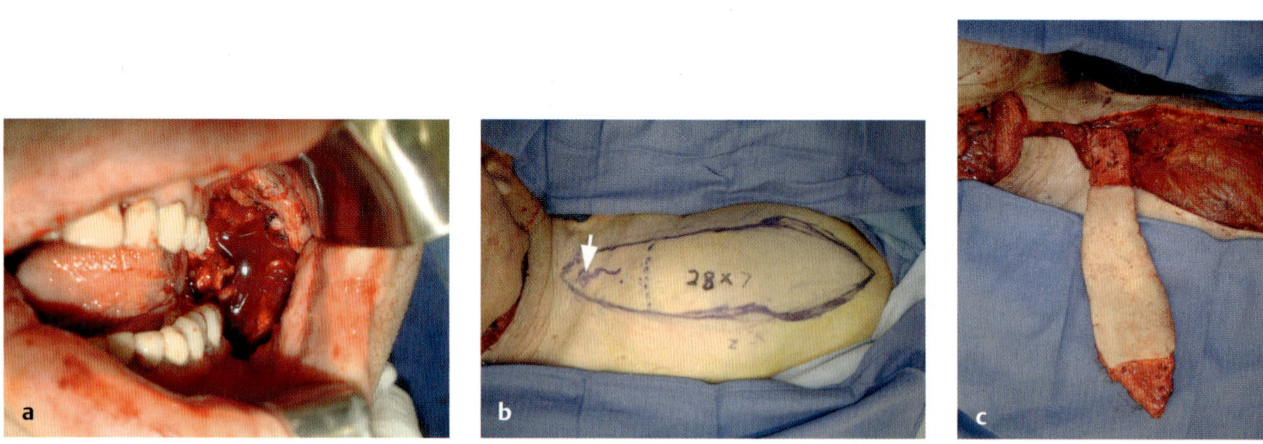


**Fig. 29.2** **(a)** An intraoral defect with exposed mandibular bone following excision of a recurrent cancer. **(b)** An SCAIF is designed on the left shoulder. A Doppler signal was noted lateral to the circle at the flap base (*arrow*). **(c)** The SCAIF has been elevated and selectively de-epithelialized.

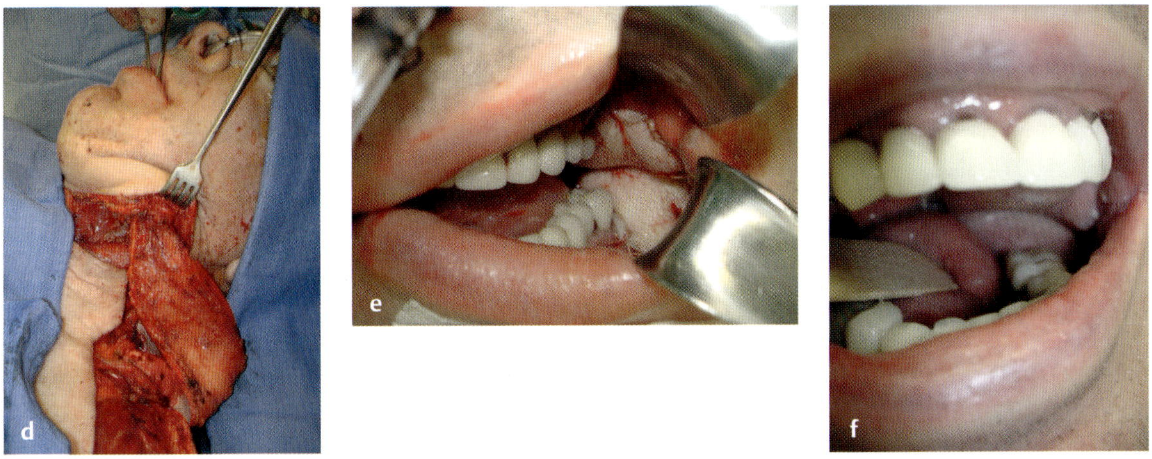


**Fig. 29.2** (*Continued*) **(d)** The flap is tunneled lateral to the mandible to reach the intraoral defect. **(e)** An intraoral photo demonstrates the flap inset. **(f)** At 12-month follow-up, the patient has a viable skin island and good mouth opening.

## Pearls and Pitfalls

- The supraclavicular artery island flap (SCAIF) is the authors' preferred head and neck regional flap option, and it is a reasonable choice for resurfacing the neck, lower one-third of the face, and lateral skull base defects.
- Men are rarely concerned about the shoulder scar. Women who wear strapless dresses should be informed preoperatively about the donor-site scar.
- A preoperative CT angiography study can confirm the position and patency of the supraclavicular artery.
- The vascular pedicle origin is left in a bed of soft tissue/fat. Vessel skeletonization is unnecessary.
- Creation of a complete skin island paddle allows greater freedom of flap inset.
- When performing flap de-epithelialization, avoid unnecessary buttonholes in the dermis to protect the microcirculation supplying the distal skin.
- The SCAIF can tolerate postoperative radiation therapy. Flap thinning and revision are performed no sooner than 6 months after the conclusion of radiation.
- When the skin island paddle remains innervated by supraclavicular nerves, referred sensation to the shoulder has been observed. Dysesthesia is uncommon. Referred sensation frequently disappears with time.
- Patients sometimes note mild restricted neck movement.

## References

1. Kazanjian VH, Converse JM. The Surgical Treatment of Facial Injuries. Baltimore, MD: Williams & Wilkins; 1949
2. Mathes SJ, Vasconez LO. The cervicohumeral flap. Plast Reconstr Surg 1978;61(1):7–12
3. Lamberty BG, Cormack GC. Misconceptions regarding the cervico-humeral flap. Br J Plast Surg 1983;36(1):60–63
4. Blevins PK, Luce EA. Limitations of the cervicohumeral flap in head and neck reconstruction. Plast Reconstr Surg 1980;66(2):220–224
5. Pallua N, Machens HG, Rennekampff O, Becker M, Berger A. The fasciocutaneous supraclavicular artery island flap for releasing postburn mentosternal contractures. Plast Reconstr Surg 1997;99(7):1878–1884, discussion 1885–1886
6. Pallua N, Magnus Noah E. The tunneled supraclavicular island flap: an optimized technique for head and neck reconstruction. Plast Reconstr Surg 2000;105(3):842–851, discussion 852–854
7. Di Benedetto G, Aquinati A, Pierangeli M, Scalise A, Bertani A. From the "charretera" to the supraclavicular fascial island flap: revisitation and further evolution of a controversial flap. Plast Reconstr Surg 2005;115(1):70–76
8. Abe M, Murakami G, Abe S, Sakakura Y, Yajima T. Supraclavicular artery in Japanese: an anatomical basis for the flap using a pedicle containing a cervical, non-perforating cutaneous branch of the superficial cervical artery. Okajimas Folia Anat Jpn 2000;77(5):149–154
9. Vinh VQ, Ogawa R, Van Anh T, Hyakusoku H. Reconstruction of neck scar contractures using supraclavicular flaps: retrospective study of 30 cases. Plast Reconstr Surg 2007;119(1):130–135
10. Vinh VQ, Van Anh T, Ogawa R, Hyakusoku H. Anatomical and clinical studies of the supraclavicular flap: analysis

of 103 flaps used to reconstruct neck scar contractures. Plast Reconstr Surg 2009;123(5):1471–1480

11. Liu PH, Chiu ES. Supraclavicular artery flap: a new option for pharyngeal reconstruction. Ann Plast Surg 2009;62(5):497–501
12. Chiu ES, Liu PH, Friedlander PL. Supraclavicular artery island flap for head and neck oncologic reconstruction: indications, complications, and outcomes. Plast Reconstr Surg 2009;124(1):115–123
13. Chiu ES, Liu PH, Baratelli R, Lee MY, Chaffin AE, Friedlander PL. Circumferential pharyngoesophageal reconstruction with a supraclavicular artery island flap. Plast Reconstr Surg 2010;125(1):161–166
14. Chan JWH, Wong C, Ward K, Saint-Cyr M, Chiu ES. Three- and four-dimensional computed tomographic angiography studies of the supraclavicular artery island flap. Plast Reconstr Surg 2010;125(2):525–531
15. Pointer DT Jr, Friedlander PL, Amedee RG, Liu PH, Chiu ES. Infratemporal fossa reconstruction following total auriculectomy: an alternative flap option. J Plast Reconstr Aesthet Surg 2010;63(8):e615–e618
16. Chen WL, Zhang DM, Yang ZH, et al. Extended supraclavicular fasciocutaneous island flap based on the transverse cervical artery for head and neck reconstruction after cancer ablation. J Oral Maxillofac Surg 2010;68(10):2422–2430
17. Anand AG, Tran EJ, Hasney CP, Friedlander PL, Chiu ES. Oropharyngeal reconstruction using the supraclavicular artery island flap: a new flap alternative. Plast Reconstr Surg 2012;129(2):438–441
18. Alves HR, Ishida LC, Ishida LH, et al. A clinical experience of the supraclavicular flap used to reconstruct head and neck defects in late-stage cancer patients. J Plast Reconstr Aesthet Surg 2012;65(10):1350–1356
19. Adams AS, Wright MJ, Johnston S, et al. The use of multislice CT angiography preoperative study for supraclavicular artery island flap harvesting. Ann Plast Surg 2012;69(3):312–315
20. Sands TT, Martin JB, Simms E, Henderson MM, Friedlander PL, Chiu ES. Supraclavicular artery island flap innervation: anatomical studies and clinical implications. J Plast Reconstr Aesthet Surg 2012;65(1):68–71

# 30 Internal Mammary Artery Perforator Flap

*Peirong Yu*

## Introduction

The most recent development or refinement in flap reconstruction has been the advent of perforator-based flaps. Many of the perforator flap applications have been for distant reconstruction as free flaps. Perforator flaps are equally valuable, however, when designed as a pedicled island flap, which can be utilized for reconstruction of defects in the trunk and extremities. These local perforator flaps often provide reliable coverage with primary closure of the donor site, resulting in excellent form and function. Pedicled perforator flaps for head and neck reconstruction have rarely been an option, however, owing to the lack of perforator flaps in this region. The newly discovered internal mammary artery perforator (IMAP) flap may be an exception.

The IMAP flap was first described in the literature in 2006 by the author for tracheostoma reconstruction.[1] Neligan et al[2] conducted injection studies and reported their clinical use of this flap in 2007. More recently Wong et al[3] reported the three-dimensional perforator anatomy using injections and three-dimensional CT scans of cadaveric specimens. More anatomical and clinical cases have been reported since then.[4,5,6]

The IMAP flap is a valuable option when used as a pedicled flap. As a free flap, however, it loses its advantages, and other fasciocutaneous flaps may be preferred because of their longer vascular pedicles and larger areas of skin provided, except that the IMAP flap may provide better a color match when it is placed on the face. For small to moderately sized defects in the lower neck or upper chest, and for tracheostoma reconstruction, an island IMAP flap provides quick and easy coverage. More importantly, it has the advantage of being a relatively thin fasciocutaneous flap, ideal for tracheostoma reconstruction.

## Anatomy

The internal mammary artery perforators, as the name implies, originate from the internal mammary artery. The internal mammary artery itself originates from the subclavian artery and travels along the sternal border on each side of the sternum. It becomes the superior epigastric artery in the upper abdomen and nourishes the upper part of the rectus abdominis muscle. In its path along the sternal border, the internal mammary artery sends out several perforators through the intercostal space to the chest skin.

The dominant IMAP is usually the one located in the second intercostal space.[3,4,5,6,7] Cadaveric studies found that the mean perforator diameter was 1.50 mm (range, 1.0 to 2.2 mm) in intercostal space 1, 1.83 mm (range, 1.3 to 2.4 mm) in intercostal space 2, and 1.47 mm (range, 1.3 to 1.7 mm) in intercostal space 3.[3] Similar findings were reported in clinical series.[8] The author's own clinical experience shows that the IMAP arteries at the second intercostal space range from 1 mm to 1.5 mm and the perforator veins are 1.5 mm to 2 mm in diameter.

Based on injection study,[3] IMAPs in the first intercostal space perfused to the level of the clavicle and lateral mammary fold in all cases and to the level of the xiphisternum one-third of the time. IMAPs in intercostal space 2 had a territory reaching the clavicle and xiphisternum in four of six cases and the lateral mammary fold in all cases. IMAPs in intercostal space 3 reached the clavicle in only 40% of cases, the xiphisternum in 60%, and the lateral mammary fold in 80% of cases. When the superior IMAPs were injected (intercostal spaces 1 and 2), the linking vessels were found to be oriented transversely. However, when the inferior IMAPs (intercostal spaces 3 to 7) were injected, the linking vessels took a more inferolateral orientation.[3] This is useful information for flap design. When the second intercostal IMAP is

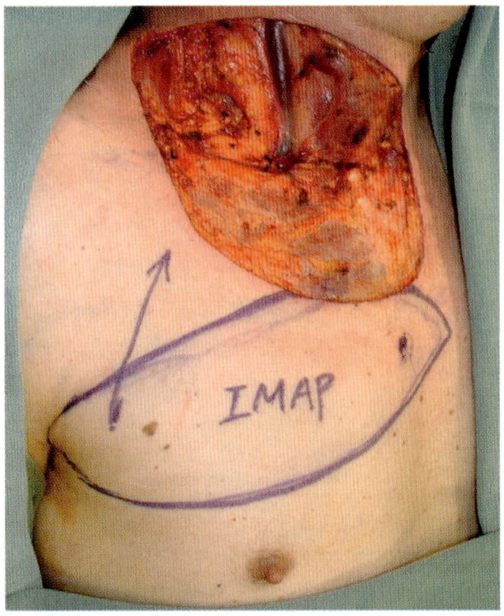


**Fig. 30.1** Design of the internal mammary artery perforator (IMAP) flap based on the perforator vessels at the second intercostal space. The Prolene suture marks the perforator. The long axis of the flap parallels the intercostal space, and the tip of the flap can extend beyond the anterior axillary line.

used, the flap design should be horizontal, whereas when the third or fourth intercostal IMAP is used, the flap should be designed in an oblique direction. In clinical practice, however, the second intercostal IMAP is most useful, since it is dominant, reaches the neck more easily, and a horizontal design results in less donor-site scarring.

## ■ Surgical Technique

Preoperative imaging studies are unnecessary. There are no contraindications except in patients with a previous coronary artery bypass graft. With the patient supine, the IMAPs at the second and third intercostal spaces along the sternal border on each side are examined with a handheld Doppler device. For head and neck reconstruction, the perforator at the second intercostal space is preferred as the basis of the flap because of its proximity to the neck defect. If the Doppler signal in the second intercostal space is significantly weaker than that at the third intercostal space, the latter should be considered. The first intercostal IMAP may be too close to the clavicle and is often smaller. The side chosen depends on the location of the defect. For a centrally located defect in the neck, the side with a stronger Doppler signal is chosen. Once the IMAP is selected, the flap is designed with its long axis parallel to the intercostal space. The medial limit of the flap is the midline of the sternum, and the length of the flap is based on the arc of rotation needed to reach the defect with the lateral limit of the flap, usually slightly beyond the anterior axillary fold (**Fig. 30.1**). When the IMAP at the second intercostal space is chosen, the long axis of the flap should be horizontal. The flap design should not extend above the clavicle or extend to the deltoid region, since the perfusion in these areas is unreliable.

The medial half of the superior incision is made first down to the fascia; subfascial dissection proceeds inferiorly with tenotomy scissors until the internal mammary perforator vessels are identified (**Fig. 30.2**). The perforator vessels do not need to be skeletonized unless the flap is to be used as a free flap. Once the perforators are located, the rest of the flap is incised (**Fig. 30.3**). If needed, the pectoralis major muscle attachments cephalad to the perforators are divided to increase the length of the vascular pedicle. The flap is then rotated to reconstruct the neck defect, either through a subcutaneous tunnel or by dividing the narrow skin bridge between the donor site and the neck defect. The viability of the very distal end of the flap is confirmed by active bleeding from the skin edge. The donor site is then closed primarily. Perforators from either the lateral thoracic artery or the intercostal artery may be encountered

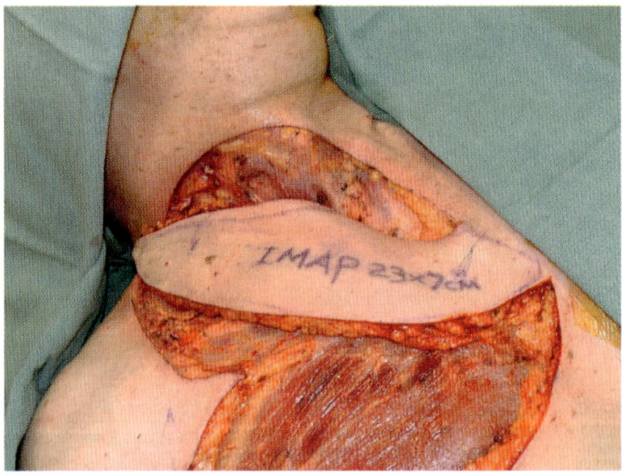


**Fig. 30.2** The superior border of the flap is incised and perforator vessels are identified via subfascial dissection before the flap is circumcised.

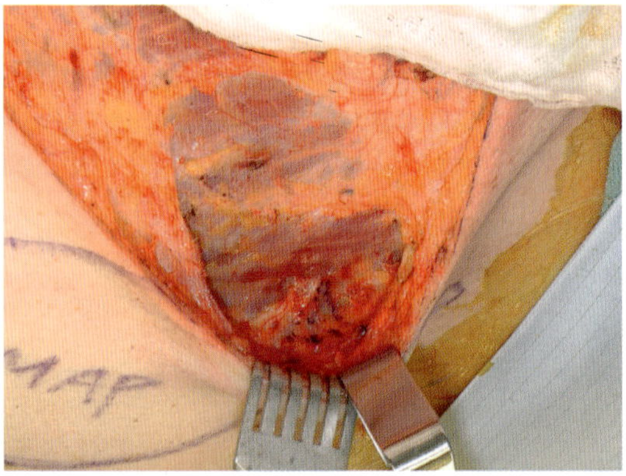

**Fig. 30.3** Once the perforators are located, the rest of the flap is incised and the flap is rotated to cover the defect.

in the lateral aspect of the flap. These perforators can be safely divided without compromising the flap perfusion. If muscle is needed, the pectoralis major muscle flap can be raised separately **(Fig. 30.4)**. This allows more freedom in flap insetting and maintains the thinness of the IMAP flap to avoid bulk around trachcostoma, advantages over the pectoralis major myocutaneous flap, especially in women.

When the flap is used as a free flap, the internal mammary artery and vein may need to be included to obtain more pedicle length and larger diameter **(Fig. 30.5)**. The rib cartilage above the perforator is removed to facilitate the dissection of the internal mammary vessels. If a large flap is needed and the donor site cannot be closed primarily, a thoracodorsal artery perforator flap can be used to close the chest donor site **(Fig. 30.6)**.

The size limit of the IMAP flap has not been clearly defined, although the above-mentioned perfusion study suggests that a single perforator can perfuse a large area of chest skin from the clavicle superiorly, lateral mammary fold laterally, to the nipple areola complex and xiphoid inferiorly.[3] A more important and clinically relevant issue is length and width ratio. A long and narrow flap is more desirable for easy reach and donor-site closure. The author's personal experience suggests that a single IMAP is able to carry a narrow (5 cm) and long (13 cm from the vascular pedicle) flap that extends 2 cm beyond the anterior axillary fold into the axilla.

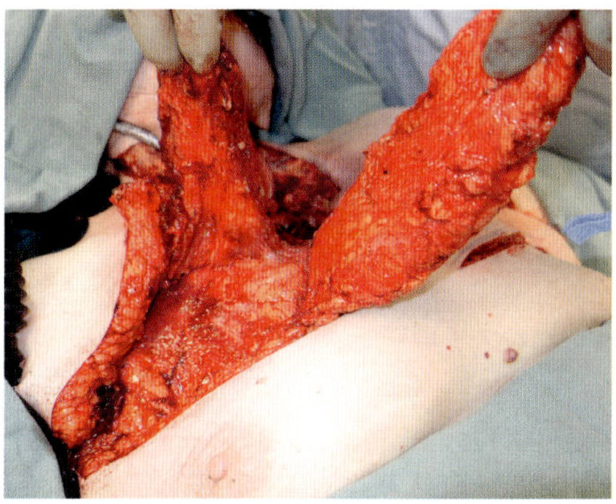

**Fig. 30.4** When muscle is also needed for the defect, the pectoralis major muscle can be harvested separately. Two separate flaps provide more freedom in flap insetting to cover the major vessels and to maintain the thinness of the IMAP flap and avoid bulk around the tracheostoma.

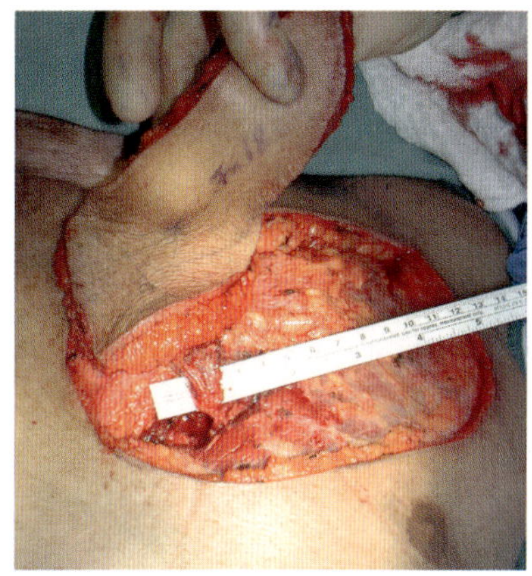

**Fig. 30.5** When the IMAP flap is used as a free flap, the main internal mammary vessels may be included to obtain a longer pedicle with a larger diameter.

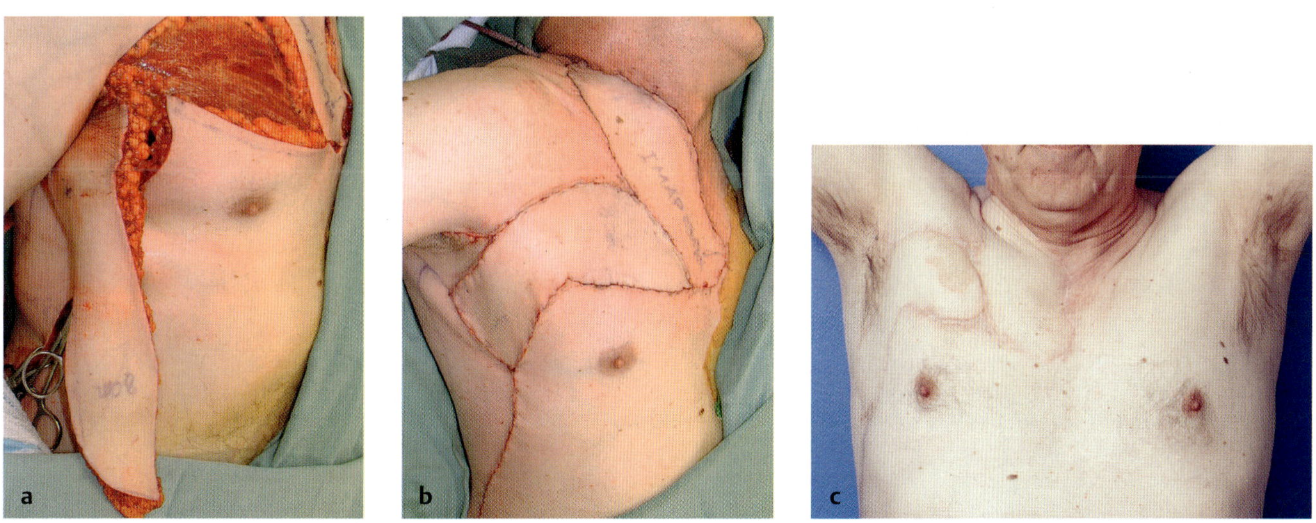

**Fig. 30.6 (a,b)** When a large IMAP flap is needed and the donor site cannot be closed primarily, a thoracodorsal artery perforator flap (TDAP flap) can be used as a pedicled island flap to cover the IMAP donor site with minimal donor-site morbidity. **(c)** Final appearance.

## Pearls and Pitfalls

- The pedicled IMAP flap is useful for small to moderately sized defects in the lower neck or upper chest, as well as for tracheostoma reconstruction, such as in patients with laryngectomy.
- The IMAP flap used as a free flap is sometimes indicated for facial reconstruction, due to its good color match with the skin of the face.
- The IMAP flap is usually based on the internal mammary perforator located in the second intercostal space, which is the dominant perforator.
- Prior coronary artery bypass graft utilizing the internal mammary artery is a contraindication to use of this flap.
- The IMAP flap based on the second intercostal space perforator should be designed with a horizontal axis for the longest reach.
- Secondary perforators from the lateral thoracic artery or an intercostal artery can be safely ligated and divided; electrocautery should be avoided to preserve the delicate subdermal plexus blood flow in this relatively thin flap.

## References


1. Yu P, Roblin P, Chevray P. Internal mammary artery perforator (IMAP) flap for tracheostoma reconstruction. Head Neck 2006;28(8):723–729
2. Neligan PC, Gullane PJ, Vesely M, Murray D. The internal mammary artery perforator flap: new variation on an old theme. Plast Reconstr Surg 2007;119(3):891–893
3. Wong C, Saint-Cyr M, Rasko Y, et al. Three- and four-dimensional arterial and venous perforasomes of the internal mammary artery perforator flap. Plast Reconstr Surg 2009;124(6):1759–1769
4. Schmidt M, Aszmann OC, Beck H, Frey M. The anatomic basis of the internal mammary artery perforator flap: a cadaver study. J Plast Reconstr Aesthet Surg 2010;63(2):191–196
5. Schellekens PP, Paes EC, Hage JJ, van der Wal MB, Bleys RL, Kon M. Anatomy of the vascular pedicle of the internal mammary artery perforator (IMAP) flap as applied for head and neck reconstruction. J Plast Reconstr Aesthet Surg 2011;64(1):53–57
6. Schellekens PP, Hage JJ, Paes EC, Kon M. Clinical application and outcome of the internal mammary artery perforator (IMAP) free flap for soft tissue reconstructions of the upper head and neck region in three patients. Microsurgery 2010;30(8):627–631
7. Munhoz AM, Ishida LH, Montag E, et al. Perforator flap breast reconstruction using internal mammary perforator branches as a recipient site: an anatomical and clinical analysis. Plast Reconstr Surg 2004;114(1):62–68
8. Hamdi M, Blondeel P, Van Landuyt K, Monstrey S. Algorithm in choosing recipient vessels for perforator free flap in breast reconstruction: the role of the internal mammary perforators. Br J Plast Surg 2004;57(3):258–265

# 31 Local Flaps in Head and Neck Reconstruction

*Edward I. Chang and Matthew M. Hanasono*

## Introduction

While free tissue transfer is quickly contradicting the traditional mantra of the "reconstructive ladder," local tissue and pedicle flaps should still be considered and integrated into the armamentarium of the reconstructive head and neck surgeon. While certain defects require a free flap, based on size, location, exposure of critical structures, and to optimize postoperative form and function, other defects are best reconstructed with "like" tissue in the form of local flaps. Smaller defects involving the oral cavity can be reconstructed with a facial artery musculomucosal flap, while external or intraoral defects can be resurfaced with a submental flap, and larger defects involving the periauricular region or orbit can be reconstructed using a temporalis muscle or fascia flap.

## Facial Artery Musculomucosal Flap

The facial artery musculomucosal (FAMM) flap was described and popularized by Pribaz et al[1] for reconstruction of intraoral defects by replacing "like with like." The flap is an axial flap based on the facial artery and incorporates the mucosa and portions of the buccinator muscle. The FAMM flap can be utilized for a variety of defects, including oronasal mucosal defects and defects involving the palate, alveolus, nasal septum, antrum, upper and lower lips, and floor of the mouth. The FAMM flap is typically used for ipsilateral defects. The size of the flap is limited by the extent that can be close primarily. It is ideally suited for smaller defects of the lips, nasal lining, and oral cavity and provides vascularized tissue that is more resistant to contracture then skin or mucosal grafts, especially in the setting of postoperative radiation.[2] The utility of the FAMM flap differs depending on whether the flap is based superiorly or inferiorly. While four FAMM flaps can potentially be harvested in any patient, a previous neck dissection precludes an inferiorly based FAMM flap on that side. Ligation of the facial artery eliminates the antegrade flow; however, a FAMM flap can still be harvested based on retrograde flow to the facial artery from the angular artery, which collateralizes with the ophthalmic artery.

### Anatomy

The facial artery arises from the external carotid artery and passes through the submandibular gland before proceeding over the mandible superficial to the buccinator muscle and deep to the risorius, zygomaticus, and other muscles of facial expression. The facial artery then continues cephalad as the angular artery that collateralizes with the distal continuation of the ophthalmic artery. The FAMM flap is an axial flap, and, therefore, the facial artery must be included in the flap to maintain its viability. Including the facial artery mandates inclusion of the buccinator muscle, which lies between the facial artery and the mucosa. While there is not a definitive vein associated with the FAMM flap, there is a rich plexus of veins that allows for adequate outflow with minimal risk for flap congestion. The FAMM flap can provide some bulk and thickness, typically between 8 to 10 mm, and it can be harvested along the entire path of the facial artery, as much as 8 cm in length. Flaps up to 3 cm wide can routinely be elevated and still allow for primary closure of the donor site.

### Preoperative Considerations

Prior to harvesting a FAMM flap, the dimensions of the defect should be confirmed, making certain that the FAMM flap will be adequate to resurface the defect and the donor site can be closed primarily. The pivot point for an inferiorly based (antegrade flow) flap is toward the retromolar trigone, while the pivot point for a superiorly based (retrograde flow) flap is toward the gingival labial sulcus near the alar margin. Attention should be paid to whether a neck dissection was performed, which would preclude harvesting an antegrade flap on the side of the neck dissection. A Doppler should be used to identify the facial artery and its trajectory so the flap can be centered over the artery.

## Operative Technique

The flap should be centered over the facial artery, which is located with the use of a handheld Doppler. The flap should be designed anterior to Stensen's duct and attention should be paid not to injure the duct orifice during the dissection. The incisions should begin distally, away from the pivot point or pedicle, and the facial artery should be identified, which requires dissection through the buccinator muscle that is incorporated into the flap **(Fig. 31.1)**. The dissection can then proceed toward the pivot point, making certain that the facial artery is included with the flap. The tortuous, serpentine course of the facial artery can be released to gain additional length on the pedicle and to allow for easier inset of the flap. The flap can then be rotated into the defect and inset, and the donor site is closed primarily.

## Case Example

A patient with a history of radiation therapy for oropharyngeal squamous cell carcinoma presented with a persistent area of gingival breakdown with mandibular bone exposure. The bone was burred down and found to be viable. A 2 cm wide, inferiorly based FAMM flap was elevated and rotated into the defect **(Fig. 31.2)**. The donor site was closed primarily.

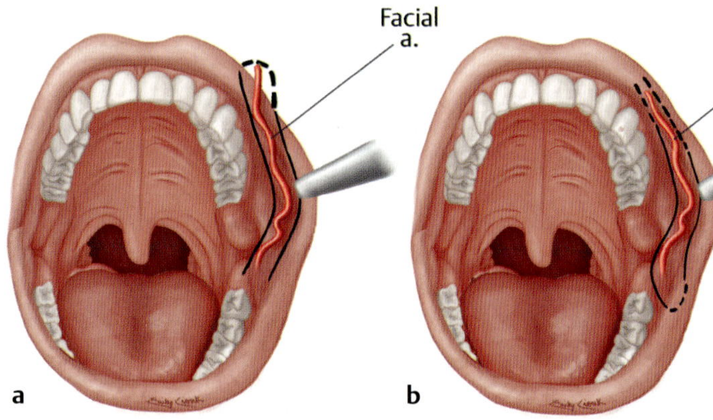


**Fig. 31.1** Anatomy of the facial artery musculomucosal (FAMM) flap. Both **(a)** inferiorly based and **(b)** superiorly based flaps are shown.

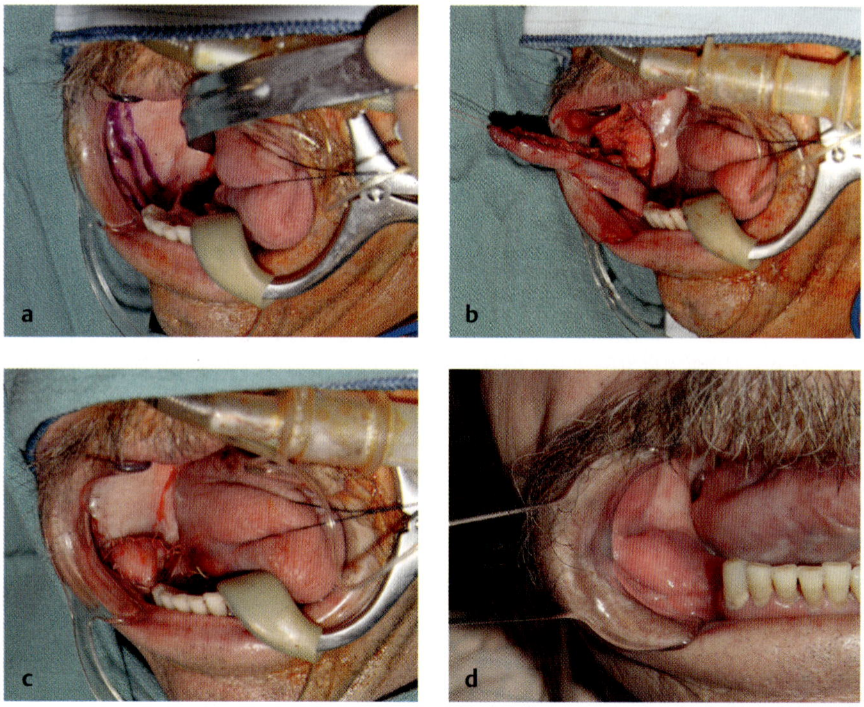


**Fig. 31.2** **(a)** Outline of the facial artery and planned FAMM flap on the right cheek buccal mucosa. **(b)** Inferiorly based FAMM flap after dissection. **(c)** FAMM flap used for reconstruction of a mandibular gingival defect with primary closure of the donor site. **(d)** Postoperative appearance.

## ■ Submental Flap

While Martin[3] is accredited with describing the submental flap in 1993, there are earlier reports documenting flaps based on the submental artery, which incorporate the underlying muscle as a platysmal myocutaneous flap.[4] The submental flap is based on branches arising from the facial artery and provides an axial blood supply to the tissue in the submental region. The tissue can then be mobilized intraorally for floor of mouth defects or utilized for resurfacing of external skin defects with exposure of the mandible.[5] The pivot point for the submental flap is roughly at the angle of the mandible, where the submental artery originates from the facial artery, although there are techniques for increasing the reach (see below). If a neck dissection has been performed, the submental flap cannot be based on that side.

### Anatomy

The submental artery is a branch of the facial artery, which is a branch of the external carotid, and emerges near the level of the insertion of the posterior belly of the digastric muscle to the hyoid bone. It then runs over the mylohyoid muscle just below the angle of the mandible before passing medial to the submandibular gland. The submental artery is deep to the anterior belly of the digastric muscle in 70% of cases and superficial in 30% of cases.[6] Between one and four perforators travel through the platysma muscle to supply the submental neck skin. Venous drainage is via the submental vein, which empties into either the facial vein or, occasionally, the external jugular vein.

### Preoperative Considerations

As with the FAMM flap, attention should be paid to whether a neck dissection was previously performed, which would preclude harvesting a submental flap on the side of the neck dissection. Flaps are designed in the skin inferior to the mandibular arch, where there is typically some redundant skin even in young patients. Placing the incision too superiorly can risk having a visible scar. The size of the flap harvested is dependent on the degree of redundancy that will allow for primary closure of the donor site; however, flaps with a width of 5 to 7 cm can routinely be closed primarily without difficulty. Dividing the distal end of the facial artery and mobilization of the distal facial artery beyond the takeoff of the submental artery can also increase the mobility of the flap and pedicle length.

### Operative Technique

A template of the defect is transposed to the submental skin, and the side of the pedicle is chosen based on the location of the defect. The inferior border of the flap is designed based on the amount of redundant skin present that will allow primary closure, estimated by a pinch test. The flap is then elevated in a subplatysmal plane from the contralateral side toward the pedicle. The submental artery is not always directly visualized distally, but it should be identified as the dissection proceeds toward the anterior belly of the digastric muscle. Many surgeons feel that including the anterior belly of the digastric with the flap makes dissection safer in terms of limiting the chances for inadvertently injuring the submental artery in this region, where it can be quite small and delicate **(Fig. 31.3)**. The length of the pedicle and arc

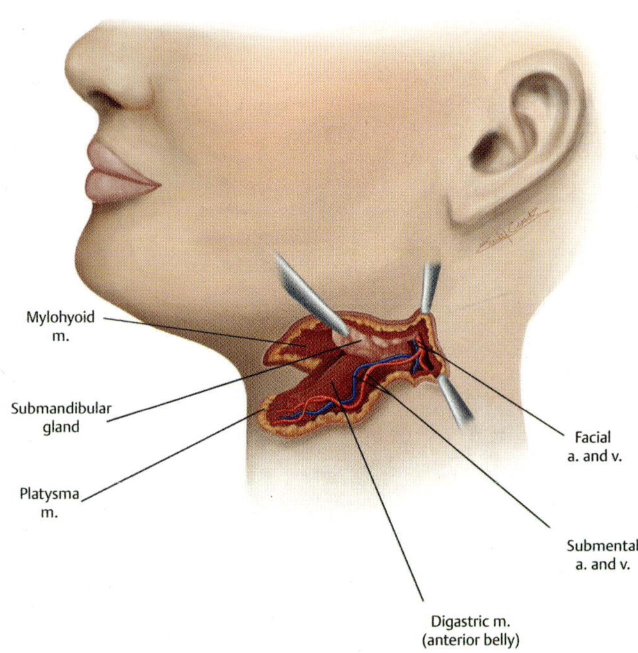


**Fig. 31.3** Anatomy of the submental artery flap.

of rotation can be increased by dissecting the pedicle proximally through the submandibular gland toward the angle of the mandible. Further length can be obtained by ligating and dividing the facial artery above the origin of the submental artery and mobilizing the facial artery up to its origin from the external carotid artery. Care should be taken not to injure the marginal mandibular nerve during the dissection. The flap is then tunneled intraorally or subcutaneously and is inset into the defect. The donor site can be closed primarily in layers over closed suction drains. As a last resort, the facial artery and vein can be divided after the take-off of the submental flap and can be either anastomosed to closer recipient vessels or lengthened with interposition vein grafts.

### Case Example

A patient presented with a recurrent basal cell cancer of the chin and underwent Mohs surgery, resulting in a 3 × 4 cm defect **(Fig. 31.4)**. A submental flap was designed based on the right submental artery. The platysma muscle was included with the skin, and the proximal portion of the skin paddle was de-epithelialized to ensure inclusion of a submental perforator, which was not visualized directly. The donor site was easily closed primarily.

## Temporalis Flap

The temporalis muscle is a useful flap, either as a muscle flap or a fascial flap if very thin, pliable tissue is needed. The earliest description of its use dates to the late 19th century, for treatment of ankylosis of the temporomandibular joint and for resurfacing of orbital exenteration defects. Since its early applications, the temporalis muscle has been described for reconstruction of orbital defects and skull base defects, coverage of mastoidectomy and temporal bone defects, palatal and oropharyngeal defects, and facial reanimation.[7] The muscle can provide bulk for parotidectomy defects to minimize contour deformities as well as act as a barrier to aberrant reinnervation of parasymphathetic nerves to prevent Frey's syndrome.

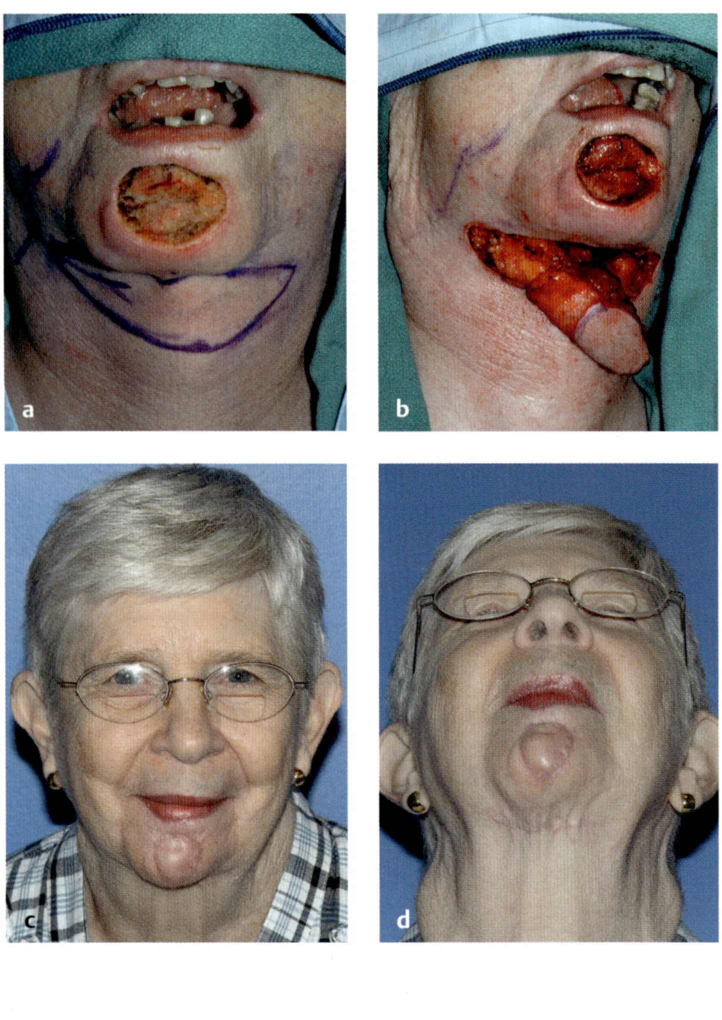


**Fig. 31.4** **(a)** Chin defect following excision of a skin cancer and planned submental artery flap. **(b)** Submental artery flap after dissection. **(c)** Postoperative appearance of the flap and **(d)** donor-site scar.

## Anatomy

The temporalis muscle is one of the muscles of mastication innervated by the trigeminal nerve. It arises from the temporal fossa and inserts on the coronoid process of the mandible and is surrounded by two layers of fascia. The superficial temporal fascia (also known as the temporoparietal fascia) is immediately deep to the scalp skin and is continuous with the subcutaneous musculoaponeurotic system (SMAS) and galea aponeurotica. The deep temporal fascia (also known as the temporalis fascia) is separated from the superficial fascia by an avascular plane of loose areolar tissue and envelops the temporalis muscle to the zygomatic arch. At the level of the arch, the deep temporal fascia is densely adherent to the periosteum of the zygomatic bone. The deep temporal fascia is supplied predominantly by the middle temporal artery, while the temporalis muscle is supplied by the anterior and posterior deep temporal vessels, which are branches of the second part of the internal maxillary artery **(Fig. 31.5)**.[8]

## Preoperative Considerations

Patients undergoing a temporalis muscle flap should be counseled regarding the possibility of a noticeable contour deformity that results from harvesting the temporalis muscle.[9] Preserving some of the anterior muscle will minimize some of the deformity anteriorly behind the lateral orbital rim, which cannot be covered with hair and will be more apparent. To gain further mobility of the flap for coverage of defects in the lower third of the face or mastoid region, the zygomatic arch can be removed, which can allow for an additional 2 to 3 cm in length. After rotation of the flap, the arch can be replaced and repaired with titanium miniplates. The frontal branch of the facial nerve typically travels along Pitanguy's line, a trajectory from 0.5 cm below the tragus to 1.5 cm above the lateral eyebrow, and should be carefully protected during the dissection of the temporalis flap.

## Operative Technique

A coronal scalp incision extended to the preauricular area affords the best exposure. The scalp is easily elevated off the superficial temporal fascia, through which the superficial temporal artery and vein and occasionally the frontal branch of the facial nerve will be visible. The superficial temporal fascia is then incised along the superior and posterior borders and is reflected anteriorly and inferiorly. The superficial temporal fat pad is elevated with the superficial temporal fascia by incising a layer of the deep temporal fascia.[10] The frontal branch of the facial nerve travels superficial to, or within, the fat pad, so keeping it with the superficial temporal fascia layer protects the nerve, and, to some extent, lessens the temporal hollowing created by harvest of the temporalis muscle flap. The temporalis muscle can be harvested in its entirety by releasing the attachments to the temporal crest. Often, including a 1 to 2 cm margin of periosteum with the flap is useful, both to extend the functional length of the flap and because it holds sutures very well. A periosteal elevator is useful in elevating the muscle from the temporal fossa, to avoid cautery injury to the deep temporal vessels, which run along the deep surface of the muscle. When the entire muscle is not needed, preservation of an anterior strip of the muscle minimizes the deformity, which can be appreciated from the frontal view.

Dissection then proceeds caudally to separate the temporalis until it passes beneath the zygomatic arch. The flap is then rotated into the defect. If further mobility is needed, the arch can be removed, allowing the muscle to be dissected more caudally. The arch can then be restored using titanium mini-plates. When the flap is

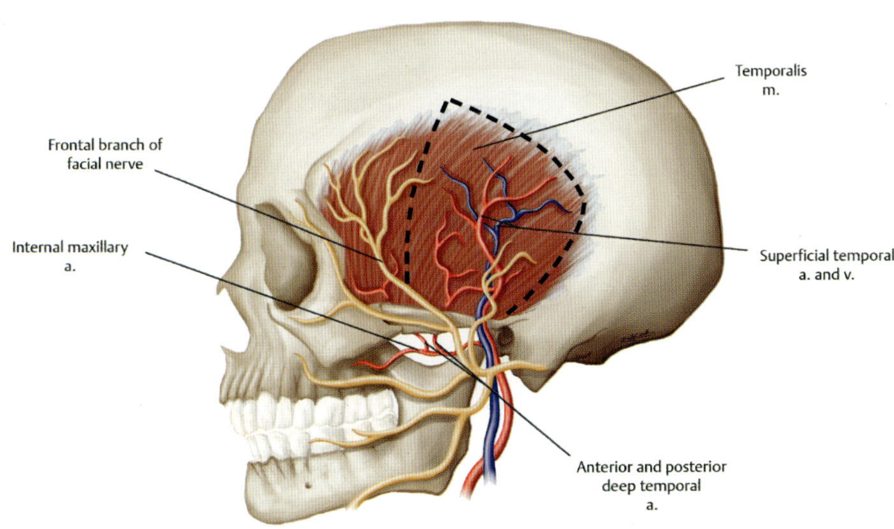


**Fig. 31.5** Anatomy of the temporalis muscle flap.

used for intraoral reconstruction, removal of the coronoid process of the mandible helps create a wide enough passage for the muscle without adding any morbidity. After the temporalis muscle flap is rotated into the defect and secured in place, the superficial temporal fascia can be replaced or can be used to help fill in the anterior donor-site temporal space and the scalp is closed in layers over drains. Some surgeons utilize acellular dermal matrix, porous polyethylene implants, or autologous fat grafting to further improve the donor-site hollowing, primarily or secondarily, as appropriate.

## ■ Case Example

A lateral temporal bone resection was performed for a deeply invasive external auditory canal squamous cell cancer. The resection involved excision of dura, with a resultant cerebrospinal fluid leak. A dermal fat graft was used to patch the dura, and the repair was then reinforced with a temporalis muscle flap **(Fig. 31.6)**. The temporalis muscle flap also eliminated the dead space and restored the contour of the mastoid region.

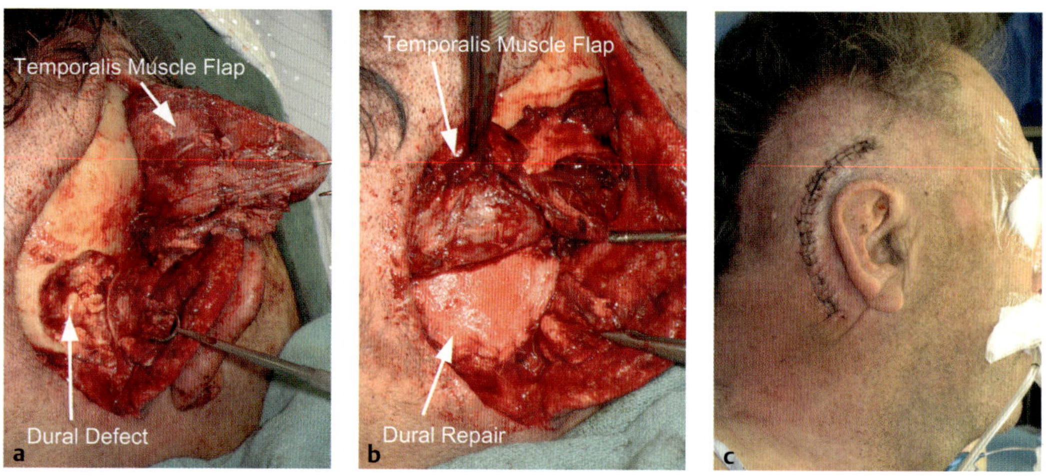


**Fig. 31.6** **(a)** A dural defect was created during resection of a temporal bone lesion. **(b)** The dural defect was repaired with a dermal fat graft and the repair was reinforced with a temporalis muscle flap. **(c)** The completed reconstruction demonstrates restoration of the mastoid region contour and elimination of dead space by the temporalis muscle flap. An anterior strip of muscle was left in place to minimize donor-site hollowing. (Photos courtesy of Melissa A. Crosby, MD.)

## Pearls and Pitfalls

- The FAMM flap is useful for a variety of small oral cavity defects, particularly those of the lips, gingiva, palate, and floor of nose.
- A handheld Doppler ultrasound is imperative for designing the FAMM flap.
- Careful dissection to keep the facial artery well attached to the musculomucosal tissue is required for the FAMM flap.
- The submental flap is a good alternative for small to medium defects, particularly in older patients with redundant neck skin.
- Including the anterior belly of the digastric muscle with the flap makes dissection less tedious and helps to ensure the integrity of the tiny branches of the submental artery in this region, which may be superficial or deep to the muscle.
- The reach of the submental flap can be increased by division of the facial artery and vein superior to the submental blood vessel take-off and by mobilizing the blood vessels.
- While the temporoparietal fascia is supplied by the superficial temporal artery, the temporalis muscle is supplied on its deep surface by the anterior and posterior branches of the deep temporal artery, which arise from the internal maxillary artery.
- A disadvantage of the temporalis muscle flap is leaving a noticeable concavity in the temporal fossa. This can be partially corrected by leaving the temporal fat pad intact, filling the space with the temporoparietal fascia, and using only the posterior portion of the temporalis muscle flap while leaving the anterior portion in situ.
- During temporalis muscle flap harvest, care must be taken to avoid the frontal branch of the facial nerve, which travels superficial to, or within, the temporal fat pad.
- Temporary removal of the zygomatic arch while transposing the temporalis muscle flap can increase the reach of the flap; the zygomatic bone is replaced after transposition and fixated with titanium mini-plates.

## References

1. Pribaz J, Stephens W, Crespo L, Gifford G. A new intraoral flap: facial artery musculomucosal (FAMM) flap. Plast Reconstr Surg 1992;90(3):421–429
2. Pribaz JJ, Meara JG, Wright S, Smith JD, Stephens W, Breuing KH. Lip and vermilion reconstruction with the facial artery musculomucosal flap. Plast Reconstr Surg 2000;105(3):864–872
3. Martin D, Pascal JF, Baudet J, et al. The submental island flap: a new donor site. Anatomy and clinical applications as a free or pedicled flap. Plast Reconstr Surg 1993;92(5):867–873
4. Coleman JJ III, Jurkiewicz MJ, Nahai F, Mathes SJ. The platysma musculocutaneous flap: experience with 24 cases. Plast Reconstr Surg 1983;72(3):315–323
5. Uppin SB, Ahmad QG, Yadav P, Shetty K. Use of the submental island flap in orofacial reconstruction—a review of 20 cases. J Plast Reconstr Aesthet Surg 2009;62(4):514–519
6. Magden O, Edizer M, Tayfur V, Atabey A. Anatomic study of the vasculature of the submental artery flap. Plast Reconstr Surg 2004;114(7):1719–1723
7. Bakamjian VY, Souther SG. Use of temporal muscle flap for reconstruction after orbito-maxillary resections for cancer. Plast Reconstr Surg 1975;56(2):171–177
8. Abul-Hassan HS, von Drasek Ascher G, Acland RD. Surgical anatomy and blood supply of the fascial layers of the temporal region. Plast Reconstr Surg 1986;77(1):17–28
9. Cordeiro PG, Wolfe SA. The temporalis muscle flap revisited on its centennial: advantages, newer uses, and disadvantages. Plast Reconstr Surg 1996;98(6):980–987
10. Hanasono MM, Utley DS, Goode RL. The temporalis muscle flap for reconstruction after head and neck oncologic surgery. Laryngoscope 2001;111(10):1719–1725

# Index

*Note:* Page numbers followed by f and t indicate figures and tables, respectively.

## U



## V



## W